Histopathology Reporting

Derek C. Allen

Histopathology Reporting

Guidelines for Surgical Cancer

Third Edition

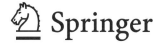 Springer

Derek C. Allen
Histopathology Laboratory
Belfast City Hospital
Belfast
UK

ISBN 978-1-4471-5262-0   ISBN 978-1-4471-5263-7   (eBook)
DOI 10.1007/978-1-4471-5263-7
Springer London Heidelberg New York Dordrecht

Library of Congress Control Number: 2013944967

Printed on acid-free paper

Springer is part of Springer Science+Business Media (www.springer.com)

To Alison, Katie, Rebecca and Amy

Preface to the Third Edition

Since the publication of the second edition of this book pathologists have further consolidated their position at the core of clinical multidisciplinary teams and their attendant meetings. These forums are pivotal nodal discussion points in patient investigation, treatment planning and prognostication. Pathologists are required to produce and comment on reports that are timely, accurate and relevant. To this end the UK Royal College of Pathologists, and other organisations (College of American Pathologists, Royal College of Pathologists of Australasia) continue to publish standards of professional practice such as the Cancer Datasets and Tissue Pathways for the handling and reporting of cancer and non-cancer specimens, respectively. Indeed, the UK Royal College of Pathologists has established key performance indicators which are to be incorporated into CPA/UKAS accreditation standards aimed at ensuring laboratory processes and outcomes are beneficial to patients. These include >90 % targets for attendance at multidisciplinary team meetings, coding of diagnoses and use of proforma histopathology reports, and diagnostic/resection report turn around times of 7–10 days. The College has also produced a standardised user satisfaction survey in metric form that should allow assessment of measureable pathology performance and team communication. This may also potentially be considered alongside colleague and user multisource feedback as part of annual appraisal and medical revalidation.

One other standard is that laboratories should aim to have a significant minority (15–30 %) of their medical and scientific staff in training grades. The structure and content of this book not only facilitates delivery of performance standards but also reflects the clinically integrated approach to the teaching of pathology as determined by the Royal College of Pathologists postgraduate training curriculum, and the General Medical Council medical student undergraduate curriculum.

Since the second edition TNM7 has been published and the WHO Classifications of Malignant Tumours are periodically revised. Other continuing trends are increasing

- Clinical and pathological specialisation
- Repertoires, techniques, sensitivity and reliability of immunohistochemistry
- Access to molecular techniques
- Use of immunohistochemistry and molecular tests as biomarkers in diagnosis, and prediction of prognosis and treatment response.

The aim of this third edition is to equip the consultant and trainee patholo-gist with a summary of the key clinical, pathological and scientific knowl-edge relevant to any particular cancer type, with the safeguarding of consistent and high quality histopathology reports.

The author gratefully acknowledges the use of illustrations from Wittekind C, Greene L, Hutter RVP, Klimfinger M, Sobin LH. TNM Atlas: Illustrated guide to the TNM/pTNM classification of malignant tumours. 5th edition. Springer-Verlag. Berlin, Heidelberg. 2005.

I would also like to express my appreciation for the support given by my colleagues in the Belfast City Hospital Histopathology Laboratory, and thanks to my co-authors in Derek C Allen, Iain R Cameron (eds) Histopathology Specimens. Clinical, Pathological and Laboratory Aspects. 2nd edition. Springer 2012.

Grateful appreciation is expressed to Melissa Morton (medical editor), Joanna Bolesworth, Beth Schad and the staff at Springer.

Belfast, UK   Derek Allen

Preface to the Second Edition

Many of the introductory comments in the first edition of this book regarding the increasingly focused approach required of pathologists to surgical cancer histopathology reports still pertain. In the intervening period a number of trends have continued to develop that have required an update.

- System-specific cancer multidisciplinary meetings with specialized clinicians and appropriate pathological, radiological and oncological support. Increasingly these meetings require fewer pathologists reporting significant numbers of relevant cases rather than a large number of pathologists reporting them only sporadically. From this has arisen cancer-specific lead pathologists encompassing a spectrum of specialist differentiation from "monospecialists" to "generalists with an interest in" and variations in between. Cancer report datasets aimed at maintaining overall standards of reporting are freely available published by various bodies, viz the Royal College of Pathologists, the Association of Directors of Anatomic and Surgical Pathology and the College of American Pathologists. In the UK the Royal College Datasets are a model for standardized reporting and their success is measured by their ongoing revision and second cycle of publication. No doubt specialist and team reporting will increase, particularly as the parameters for each cancer type report become more complex. Datasets with their notes and attendant information are required not only to update pathologists but also to keep them aware of significant pathology in other areas that might impact on their own specialization, e.g. metastatic carcinoma. Availability as PC-based templates also facilitates reporting, audit and download to cancer registries.
- In immunohistochemistry there is an ever-expanding range of increasingly robust antibodies which, with antigen retrieval methods, are applicable to surgical histopathology material. Panels of these antibodies not only help to identify the tumour type and subtype but can also give prognostic information as to the likely biological outcome and response to hormonal or chemotherapy. The data change rapidly, often with supposedly cancer type-specific antibodies becoming less so with time but still useful in combination with other putatively positive and negative markers in a panel. It can be difficult for the pathologist to keep abreast of current information in this field and which antibodies to use that will give reliable results.
- Increasing multi-professional team working in the laboratory necessitates provision of core information to Biomedical Scientists as a basis for why

we do what we do and how we do it in reporting surgical cancer histopathology specimens, particularly in relation to supervised role delegation such as specimen dissection. This knowledge base is also necessary to students and trainees, given the changes that have occurred in the undergraduate medical curriculum, in postgraduate medical training and the pressures on academic pathology.

- The 6th edition UICC TNM Classification of Malignant Tumours and the 5th edition UICC TNM Atlas have been published.

This text aims to augment and complement dataset reporting for surgical cancer histopathology specimens. Hopefully it highlights the main diagnostic and prognostic criteria for the common cancer types but also provides diagnostic clues for differential diagnoses and characterizes typical immunophenotyping. The author gratefully acknowledges the use of illustrations from Wittekind C, Greene FL, Hutter RVP, Klimpfinger M, Sobin LH (eds) TNM Atlas: Illustrated Guide to the TNM/pTNM Classification of Malignant Tumours. 5th edition. Springer. Berlin Heidelberg 2004.

I would also like to express my appreciation of the support from my colleagues at the Belfast City Hospital Histopathology Laboratory and thanks to my co-authors in Derek C Allen, R Iain Cameron (eds) Histopathology Specimens. Clinical, Pathological and Laboratory Aspects. Springer. London 2004 – Tong Fang Lioe, Seamus Napier, Roy Lyness, Glenn McCluggage, Declan O'Rourke, Maurice Loughrey, Damian McManus, Maureen Walsh, Kathleen Mulholland, Richard Davis, Lakshmi Venkatraman and Peter Hall. Thanks also to Melissa Morton, Eva Senior and the staff at Springer, my secretary Michelle McLaughlin (I don't know how you read the writing!), and, last but most of all, my wife Alison and our girls Katie, Rebecca and Amy.

Belfast, UK   Derek Allen

Preface to the First Edition

Current reorganization of cancer services has emphasized the need for higher quality standardized histopathology reports on surgical cancer specimens. Increasing clinical subspecialization is demanding detailed histopathology reports which are inclusive of multiple diagnostic and prognostic data directly relevant to the clinical management of each cancer type in individual patients. It is increasingly difficult for the consultant or trainee pathologist, surgeon or oncologist to recall those facts most salient to each cancer type, particularly if they are practising across a number of subspecialties and are generalist in remit. From this have arisen standardized or minimum dataset reports as a practical educative and reporting aid for surgical histopathology specimens. This approach is being actively pursued by various national bodies such as the Royal College of Pathologists (UK) and the Association of Directors of Anatomic and Surgical Pathology (USA). This book aims to supplement and complement this trend by acting as an educative and practical tool for both trainees and consultants. It provides an easily understood and memorized framework for standardized histopathology reports in surgical cancer. It notes the gross description, histological classification, tumour differentiation, extent of local tumour spread, involvement of lymphovascular channels, lymph nodes and excision margins of the common carcinomas and summarizes non-carcinomatous malignancies. It incorporates the fifth edition TNM classification of cancer spread, comments on any associated pathology and gives diagnostic clues and prognostic criteria. The staging information is supplemented visually by line diagrams. It emphasizes those features of a particular cancer that are relevant to clinical management and prognosis. It aims to give the reader a more systematic and analytical approach to the description of surgical pathology specimens, resulting in reports that are consistent and inclusive of the data necessary for the surgical and oncological management of patients. Its format acts as an aide-memoire for routine reporting of the common cancers, but it also lists diagnostic options and summary features of rarer cancers as a pointer to their diagnosis and consultation of specialist texts, as listed in the Bibliography. Reports inclusive of the data herein should also facilitate demographic, research, quality control and audit procedures. I hope that you find the information in this book to be interesting, relevant and of practical use.

The author gratefully acknowledges the use of illustrations from Hermanek P, Hutter RVP, Sobin LH, Wagner G, Wittekind Ch (eds). TNM

Atlas: Illustrated Guide to the TNM/pTNM Classification of Malignant Tumours, 4th edn. Springer. Berlin Heidelberg New York 1997.

I would like to express my grateful appreciation to Nick Mowat, Phil Bishop, Nick Wilson and the staff at Springer, my colleagues at the Belfast City Hospital Histopathology Laboratory and Mrs Debbie Green and Miss Kim Turkington for their secretarial expertise. Thanks also to my wife Alison and our girls, Katie, Rebecca and Amy, who often kept quiet when "Mr Grumpy" wanted them to.

Belfast, UK   Derek Allen

Contents

Part III Respiratory and Mediastinal Cancer

Part IV Skin Cancer

Part V Breast Cancer

Part VI Gynaecological Cancer

Part VII Urological Cancer

Part VIII Lymph Node Cancer

Introduction

Histopathology reports on surgical cancer specimens are becoming increasingly complex for many reasons. With closer clinicopathological correlation and the use of novel immunohistochemical and molecular techniques new entities and classifications of tumour emerge that are linked to prognosis and response to various treatment modalities. Increasingly the surgical oncologist wants tissue biopsy proof of cancer diagnoses so that patients may be recruited to suitable treatment protocols and clinical trials. No longer is it sufficient to simply say what it is but this must be qualified by assessment of prognostic indicators such as tumour grade, extent of organ spread, relationship to primary excision margins, lymph node and vascular spread. A useful maxim when reporting any surgical cancer is "type it, grade it, stage it, is it in vessels, and is it out?" Accurate classification and information on tumour stage and prognosis requires increased time and detail on surgical pathology dissection and reporting. These necessary, but stringent demands are met by diagnostic surgical pathologists with varying degrees of success and standards of reporting. For example, an audit of colorectal cancer pathology reports in one National Health Service region of the United Kingdom showed that only 78 % of colonic cancer reports and 47 % of rectal cancer reports met previously agreed criteria in providing the prognostically important information.

This study arose prior to the routine use of *standardised cancer datasets* which not only itemise core and non-core factors relevant to patient management, but also include key audit criteria as a means to improving quality standards e.g. for colorectal cancer the mean lymph node harvest and percentage case involvement of the serosa and extramural vessels. This approach in the United Kingdom is sponsored by the Royal College of Pathologists second and third edition Cancer Datasets which are readily available on-line. Tissue Pathways for non-cancer specimens are also published. Both are available at http://www.rcpath.org/publications-media/publications/datasets/datasets-TP.htm. It also forms the basis of an international collaboration for standardised cancer reporting referencing the College of American Pathologists Cancer Protocols and Checklists (http://cap.org/apps/cap.portal?_nfpb=true&pagelabel-home) and the Royal College of Pathologists of Australasia Structured Reporting Cancer Protocols (http://www.rcpa.edu.au/Home.htm). Furthermore the UK Royal College of Pathologists has published a series of Key Performance Indicators in Pathology (available at http://www.rcpath.org/rcpath-consulting) to enhance and provide a metric assessment of quality standards in the end-to-end laboratory service. They include timeframe and percentage achievement targets for: availability and timeliness of clinical advice, participation in multidisciplinary meetings, coding of histopathology reports, use of cancer biopsy and resection report proformas, documentation of second opinions, critical results communication, reporting turn around times, monitoring of outstanding reports, appraisal, continuing professional development, participation in appropriate interpretive EQA schemes, user satisfaction surveys (accessed at http://rcpath.org/rcpath-user-satisfaction-survey), teaching, training, supervision and succession planning. This raft of standards are enabling ISO 15189 process focused CPA UK (Ltd) laboratory accreditation to evolve by developing a more holistic patient/outcome based approach. Along with contemporary guidelines on staffing and workload levels (available at http://www.rcpath.org/publications-media/publications#histo) they also form a basis for annual medical staff appraisal and revalidation in the UK. Similarly the RCPath has a code of practice for histopathologists and histopathology services, also available at the same web address.

From the pathologist's point of view standard reports act as an important aide-memoire for the inclusion of necessary data and audit shows that quality standards of information increase accordingly. Also, once the pathologist is familiarised with them such reports are relatively time-efficient to dictate and transcribe. The clinician (surgeon or oncologist) can extract from them the relevant data with ease and cancer registries can be facilitated – supplemented by automated download and the capacity for search of key audit criteria if the database is suitably computerised.

The approach taken herein is aimed at fostering the use of standard format reports in surgical cancer. The headings used are common to all cancers, and can be preset onto a computer field or, if this is not available, easily memorised, dictated and typed in a listed format. The end product is concise, clear and relevant to patient management. The format is:

1. Gross description
   Specimen: description
   Tumour:
     Site
     Size
     Appearance
     Edge
2. Histological type
3. Differentiation/grade
4. Extent of local tumour spread
5. Lymphovascular invasion
6. Lymph nodes
7. Excision margins
8. Other pathology
9. Other malignancy
   These criteria are chosen for the following reasons:

1.   Gross Description

Specimen

Specimen type; *biopsy or resection*. Full standard format reports are most relevant to resection specimens although the principles and abridged forms are applicable to biopsies. Sometimes a resection is more conveniently reported as free text, or, in standard format but requiring clarification in the further comments section. If dictated as free text care must be taken to include the required diagnostic and prognostic parameters. Biopsy reports should at least comment on the following (if the data are available): tumour point of origin, type of cancer, differentiation or grade, extent of mucosal or submucosal spread, adjacent dysplasia or carcinoma in situ and involvement of lymphovascular channels. The proportion of tissue involved by tumour can be useful, e.g. prostate cancer. It is important epidemiologically that cancer registries can distinguish between biopsy and resection specimens to avoid duplication of statistical data leading to overestimates of cancer incidence and prevalence. This can be achieved by unique patient identification and careful indexing of SNOMED T (topography) and P (procedure) codes. This also facilitates audit of biopsy and resection proven cancer numbers and correlation with other techniques such as exfoliative or fine needle aspiration cytology, radiological imaging and serum marker levels (e.g. prostate specific antigen, PSA).

Specimen type also has implications for excision margins and clinical adjuvant treatment and follow up e.g. breast sparing excision biopsy versus mastectomy, diathermy snare polypectomy versus colonic resection.

Specimen weight and size. This may also be an indicator of the underlying pathology, e.g. primary adrenal cortical neoplasms >50 g are usually carcinoma rather than adenoma, and abundant vesicular uterine curettings up to 100 g suggests complete hydatidiform mole with subsequent potential for persistent trophoblastic disease and choriocarcinoma.

Tumour

Site

Location of tumour within the mucous membrane or wall can often give clues as to its nature. Mucous membrane lesions are often primary and epithelial or sometimes lymphoid in character. Mural lesions may be primary and mesenchymal or, similar to serosal disease, secondary and extrinsic. Site dictates which adjacent tissues are involved by direct spread (e.g. cervix carcinoma–ureter) and can indicate variable tumour differentiation and prognosis within a given structure (e.g. multifocal neoplasia within the urinary tract). It can also be used as an audit tool to monitor resection rates as in anterior resection versus abdominoperineal resection for rectal carcinoma. It can influence the diagnosis, e.g. epiphyseal versus diaphyseal bone tumours, renal pelvis (transitional cell) carcinoma versus renal cortical (clear cell) carcinoma. Laterality (right or left) is obviously extremely important in patient management. Some cancers also have a tendency for multifocal growth, e.g. transitional cell carcinoma of the urinary tract or thyroid papillary carcinoma.

Size

Size influences the diagnosis (gastrointestinal stromal tumours >5 cm are more likely to be malignant) and the prognosis (renal cell carcinoma: ≤ 7 cm = pT1, >7 cm = pT2; sarcoma: prognosis relates to tumour grade, size and adequacy of excision; breast carcinoma: Nottingham Prognostic Index = 0.2 × size (cm) + grade + lymph node stage). Gross measurements should ideally be made on the fresh tissue and checked against the histological slide allowing for tissue shrinkage with fixation and processing (e.g. 30 % for oesophageal resections). Small measurements are done with a dome magnifier, the stage micrometer or an eyepiece graticule. Guidelines are given (National Health Service Breast Screening Programme) to distinguish between size of invasive tumour from whole size (+ in situ change) tumour measurements and a radiological performance indicator is the percentage yield of invasive tumours <1 cm in diameter.

Appearance

Characteristic appearances are:

Luminal and polypoid
- Oesophageal spindle cell carcinoma.
- Uterine malignant mixed mesodermal tumour (carcinosarcoma).
- Gastrointestinal multiple lymphomatous polyposis or familial adenomatous polyposis.

Nodular
- Carcinoid tumour of bronchus or ileum.
- Malignant melanoma.

Sessile/plaque
- Early gastrointestinal carcinoma (stomach, oesophagus, colorectum).
- Lymphoma of gut.
- High-grade bladder carcinoma.

Ulcerated
- Usual carcinoma morphology.

Fleshy
- Malignant lymphoma, seminoma.

Pigmented
- Malignant melanoma.

Haemorrhagic
- Choriocarcinoma (gestational or testicular), renal cell carcinoma.

Cystic
- Ovarian carcinoma.
- Renal cell carcinoma.
- Thyroid papillary carcinoma.
- Secondary squamous carcinoma of head and neck.

Edge

Circumscribed	Mucinous carcinoma, medullary carcinoma and phyllodes tumour of breast, pancreatic endocrine tumours, some gut cancers.
Irregular	Infiltrating carcinoma. In general an irregularly infiltrating tumour margin is more aggressive than a pushing margin.

2.   Histological Type

For the most part this mirrors the World Health Organization (WHO) International Classification of Tumours but refers to other classifications where appropriate. The classifications have also been partially edited to reflect those diagnoses that are more commonly encountered or discussed as differential diagnoses.

Histological type influences:

1. Prognosis – breast carcinoma
   - Excellent: tubular, cribriform, mucinous.
   - Good: tubular mixed, alveolar lobular.
   - Intermediate: classical lobular, invasive papillary, medullary.
   - Poor: ductal (no special type), mixed ductal and lobular, solid lobular.
2. Management – lung carcinoma
   - Non-small cell carcinoma: surgery ± radio-/chemotherapy depending on stage.
   - Small cell carcinoma: chemo-/radiotherapy.
3. Tumour distribution
   - Thyroid papillary carcinoma: potentially multifocal.
   - Ovarian epithelial borderline tumours: bilaterality, peritoneal implants, pseudomyxoma peritonei, appendiceal mucinous neoplasia.
4. Associated conditions
   - Thyroid medullary carcinoma: multiple endocrine neoplasia syndromes (MEN).
   - Duodenal periampullary carcinoma: familial adenomatous polyposis (FAP).

3.   Differentiation/Grade

Three tier systems (well/moderate/poor differentiation or Grade 1/2/3, bladder carcinoma WHO I/II/III) have traditionally been used based on subjective assessment of similarity to the ancestral tissue of origin (e.g. keratinisation and intercellular bridges in squamous carcinoma and tumour gland formation in adenocarcinoma), cellular pleomorphism,[1]

---

[1]Cellular pleomorphism: this largely relates to nuclear alterations in size, shape, polarity, chromasia, crowding and nucleolar prominence. Cytoplasmic differentiation may also be taken into account (e.g. breast carcinoma – tubule formation).

mitoses[2] and necrosis.[3] This is strengthened when the individual criteria are formally evaluated and assimilated into a score that gives strong prognostic information (breast carcinoma, sarcoma). However a subjective three tier system is not advantageous when the majority of lesions fall into one category (e.g. colorectal carcinoma is predominantly moderately differentiated) and there is a lack of prognostic stratification. It is also compounded by poor reproducibility and tumour heterogeneity. This has resulted in emergence of two tier systems to identify prognostically adverse cancers (poorly differentiated/high-grade versus well to moderately differentiated/low-grade in colorectal carcinoma). In addition specific grading systems exist, e.g. Fuhrman nuclear grade in renal cell carcinoma and the Bloom and Richardson grade in breast cancer. Poor differentiation (G3) overlaps with and is sometimes combined with the undifferentiated (G4) category. Mixed differentiation with regard to tumour subtype and grade is relatively common. Carcinosarcoma (syn sarcomatoid carcinoma, spindle cell carcinoma) represents carcinoma with spindle cell change, and variable monophasic/biphasic and homologous or heterologous mesenchymal differentiation arising from malignant pluripotential stem cells and the process of epithelial-mesenchymal transition (EMT).

4.   Extent of Local Tumour Spread

Blocks

Due to tumour heterogeneity and variation in direct extension multiple blocks of tumour and adjacent structures should be taken to ensure a representative sample. A useful general principle is one block per centimetre diameter of tumour mass with targeting of specific areas, e.g. solid foci in ovarian tumours, haemorrhagic foci in testicular tumours (choriocarcinoma).

Colorectal carcinoma: 4 or 5 blocks to show the tumour in relation to mucosa, wall, serosa, mesentery and extramural vessels.

Thyroid nodule: 8–10 blocks including the capsule to distinguish follicular adenoma from minimally invasive follicular carcinoma.

Ovarian tumours: 1 block/centimetre diameter to account for the spectrum of benign, borderline and malignant changes in one lesion, particularly mucinous tumours.

---

[2]Mitoses: the assessment of mitotic activity either as a stand-alone mitotic activity index or as part of a grading system is a strong prognostic factor as in breast carcinoma. However, care must be taken: (a) delayed fixation may significantly alter numbers of mitoses but also makes them more difficult to identify. (b) hyperchromatic, pyknotic, apoptotic bodies should be ignored and only clearly defined mitotic figures counted. Strict criteria should be used such as absence of the nuclear membrane and clear hairy extension of nuclear material ± increased basophilia of the cell cytoplasm. (c) counts should be related to a fixed field area against which various high power microscope objectives can be calibrated. In general a × 40 objective is used.

[3]Tumour necrosis: apoptotic (single cell) or coagulative (confluent with pyknotic nuclear material in eosinophilic debris).

Border

Pushing/infiltrative.

Lymphocytic Reaction

Prominent/sparse.

Carcinomas with a pushing border and prominent lymphocytic reaction are regarded as having a better prognosis than those with a diffusely irregular infiltrating margin and sparse lymphocytic reaction e.g. colorectal carcinoma, head and neck carcinoma, malignant melanoma, medullary carcinoma of breast, advanced gastric carcinoma.

Perineural Spread

Carcinoma prostate, gall bladder and extrahepatic bile duct, pancreas and salivary gland adenoid cystic carcinoma where it is also a useful diagnostic feature of malignancy. In prostatic cancer there is some evidence that perineural invasion relates to the presence of extracapsular spread of disease and in other cancers it increases the likelihood of local recurrence.

Breslow Depth/Clark Level

Malignant melanoma. Direct linear measurement (mm) and anatomical level of invasion of the vertical component are strong prognostic indicators.

TNM (Tumour Node Metastasis) Classification

The TNM classification is an international gold standard for the assessment of spread of cancer and the revised 7th edition has been published by the UICC (International Union Against Cancer) taking into account new prognostic information, investigations and treatments. The system has evolved over 60 years as a tool for the careful collection of accurate data pertaining to cancer spread which can then be consistently related to planning of treatment, prognosis, evaluation of treatment and exchange of information between clinicians and centres. Virtues are that it translates into hard data some of the subjective language used in descriptive pathology reports and also encourages the pathologist to be more analytical in approach. It also improves pathologist to clinician communication. The post-surgical histopathological classification is designated pTNM and is based on pre-treatment, surgical and pathological information.

pT	Requires resection of the primary tumour or biopsy adequate for evaluation of the highest pT category or extent of local tumour spread
pN	Requires removal of lymph nodes sufficient to evaluate the absence of regional node metastasis (pN0) and also the highest pN category

| pM | Requires microscopic examination of distant metastases which is often not available to the pathologist and therefore designated on clinical or radiological grounds. If available (e.g. a multidisciplinary meeting) the TNM categories can be stratified into clinical stage groupings which are used to select and evaluate therapy, e.g. carcinoma in situ is stage 0 while distant metastases is stage IV. However for the most part the pathologist concentrates on pT and pN which gives reasonably precise data to estimate prognosis and calculate end results. Stage grouping is mostly based on the anatomical extent of disease but for some tumour sites or entities other factors are included: histological type (thyroid), age (thyroid), grade (bone, soft tissue, prostate), tumour markers (testis) and risk factors (gestational trophoblastic tumour). |

Multiple synchronous tumours (diagnosis within 2 months of each other): classify the tumour with the highest pT category and indicate the number of tumours in brackets, e.g. pT2 (4). In simultaneous bilateral cancers of paired organs each tumour should be classified independently. Systemic or multi-centric cancers potentially involving many discrete organs are categorised only once in any individual e.g. malignant lymphoma, leukaemia, Kaposi's sarcoma and mesothelioma. If there is doubt about the assigned T, N or M category in a particular case then the lower (i.e. less advanced) category is chosen. Note that in practice the multidisciplinary meeting may choose to upgrade the category to ensure that the patient receives adequate therapy, particularly in younger and fit individuals. When size is a criterion for the pT category, it is a measurement of the actual unfixed invasive component. Adjacent in situ change is not counted and if the fixed specimen shows a significant discrepancy with the clinical tumour measurement the latter is chosen.

Direct spread into an adjacent organ is recorded in the pT classification and is not considered distant metastasis whereas direct spread into a regional lymph node is considered in the pN category. The number of resected and positive nodes is recorded. Metastasis in a non-regional node is pM disease.

pT	Primary tumour
pTX	Primary tumour cannot be assessed histologically
pT0	No histological evidence of primary tumour
pTis	Carcinoma in situ
pT1, pT2, pT3, pT4	Increasing size and/or local extent of the primary tumour histologically.
pN	Regional lymph nodes
pNX	Regional lymph nodes cannot be assessed histologically – not submitted. If submitted but less than the recommended number for a regional lymphadenectomy designate as uninvolved with the number harvested in brackets e.g. pN0(6)
pN0	No regional lymph node metastasis histologically
pN1, pN2, pN3	Increasing involvement of regional lymph nodes histologically.

Main categories can be subdivided for further specificity, e.g. pT1a or pT1b to signify unifocality or multifocality.

Note than an X classification does not necessarily signify inadequate staging e.g. known metastatic disease (pM1) supercedes the pN category, or, pNX may arise because of a correct decision to treat by local excision e.g. thera-peutic polypectomy in the colorectum.

The TNM classification is applied to carcinoma only in the majority of tissues. Other qualifying malignant tumours are malignant mesothelioma, malignant melanoma, gastrointestinal endocrine and stromal tumours, gesta-tional trophoblastic tumours, germ cell tumours and retinoblastoma.

TNM Optional Descriptors

L	Lymphatic invasion
LX	Cannot be assessed
L0	Not present
L1	Present

V	Venous invasion
VX	Cannot be assessed
V0	Not present
V1	Microscopic
V2	Macroscopic (lumen or wall alone)

Note that lymphovascular invasion does not qualify as local spread of tumour in the pT classification (except liver and testis)

Pn	Perineural invasion
PnX	Cannot be assessed
Pn0	Not present
Pn1	Present

Prefix

y	Tumour is classified during or after initial multimodality therapy
r	Recurrent tumour, staged after a disease free interval
a	Classification first determined at autopsy

Suffix

m	Multiple primary tumours at a single site
mi	Nodal micrometastasis $\leq$2 mm.
i	Nodal isolated tumour cells (ITC) $\leq$0.2 mm
sn	Sentinel nodes
cy	Positive pleural or peritoneal washings e.g. pM1 (cy+). An exception is primary ovarian carcinoma where cy+ is part of the pT or pM categories.

Where appropriate other internationally recognised staging systems are also given, e.g.

Malignant lymphoma	Ann Arbor
Gynaecological cancers	International Federation of Gynaecology and Obstetrics (FIGO)

5.   Lymphovascular Invasion (LVI)

Definition

LVI usually relates to microscopic tumour emboli within small thin walled channels in which distinction between post-capillary venule and lymphatic channel is not possible – hence the general term LVI is used. It is important to identify an endothelial lining to differentiate from retraction space artifact, which often comprises a rounded aggregate of tumour sited centrally and free within a tissue space. Other helpful features of LVI are the presence of red blood cells, thrombosis and a point of attachment to the endothelium. In difficult cases endothelial markers (CD 34, CD 31, D2-40(podoplanin)) may be helpful, but in general adherence to strict morphological criteria is recommended.

Significance

There is controversy as to the significance of LVI but in practice most pathologists view tumours with prominent LVI as those that are most likely to show longitudinal submucosal spread/satellite lesions and lymph node involvement. Extratumoural LVI is regarded as more significant than intratumoural LVI and is most frequently encountered at the invasive edge of the tumour. LVI in tissue well away from the tumour is a strong marker of local and nodal recurrence in breast carcinoma, and is a criterion indicating the need for postoperative adjuvant therapy. When present in the overlying skin it denotes the specific clinicopathological entity of inflammatory breast carcinoma which is staged pT4. LVI is a strong determinant of adjuvant chemotherapy in testicular germ cell tumours. LVI also forms part of the pT classification for testicular and liver tumours, and, if present in a distant organ (e.g. lymphangitis carcinomatosa of the lung in pancreatic cancer) it is classified as disseminated disease (pM1).

Vascular Involvement

Some tumours (hepatocellular carcinoma, renal cell carcinoma) have a propensity for vascular involvement and care should be taken to identify this on specimen dissection and microscopy as it also alters the tumour stage. Extramural vascular invasion is a significant adverse prognostic factor in colorectal carcinoma but can be difficult to define. Sometimes one is reliant on circumstantial evidence of a tumour filled longitudinal structure with a wall partly formed of smooth muscle, lying at right angles to the muscularis propria and adjacent to an arteriole. Widowed arteries can be a useful indicator of venular involvement in a number of situations. The significance of vessel wall infiltration without luminal disease is uncertain but probably indicates potential access to the circulation.

6.   Lymph Nodes

As discussed above the assessment of regional lymph nodes in a surgical cancer resection requires sufficient numbers to be able to comment on the absence of regional metastases and also the highest pN category i.e. the total node yield and the number involved are important. In gastric carcinoma this means sampling and examining up to 15 regional nodes. Thus lymph node yields can be used to audit both care of dissection by the pathologist, adequacy of resection by the surgeon and the choice of operation e.g. axillary node sampling versus clearance. This is also influenced by use of preoperative neoadjuvant treatment. All nodes in the specimen should be sampled and although ancillary techniques exist (e.g. xylene clearance, revealing solutions) there is no substitute for time spent at careful dissection with a readiness to revisit the specimen after discussion at the multidisciplinary meeting. Care should be taken not to double count the same lymph node. The TNM target numbers recommended for a regional lymphadenectomy appropriate to a particular site should be kept in mind on dissecting the specimen. The pathologist should also remember to count those nodes in the histological slides that are immediately adjacent to the tumour as they are sometimes ignored yet more likely to be involved.

What Is a Node?

- A lymphoid aggregate ≥1 mm diameter with an identifiable subcapsular sinus.
- Direct extension of the primary tumour into lymph nodes is classified as a lymph node metastasis (TNM rule).
- A tumour nodule (satellite) in the connective tissue of a lymph drainage area without histological evidence of residual lymph node is classified in the pN category as a regional lymph node metastasis if the nodule has the form and smooth contour of a lymph node (having first ensured that it does not represent tumour in a venule). A tumour nodule with an irregular contour is classified in the pT category i.e. as discontinuous extension. It presumably arises as a result of extramural lymphovascular seedlings.

Note that this differs from the 5th edition TNM classification in which a connective tissue drainage area tumour nodule <3 mm was designated as discontinuous extension and ≥3 mm as a nodal metastasis. Although the TNM6/7 rule change probably more accurately reflects biological events it has caused discussion in the UK with concerns over observer reproducibility and inconsistency with on-going international trials. The resolution of this issue awaits further studies.

When size is a criterion for pN classification, e.g. breast carcinoma, measurement is of the metastasis, not the entire node (TNM rule). Size is also the whole measurement of a conglomerate of involved lymph nodes, and, includes perinodal tumour.

Micrometastases

The significance of nodal micrometastases ≤2 mm (designated (mi) e.g. pN1 (mi)), and, isolated tumour cells (ITC) ≤0.2 mm (designated (i+) e.g. pN0 (i+)) demonstrated by immunohistochemistry is not resolved. In practical terms an accommodation within available resources must be made. Most busy general laboratories will submit small nodes (<5 mm) intact or bisected, and a mid-slice of larger ones. Additional slices may be processed as required if the histology warrants it. Sometimes there is circumstantial evidence of occult metastases, e.g. a granulomatous response that will promote the use of immunohistochemistry in the search for micrometastases/ITCs. The prognostic significance of micrometastases has yet to be clarified for the majority of cancers, e.g. a search for micrometastases is advocated by some in breast and colorectal carcinoma but considered to be of equivocal significance in oesophageal carcinoma. This area needs further clarification from large international trials which examine clinical outcome related to the immunohistochemical and molecular (RT-PCR) detection of minimal residual disease in lymph nodes and bone marrow samples considered tumour negative on routine examination. Detection by non-morphological techniques such as flow cytometry or DNA analysis is designated (mol+) e.g. pN0 (mol+) or pM0 (mol+) in lymph node or bone marrow respectively. In the interim the rationale behind asigning (i+) and (mol+) to the pNO category is because they do not typically show evidence of metastatic activity e.g. proliferation, stromal reaction or penetration of vascular or lymphatic sinus walls.

Sentinel Node

The sentinel lymph node is the first lymph node to receive lymphatic drainage from a primary tumour. If it is tumour positive other regional lymph nodes are likely to be involved, but not involved if the sentinel node is negative. It is tracked by vital dye or radioactive colloid mapping. It is cut into 2 mm serial slices perpendicular to the nodal long axis, all processed and examined histologically. This may be supplemented by appropriate immunohistochemistry e.g. cytokeratins, melanoma markers.

Limit Node

The limit node is the nearest node(s) to the longitudinal and/or apical resection limits and suture ties. Some specimens e.g. transverse colon, will have more than one and they should be identified as such.

Extracapsular Spread

Extracapsular spread is an adverse prognostic sign and an indicator for potential local recurrence (e.g. bladder cancer), particularly if the spread is near to or impinges upon a resection margin e.g. axillary clearance in breast carcinoma. Perinodal tumour is also included in measurement of metastasis maximum dimension.

7.   Excision Margins

The clearance of excision margins has important implications for patient follow up, adjuvant therapy and local recurrence of tumour. Positive resection margins in a breast cancer may mean further local excision, conversion to a total mastectomy and/or radiotherapy to the affected area. Measurements should be made on the gross specimen, checked against the histological slide and verified using the stage micrometer or eyepiece graticule. A very useful practical aid is a hand-held perspex dome magnifier that contains an in-built graduated linear scale. Painting of the margins by ink supplemented by labeling of the blocks is important. Paint adheres well to fresh specimens but also works on formalin fixed tissue. India ink or alcian blue are commonly used. Commercially available multicoloured inks are helpful, particularly if there are multiple margins as in breast carcinoma. The relevance of particular margins varies according to specimen and cancer type.

1. *Longitudinal margins*. Involvement can be by several mechanisms:
   (a) *Direct spread*. In rectal carcinoma the longitudinal margin in an anterior resection is considered satisfactory if the anastomosis is 2–3 cm beyond the macroscopic edge of the tumour, i.e. direct longitudinal spread is minimal. However, there may be involvement if the tumour is extensively infiltrative, poorly differentiated or of signet ring cell type, or shows prominent LVI. Appropriate limit blocks should be taken. In addition to the resection specimen limits separate anastomotic rings are also usually submitted.
   (b) *Discontinuous spread*. In oesophageal and gastric carcinoma there is a propensity for discontinuous lymphovascular submucosal and mural spread, and margins should be checked microscopically even if some distance from the primary tumour.
   (c) *Multifocal spread*. In transitional cell carcinoma of the urinary tract, malignant lymphoma of the bowel and papillary carcinoma of the thyroid potential multifocality must be borne in mind.
2. *Circumferential radial margin (CRM)*. An often ignored measurement these margins are assuming increasing importance in relation to local recurrence and morbidity e.g. mesorectal CRM and rectal carcinoma. It is recommended practice to measure how far the carcinoma has spread beyond the organ wall and how far it is from the CRM. Other examples are: oesophageal carcinoma and the adventitial margin, cervical carcinoma and the paracervical/parametrial margin, renal carcinoma and the perinephric fat/fascial margin. Lymph node mestastasis at a CRM is also considered positive. The significance of some other examples is less well defined but comment should be made e.g. the mesenteric edge in colonic carcinoma.
3. *Quadrant margins*. Examples are a skin ellipse for carcinoma or malignant melanoma. Usually the longitudinal axis margins are well clear and

the nearest to the tumour are the transverse axis and deep aspects. It is important to check clearance not only of the infiltrating tumour but also adjacent field change, e.g. epidermal dysplasia or radial spread of a malignant melanoma. Actual measurement of margin clearance can be important in assessing the need for further local excision e.g. malignant melanoma. An alternative technique is multiple serial transverse slices demonstrating the entirety of the transverse axis margins with the longitudinal axis tips also embedded in-toto ("toast-racking").

4. *Serosa or peritoneum.* This is a visceral "anatomical margin" and breech of it allows carcinoma to access the abdominal and pelvic cavities. Its importance has been re-emphasised, as for example at the upper anterior aspect of the rectum where there is potential for peritoneal disease as well as local mesorectal recurrence posterolaterally. Standard practice may for some cancers also involve measuring the distance from the invasive edge of the tumour to the serosa e.g. uterine adenocarcinoma.

   Colonic carcinoma: prognostic distinction is made between carcinoma in a subserosal inflammatory (pT3) and carcinoma being at and ulcerating the serosal surface (pT4). The serosa is considered involved if tumour is actually at or ulcerating the lining of mesothelial cells.

   Lung carcinoma: pleural involvement is infiltration of the inner elastin layer or beyond.

5. *Multiple margins.* As in breast carcinoma (lateral/medial, superior/inferior, superficial/deep) this requires differential painting and block labelling, according to a previously agreed protocol for specimen orientation markers, e.g. surgical sutures or clips. Alternatively the surgeon may submit multiple site orientated shave margins marked as to their inner and outer (new in-vivo margin) aspects.

6. *Involvement.* Inadequate clearance of excision margins varies according to the tissues and tumours concerned:

   Breast carcinoma: invasive <5 mm; in situ (ductal) <10 mm. In clinical practice a non-involved margin of 1–2 mm is acceptable.

   Rectal carcinoma: mesorectum; ≤1 mm (either by direct extension or discontinuous in a node or lymphovascular channel)

TNM Resection Classification

R	Residual tumour
Rx	Presence of residual tumour cannot be assessed
R0	No residual tumour
R1	Microscopic residual tumour (proven by tumour bed biopsy or cytology) and in effect if tumour involves (to within ≤1 mm) the resection margin
R2	Macroscopic residual tumour.

Residual disease takes into consideration not only locoregional tumour but also any remaining distant metastases. It can also be applied following surgery, radiotherapy, or chemotherapy, alone or in combination. For a number of tumour sites there are semiquantitative histological regression grading systems applicable to post multimodal treatment e.g. oesophageal and rectal cancers, and bone and soft tissue sarcomas. Due to the variation in these schemes it is recognized that there is a need for an internationally standardized grading system that is reproducible and clinically relevant. The gauge of response to therapy should be the amount of residual tumour tissue present rather than the fibrosis, as the latter may not be a consequence of treatment, but tumour related stromal desmoplasia. It should be noted that clinical response to neoadjuvant therapy does not always directly correlate with evidence of tumour regression in the resection specimen.

8.   Other Pathology

This heading reminds the pathologist to look for and comment on relevant predisposing and concurrent lesions, associated conditions and useful markers.

Some examples are:

- Gastric carcinoma, incomplete (type IIb) intestinal metaplasia, gastric atrophy, dysplasia, synchronous MALToma, *Helicobacter pylorii*.
- Colorectal carcinoma, adenomatous polyps, familial adenomatous polyposis, periampullary carcinoma and duodenal adenoma.
- Thyroid medullary carcinoma, multiple endocrine neoplasia (MEN) syndromes.
- Hepatocellular carcinoma, hepatitis B/C infection, cirrhosis, Budd–Chiari syndrome, varices.

Other general comments are included such as diagnostic criteria, immunophenotype, prognostic indicators, clinical and treatment parameters. Local recurrence and survival rates are both specific to individual sources and broadly indicative of the data available in the bibliography references.

9.   Other Malignancy

The TNM classification is targeted primarily at carcinoma but also includes malignant mesothelioma, malignant melanoma, gastrointestinal endocrine and stromal tumours, gestational trophoblastic tumours, germ cell tumours and retinoblastoma. This section notes the commoner non-carcinomatous cancers such as uterine smooth muscle/stromal tumours, malignant lymphoma/leukaemia and sarcoma. Summary diagnostic and prognostic criteria are given where relevant.

Ancillary Techniques

Various ancillary techniques are important in the histopathology of surgical cancer and should be employed as appropriate. Some of these are commented on at various points in the protocols e.g. under sections "Histological Type" and "Other Pathology".

Photography

At the bench line diagrams and specimen digital macrophotography are crucial means of correlating block samples, disease stage and margin status, and, communication between dissector, reporting pathologist and the clinical multidisciplinary team.

Cytology

Fine needle aspiration cytology (FNAC): using 25-22 gauge needles has become the first order investigation in many cancers due to its speed, cost effectiveness, proficiency and convenience for both clinician and patient. It can not only provide specific inflammatory (e.g. Hashimoto's thyroiditis) and malignant diagnoses (e.g. thyroid papillary carcinoma), but can sort patients into various management groups: viz., inflammatory and treat, benign and reassure, atypical and further investigation (by core/open biopsy or excision), or malignant with specific therapy (surgery, chemotherapy, radiotherapy). It can be used to refute or confirm recurrence in patients with a known previous diagnosis of malignancy and to monitor response to therapy or change in grade of disease. It provides a tissue diagnosis of cancer in patients unfit for more invasive investigations or when the lesion is relatively inaccessible e.g. in the lung periphery, mediastinum, abdomen, pelvis and retroperitoneum. It must be integrated with the clinical features and investigations (serology, radiology) and can be complemented by other techniques e.g. core biopsy. It potentially provides material for routine morphology, histochemical and immunocytochemical techniques, electron microscopy, cell culture and flow cytometry. The direct smear and cytospin preparations can be augmented by formalin fixed paraffin processed cell blocks of cell sediments and needle core fragments (mini-biopsies) which can combine good morphology (the cores providing a tissue pattern) and robust immunohistochemistry. It can be applied to many organs: salivary gland, thyroid gland, palpable lymphadenopathy, breast, skin, prostate, subcutaneous tissues and deep connective tissues although in some cases e.g. breast cancer, a lack of locally available cytopathological expertise has in part resulted in a trend back towards core needle biopsy. Radiologically guided FNAC is useful for non-central respiratory cancers and tumours in the mediastinum, liver, pancreas, kidney, retroperitoneum, abdomen and pelvis. Endoscopic FNAC is also being used more frequently e.g. transbronchial, transrectal, transduodenal and transgastric/transoesophageal for lymph node staging or tumours covered by intact mucosa. Body cavity fluid cytology (both aspirates of free pleural, pericardial and peritoneal fluid and peritoneal/pelvic washings) continues to play an active role in the diagnosis, staging and monitoring of cancer. Yield of information is maximised by a combination of morphology and immunohistochemistry on direct smear/cytospin preparations (using air dried Giemsa and wet fixed Papanicolaou/H and E stains) and cell blocks (cell sediments and fragments).

Exfoliative cytology: along with cytological brushings and washings is also pivotal in the assessment of various cancers e.g. lung cancer, where the information obtained is complementary to that derived from direct biopsy and aspiration cytology. It can provide diagnostic cells not present in the biopsy specimen (for reasons of sampling error, tumour type or accessibility), correlate with it or allow subtyping that is otherwise obscured in artifacted biopsy material. Common sites of application are bronchus, mouth, oesophagus, stomach, bile duct, large intestine, bladder, renal pelvis and ureter.

Liquid based preparations: with good morphology and preservation of immunogenicity are increasingly complementing or replacing traditional cytological methods.

Frozen Sections

There has been a dramatic reduction in breast pathology due to the triple approach of clinical, radiological and cytological examination (supplemented by wide core needle biopsy) resulting in preoperative diagnosis and appropriate planning of treatment. Frozen section is contraindicated in impalpable screen detected lesions. Other uses are:

- Check excision of parathyroid glands versus thyroid nodules or lymph nodes in hyperparathyroidism.
- Operative margins in gastric carcinoma, partial hepatectomy, head and neck and urinary cancers.
- Cancer versus inflammatory lesions at laparotomy.
- Lymph node metastases in head and neck, urological, and gynaecological cancers prior to radical dissection.
- Mohs' micrographical surgery in resection of basal cell carcinoma of the face.
- Frozen sections should be used sparingly due to problems of interpretation and sampling in the following cancers: malignant lymphoma, ovarian carcinoma, minimally invasive thyroid carcinoma, pancreas and extrahepatic bile duct carcinoma.

Histochemical Stains

Histochemical stains are appropriately mentioned and can be valuable, examples being: PAS ± diastase or mucicarmine for adenocarcinomatous differentiation, PAS-positive inclusion bodies in malignant rhabdoid tumours and alveolar soft part sarcoma, PAS-positive glycogen in renal cell carcinoma.

Immunohistochemistry

Immunohistochemistry: has become the surgical pathologist's "second H&E" and is invaluable in assessing tumour type, prognosis and potential response to treatment i.e. as *diagnostic, prognostic and predictive biomarkers*. It also has a role as a surrogate marker of an inherited mutation e.g. demonstration of defective mismatch repair proteins in hereditary non-polyposis colorectal cancer (HNPCC).

Tumour Type

- Further detail is given in their respective chapters but typical cancer type immunoprofiles are given in Table 1.
- Select antibody panels are also of use in differential diagnosis in a number of circumstances (Table 2).
- The cytokeratin subtypes CK7 and CK20 have an important role to play in tumour characterisation (Table 3).

Prognosis

- Her-2, p53 oncogene expression, Ki-67 (MIB-1) proliferation index.

Potential Treatment Response

- Oestrogen/androgen expression and hormonal response in breast (e.g. Tamoxifen) and prostate cancer.
- Her-2 expression and Herceptin (trastuzumab) therapy in breast cancer and gastric cancer.
- CD 20 expression and Rituximab therapy in non-Hodgkin's malignant lymphoma.
- CD117 expression and Imatinib (Glivec) therapy in GISTs.

Antibodies should not be used in isolation but a panel employed with positive and negative in-built and external controls. This is due to a spectrum of co-expression seen with a number of antibodies e.g. EMA (carcinoma, plasmacytoma, Hodgkin's disease and anaplastic large cell lymphoma) and CD 15 (Hodgkin's disease and lung adenocarcinoma). *Interpretation should also be closely correlated with the morphology.* The antibodies in Table 1 are only part of a rapidly enlarging spectrum of new generation, robust antibodies that can be used with formalin fixed, paraffin embedded tissues, and show enhanced demonstration of expression by heat mediated antigen retrieval techniques such as microwaving and pressure cooking, and, highly sensitive polymer based detection systems. It is important to determine that the immunopositive reaction is in an appropriate location (e.g. membrane staining for Her-2, nuclear staining for ER, TTF-1), is not simply related to entrapped normal tissues (e.g. infiltration of skeletal muscle fibres), and is of appropriate staining intensity. In some circumstances the number of positive cells is important e.g. Ki-67 index.

A collaborative guide to the use of corresponding clinical serum tumour markers can be found at http://www.pathologyharmony.co.uk/harmony-bookmark-v7.pdf

Electron Microscopy

Electron microscopy has a diagnostic role to play where morphology and immunochemistry are inconclusive. It requires specialized equipment and expertise and may be more appropriately provided on a regional or network basis. Specific features can be sought in:

Table 1 Immunoprofile of cancer types

System	Tumour/condition	Marker panel
Head and Neck	Salivary gland tumours	Epithelium: AE1/AE3 and myoepithelium: S100, calponin, CK 5/6, p63. Grade: Ki-67
	Thyroid gland carcinoma	Papillary and follicular: thyroglobulin, TTF-1, CK19, galectin 3. Medullary: calcitonin, CEA, chromogranin, Ki-67
	Squamous cell carcinoma	AE1/AE3, CK5/6, p63, p16 (HPV related oropharyngeal). EBER (EBV related nasopharyngeal)
Gastrointestinal	Oesophageal carcinoma	Squamous: AE1/AE3, CK5/6, p63
		Adenocarcinoma: CAM5.2, CK7, ± CK20 (>50 %)
	Barrett's dysplasia	p53, Ki-67, AMACR
	Gastric adenocarcinoma	CEA, EMA, CK7, ± CK20 (>50 %), CDX-2. E cadherin+/Her-2 ± (intestinal type), E cadherin/Her-2 − (diffuse type)
	Small bowel adenocarcinoma	CEA, EMA, CK20, ± CK7 (50 %)
	Colorectal adenocarcinoma	CEA, EMA, CK20, CDX-2, β catenin ± CK7 (5–10 % poor differentiation or MSI-H). MMR abs
	Hepatocellular carcinoma	AFP, Hep Par1, CEA (polyclonal/canalicular), CD10, CAM5.2, CK8, CK18
	Pancreaticobiliary carcinoma	CEA, CA19-9, CA125, CK7, CK19, p53 ± CK20, CDX-2. Loss of DPC4
	Gastrointestinal stromal tumours	DOG1, CD117, CD34, Ki-67, ± Sm actin, desmin, S100, protein kinase c theta
	Gastrointestinal endocrine tumours	Chromogranin, synaptophysin, CD56, CDX-2, Ki-67 ± CAM 5.2, gastrin, insulin, glucagon
	Anal squamous carcinoma	AE1/AE3, CK5/6, p63, p16
Respiratory	Small cell carcinoma	CAM 5.2 (paranuclear dot), CD56, synaptophysin, TTF-1, Ki-67. Chromogranin – carcinoid.
	Non-small cell carcinoma	Adenocarcinoma: CAM 5.2, Ber EP4, CK7, TTF-1, napsinA, CD15, MOC 31
		Squamous cell: AE1/AE3, CK5/6, p63, 34βE12
	Malignant mesothelioma	Positive: CAM 5.2, AE1/AE3, CK5/6, CK7, calretinin, WT1, thrombomodulin, HBME1, p53, EMA.
		Negative: CEA, BerEP4, CD15, MOC 31, desmin

(continued)

Table 1 (continued)

System	Tumour/condition	Marker panel
Gynaecological	Ovarian carcinoma	Serous: CK7, CA125, WT1, Ki-67, ER, p16
		Mucinous/endometrioid: CEA, CK7, ± ER, CK20, CDX-2
	Sex cord stromal (also testicular tumours)	Inhibin, melan-A, vimentin, calretinin, CD99, ± CAM 5.2, AE1/AE3, EMA, Ber EP4, Ki-67
	Uterus, mesenchymal	Leiomyomatous: desmin, h-caldesmon, Sm actin, ± CD10, Ki-67, ER
		Stromal: CD10, Ki-67, ± desmin, h-caldesmon, Sm actin, ER
	Endometrial carcinoma	Endometrioid: ER, vimentin, CAM 5.2, AE1/AE3, CK7 ± CK 20, CD10.
		Serous: p53, Ki-67, p16, HMGA2, PTEN
	Cervix – CGIN	Ki-67, p16, bcl-2±
	Cervical adenocarcinoma	CEA, CK7, ± CK20 (ER/vimentin negative), p16
	Cervical squamous carcinoma	AE1/AE3, CK5/6, p63, p16
	Hydatidiform mole	p57 ^{kip2} in partial/complete moles (present/absent)
Genitourinary	Renal clear cell carcinoma	CAM 5.2, AE1/AE3, CD10, EMA, vimentin, CD15, RCC ab
	Renal papillary carcinoma	CK7, Ber EP4. CD117 negative
	Renal chromophobe carcinoma	CK7, Ber EP4, E-cadherin, MOC 31 (decreased CD10, vimentin, RCC ab). CD117 positive
	Transitional cell carcinoma	34βE12, AE1/AE3, CK7, CK20, p53, uroplakin III
	Prostate carcinoma	PSA (polyclonal), PSAP, AMACR, and CK7/20, 34βE12, p63 basal cell negative
	Testicular germ cell tumour	Seminoma: PLAP, CD117, OCT3/4, SALL 4, D2-40, HCG, inhibin (syncytiotrophoblast giant cells), cytokeratins±
		Embryonal carcinoma: CAM 5.2, CD30, OCT3/4, SALL 4, D2-40, ± PLAP
		Yolk sac tumour: CAM 5.2, AFP, SALL 4, glypican-3, ±PLAP. Negative for CD30, CD117, OCT3/4, D2-40
		Choriocarcinoma: HCG, CK7 (cytotrophoblast). OCT3/4 negative
Breast	Breast carcinoma	ER, PR, Her-2, CK7. Also Sm actin, CK5/6, p63, CK14, CK8/18, E-cadherin (see Chap. 22)

Soft tissue	Spindle cell sarcoma	Vimentin, CD34, Sm actin, desmin, h-caldesmon, CAM 5.2, AE1/AE3, EMA, S100, CD99, TLE1, HHV8, DOG1, CD117, β catenin, ALK. HMB45
	Small round blue cell tumours	CD45, tdt, S100, CD99, Fli1, desmin, myogenin, WT1, NB84, CAM 5.2, CD56, CK20
	Adrenal carcinoma	Inhibin, melan-A, synaptophysin, Ki-67, cytokeratin±, and EMA, CEA negative
	Phaeochromocytoma	Chromogranin, synaptophysin, S100 sustentacular cells, Ki-67, cytokeratins±
Skin	Cutaneous carcinoma	Basal cell: Ber EP4+/EMA-
		Squamous cell: Ber EP4-/EMA+
	Malignant melanoma	S100, melan-A, HMB 45, Ki-67
	Merkel cell carcinoma	Synaptophysin, CD56, CK20, CAM 5.2, Ki-67. TTF1 negative
Haemopoietic	Malignant lymphomas and leukaemias	CD45, CD20, CD3 and CD4, CD5, CD8, CD10, CD15, CD21, CD23, CD30, CD34, CD43, CD56, CD57, CD61, CD68, CD117, κ and λ, cyclin D1, bcl-2, bcl-6, bcl-10, ALK, Ki-67, LMP1, EBER, granzyme B, myeloperoxidase, mum1, Pax5, Oct2, BoB1, EMA, TIA1, Factor VIII, chloroacetate esterase, neutrophil elastase

Adapted from McManus DT. Miscellaneous specimens. In: Allen DC, Cameron RI, editors. Histopathology specimens. Clinical, pathological and laboratory aspects. 2nd ed. London: Springer; 2012

Queries about immunohistochemical staining may be answered at http://www.immunoquery.com and http://e-immunohistochemistry.info/

Sm actin smooth muscle actin, *TTF-1* thyroid transcription factor, *CK* cytokeratins: specific (e.g. CK7, 20) or cocktails (CAM 5.2: CKs 8, 18, 19; 34βE12: CKs 1, 5, 10,14; AE1/AE3: CKs 10, 15, 16, 19/1-8). *AFP* α-fetoprotein, *HCG* human chorionic gonadotrophin, *PLAP* placental alkaline phosphatase, *Hep Par1* hepatocyte antibody, *RCC ab* renal cell carcinoma antibody, *CD56* neural cell adhesion molecule (NCAM). *Ki-67* MIB 1, *ER* oestrogen receptor, *PR* progesterone receptor, *PSA* prostate specific antigen, *PSAP* prostate specific acid phosphatase, *AMACR (P504S)* alpha-methylacyl co-enzyme A racemase, *tdt* terminal deoxynucleotidyltransferase, *ALK* anaplastic lymphoma kinase, *LMP1* latent membrane protein (EBV), *EBER* EBV encoded RNA (in-situ hydridisation), *MSI-H* high level of microsatellite instability, *MMR abs* mismatch repair antibodies MLH1, PMS2, MSH2, MSH6, *DPC4* deleted in pancreatic cancer, *DOG1* discovered on gastrointestinal stromal tumours 1, *CDX-2* caudal homeobox gene

Table 2 Select antibody panels in differential diagnosis

Differential diagnosis	Antibody panel
Poorly differentiated tumour	
Carcinoma/melanoma/lymphoma[a]/germ cell tumour/GIST/PEComa/sarcoma (epithelioid variants)/granulocytic sarcoma	CAM 5.2, AE1/AE3, S100, melan-A, HMB-45, CD45, CD30, ALK, PLAP, OCT3/4, SALL 4, CD117, DOG-1, desmin, CD34, CD68
Mesothelioma/pulmonary adenocarcinoma	CK7, CK5/6, calretinin, WT1, EMA, CEA, Ber EP4, MOC 31, TTF-1
Small round cell tumour	
Small cell carcinoma/Merkel cell carcinoma/melanoma/lymphoma/leukaemia (lymphoblastic)/Ewing's: PNET/rhabdomyosarcoma/neuroblastoma/intra-abdominal desmoplastic small cell tumour	CAM 5.2, synaptophysin, CD56, TTF1, CK20, S100, CD45, tdt, CD99, Fli1, desmin, myogenin, NB84, WT1, Ki-67
Bladder/prostate carcinoma	CK7, CK20, 34βE12, uroplakin III, PSA, PSAP, AMACR
Renal carcinoma/adrenal cortical neoplasm/phaeochromocytoma	CAM 5.2, AE1/AE3, CD10, EMA, RCC ab, inhibin, melan-A, synaptophysin, S100, chromogranin
Hepatocellular carcinoma/cholangiocarcinoma/metastatic colorectal carcinoma	CAM 5.2, AE1/AE3, AFP, Her Par 1, CEA (polyclonal/canalicular), CD10, CK7, CA19-9, CK20, CDX-2
Paget's disease of nipple/melanoma/Bowen's disease	CAM 5.2, AE1/AE3, EMA, CK7, Her-2, p63, S100, melan-A (CK20 for anovulval Paget's)
Metastatic carcinoma of unknown primary site: site indicative antibodies	Thyroglobulin, TTF-1, CK19, galectin3: differentiated thyroid carcinoma
	CEA, calcitonin: medullary carcinoma thyroid
	TTF1, napsin A: lung adenocarcinoma
	PSA (polyclonal), PSAP, AMACR: prostate carcinoma
	CDX-2: gastrointestinal carcinoma
	CA19-9: pancreas, upper gastrointestinal carcinoma
	CA125: ovarian serous (also WT1) and sometimes pancreas, breast carcinoma
	GCDFP-15, ER, PR: breast carcinoma
	PLAP, CD117, OCT3/4, SALL 4, CD30, AFP, HCG: germ cell tumour
	AFP, Hep Par 1, CD10, CEA (polyclonal/canalicular): hepatocellular carcinoma
	RCC ab, CD10, vimentin, EMA: renal cell carcinoma
	CK7, CK20: see Table 3
Neuroendocrine tumours	Chromogranin, synaptophysin, CD56, Ki-67. Synaptophysin is a robust panmarker of neuroendocrine tumours. Chromogranin stains low-grade/well differentiated endocrine (carcinoid) tumours more strongly, and high-grade endocrine (small cell/large cell) carcinoma weakly. CD56 and Ki-67 are the converse of this.

[a]Including anaplastic large cell lymphoma (ALCL)

Table 3 CK7, CK20 tumour expression

Immunoprofile	Carcinoma
CK7+CK20+	Gastric/oesophageal adenocarcinoma
	Pancreatic adenocarcinoma
	Transitional cell carcinoma
	Ovarian mucinous adenocarcinoma
CK7+CK20−	Lung adenocarcinoma
	Breast adenocarcinoma
	Ovarian serous and endometrioid adenocarcinoma
	Endometrial/endocervical adenocarcinoma (usually CK20 negative)
	Mesothelioma
CK7 − CK20+	Colorectal adenocarcinoma
CK7 − CK20−	Prostate adenocarcinoma
	Renal clear cell adenocarcinoma
	Hepatocellular carcinoma
	Lung carcinoma (non-adenocarcinoma types)

- Carcinoma (tight junctions, short microvilli, secretory vacuoles, intermediate filaments).
- Melanoma (pre-/melanosomes).
- Vascular tumours (intra-cytoplasmic lumina, Weibel-Palade bodies).
- Neuroendocrine carcinoma (neurosecretory granules).
- Mesothelioma (long microvilli).
- Smooth muscle/myofibroblastic tumours (longitudinal myofilaments with focal dense bodies).
- Rhabdomyosarcoma (basal lamina, sarcomere Z line formation).
- Perineural/meningeal lesions (elaborate complex cytoplasmic processes).

Molecular and Chromosomal Studies

Evolving areas of diagnostic use of molecular and chromosomal studies are *clonal immunoglobulin heavy/light chain restriction* and *T cell receptor gene rearrangements* in the confirmation of malignant lymphoma, and, the characterisation of various cancers (particularly malignant lymphoma, sarcoma and some carcinomas, e.g. renal) by *specific chromosomal translocation changes*. Gene rearrangement studies can be carried out on formalin fixed paraffin embedded material but fresh tissue put into suitable transport medium is required for metaphase cytogenetic chromosomal analysis – although reverse transcriptase polymerase chain reaction (RT-PCR) methods are being developed for paraffin material. Genotypic subtypes of various malignancies, e.g. rhabdomyosarcoma, have been defined with differing clinical presentation, prognosis and response to therapy. *Detail is given in* Table 4 but some examples are:

Follicle centre lymphoma, follicular	t(14 ; 18)
Mantle cell lymphoma	t(11 ; 14)
Synovial sarcoma	t(X : 18) (p 11.2; q 11.2)
Myxoid liposarcoma	t(12 ; 16) (q 13 ; p 11)
Alveolar rhabdomyosarcoma	t(2;13) (q 35; q 14)

Table 4 Translocations in cancer types

Translocation	Tumour type	Testing methods	Clinical utility
t(11;22)(q24;q12) EWS-FLI 1 fusion t(21;22)(q12;q12) EWS-ERG fusion also t(2,7,17;22)	Ewing's Sarcoma/PNET	Breakapart FISH assay for EWS target; rt-PCR for specific fusion partners	Diagnosis
t(11;22)(p13;q12) EWS-WT1 fusion	Intra-abdominal Desmoplastic Small Round Cell Tumour	Breakapart FISH assay for EWS target; rt-PCR for specific fusion partners	Diagnosis
t(12;22)(q13;q12) EWS-ATF1 fusion	Clear Cell Sarcoma	Breakapart FISH assay for EWS target; rt-PCR for specific fusion partner	Diagnosis
t(X;18)(p11;q11) SYT-SSX1 or SYT-SSX2 fusion	Synovial Sarcoma	FISH translocation assay or rtPCR for specific fusion partners	Diagnosis ?Prognosis
t(2;13)(q35;q14) PAX-3 FKHR fusion t(1;13)(p36;q14) PAX-7-FKHR fusion	Alveolar Rhabdomyosarcoma	FISH translocation assay or rtPCR for specific fusion partners	Diagnosis
t(12;16)(q13;p11) TLS-CHOP fusion t(12;22)(q13;q12) EWS-CHOP fusion	Myxoid Liposarcoma	FISH translocation assay or rtPCR for specific fusion partners	Diagnosis
t(17,22)(q21;q13) COL1A1-PDGFR βfusion	Dermatofibrosarcoma Protuberans	FISH translocation assay or rt-PCR	Diagnosis/Predictive of response to imatinib
t(8,14) (q24;q32) & variants C-myc translocated to Ig heavy chain and deregulated expression	Burkitt's Lymphoma	Breakapart c-myc FISH assay, Southern Blot of hmwDNA,	Diagnosis of Burkitt's but also found in subset DLBCL where it has prognostic implications
t(14,18)(q32;q21) & variants BCL2 translocated to Ig heavy chain and deregulated expression	Follicular Lymphoma	FISH, PCR BCL2 immunohistochemistry	Diagnosis of follicular lymphoma but also seen in subset DLBCL where it has prognostic implications
t(11,14)(q13;q32) & variants Cyclin D1 translocated to Ig heavy chain and deregulated expression	Mantle Cell Lymphoma	FISH, PCR Cyclin D1 immunohistochemistry	Diagnosis of mantle cell lymphoma

Translocation	Tumour type	Testing methods	Clinical utility
T(2,5)(p23;q35) NPM –ALK fusion	Anaplastic Large Cell Lymphoma	FISH breakapart ALK probe rt-PCR	Diagnosis of Anaplastic Large Cell Lymphoma /inflammatory myofibroblastic tumour
TPM3 clathrin or other gene fusion targets	Inflammatory Myofibroblastic Tumour	Immunohistochemistry ALK	Potentially predictive of response to crizotinib in non-small cell lung cancer
TMPRSS2–ERG or other ETS family members	Prostatic Adenocarcinoma	FISH translocation assay or rt-PCR	??Prognostic

From McManus DT. Miscellaneous specimens and ancillary techniques. In: Allen DC, Cameron RI, editors. Histopathology specimens: clinical, pathological and laboratory aspects. 2nd ed. London: Springer; 2012

Reciprocal translocations are particularly associated with lymphomas and sarcomas but more recently have also been detected in some carcinomas as well. Translocations may result in altered/over expression of gene products (most lymphomas e.g. cyclinD1or BCL2), or result in a novel chimaeric fusion gene product (most sarcomas e.g. EWS-FLI 1). Translocations can be detected by dual colour interphase FISH assays to a single target gene with breakapart probes designed to span the breakpoint or by using dual target probes to detect fusion signals. Mutliplex Rt-PCR may be used to detect different fusion gene products and in some instances immunohistochemistry can be employed to detect increased expression (e.g. cyclin D1) /abnormal localisation of gene products (e.g. ALK) with appropriate antibodies. Although such techniques are applicable to conventional formalin fixed paraffin embedded tissue sections, submission of fresh tissue allows preparation of touch imprints for FISH and extraction of higher molecular weight and better preserved nucleic acid. Translocations are of particular use in diagnosis as detection of such translocations can help corroborate difficult or rare diagnoses in these tumour types. Some translocations are associated with constitutive activation of tyrosine kinases (e.g. ALK) and also have a role as predictive biomarkers for novel targeted therapies

Somatic mutation analysis has a number of applications in *differential diagnosis, prediction of prognosis and treatment response. Detail is given in* Table 5 but some examples are:

Colorectal cancer	K-RAS, microsatellite instability levels, BRAF
Melanoma, thyroid cancer	BRAF
Lung adenocarcinoma	EGFR, ALK
GISTs	c-kit, PDGFR
Renal cancer	Xp11

In situ hybridisation techniques may be used to detect viral nucleic acid (e.g. EBV in post transplant lymphoproliferative disorders, HPV subtyping in cervical biopsies), lymphoid clonality (κ, λ light chain mRNA), and karyotypic abnormalities such as Her-2/neu amplication in breast cancer and n-myc in neuroblastoma.

Flow cytometry has a diagnostic role in subtyping of leukaemia and malignant lymphoma, and may help distinguish between partial and complete hydatidiform moles.

Quantitative Methods

There is a role for the use of quantitative methods as diagnostic aids. These include stereology, morphometry, automated image analysis, DNA cytophotometry and flow cytometry. In general adverse prognosis is related to alterations in tumour cell nuclear size, shape, chromasia, texture, loss of polarity, mitotic activity index, proliferation index (Ki-67 or S-phase fraction on flow cytometry), DNA aneuploidy and spatial density. Most of these techniques show good correlation with carefully assessed basic histopathological criteria and, rather than replacing the pathologist and microscope, serve to emphasise the importance of various parameters and sound morphological technique. Areas of incorporation into pathological practice are:

- Morphometric measurement of Breslow depth of melanoma invasion, osteoid seams in osteomalacia, and muscle fibre type and diameter in myopathy.
- Mitotic activity index in breast carcinoma, GISTs, gynaecological and soft tissue sarcomas.
- DNA ploidy in partial versus complete hydatidiform mole.

With the advent of more sophisticated computers and machine driven technology, artificial intelligence and automated tissue analysis are being explored:

- Automated cervical cytology.
- Inference and neural networks in prostatic cancer and colonic polyps.
- Bayesian belief networks and decision support systems in breast cytology.
- MACs (malignancy associated changes) in prostate cancer based on alterations in nuclear texture.

Table 5 Genetic based predictive tests in cancer types

Somatic genetic change	Cancer type	Methodology	Clinical relevance
K-RAS mutations	Colon Cancer	PCR/direct sequencing	Predictive: mutation positive less likely to respond to anti-EGFR treatment
BRAF mutations	Melanoma	PCR/direct sequencing or tests for V600E mutation	Predictive of response to vemurafinib.
	Thyroid Carcinoma		Diagnosis? Predictive of stage
EGFR mutations	Lung Adenocarcinoma	PCR/direct sequencing	Predictive: mutation positive more likely to respond to gefitinib treatment
c-kit/PDGFRA mutations	Gastrointestinal Stromal Tumours	PCR/direct sequencing	Predictive: exon 11 mutations more likely to respond than exon 9 to imatinib
HER2 over expression/ amplification	Breast Carcinoma, Gastric Carcinoma	Algorithmic IHC /FISH, CISH or DDISH	Predictive: strong (+++) IHC and moderate IHC(++)/ISH positive more likely to respond to trastuzamab
EML4-ALK translocations	Lung Adenocarcinoma	IHC, ALK breakapart FISH assay	Predictive of response to erlotinib
Mismatch repair gene immunohistochemistry	Colorectal Carcinoma, Endometrial	IHC	In context of family history /fulfilment of revised Bethesda criteria suggests HNPCC.
MSI testing	Carcinoma	PCR, electrophoresis	Some evidence as prognostic marker (good) and detrimental effect on response to conventional fluoropyrimidine based adjuvant treatment
XP11 translocations	Renal Cell Carcinoma	FISH for translocation/TFE3 immunohistochemistry	Diagnosis of subtype of renal carcinoma

From McManus DT. Miscellaneous specimens and ancillary techniques. In: Allen DC, Cameron RI, editors. Histopathology specimens: clinical, pathological and laboratory aspects. 2nd ed. London: Springer 2012

Carcinomas are often associated with more genetic complexity and heterogeneity than lymphomas and sarcomas. Fewer translocations have been detected. However, the introduction of targeted therapies has led to clinical demand for predictive biomarkers of response. Whilst algorithmic testing by IHC and FISH has been successful in predicting response to trastuzamab, EGFR IHC has been less successful in predicting response to anti-EGFR therapy. Indeed recently RAS mutations have emerged as a negative predictive marker for response to cetuximab therapy in colorectal carcinoma as it lies "downstream" to the EGFR in the phosphorylation cascade signalling mechanism. Activating point mutations in receptors with tyrosine kinase domains have been associated with response to novel tyrosine kinase inhibitors

The sharp rise in demand for such predictive tests has not always been accompanied by a concomitant increase in capacity in pathology laboratories and such assays tend to be performed in larger centres with multiprofessional input and suitable volumes. More targeted therapies (esp tyrosine kinase inhibitors) are under development/in trials and this area is set for significant expansion in coming years, acknowledged by initiatives such as CR UK's Stratified Medicine Programme. It is also possible that the falling costs and increased availability of next generation /massively parallel sequencing platforms will permit the development of predictive assays based on activation or disruption of signalling networks rather than individual target genes

- Bioinformatics facilitates analysis of gene and tissue microarrays used to test the level of expression for multiple genes in relatively few samples, or, the staining pattern of relatively few markers on a large number of samples, respectively. This allows more standardised scoring of current prognostic markers on samples from multiple patients, and also leads to the discovery of new prognostic cancer biomarkers.

This whole area of translational research is rapidly developing and evolving and it remains to be resolved as to which facets will eventually be incorporated into routine practice.

Error, Audit, Quality Assurance, Clinical Governance and Digital Microscopy

Errors in a subjective discipline such as diagnostic pathology are inevitable but rates are surprisingly low (1–2 %). Whether cognitive (oversight or interpretational) or operative (non-analytical) they may be purely academic (e.g. a difference in nomenclature) or clinically significant (e.g. a false positive diagnosis of cancer). Any surgical pathologist hopes to avoid the latter and the potential consequences for the patient. Errors are discovered by various routes: inconsistency in clinical outcome with individual case review, review at regular multidisciplinary cancer meetings, topic related audit, systematic selective surgical case review, or, prospective in-house or external case referral for opinion. Clinical governance defines standards of care with open acknowledgement, communication and correction of errors. Professionals are encouraged to quality assure, sometimes double report, check their work in a team context supporting colleagues, and identify any indicators of underperformance. Advice from the Royal College of Pathologists is that pathologists should not report outside their field of expertise, and that there should be judicious use of various forms of double reporting e.g. to address particular local needs, in the context of review for multidisciplinary team meetings, and for some diagnoses where mandated by specialist organisations (available at www.rcpath.org/publications-media/publications). In the UK the Royal College of Pathologists Professional Standards Unit publishes protocols and advises on issues of professional performance with the capacity to investigate and recommend remedial action in individual cases. Consequently most pathologists adopt several strategies to maintain standards including participation in continuing professional development (CPD) and interpretive external quality assurance (EQA) schemes. CPD entails attendance at local, national and international conferences and seminars, journal reading and other educational activities relevant to the pathologist's practice with reinforcement of strengths and identification of knowledge gaps. This approach is inherent to annual appraisal and medical revalidation which should be consolidative and developmental in nature. EQA schemes are general or specialist in type with pre-circulation of slides or access to web-based digitally scanned images and clinical clues. The pathologist submits diagnostic answers which are marked in comparison to the participants' consensus diagnoses. Results are confidential to the pathologist but an individual with repeated outlying marks will be flagged up to the scheme co-ordinator so that appropriate advice can be given. Definition of what constitutes a specialist pathologist is complex but at least involves spending a significant amount of professional time practising in the relevant area and participation in the relevant multidisciplinary team meeting and an appropriate EQA scheme. Pragmatic experience tells who to send the referral case to and just "who can do the business". The rapidly improving technology of digitised virtual microscopy with scanning of whole slide images is developing roles as an alternative to slide circulation in EQA schemes, case referral to experts, live remote diagnostic reporting, image incorporation into diagnostic reports, facilitation of cross site multidisciplinary meetings, education and training, and in research and archiving. Automated immunohistochemistry, multiblocks and scanning of tissue microarrays will augment morphology by assessment of multiple prognostic markers. Thus the way ahead is charted for the surgical pathologist building on the foundation of clinical knowledge allied to morphological expertise, supplemented by various ancillary techniques, and showing a slide around to colleagues whose opinion you value.

Bibliography

Allen DC. The W5, how and what next of BMS specimen dissection. Curr Diagn Pathol. 2004;10:429–34.

Allen DC. Histopathology reporting. Guidelines for surgical cancer. 2nd ed. London: Springer; 2006.

Al-Janabi S, Huisam A, Van Diest PJ. Digital pathology: current status and future perspectives. Histopathology. 2012;61:1–9.

American Registry of Pathology. AFIP atlas of tumor pathology series I-IV. Accessed at http://www.pathologyoutlines.com/booksAFIP.html.

Ashton MA. The multidisciplinary team meeting: how to be an effective participant. Diagn Histopathol. 2008;14:519–23.

Bahrami A, Truong LD, Ro JY. Undifferentiated tumor: true identity by immunohistochemistry. Arch Pathol Lab Med. 2008;132:326–48.

Carbone A, De Paoli P. Cancers related to viral agents that have a direct role in carcinogenesis: pathological and diagnostic techniques. J Clin Pathol. 2012;65:680–86.

Chetty R, Gill P, Bateman AC, Driman DK, Govender D, Bateman AR, Chua YJ, Greywoode G, Hemmings C, Imat I, Jaynes E, Lee CS, Locketz M, Rowsell C, Rullier A, Serra S, Szentgyorgyi E, Vajpeyi R, Delaney D, Wang LM. Pathological grading of regression: an International Study Group perspective. J Clin Pathol. 2012; 65:865–66.

College of American Pathologists. Cancer protocols and checklists. Accessed at http://www.cap.org/apps/cap.portal?_nfpb=true&_pagelabel=home.

Connolly JL, Fletcher CDM. What is needed to satisfy the American College of Surgeons Commission on Cancer (COC) requirements for the pathologic reporting of cancer specimens? Hum Pathol. 2003;34:111.

Domizio P, Lowe D. Reporting histopathology sections. London: Chapman and Hall; 1997.

Du Boulay C. Error trapping and error avoidance in histopathology. In: Lowe DG, Underwood JCE, editors. Recent advances in histopathology, vol. 20. London: RSM Press; 2003. p. 103–14.

Fletcher CDM, editor. Diagnostic histopathology of tumours. 3rd ed. Philadelphia: Churchill Livingstone; 2007.

Furness P. Developing and running an EQA scheme in diagnostic histopathology. Curr Diagn Pathol. 2004;10:435–43.

Govender D, Chetty R. Gene of the month: BRAF. J Clin Pathol. 2012;65:986–8.

Groenen PJTA, Blokx WAM, Diepenbroek C, Burgers L, Visinoni F, Wesseling P, van Krieken JHJM. Preparing pathology for personalized medicine: possibilities for improvement of the pre-analytical phase. Histopathology. 2011;59:1–7.

Hall PA. DNA ploidy studies in pathology – a critical appraisal. Histopathology. 2004;44:614–20.

Hirschowitz L, Wells M, Lowe J. On behalf of the Royal College of Pathologists Specialty Advisory Committee on Histopathology. Double-reporting in histopathology. Accessed at www.rcpath.org/publications-media/publications.

Jasani B, Rhodes A. The role and mechanism of high temperature antigen retrieval in diagnostic pathology. Curr Diagn Pathol. 2001;7:153–60.

Lester SC. Manual of surgical pathology. 3rd ed. New York: Elsevier/Saunders; 2010.

McCourt CM, Boyle D, James J, Salto-Tellez M. Immunohistochemistry in the era of personalised medicine. J Clin Pathol. 2013;66:58–61.

McKay B. Electron microscopy in tumour diagnosis. In: Fletcher CDM, editor. Diagnostic histopathology of tumours, vol. 2. 3rd ed. London. Churchill Livingstone; 2007. p. 1831–59.

McKee PH, Chinyama CN, Whimster WF, Bogomoletz WV, Delides GS, de Wolf CJM, editors. Comprehensive tumour technology handbook. UICC. New York: Wiley-Liss; 2001.

Nocito A, Kononen J, Kallioniemi OP, Sauter G. Tissue microarrays for high-throughput molecular pathology research. Int J Cancer. 2001;94:1–5.

Rosai J. Rosai and Ackerman's surgical pathology. 10th ed. Edinburgh: Elsevier; 2011.

Sanders SA, Smith A, Carr RA, Roberts S, Gurusamy S, Simmons E. Enhanced biomedical scientist cut-up role in colonic cancer reporting. J Clin Pathol. 2012;65:517–21.

Silverberg SG, DeLellis RA, Frable WJ, Li Volsi VA, Wick R, editors. Silverberg's principles and practices of surgical pathology and cytopathology. 4th ed. Philadelphia: Churchill Livingstone; 2006.

Simmons EJV, Saunders DSA, Carr RA. Current experience and attitudes to biomedical scientist cut-up: results of an online survey of UK consultant histopathologists. J Clin Pathol. 2011;64:363–6.

Sobin LH, Gospodarowicz M, Wittekind Ch, editors. TNM classification of malignant tumours. UICC. 7th ed. Chichester/Hoboken: Wiley-Blackwell; 2010.

Spence RAJ, Johnston PG, editors. Oncology. Oxford: Oxford University Press; 2001.

Stricker T, Catenacci DVT, Seiwert TY. Molecular profiling of cancer – the future of personalized medicine: a primer on cancer biology and the tools necessary to bring molecular testing to the clinic. Semin Oncol. 2011;38:173–85.

Sturgeon CM, Lai LC, Duffy MJ. Serum tumour markers: how to order and interpret them. BMJ. 2009;339:852–8.

Teruya-Feldstein J. The immunohistochemistry laboratory: looking at molecules and preparing for tomorrow. Arch Pathol Lab Med. 2010;134:1659–65.

The Royal College of Pathologists: Cancer datasets and tissue pathways. Accessed at http://www.rcpath.org/index.asp?PageID=254.

The Royal College of Pathologists of Australasia. Structured reporting cancer protocols. Available at http://rcpa.edu.au/Publications/StructuredReporting/CancerProtocols.htm.

Troxel DB. Error in surgical pathology. Am J Surg Pathol. 2004;28:1092–5.

The Royal College of Pathologists, Institute of Biomedical Science, Association of Clinical Biochemistry. Tumour marker requesting. Guidance for non specialists. Accessed at http://www.pathologyharmony.co.uk/harmony-bookmark-v7.pdf.

Van den Rijn M, Gilks CB. Applications of microarrays to histopathology. Histopathology. 2004;44:97–108.

Vollmer RT. Pathologists' assistants in surgical pathology. The truth is out. Am J Clin Pathol. 1999;112:597–8.

Westra WH, Hruban RH, Phelps TH, Isacson C. Surgical pathology dissection: an illustrated guide. 2nd ed. New York: Springer; 2003.

WHO Classification of Tumours. Lyon: IARC press. Accessed at http://www.iarc.fr/en/publications/pdfs-online/pat-gen/.

Wittekind C, Greene FL, Hutter RVP, Klimpfinger M, Sobin LH. TNM atlas: illustrated guide to the TNM/pTNM classification of malignant tumours. UICC. 5th ed. Berlin: Springer; 2004.

Part I

Gastrointestinal Cancer

- Oesophageal Carcinoma
- Gastric Carcinoma
- Ampulla of Vater and Head of Pancreas Carcinomas
- Small Intestinal Carcinoma
- Colorectal Carcinoma
- Vermiform Appendix Tumours
- Anal Canal Carcinoma (with Comments on Pelvic Exenteration)
- Gall Bladder Carcinoma
- Extrahepatic Bile Duct Carcinoma
- Liver Carcinoma

Geographical incidence of oesophageal cancer varies greatly with high risk areas in China and Asia where the predominant tumour type is squamous cell carcinoma. This contrasts with the sharp increase in distal oesophageal adenocarcinoma in low risk areas in the Northern and Western hemispheres. Risk factors are male gender, smoking, alcohol ingestion, obesity, metabolic syndrome, gastrooesophageal reflux, fungal and Human Papilloma Virus (HPV) infections.

Oesophageal cancer usually presents with progressive dysphagia initially for solids and ultimately liquids. Investigation is by endoscopy and biopsy, and chest x-ray to detect any enlargement of the heart, mediastinal lymph nodes or lung lesion that may be causing extrinsic compression. For biopsy proven cancer, staging for local and distant disease includes ELUS (endoluminal ultrasound for tumour depth and lymph node spread), CT (computerized tomography) scan chest and abdomen and combined CT/PET (positron emission tomography) scan for locoregional and non-regional metastases. Oesophagogastric junctional adenocarcinoma and select cases of distal oesophageal adenocarcinoma have laparoscopy with peritoneal staging washings. Bronchoscopy may be undertaken in patients with clinical or radiological features suspicious of tracheobronchial invasion. Thoracoscopy may be required to sample suspect mediastinal lymph nodes. The potential for synchronous upper aerodigestive tract tumours is borne in mind. Patients with identified distant metastases or involved lymph nodes in three compartments (neck, mediastinum, abdomen) are not suitable for curative treatment.

Treatment of oesophageal cancer may be palliative (chemoradiotherapy, laser ablation, stent) in bulky high stage disease, or, curative in intent with earlier lesions. The latter may involve neoadjuvant therapy (chemoradiation for squamous cell carcinoma: chemotherapy for adenocarcinoma) to downstage the tumour, followed by radiological restaging, and then surgery, or either modality alone. Postoperative chemotherapy may be used for adenocarcinoma depending on patient fitness and the pathological stage of disease in the surgical specimen, but not usually for squamous cell carcinoma. Choice of operative procedure depends on the general health of the patient, the tumour site and extent, the choice of planned oesophageal substitute (stomach, jejunum, colon), and preference of the surgeon. Ideally longitudinal clearance margins of 5–10 cm should be achieved and an appropriate two field lymphadenectomy performed to improve staging and local disease control. Transthoracic or transdiaphragmatic hiatal approaches are available with the latter particularly suitable for localised distal oesophageal lesions and resulting in less operative morbidity than thoracotomy. Minimally Invasive Oesophagectomy (MIO) procedures are being developed using combined thoracoscopic and laparoscopic techniques. There is currently no preferred evidence based method of choice. Early lesions confined to the mucosa may be amenable to local surgical techniques e.g. endoscopic mucosal resection (EMR) or endoscopic submucosal dissection (ESD). It is recognized that these "big biopsy" specimens have a triple purpose: diagnostic, staging and potentially therapeutic. Follow up radical surgery may be necessary if there is submucosal, lymphovascular or margin involvement in the histopathology specimen.

1.1   Gross Description

Specimen

- Biopsy/EMR/ESD/partial oesophagectomy/ total thoracic oesophagectomy (TTO)/ oesophagectomy with limited gastrectomy/ oesophagogastrectomy.
- Procedure: endoscopic/MIO/transthoracic or transhiatal.
- Number of fragments (a minimum of eight is recommended)/EMR/ESD dimensions(mm)/ length of oesophagus and proximal stomach (cm). Measurements are better assessed on the fresh specimen as formalin fixation causes up to 30 % contraction. The external surface is also inspected for the presence of adventitial fat, lateral mediastinal pleura, pericardium and distally abdominal peritoneum.

Tumour

Site

- Mid/lower oesophagus/oesophagogastric junction/cardia (Fig. 1.1).
- Distances (cm) to the proximal and distal resection limits and the oesophagogastric junction. The junction can vary in location or be obscured by tumour. Anatomically distal oesophagus has an external layer of adventitia or abdominal peritoneum whereas proximal stomach is orientated to serosa. Tumour is clearly oesophageal if its bulk or epicentre is above the oesophagogastric junction as defined by internal or external landmarks e.g. the mucosal squamocolumnar Z line, where the tubular oesophagus

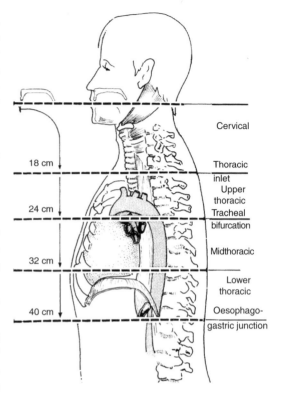

Fig. 1.1 Oesophagus (Reproduced, with permission, from Wittekind et al. (2005), © 2005)

ends and the saccular stomach begins, or orientation to adventitial fat. This may also be corroborated histologically with the finding of Barrett's metaplasia/dysplasia or squamous epithelium/dysplasia in the oesophagus. Note that under TNM7 tumours of the oesophagogastric junction, and those in the proximal stomach with an epicenter within 5 cm of the junction and involving the oesophagus, are staged as an oesophageal cancer. Those within 5 cm of the junction but not involving the oesophagus are considered gastric in origin. From a clinical point of view tumours involving the junction are classified as Siewert I (distal oesophagus growing down), II (truly junctional) or III (gastric cardia growing up). In addition squamous cell, small cell and undifferentiated carcinomas involving the junction are regarded as oesophageal in origin.

Size

- Length × width × depth (cm) or maximum dimension (cm).
- Superficial carcinoma is often small (<2–3 cm long) but advanced carcinoma frequently involves long segments of oesophagus.

Appearance

- Polypoid: spindle cell carcinoma with good prognosis.
- Warty/verrucous: verrucous carcinoma.
- Nodular/plaque: superficial carcinoma (the gross and endoscopic appearances may be classified similar to that of early gastric cancer; see Chap. 2).
- Fungating/stricture/ulcerated/infiltrative: usual types.
- Multifocal (10 %).
- Regression and scarring post adjuvant chemo-/radiotherapy.

Edge

- Circumscribed/irregular.

Other Pathology

- Fistula/perforation either spontaneous, post neoadjuvant therapy or post endoscopy.
- Diverticulum.
- Achalasia.
- Barrett's metaplasia: velvety mucosa distinct from the pale squamous mucosa and proximal to the junction.
- Male preponderance (3:1).

1.2   Histological Type

Adenocarcinoma

- *50–60 % of cases.*
- In the *distal oesophagus/oesophagogastric junction* on the basis of specialised enteric type *Barrett's metaplasia* and *dysplasia*. The incidence of this tumour has greatly increased (×3–5 in the last 20 years). Various suggested factors are heredity, improved socio-economic conditions with obesity from a Western diet rich in processed foods, antibiotic eradication of acid suppressing pangastric cag-A (cytotoxin associated gene product) positive *Helicobacter pylorii* with restoration of gastric acidity and increased gastro-oesophageal reflux disease, proton pump inhibitor therapy and bile reflux. Most are tubular or papillary and of *intestinal type*, some are signet ring cell or mucinous. There is *poor prognosis* as presentation is at a late stage, typically with adventitial, lymph node and perineural invasion.

Squamous Cell Carcinoma

- *30–40 % of cases.*
- *Mid-oesophagus*, older age. Risk factors are smoking and excess alcohol.
- Usually moderately differentiated and keratinising.
- *Verrucous*: exophytic and keratotic with a pushing deep margin of cytologically bland bulbous processes. Slow growing but anecdotally may become more aggressive especially after radiation.
- *Basaloid*: poor prognosis and *aggressive*. Deeply invasive nested pattern of palisaded basaloid cells with central necrosis, atypia and mitoses.

Spindle Cell Carcinoma (Polypoid Carcinoma/Carcinosarcoma)

- A spindle cell squamous carcinoma that undergoes varying degrees of stromal mesenchymal homologous or heterologous differentiation.
- Men, sixth decade.

Adenosquamous Carcinoma

- Mixed glandular and squamous cell differentiation, *aggressive*.

Undifferentiated Carcinoma

- Absent squamous cell or glandular differentiation and a *high-grade lesion*.
- In poorly differentiated lesions, adenocarcinoma may be CK7/CAM5.2 positive, and squamous cell carcinoma negative for these markers but CK5/6, p63 positive. However, there can be considerable overlap in immunophenotypic expression. Characterisation is of use as squamous cell carcinomas are often more responsive to neoadjuvant chemoradiation (adenocarcinoma receives chemotherapy only), and can be associated with synchronous or metachronous upper aerodigestive tract tumours.

Mucoepidermoid/Adenoid Cystic Carcinoma

- Of oesophageal submucosal duct origin with a tendency to local recurrence and metastases in 50 % of cases.

Small Cell Carcinoma

- A poorly differentiated/high-grade neuroendocrine carcinoma, either primary or secondary from lung, or as part of a mixed differentiation oesophageal cancer. It is of *poor prognosis*. Distinguish from poorly differentiated basaloid squamous cell carcinoma or adenocarcinoma by synaptophysin/CD56/TTF-1 and paranuclear dot CAM 5.2 expression in small cell carcinoma.

Malignant Melanoma

- Primary or secondary. Primary requires adjacent mucosal junctional atypia. Comprises *0.1 % of oesophageal malignancy* – polypoid, ulcerated, satellite nodules, pigment, *poor prognosis*.

Metastatic Carcinoma

- *Direct spread*: stomach, thyroid, hypopharynx, bronchus and lung
- *Distant spread*: breast, malignant melanoma.

1.3 Differentiation

Well/moderate/poor/undifferentiated, or Grade 1/2/3/4.
- Influence on prognosis is uncertain unless the tumour is anaplastic e.g. undifferentiated carcinoma, small cell carcinoma or basaloid carcinoma.
- For squamous cell carcinoma differentiation features are keratinisation and intercellular bridges, and, for adenocarcinoma the percentage tumour gland formation (well/G1 >95 %: moderate/G2 50–95 %: poor/G3 <50 %). Undifferentiated carcinomas cannot be categorised as either squamous cell or adenocarcinoma and are classified as Grade 4 (as is small cell carcinoma).
- Heterogeneity of grade and differentiation within individual tumours is not uncommon e.g. mixed intestinal and signet ring patterns.

1.4 Extent of Local Tumour Spread

Border: pushing/infiltrative.
Lymphocytic reaction: prominent/sparse.
Depth (pT stage) and distance (mm) to the nearest painted perioesophageal circumferential resection margin (CRM) (Fig. 1.2).
Superficial ("*early*") *squamous cell carcinoma* of the oesophagus is defined as intraepithelial or invasive squamous cell carcinoma confined to the mucosa or submucosa, with or without lymph node spread (pTis, pT1). It is of more *favourable prognosis* than the usual muscle invasive deep or "*advanced*" carcinoma (*beyond the muscularis propria*) with differing 5 year survival rates: 60–90 % versus 5–10 %. Carcinoma invading *submucosa* does less well (25–35 %

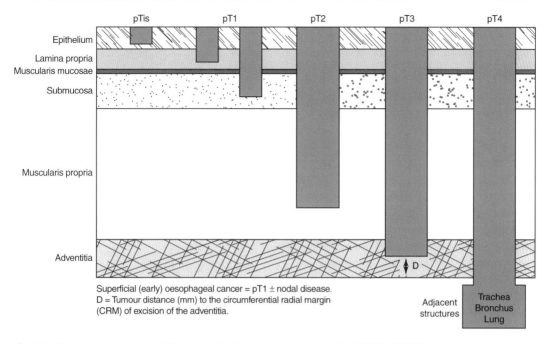

Fig. 1.2 Oesophageal carcinoma (Reproduced, with permission, from Allen (2006), © 2006)

lymph node metastases, 55 % 5 year survival) than that confined to the mucosa alone (88 % 5 year survival irrespective of lymph node status). *Depth of invasion* is the most important *prognostic indicator* on multivariate analysis and requires histological assessment as there is variable correlation with gross, radiological and endoscopic appearances. Note that on biopsy distinction between dysplastic glands or squamous epithelium abutting an irregular muscularis mucosae and true invasion can be difficult: look for single cells and nests of infiltration (± a desmoplastic stromal reaction). This is further complicated by the relatively common finding of duplication of the muscularis mucosae in Barrett's metaplasia. The edge of a well differentiated adenocarcinoma may manifest only as mildly atypical glands devoid of stromal reaction but undermining oesophageal squamous epithelium. However, the pitfall of squamous re-epithelialisation overlying Barrett's mucosa (± dysplasia) related to ablation treatment must also be borne in mind.

The TNM7 classification applies only to carcinomas.

pTis	Carcinoma in situ/high-grade dysplasia
pT1	Tumour invades lamina propria (pT1a) or submucosa (pT1b)
pT2	Tumour invades muscularis propria
pT3	Tumour invades adventitia
pT4	Tumour invades adjacent structures:
pT4a	Pleura, pericardium or diaphragm, and
pT4b	Aorta, vertebral body, trachea.

About 50 % of distal oesophageal carcinomas spread into the proximal stomach with potential for serosal involvement. Junctional and gastric tumour components are regarded as oesophageal in site for TNM7 staging.

In cases with post neoadjuvant therapy tumour regression, ypT is determined by the *deepest residual viable tumour* and not more deeply placed acellular keratin debris where tumour may have been. A *three grade classification of tumour response to neoadjuvant therapy* (no or minimal residual tumour/moderate residual tumour/no response) is a *prognostic indicator* with complete regression and absence of lymph node or distant metastases being favourable signs. Histological tumour regression shows variable correlation with other measures of clinical response such as improvement in dysphagia, or decrease in tumour metabolic FDG (fluorodeoxyglucose) avidity on PET scan.

1.5   Lymphovascular Invasion

Present/absent.
Intra-/extratumoural.

The presence of lymphovascular invasion (LVI) is a *strong prognostic indicator*. In advanced carcinoma lamina propria and submucosal LVI are not infrequent, resulting in carcinomatous emboli several centimetres beyond the gross tumour edge. These skip metastases (15 % of cases) are not classified separately under TNM7. Perineural invasion is also characteristic.

1.6   Lymph Nodes

The significance of lymph node micrometastases (≤2 mm diameter) is uncertain but *involvement of lymph nodes*, particularly if multiple, is a *strong prognostic indicator*. Lymph node metastases occur *early in the disease course* (60 % at the time of presentation) and are the commonest cause of treatment failure. Histological assessment is required as specificity of lymph node involvement on ELUS is limited. Involvement of stomach and later liver, lungs and adrenal gland is not infrequent. Up to *30 % of metastases are clinically occult* and discovered at CT/PET examination.

Site/number/size/number involved/limit node/ extracapsular spread.

Regional nodes: perioesophageal including coeliac axis nodes and paraoesophageal lymph nodes in the neck, but not supraclavicular lymph nodes. A mediastinal lymphadenectomy will ordinarily include a minimum of six regional lymph nodes.

pN0	No regional lymph node metastasis
pN1	Metastasis in 1–2 regional lymph node(s)
pN2	Metastasis in 3–6 regional lymph nodes
pN3	Metastasis in seven or more regional lymph nodes
pM1	Distant metastasis
	Commonest sites are mediastinum, lung and liver (Fig. 1.3)

1.7   Excision Margins

Distances (cm) to the proximal and distal limits of excision.

Distance (mm) to the painted perioesophageal CRM. Involvement (tumour present to within 1 mm) is an index of the degree of tumour spread and extent of surgical resection with potential for local recurrence or residual mediastinal disease and decreased survival.

Oesophageal carcinoma may show *multifocality* (10–25 %), direct or discontinuous submucosal and lymphovascular spread and *intramural metastasis* (15 %). This has obvious implications for examination of resection margins (sometimes by intraoperative frozen section) and potential for local recurrence.

1.8   Other Pathology

Diverticula, achalasia, coeliac disease and Plummer-Vincent syndrome (middle aged to elderly females, iron deficiency anaemia, post cricoid pharyngo-oesophageal web) have an increased incidence of oesophageal carcinoma. Squamous cell carcinoma is usually in the mid-thoracic oesophagus while Barrett's related adenocarcinoma is commoner, being the most frequent malignant tumour of the distal oesophagus. The *incidence* of *Barrett's related adenocarcinoma* and *oesophagogastric junctional tumours* has markedly *increased*.

Barrett's metaplasia: defined as replacement of the lower oesophageal squamous mucosa by metaplastic glandular epithelium due to *gastrooesophageal reflux disease*. The Barrett's segment can be *classical* (*>3 cm long*) or *short* (*<3 cm long*), with in particular long segment disease having an increased risk of malignancy. The clinical extent of the Barrett's change is described according to its length of circumferential disposition and total segment length i.e. C2M6 is circumferential over 2 cm in a 6 cm long segment. Ultra-short segment Barrett's is now regarded as junctional metaplasia, a separate condition related to helicobacter pylorii infection or acid reflux. An approximate guide is that 10 % of patients with hiatus hernia and/or gastrooesophageal reflux develop Barrett's metaplasia.

Fig. 1.3 Oesophagus: regional lymph nodes (Reproduced, with permission, from Wittekind et al. (2005), © 2005)

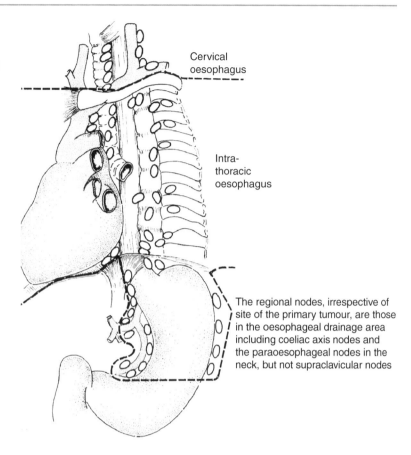

Cervical oesophagus

Intra-thoracic oesophagus

The regional nodes, irrespective of site of the primary tumour, are those in the oesophageal drainage area including coeliac axis nodes and the paraoesophageal nodes in the neck, but not supraclavicular nodes

Of these about 10 % subsequently have *dysplasia* or *adenocarcinoma* with ×30 risk that of the general population, although this may be an overestimate. The *specialised intestinal* or *enteric variant of Barrett's metaplasia* is the usual precursor to dysplasia rather than the atrophic gastric fundic or non-specialised cardia types.

The *biological behaviour* of *low-grade dysplasia* is uncertain with potential for regression after high dose proton pump inhibitor (PPI) treatment, or progression. It requires reassessment and if a higher grade lesion is excluded, PPI treatment is instigated with subsequent 6 monthly endoscopic surveillance. There is a *strong (30%) association* between *high-grade dysplasia* and concurrent or subsequent *adenocarcinoma*, indicating the need for immediate clinicopathological reassessment, short-term follow up, and consideration given to its eradication (see below). The recognition of significant dysplasia requires *confirmation* by a second experienced pathologist or positive repeat biopsy. Useful clues to the presence of dysplasia are mucosal villousity and persistence of cytological dysmaturation into the surface epithelium. Features suggestive of *adenocarcinoma* include cribriform architecture and high-grade dysplastic epithelium with any or several of: superficial ulceration, infiltration by polymorphs, necrotic eosinophilic lumenal and nuclear debris, and undermining of squamous mucosa. Infiltration of lamina propria and stromal desmoplasia indicate established malignancy. Observer agreement rates are reasonably good for high-grade dysplasia. However, it is important to distinguish *florid regenerative changes* in oesophageal squamous and glandular mucosae from dysplasia. This must take into account erosion, ulceration and the degree of inflammation that is present, as well as cytoarchitectural changes e.g. nuclear enlargement with nucleolar prominence and basal cell hyperplasia. *Squamous epithelial regrowth* after anti-reflux, laser or photodynamic ablative therapy can produce variably atypical and confusing cytoarchitectural changes, as does chemoradiation therapy. Maturation towards the epithelial surface is reassuring. Over expression of p53 or AMACR and a high Ki-67 proliferation index (especially in the surface epithelium) can sometimes help to confirm mucosal dysplasia and its potential for progression to adenocarcinoma in dysplastic Barrett's mucosa. It should be noted that the *primary diagnosis of Barrett's metaplasia* (CLO – Columnar Lined Oesophagus) is heavily dependent on the *endoscopic findings* and *site of biopsy* i.e. an origin from the anatomical oesophagus. Pathognomonic histological features are metaplastic glandular epithelium associated with native oesophageal structures e.g. submucosal glands or ducts. Glandular mucosa with squamous epithelial islands is also a useful clue. Specialised enteric differentiation is reasonably distinctive whereas fundic gastric mucosa is more often associated with hiatus hernia.

Surveillance for dysplasia in Barrett's mucosa is recommended as annual or biennial endoscopy with quadrantic, segmental (every 2 cm) biopsies. More sophisticated endoscopic techniques are now more commonly available e.g. magnification/ chromoendoscopy, spectroscopy. *Target biopsy* of any gross lesion (ulcers, nodules, plaques, strictures) is important as this is more likely to yield significant pathology. In the absence of tumour, or in a medically unfit patient with an early mucosal lesion, *local ablative therapy* can be used e.g. EMR of any mucosal nodule, and high radiofrequency (HALO), laser or photodynamic therapy to the background Barrett's segment. In general, mucosa confined disease can be managed by endosopic treatment and subsequent surveillance. Detailed multidisciplinary team discussion and *careful patient selection* are crucial when considering organ conserving treatment. Adverse histological prognostic factors in any EMR specimen or signs of clinical progression may signify the need to proceed to radical surgery. Close patient follow up is required. *Oesophagectomy* tends to be reserved for cases with submucosal invasion as it has up to a 25 % risk of lymph node metastases, where there are clinically suspected regional lymph node metastases, or there has been unsuccessful endoscopic therapy, or high-grade dysplasia that is beyond treatment by HALO. Non-regional disease precludes radical surgery.

Field change squamous cell dysplasia/carcinoma in situ: often encountered adjacent to or overlying squamous cell carcinoma. A precancerous phase and the biological course of these premalignant changes is uncertain but better established in countries such as China and Japan where the incidence of oesophageal carcinoma is greater. This has led to the establishment of endoscopic and cytological screening programmes targeted at the detection of early stage carcinoma (10–15 % only of cases in the West). As with glandular dysplasia a two-tiered system of *low-grade* (≤50 % of the epithelial width) and *high-grade dysplasia* is used. Dysplasia is found more frequently overlying and adjacent to superficial than advanced squamous cell carcinoma. It may be identified at endoscopy as friable, erythematous plaques or nodules. *Some 25 % of high-grade dysplasia lesions progress to carcinoma.* If confined to the mucosa at endoscopy and ELUS, *local mucosal resection* (EMR) or *ablation* (HALO, laser) may be used. Histologically it must be distinguished from inflammatory regenerative or reflux changes, viral infection (herpes simplex, CMV), pseudoepitheliomatous hyperplasia (e.g. overlying a granular cell tumour), chemoradiotherapy changes and established cancer. A further diagnostic clue is that squamous dysplasia lifts off with the biopsy forceps in intact strips bound by basement membrane whereas squamous cell cancer fragments.

Concurrent squamous cell carcinoma: of bronchus and oropharyngolaryngeal ring has an *incidence of 10–15 %.* Bronchoscopy and upper airways endoscopy may be required prior to radical treatment to exclude a lung cancer spreading to involve the oesophagus. Conversely careful scrutiny of the chest CT scan is also necessary to identify any evidence of spread of an oesophageal cancer to contiguous mediastinal structures (pT4 disease) that might exclude consideration of radical surgery.

Chemo-/radiotherapy necrosis and tumour regression: cell apoptosis, vacuolation and degeneration, necrosis, inflammation, fibrosis, residual aggregates of keratin with a giant cell reaction, and perforation may all be seen leaving only residual microscopic tumour. The degree of *tumour response to treatment is graded* according to the five tier *Mandard score*. As discussed above a three grade scoring system is easier to use in practice and more reproducible. Post surgical pathological staging is determined by the *deepest focus of residual tumour*, and not tissue reaction or acellular keratin where tumour may have been present pretreatment. *Chemoradiation* is the main treatment for extensive squamous cell carcinoma of the middle third of the oesophagus, and, *chemoradiation±surgery* for medically fit patients with locally confined lesions <5 cm in length, and cancers of the distal third. Preoperative chemoradiation is being increasingly used in an attempt to *downstage the tumour* and achieve better *operative resectability*. Distal oesophageal and junctional adenocarcinomas receive *preoperative chemotherapy*, and *postoperative adjuvant chemotherapy* depending on the pathological staging of the resection specimen. Postoperative chemotherapy is generally not used for squamous cell carcinoma. It is estimated that some *50–60 % of tumours show quite marked morphological changes of regression*, with squamous cell carcinoma being more radiotherapy and chemoresponsive than adenocarcinoma. More sophisticated preoperative staging (e.g. CT/PET scan and ELUS with FNAC) is being assessed as a means of predicting those patients likely to benefit from preoperative neoadjuvant therapy, and in selecting patients with locoregional confined disease for primary resection. Patients are restaged radiologically after neoadjuvant therapy is completed prior to curative intent radical surgery. This is in case there has been non-response and tumour progression in the interim. Ablative laser therapy and insertion of an expansile metal stent are additional *palliative measures* for bulky obstructive non-resectable tumour.

  Spindle cell carcinoma: cytokeratin and mesenchymal markers (vimentin, desmin, actin) are helpful in spindle cell carcinoma (syn. carcinosarcoma). These tumours show a *biphasic spectrum of differentiation* viz malignant epithelial (squamous) and mesenchymal (usually sarcoma not otherwise specified, sometimes cartilage, bone, striated muscle). There is either intimate intermingling or juxtaposition of the components which are present in variable amounts (the epithelial component may be microscopic or in situ). *Prognosis is intermediate to good* because they are exophytic intraluminal lesions which present at a relatively early stage despite their size (50 % 5 year survival).

Prognosis

Prognosis of oesophageal cancer is poor (5 year survival 5–10 % in the Western Hemisphere), and relates to *tumour type* (small cell carcinoma, basaloid carcinoma are adverse), *grade* (equivocal), *diameter* (in superficial carcinoma), but most importantly *depth of invasion* and *stage*. *Lymph node status* and whether the *longitudinal* and *circumferential radial margins* are positive (55 % recurrence rate, 25 % 5 year survival) or negative (13 % recurrence rate, 47 % 5 year survival in one series) are important prognostic variables. Early oesophageal squamous cell carcinoma does significantly better than advanced disease. Early (pT1) adenocarcinoma may show less lymph node disease and local recurrence than equivalent squamous cell lesions. However, for the majority of cases, although adenocarcinoma may have slightly better overall 5 year survival (25 %), the two main pathological types have little differential influence on prognosis.

1.9   Other Malignancy

Malignant Lymphoma/Leukaemia

- Rare. More usually secondary to gastric or systemic/mediastinal lymph node disease.
- Primary lymphoma is large B cell in type, or extranodal marginal zone lymphoma (MALToma).
- Consequences of immunosuppression due to the tumour or its treatment may be seen e.g. CMV, herpetic or fungal oesophagitis.

Leiomyoma/ Leiomyosarcoma/GISTs

- *Leiomyomas* greatly outnumber *leiomyosarcomas* (malignancy: >5 cm diameter, necrosis, mitoses >5/50 high-power fields, cellular atypia, infiltrative margins). Most leiomyomas are small, identified by endoscopy and arise from the muscularis mucosae or inner muscularis propria. They can be multiple, intraluminal or intramural. Oesophageal gastrointestinal stromal tumours (*GISTs*) are rare (DOG1/CD117/CD34 positive, desmin negative) and potentially malignant with liver metastases.

Sarcoma

- Rare. 90 % are *leiomyosarcoma* (desmin, h-caldesmon positive).
- Embryonal rhabdomyosarcoma (childhood: desmin/myo D1/myogenin positive).
- Kaposi's sarcoma (AIDS): human herpes virus 8 (HHV 8) positive.
- Synovial sarcoma : children/adults, polypoid mass in upper oesophagus.
- Exclude the more common possibility of a spindle cell carcinoma (polypoid carcinoma/carcinosarcoma) with cytokeratin positive spindle cells and varying degrees of homologous or heterologous mesenchymal differentiation.

Others

- Rare: granular cell tumour (S100 positive, overlying pseudoepitheliomatous hyperplasia), well differentiated neuroendocrine (carcinoid) tumour: chromogranin, synaptophysin, CD56 positive, Ki-67 ≤2 %, good prognosis.

Bibliography

Allen DC. Histopathology reporting: guidelines for surgical cancer. 2nd ed. London: Springer; 2006.

Allum WH, Blazeby JM, Griffin SM, Cunningham D, Jankowski JA, Wong R, On behalf of the Association of Upper Gastrointestinal Surgeons of Great Britain and Northern Ireland, the British Society of Gastroenterology and the British Association of Surgical Oncology. Guidelines for the management of oesophageal and gastric cancer. Gut. 2011;60: 1449–72.

Barr H. The pathological implications of surveillance, treatment and surgery for Barrett's oesophagus. Curr Diagn Pathol. 2003;9:242–51.

Bogomeletz WV. Early squamous cell carcinoma of oesophagus. Curr Diagn Pathol. 1994;1:212–5.

Bosman FT, Carneiro F. WHO classification of tumours of the digestive system. 4th ed. Lyon: IARC press; 2010.

Chandrasama P, Wickramasinghe K, Ma Y, DeMeester T. Adenocarcinomas of the distal esophagus and "gastric cardia" are predominantly esophageal carcinomas. Am J Surg Pathol. 2007;31:569–75.

Coad RA, Shepherd NA. Barrett's oesophagus: definition, diagnosis and pathogenesis. Curr Diagn Pathol. 2003; 9:218–27.

Cotton P, Williams C. Practical gastrointestinal endoscopy. 4th ed. London: Blackwell Science; 1996.

Day DW, Jass JR, Price AB, Shepherd NA, Sloan JM, Talbot IC, Warren BF, Williams GT. Morson and Dawson's gastrointestinal pathology. 4th ed. Oxford: Blackwell Sciences; 2003.

Flejou J-F, Svrcek M. Barrett's oesophagus – a pathologist's view. Histopathology. 2007;50:3–14.

Galmiche JP, Pallone F. Barrett's oesophagus and oesophageal adenocarcinoma. Gut. 2005;54(S1): i1–42.

Hage M, Siersema PD, van Dekken H. Oesophageal pathology following ablation of Barrett's mucosa. Curr Diagn Pathol. 2006;12:127–35.

Ibrahim NBN. Guidelines for handling oesophageal biopsies and resection specimens and their reporting. J Clin Pathol. 2000;53:89–94.

Jankowski J, Barr H, Wang K, Delaney B. Diagnosis and management of Barrett's oesophagus. BMJ. 2010;341: 597–602.

Lagergren J, Lagergren P. Oesophageal cancer. BMJ. 2010;341:1207–11.

Lewin KJ, Appelman HD. Tumors of the esophagus and stomach. Atlas of tumor pathology. 3rd series. Fascicle 18. Washington: AFIP; 1996.

Logan RPH, Harris A, Misciewicz JJ, Baron JH, editors. ABC of the upper gastrointestinal tract. London: BMJ Books; 2002.

Mandard AM, Dalibard F, Mandard JC, Marnay J, Henry-Amar M, Petiot JF, Roussel A, et al. Pathologic assessment of tumour regression after preoperative chemoradiotherapy of oesophageal carcinoma. Cancer. 1994;73:2680–96.

Moyes LH, Going JJ. Still waiting for predictive biomarkers in Barrett's oesophagus. J Clin Pathol. 2011;64: 742–50.

Odze RD, Goldblum JR. Surgical pathology of the GI tract, liver, biliary tract and pancreas. 2nd ed. Philadelphia: Saunders Elsevier; 2009.

Pech O, May A, Rabenstein T, Ell C. Endoscopic resection of early oesophageal cancer. Gut. 2007;56: 1625–34.

Schlemper RJ, Riddell RH, Kato Y, et al. The Vienna classification of gastrointestinal epithelial neoplasia. Gut. 2000;47:251–5.

The Royal College of Pathologists: Cancer Datasets (Oesophageal Carcinoma, Gastric Carcinoma, Carcinomas of the Pancreas, ampulla of Vater and Common Bile Duct, Colorectal Cancer, Gastrointestinal Stromal Tumours (GISTs), Liver Resection Specimens and Liver Biopsies for Primary and Metastatic Carcinoma, Endocrine Tumours of the Gastrointestinal Tract including Pancreas) and Tissue Pathways

(Gastrointestinal and Pancreatobiliary Pathology, Liver Biopsies for the Investigation of Medical Disease and for Focal Liver Lesions). Accessed at http://www.rcpath.org/index.asp?PageID=254.

Wang LM, Sheahan K. Pathological assessment of post-treatment gastrointestinal and hepatic resection specimens. Curr Diagn Pathol. 2007;13:222–31.

Wittekind CF, Greene FL, Hutter RVP, Klimpfinger M, Sobib LH. TNM atlas: illustrated guide to the TNM/pTNM classification of malignant tumours. 5th ed. Berlin: Springer; 2005.

Yantis RK, Odze RD. Neoplastic precursor lesions of the upper gastrointestinal tract. Diagn Histopathol. 2008;14:437–52.

Gastric Carcinoma

Gastric cancer accounts for 8 % of cancers worldwide with high incidence (Eastern Asia and Eastern Europe, Central/Latin America) and low incidence (North America and Northern Europe, Africa) areas. The former tends to distal tumours of intestinal type, the latter to more proximal tumours with a significant proportion of diffuse cancers. Risk factors are smoking, diet (high in salt-preserved/smoked foods – low in fresh fruit/vegetables), bile reflux and Helicobacter pylorii infection. About 10 % show familial clustering and 1–3 % are on a direct hereditary basis.

Gastric cancer can present with anaemia, haematemesis, weight loss, abdominal pain or dyspeptic symptoms. Investigation is by endoscopy with biopsy. Decreased distensibility and wall motility either on endoscopy or barium meal examination are suspicious of linitis plastica (diffuse carcinoma). Multiple biopsies (a minimum of eight) are required as up to 10 % of endoscopically suspicious lesions will require re-biopsy. Staging for local and distant disease includes endoluminal ultrasound (ELUS: tumour depth and lymph node spread), CT scan chest, abdomen and pelvis, PET scan, and, peritoneal laparoscopy with cytological washings and biopsy of any nodules or plaques in the serosa or omentum.

Non-regional disease is an indicator for palliative treatment including chemotherapy, and surgery if there is anatomical dysfunction e.g. gastric outlet obstruction or anaemia. Curative intent surgery can be localised (EMR/ESD) or radical, the extent of the latter depending on the patient's age, fitness, tumour type, stage and location. Distal (antral) tumours are treated by subtotal gastrectomy and proximal tumours by total gastrectomy. The aim is to achieve a complete (R0) resection with proximal, distal and circumferential margin clearance. Limited gastric resection is used for palliation or in the very elderly. Extent of lymphadenectomy is tailored accordingly. Surgery is often preceded by a course of neoadjuvant chemotherapy and radiological re-staging. Postoperative adjuvant chemotherapy may be indicated following full clinicopathological staging of the surgical specimen and multidisciplinary team discussion. A minority of patients with locally advanced or recurrent disease are suitable for trastuzumab therapy.

2.1 Gross Description

Specimen

- Cytological brushings, washings or aspirate/endoscopic biopsy/EMR(endoscopic mucosal resection)/ESD(endoscopic submucosal dissection)/partial (proximal or distal) or total gastrectomy/oesophagogastrectomy/lymphadenectomy ± omentectomy.
- Number of biopsy fragments/EMR/ESD dimensions (mm).
- Length (cm) along greater curvature.
- Length (cm) of oesophagus and duodenum.

Fig. 2.1 Stomach
(Reproduced, with
permission, from Wittekind
et al. (2005), © 2005)

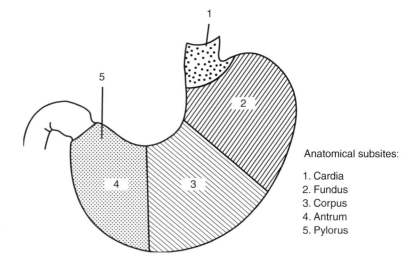

Anatomical subsites:

1. Cardia
2. Fundus
3. Corpus
4. Antrum
5. Pylorus

Tumour

Site

- Distal oesophagus/cardia/fundus/ corpus/ antrum/pylorus/duodenum (Fig. 2.1).
- Lesser curve/greater curve.
- Anterior/posterior wall.
- Antrum (50 %) and lesser curve (15 %) are traditionally the most frequent sites. However, the incidence of *distal gastric carcinoma is decreasing* while that of the *proximal stomach and cardia is markedly increasing*. This is in part due to eradication of helicobacter pylorii infection and loss of its acid suppression effect with more reflux changes. *Proximal cancer* presents at a more *advanced stage* than equivalent-size distal lesions with a *worse prognosis* and similarities in behaviour to distal oesophageal adenocarcinoma. Adenocarcinomas in the vicinity of the oesphagogastric junction are clinically designated as either Siewert I: distal oesophagus coming down, Siewert II: junctional, or Siewert III: gastric cardia going up. Note that under TNM7 tumours of the oesophagogastric junction, and those in the proximal stomach with an epicenter within 5 cm of the junction and involving the oesophagus are staged as an oesophageal cancer. Those within 5 cm of the junction but not involving the oesophagus are considered gastric in origin.
- Multifocal 6 %: in particular early gastric cancer and malignant lymphoma.

Size

- Length × width × depth (cm) or maximum dimension (cm).

Appearance

- Polypoid/plaque/ulcerated/infiltrative/ mucoid/linitis plastica (leather bottle stomach)/scirrhous/fleshy.

Advanced (muscle invasive) gastric cancer is classified macroscopically according to Borrmann type as:

I	Polypoid
I	Fungating
III	Ulcerated
IV	Infiltrative

Types I, II/III and IV tend to correspond to tubulo/papillary, intestinal, and signet ring cell (linitis plastica) adenocarcinomas respectively, although there is overlap between the categories. Polypoid/exophytic tumours are regarded as being of better prognosis than ulcerated/deeply infiltrative cancers.

Edge

• Circumscribed/irregular.

2.2   Histological Type

An amalgam of the WHO and Lauren classifications is used.

Adenocarcinoma

Intestinal	50 %	Antrum
Diffuse	20 %	Body of stomach, young or elderly patients
Mixed	25 %	
Solid	5 %	

The WHO system classifies gastric cancer as: tubular, papillary, mucinous, poorly cohesive (including signet ring cell and its variants), and mixed carcinomas.

Intestinal carcinomas: have tubuloacinar (common), papillary or mucinous (colloid) patterns, and form polypoid or ulcerative lesions with expansile margins. They are associated with *atrophic gastritis*, *intestinal metaplasia* and *dysplasia*. By definition tubular adenocarcinoma is well differentiated and may be difficult to diagnose due to wide separation of glands in a non-desmoplastic stroma. Undermining of structures can be helpful e.g. muscularis mucosae or oesophagogastric junction squamous epithelium. Equally, papillary adenocarcinoma is exophytic with well differentiated epithelial fronds supported by fine fibrovascular stroma. Biopsies may only sample its surface component and distinction from high-grade dysplasia can be problematic. Its endoscopic and ELUS/CT appearances and sharp demarcation from adjacent mucosa must be taken into account. The definition of a mucinous adenocarcinoma, whether glandular, colloid or signet ring cell requires mucin production in >50 % of the tumour cells or area.

Diffuse carcinomas: comprise single cells with clear or eosinophilic *signet ring cell* cytonuclear appearances, and form *linitis plastica* with infiltrating margins. A point of origin from dysplasia is often difficult to demonstrate as the tumour emanates from the mid-mucosal proliferative zone (from non-metaplastic foveolar or mucous neck cells), or, deep lamina propria invading submucosa, muscularis, serosa and with *transperitoneal spread*. The cells do not express the adhesion protein E-cadherin. A minority (8–10 %) of gastric cancers are hereditary. In a young patient occult presentation with an inherited autosomal dominant (germline mutation in E-cadherin CDH1) diffuse gastric cancer, which in females can be associated with breast lobular carcinoma, should be considered. Alternatively intestinal gastric cancer can develop in a young patient as part of the hereditary non-polyposis colon cancer syndrome (HNPCC) and rarely Familial Adenomatous Polyposis (FAP).

Adenocarcinoma Variants

Invasive micropapillary carcinoma: small clusters of cells in clear spaces simulating vascular channels. It shows a high propensity for lymphovascular and lymph node metastases.

Hepatoid carcinoma: glandular and hepatocellular differentiation with marked vascular invasion and poor prognosis. ± AFP immunoexpression, polyclonal CEA positive.

Parietal cell carcinoma: rare, solid sheets of cells with eosinophilic granular cytoplasm.

Medullary carcinoma, lymphoepithelial carcinoma: medullary carcinoma has a solid syncytial morphology, regular vesicular nuclei with pinpoint nucleoli, and a pushing circumscribed margin associated with a dense peritumoural lymphoplasmacytic infiltrate. It has a high level of microsatellite instability (MSI-H), and is similar to the right sided colonic cancers found in HNPCC. Conversely, lymphoepithelial carcinoma has single cells, small clusters and glands and an infiltrating margin with numerous intratumoural or tumour infiltrating lymphocytes (TILs). It has a 77 % 5 year survival and can be associated with Epstein-Barr virus infection. Anecdotally these EBV positive cases are more chemoresponsive than usual gastric cancer.

Adenosquamous Carcinoma and Squamous Cell Carcinoma

- Rare: need gland formation, keratinisation and intercellular bridges. They show vascular invasion and are *aggressive*.

Undifferentiated Carcinoma

- Cytokeratin positive but no glandular or squamous cell differentiation.

Neuroendocrine Tumours

- Well differentiated/low-grade neuroendocrine (carcinoid) tumour, or, poorly differentiated/high-grade neuroendocrine (small cell/large cell) carcinoma. See Sect. 2.9.

Malignant Lymphoma

- Low-grade MALToma with potential for high-grade transformation.
- Less commonly: diffuse large B cell lymphoma, follicle centre cell lymphoma, mantle cell lymphoma, T cell lymphoma.

Metastatic Carcinoma

- *Direct spread*: pancreas, oesophagus, transverse colon.
- *Distant spread*: small cell carcinoma lung, malignant melanoma, breast, kidney, choriocarcinoma, ovary, germ cell tumour.
- Metastatic infiltrating lobular carcinoma of breast can mimic signet ring cell carcinoma of stomach and a known clinical history of a previous breast primary is crucial to the diagnosis. Breast cancer may also be ER/PR/GCDFP-15/CK7 positive and CK20 negative. Note that a significant minority of gastric adenocarcinomas may also be oestrogen receptor positive but do not show the diffuse strong positivity seen in breast lobular cancer.

2.3 Differentiation

Well/moderate/poor/undifferentiated, or, Grade 1/2/3/4

For adenocarcinoma based on the percentage tumour gland formation (well/G1 >95 %: moderate/G2 50–95 %: poor/G3 <50 %).

Undifferentiated gastric carcinoma (grade 4) shows no glandular differentiation and requires positive cytokeratin stains to distinguish it from malignant lymphoma or sarcoma. Signet ring cell carcinoma is regarded as poorly differentiated (grade 3) and small cell carcinoma as undifferentiated (grade 4).

Goseki grade – based on mucin secretion and tubule formation:

I	Tubules well differentiated, mucin poor
II	Tubules well differentiated, mucin rich
III	Tubules poorly differentiated, mucin poor
IV	Tubules poorly differentiated, mucin rich.

Well differentiated mucin poor cancers have better 5 year survival rates (50–80 %) than moderately or poorly differentiated mucin rich tumours (18–46 %). Mucin subtyping into gastric (MUC5a, MUC6) and intestinal (MUC2, CDX2, CD10) may be able to identify more aggressive cancers although this is not yet fully clarified.

2.4 Extent of Local Tumour Spread

Border: pushing/infiltrative.

Well circumscribed tumours have longer patient survival than infiltrating cancers (except in early gastric cancer).

Lymphocytic reaction: prominent/sparse.

Gastric cancer is considered as either *early* (*pT1*) or *advanced* (≥*pT2*) as there is *prognostic discrepancy* between the various levels of invasion. Five year survival figures are: pT1(85– 95 %), pT2(60–80 %), pT3(40–50 %).

The TNM7 classification applies only to carcinomas (Fig. 2.2).

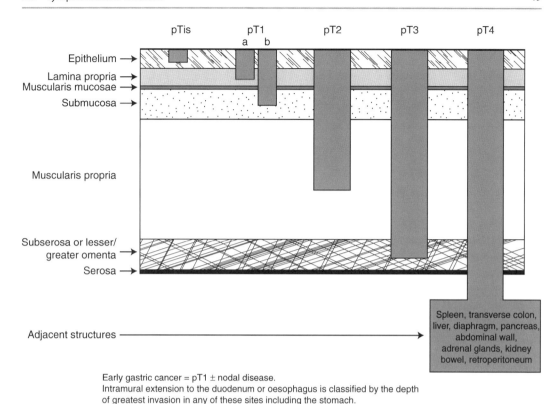

Early gastric cancer = pT1 ± nodal disease.
Intramural extension to the duodenum or oesophagus is classified by the depth
of greatest invasion in any of these sites including the stomach.

Fig. 2.2 Gastric carcinoma (Reproduced, with permission, from Allen (2006), © 2006)

pTis	Carcinoma in situ: intraepithelial tumour without invasion of the lamina propria/ high-grade dysplasia
pT1	Tumour invades lamina propria (pT1a) or submucosa (pT1b)
pT2	Tumour invades muscularis
pT3	Tumour invades subserosa or mesenteric/ omental fat
pT4	Tumour perforates serosa or invades adjacent structures (spleen, transverse colon, liver, diaphragm, pancreas, abdominal wall, adrenal gland, kidney, small intestine, retroperitoneum).

The lesser omentum includes the gastrocolic and gastrohepatic ligaments, and involvement of their peritoneal covering constitutes pT4 disease. *Discontinuous greater omental or peritoneal tumour nodules, or positive peritoneal cytology are classified as metastatic disease (pM1).*

Intramural extension to the oesophagus or duodenum is classified by the depth of greatest invasion in any of these sites.

Diffuse gastric carcinoma may not elicit a desmoplastic stroma and the depth of mural invasion, which is often extensive and can be characterised by small, inapparent non-mucinous tumour cells in the muscularis propria and adventitia, may be underestimated. Equally margin status can be incorrectly assessed. Stains (PAS ± diastase, cytokeratins, CEA, EMA) should be used to show its full extent and also to distinguish tumour cells from histiocytes in both the mucosa and lymph node sinus network. Tumour regression following neoadjuvant chemotherapy can also markedly alter the volume of residual viable cancer making accurate pathological staging problematic.

2.5 Lymphovascular Invasion

Present/absent.

Intra-/extratumoural.

Venous, lymphatic and perineural invasion are adverse prognostic factors.

Fig. 2.3 Stomach: regional lymph nodes (Reproduced, with permission, from Wittekind et al. (2005), © 2005)

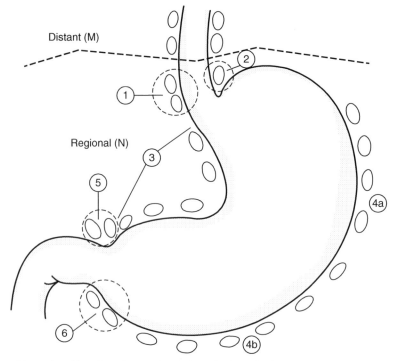

The regional lymph nodes are the perigastric along the lesser (1,3,5) and greater (2,4a,4b,6) curvatures, the nodes located along the left gastric (7), common hepatic (8),splenic (10,11) and coeliac arteries (9) and the hepatoduodenal nodes (12). Involvement of the other intra-abdominal lymph nodes such as retropancreatic, mesenteric and para-aortic is classified as distant metastasis.

Intestinal gastric adenocarcinoma tends to *venous invasion* with spread to liver, lung, adrenal glands and bone. *Diffuse gastric carcinoma* favours *lymphatic* and *direct transperitoneal spread*. Bilateral ovarian metastases from diffuse gastric cancer comprise the majority of *Krükenberg tumours*. Uterine body, cervix and colorectum can also be involved by metastatic disease. About 50 % of patients present with extragastric spread of tumour.

2.6 Lymph Nodes

Site/number/size/number involved/limit node/ extracapsular spread (Figs. 2.3 and 2.4).

Regional nodes: perigastric, hepatoduodenal, lymph nodes along the left gastric, common hepatic, splenic and coeliac arteries. Other intra-abdominal lymph nodes (retropancreatic, mesenteric, paraaortic) are distant metastases (pM1). A regional lymphadenectomy will ordinarily include a minimum of 16 lymph nodes but numbers depend on the extent of surgery. In a *D1 resection* only perigastric lymph nodes are excised. In a *D2 (radical) gastrectomy* there is additional lymph node dissection along the hepatic artery, coeliac plexus, greater omentum, gastrosplenic omentum, portal vein, and splenic artery. A *D3 resection* includes lymph nodes from the hepatoduodenal ligament, superior mesenteric vein, aorta/vena cava to the inferior mesenteric artery and retropancreatic area. D2 nodes are generally located >3 cm from the tumour. The surgeon may choose to submit these in separately labelled containers and a minimum yield of 25 nodes is commonly targeted.

Fig. 2.4 Stomach: regional lymph nodes (Reproduced, with permission, from Wittekind et al. (2005), © 2005)

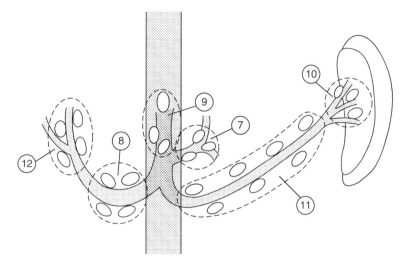

pN0	No regional lymph node mestatasis
pN1	1–2 involved regional nodes
pN2	3–16 involved regional nodes
pN3	More than 16 involved regional nodes.

Survival at 5 years decreases with increasing numbers of involved lymph nodes – N1/N2: 46 % to N3: 30 % of patients.

2.7   Excision Margins

Distances (mm) to the radial, proximal and distal limits of excision and serosa.

Gastric carcinoma (especially diffuse signet ring cell) may show a *multifocal distribution* and submucosal skip lesions. Margins need to be checked histologically even if well away from the main tumour mass on gross examination. Diffuse carcinoma present to within 5 cm of the resection margin has an adverse prognosis. Distal intestinal cancers tend to stop at the pylorus while diffuse carcinoma may involve the first part of the duodenum. Proximal (cardia) tumours often involve distal oesophagus (Siewert III).

The radial margin is the non-peritonealised lesser or greater omental margin closest to the tumour. It can be inspected and inked prior to blocking although it can be difficult to identify in individual cases.

2.8   Other Pathology

Early Gastric Cancer (EGC)

Forming *10–15 % of gastric cancers* in the Western hemisphere and limited to the mucosa ± submucosa ± lymph node involvement. The *5 year survival is 85–95 %* compared with 20–35 % for advanced gastric cancer. Designation as EGC is on a resection specimen as endoscopic biopsies are constrained by sampling limitations.

Macroscopic/Endoscopic Classification of EGC

Type I	Protruded	10 %
Type IIa	Raised	Superficial 80 %
Type IIb	Flat	
Type IIc	Depressed	
Type III	Excavated	10 %

Mixed types are common. Types I and IIa tend to be well differentiated (tubular, papillary) whereas types IIb, IIc and III also include ulcerated intestinal, poorly differentiated and signet ring cell tumours, although there is considerable overlap between macroscopic and microscopic appearances.

Lesser curve is the commonest site but *10 % are multifocal* and require mapping of the resection specimen.

Tumours with lymph node metastases do worse than those without and tend to be large (>5 cm 80 % positive lymph nodes), or show *submucosal invasion (19% positive lymph nodes)* rather than being confined to the mucosa (4 % positive nodes).

Two prognostic paradoxes contrast with advanced gastric carcinoma:

1. Diffuse type EGC has a better prognosis than intestinal type EGC due to vascular spread in the latter
2. EGC with a broad, expansile deep margin destroying muscularis mucosae (pen A) is more aggressive than EGC with an irregular infiltrating margin fenestrating the muscle (pen B). The tendency for pen A tumours to progress to advanced carcinoma is thought to relate to higher DNA aneuploidy rates. Pen A tumours form a minority (10 %) of EGC but have higher rates of lymphovascular invasion, lymph node metastases (25 %) and lower 10 year survival rates (65 %)
3. i.e. well differentiated cancers with a pushing margin do worse than poorly differentiated tumours with an infiltrating margin.

Treatment is usually by *partial gastrectomy* but after appropriate clinicopathological staging *local excision by EMR/ESD is possible. Risk factors* predictive of lymph node metastases and the need for *further surgery* are: size >3 cm, surface ulceration (>50 %), poor differentiation, deep submucosal (sm2/sm3) invasion, lymphovascular invasion and incomplete excision with deep margin involvement.

Predisposing Lesions

Gastritis[1]: ± *Helicobacter pylorii (HP)*. Demonstrated by histochemical (cresyl violet, Giemsa, Warthin-Starry) or antibody stains. HP can assume a coccoid rather than spiral form in resection specimens. HP positive patients have

×3–6 increased cancer risk especially those with the cytotoxic (cag-A) genotype of HP.

Intestinal metaplasia[2]: type IIb/III (sulphomucin rich). Demonstrated by high iron diamine alcian blue or Gomori's aldehyde fuchsin alcian blue stains. The large intestinal variant of metaplasia is more strongly associated with mucosal dysplasia and intestinal pattern gastric adenocarcinoma. Mucin subtyping is not routinely done as it is not considered a sufficiently strong predictive factor although the extent of intestinal metaplasia is broadly indicative.

Atrophy[3]: ± pernicious anaemia with gastric parietal cell and intrinsic factor antibodies. *Ten to twenty percent develop carcinoma.*

Dysplasia: *low/high-grade*, either in flat (commonest), sessile or polypoid mucosa, and in metaplastic (intestinal) or non-metaplastic (gastric foveolar) mucosa. Gastrointestinal epithelial neoplasia is categorised according to the Vienna Consensus Classification (Table 2.1)

There is a *strong association (30–80%)* between *high-grade dysplasia* and *adenocarcinoma* either concurrently or within 1–2 years of diagnosis. Distinction between high-grade dysplasia/carcinoma in situ and lamina propria invasion can be difficult. In Europe and the USA there needs to be invasion of the lamina propria or muscularis mucosae before the term (intramucosal) adenocarcinoma is used i.e. both cytological and architectural derangement. Eastern hemisphere pathologists require less stringent criteria. In practice an array of histological features indicates progression to *adenocarcinoma*. These include singles or clusters of atypical cells in the lamina propria, glandular complexity (cribriform or laterally anastomosing epithelium), or stromal desmoplasia. Diagnosis of dysplasia in a biopsy should be followed by *reassessment* with multiple biopsies to exclude concurrent adenocarcinoma. Dye spraying can facilitate endoscopic identification. Imaging e.g. ELUS may help define a mass or infiltrative lesion. If this is absent flat low-grade dysplasia may be *monitored endoscopically*, while polypoid low-grade dysplasia and high-grade dysplasia in flat or polypoid mucosa

---

[1] Classified and semi-quantitatively graded (none/mild/moderate/marked) using the Sydney classification. It classifies and grades chronic gastritis based on an assessment of *histological* (neutrophils, chronic inflammation, atrophy, intestinal metaplasia), *topographical* (antral/corpus predominant or pangastritis) and *aetiological* (HP, drugs) factors.

[2] See footnote 1.

[3] See footnote 1.

Table 2.1 Vienna consensus classification of gastrointestinal neoplasia

Category	Neoplasia/dysplasia
1.	Negative
2.	Indefinite
3.	Non-invasive low grade
	Low grade adenoma/dysplasia
4.	Non-invasive high grade
4.1	High grade adenoma/dysplasia
4.2	Non-invasive carcinoma (carcinoma in-situ)
4.3	Suspicious of invasive carcinoma
5.	Invasive – either intramucosal[a], submucosal or beyond

The WHO (2010) classification uses the term intraepithelial neoplasia interchangeably with dysplasia and the categories: negative, indefinite, low-grade, high-grade/intramucosal neoplasia (carcinoma) and invasive neoplasia (carcinoma)

[a]A more recent proposed modification suggests categorising intramucosal carcinoma as 4.4 as these sub-categories show poor intra-/inter observer reproducibility and all require at least endoscopic or surgical local resection. Choice of procedure will depend on the lesion size, depth of invasion (as assessed by endoscopy, radiology and endoscopic ultrasound), histological grade and general features (age, fitness)

should be considered for either *local endoscopic* or *formal surgical resection*. With local resection careful histological assessment of the specimen and discussion at the multidisciplinary meeting are needed to exclude any requirement to proceed to more radical surgery. Care must be taken to distinguish dysplasia from regenerative change in inflammation and ulceration, reactive gastropathy e.g. foveolar hyperplasia in bile reflux and drug ingestion (NSAIDs, aspirin), and crypt juxtaposition in small intestinal metaplasia. A lack of surface epithelial maturation, budding/branching and cystically dilated deep glands are useful pointers to dysplasia.

Polyps

- *Hyperplastic*: often antral and regenerative in nature. A 1–3 % risk of malignancy (either within the polyp or elsewhere in the stomach), particularly if large (>2 cm) and multiple.
- *Fundic gland cyst*: the commonest gastric polyp. Associated with FAP in a young

patient, but usually in older patients receiving proton pump inhibitor therapy (due to parietal cell hyperplasia consequent upon secondary hypergastrinaemia). Rarely the polyps show surface dysplasia in FAP.
- *Adenomatous*: 8 % of cases with a 30–40 % risk of malignancy related to the size (>2 cm), villous architecture and grade of dysplasia.
- *Rare*: FAP, Peutz-Jeghers, Cowden's syndromes, inflammatory fibroid polyp.

Ménétrier's disease and lymphocytic gastritis: hyperplastic gastropathy can be associated with adenocarcinoma.

Synchronous gastric lymphoma of mucosa associated lymphoid tissue (MALToma): also *Helicobacter* related.

Tumours covered by intact mucosa: such as diffuse gastric carcinoma (signet ring cell) or stromal tumours, can be difficult to demonstrate by routine biopsy and multiple biopsies with jumbo forceps may be required. Cytological brushings and washings or endoscopic FNAC may be helpful.

Gastrointestinal cytology: may yield positive information in the following situations

(a) FNAC of submucosal/mural/extrinsic lesions including enlarged locoregional lymph nodes found on staging CT/ELUS

(b) FNA of pancreatic mass lesions and brushings of common bile duct/pancreatic duct strictures

(c) Brush cytology of oesophageal and colonic strictures not amenable to usual biopsy.

Endoscopic biopsies: multiple (a minimum of eight) biopsies should be taken from ulcerated carcinomas including the ulcer base and mucosal edges. Distinction must be drawn between adenocarcinoma and pseudomalignant changes in glandular epithelium, endothelial cells and stromal cells in erosions and ulcer base tissue. Biopsy from the base of a deeply penetrating benign peptic ulcer may yield hepatocytes or pancreatic acinar cells not to be misinterpreted as gastric adenocarcinoma. Gastric xanthoma (CD 68 positive, cytokeratin and mucin negative) can also mimic diffuse gastric carcinoma and immunohistochemistry is helpful in these situations.

Immunophenotype

Gastric carcinoma is variably neutral and acidic mucin positive (PAS-AB, mucicarmine), cytokeratin (CAM 5.2, CK7/± 20), EMA and CEA positive, ± CDX-2. Diffuse carcinoma is E-cadherin negative and intestinal pattern adenocarcinoma is positive. In cases with *advanced stage or recurrent disease* biopsy or resection tissues are assessed for *Her-2 over expression* as a guide to potential response to monoclonal antibody *Herceptin (trastuzumab) therapy*. As for breast carcinoma, immunohistochemistry (supplemented by fluorescent, chromogenic or dual colour/dual hapten in situ hybridization for equivocal 2+ cases) is used with a positive result indicated by strong membrane staining in >30 % of the cells. Expression can be heterogeneous within a tumour requiring adequate sampling, and staining can be limited to the basolateral membranes. There can also be false positives and variation with the staining platform that is used. About 20 % of gastric cancers are positive (intestinal type 33 %, diffuse type 5 % only).

Prognosis

Prognosis of gastric cancer is poor, the majority of cases presenting with advanced disease. It relates to *histological type*, *grade* and crucially, *stage*. Intestinal gastric carcinoma has higher 5 year survival rates than diffuse gastric carcinoma, e.g. for pT3 lesions 42 % versus 17 %. Intestinal gastric carcinoma may be considered for partial gastrectomy because of its expanding margins, whereas total gastrectomy is advised for diffuse carcinoma. Additional important prognostic indicators are lymph node status, lymphovascular invasion, peritoneal and resection line involvement, and an infiltrative versus an expansive tumour margin. These factors tend to outweigh other parameters such as the Lauren and Ming classification or Goseki grade. *Prior to proceeding to radical surgery complete clinical staging is necessary to exclude any non-regional disease*. This involves CT ± PET scan and peritoneal laparoscopy with cytology and biopsy. Preoperative neoadjuvant and palliative

chemotherapy have roles to play. EGC does considerably better (see above) and may be amenable to endoscopic mucosal resection or submucosal dissection (EMR/ESD).

2.9   Other Malignancy

Gastric Carcinoid Tumours

A well differentiated/low-grade neuroendocrine tumour, and chromogranin, synaptophysin positive, CD56±. Mitoses are usually <2 per 10 high power fields (hpfs) and Ki-67 index is ≤2 % (i.e. a grade 1 (G1) tumour).

They are either small and multiple (types 1 and 2), or larger, solitary and sporadic (type 3).

1. *Multiple (benign)*: commonly type 1 lesions associated with autoimmune atrophic gastritis and endocrine cell hyperplasia (nodules <150 μm). Rarely Zollinger Ellison syndrome and MEN 1 (type 2 lesions). Gastric atrophy → hypochlorhydria → hypergastrinaemia → ECL (enterochromaffin like) cell hyperplasia → microcarcinoidosis (multiple, mucosal, 1–3 mm). Can be *monitored by endoscopy* and treated conservatively with biopsy excision of small polyps up to 1 cm diameter. Polyps 1–2 cm in size are treated by *polypectomy* or *local resection* as they are of uncertain or low malignant potential with an overall metastatic rate of approximately 2–5 %.

2. *Single (type 3 lesions/aggressive)*: 13 % of cases overall with a 22–75 % metastatic rate and 25 % mortality. If the lesion is large (>2 cm) or ulcerated consider definitive *surgical resection*.

   Malignancy relates to:
   - Any functioning tumour
   - Angioinvasion
   - Non-functioning tumour ≥2 cm diameter and with invasion beyond the submucosa
   - Atypical features (atypia, necrosis, increased mitoses (≥2/10 hpfs) and/or Ki-67 index (>2 %)) i.e. a G2/G3 tumour
   - *70–80 % 5 year survival*.
   - Indolent growth with spread to nodes, liver, bone and skin.

TNM7: carcinoid in situ ≤0.5 mm, pT1 ≤1 cm, pT2 >1 cm or into muscularis propria, pT3 into subserosa, pT4 involves serosa or adjacent structures.

The European Neuroendocrine Tumour Society designates subserosa as pT2 and serosa as pT3.

Gastrointestinal neuroendocrine tumour cells express functional somatostatin receptors and tumours can be detected by octreotide (somatostatin antagonist) scan, and treated with similar agents.

Gastrointestinal Mesenchymal or Stromal Tumours (GISTs)

Site: stomach (60–70 %), small intestine (25–35 %), colorectum and oesophagus (10 %). Submucosal, mural or serosal subsites.

Myogenic: 10 % of cases are desmin/h-caldesmon/smooth muscle actin positive and DOG-1/CD117 (c-kit) negative, representing true leiomyoma or leiomyosarcoma (rare).

Neural: 10 % of cases are S100/synaptophysin positive and DOG-1/CD117 (c-kit) negative, representing Schwannoma (has a characteristic peritumoural lymphoid infiltrate), granular cell tumour, neurofibroma (can be associated with von Recklinghausen's disease, MEN syndrome and GISTs elsewhere in the gastrointestinal tract).

Stromal: *DOG-1*, *CD 117* (c-*kit*: tyrosine kinase receptor), CD34 positive, and absent or incomplete myogenic/neural differentiation. Putative precursors are the interstitial cells of Cajal, which are gastrointestinal pacemaker cells located in the deep submucosa and myenteric plexus. Note that there can be heterogeneity and focal expression of antigens. In general, antigen positivity is DOG-1 and CD117 (>95 %), CD34 (70–85 %), smooth muscle actin (20–40 %), h-caldesmon (60–80 %) and nestin (90–100 %). DOG-1/CD117 negative GISTs may be identified by positive protein kinase c theta and PDGFR (platelet derived growth factor receptor) positive mutation analysis. *C-kit mutation analysis* (exon 11 in 70 % of cases) is also helpful in confirming the *diagnosis*, *prediction of progression* and *response to drug treatment* (exon 11 is more responsive than exon 9). Mutation analysis is generally recommended if immunohistochemistry is equivocal, and in cases of borderline/malignant GISTs. Note that other malignant tumours can also be CD117 positive e.g. seminoma, malignant melanoma and some metastatic carcinomas e.g. breast, ovary, colorectal, small cell carcinoma. DOG-1 (transmembrane protein Discovered On GIST1) is a highly sensitive and specific marker for GIST but may also show weak to moderate expression in some other tumours e.g. colorectal, endometrioid and acinic cell carcinomas, spindle cell malignant melanoma and malignant peripheral nerve sheath tumours. GANT (gastrointestinal autonomic nerve tumour) is now regarded as a variant of GIST and assessed accordingly. A small minority of patients with GISTs have a positive family history of these tumours, Carney triad (gastric GIST, pulmonary chondroma, extraadrenal paraganglioma) or type 1 neurofibromatosis. Malignancy, which is less frequent than in small intestinal stromal tumours, cannot be accurately predicted from the histology. However, *indicators of malignancy* (strongest asterisked) are:

- Size (>5 cm)*
- Cellularity (cell density increases in sarcoma)
- Atypia
- Cell type (epithelioid is worse than spindle cell)
- Necrosis (coagulative in type)*
- Margins (circumscribed versus infiltrative, e.g. invasion into mucosal lamina propria)*
- Mitoses >5/50 high power fields*
- Location in fundus or gastro-oesophageal junction.
- Loss of CD 117/DOG-1 expression and over expression of p53.

Clinical risk: gastric GISTs are categorized as no, very low, low, moderate or high *metastatic risk* on the basis of *size* and *mitoses* (Table 2.2). Treatment is *complete surgical* (*open or laparoscopic*) *resection* by either local (sleeve) or radical gastric resection depending on the tumour size and location. Neoadjuvant therapy is not licensed in the UK but is sometimes used on an individual basis to produce tumour regression to facilitate choice and ease of operative technique e.g. anorectal, oesophagogastric or duodenal GISTs.

Table 2.2 Risk factors in gastric GISTs – risk of progressive disease, metastases or tumour related death

	Tumour dia (cm)	Mitoses/50 hpfs	Percentage risk
No risk	≤2	<5	0
Very low risk	>2–5	<5	1.9
Low risk	>5–10	<5	3.6
Moderate risk	>10	<5	10
	>2–5	>5	16
High risk	>5–10	>5	55
	>10	>5	86

Metastases: histological grading of established sarcoma is contentious and tumour size is a suggested index of metastatic risk. *Metastases are commonly to peritoneum, liver, pancreas, retroperitoneum* and *lungs*. Metastases are CT/PET scan positive but become negative on treatment. Metastatic disease responds well to *medical therapy (Glivec (imatinib))* resulting in hyalinization, myxoid and cystic degeneration. It gives several disease free years but usually therapeutic escape occurs with *recurrent peritoneal disease or size progression of liver metastases*. This may relate to the cytostatic rather than tumouricidal effects of the treatment, or newly acquired mutations in the tumour cells. Up to 13 % of patients show no primary response to therapy and disease progression within 6 months.

Biopsy proof can be difficult as GISTs are extramucosal lesions (submucosal and mural) often with surface ulceration. FNAC at endoscopy may be helpful in establishing a diagnosis of a spindle cell lesion. The biopsy forceps may also be directed to the base of the ulcer where there is already mucosal loss.

See Chap. 4, Sect. 4.9.

Malignant Lymphoma

• Secondary to systemic/lymph node disease or primary (commoner) in the stomach, it is the *commonest site* for *extranodal non-Hodgkin's malignant lymphoma* (40 % of cases). Primary disease bulk is centred on the stomach and its regional lymph nodes.

Gastric malignant lymphoma: can present as single or multiple lesions, a sessile plaque or thickened folds found incidentally at endoscopy, an ulcerated tumour or a thickened non-expansile stomach. The majority are of B cell MALT (mucosa associated lymphoid tissue) type, the low-grade variant being characterised by a proliferation of small to medium sized centrocyte like cells, destructive lymphoepithelial lesions, monotypic immunoglobulin expression in surface plasma cells, invasion between or into reactive follicles (follicular colonisation) and/or immunoglobulin gene rearrangements on PCR. There is evidence that *localized low-grade lesions* (i.e. without deep submucosal or muscle invasion) may regress on *anti-Helicobacter medication* and they usually pursue an *indolent time course* with potential metastases to other extranodal sites e.g. gastrointestinal tract and Waldeyer's ring. They may also transform to or present as *high-grade lesions* necessitating *chemotherapy and/or surgery*, which are also applicable to extensive low-grade disease. Potential *resistance to anti-helicobacter treatment* is indicated by tumour cell bcl-10 expression, presence of the t11:18 translocation (30 % of cases), large cells or disease in the deep submucosa or beyond. ELUS may help to define the latter. Advanced stage disease and t11:18 tumours should be considered for radiotherapy or chemotherapy. The cytological composition of MALToma can be heterogeneous and clear distinction between a mucosal or lymph node origin can be arbitrary, especially in high-grade disease. From a practical point of view establishing *a diagnosis of malignant lymphoma, B cell phenotype, low- or high-grade character* and *full clinicopathological staging* are the salient features relevant to management.

Immunohistochemistry may also be helpful in establishing *monoclonality* (κ, λ light chain restriction), demonstrating *lymphoepithelial* lesions (cytokeratins), and *lymphoma subtype*. For example, low-grade MALToma is CD 45/CD 20 positive but CD 5, CD 10, CD 23 and bcl-2 negative, separating it from other low-grade B cell lymphomas. Cytokeratins and common lymphoid antigen (CD 45) are also necessary to distinguish high-grade lymphoma from undifferentiated carcinoma, and signet ring or plasmacytoid change in malignant lymphoma from signet ring cell gastric adenocarcinoma. Low- and high-grade areas may coexist in gastric lymphoma and there can be adjacent synchronous or metachronous (up to several years later) adenocarcinoma associated with MALToma. About 40–60 % of gastric malignant lymphomas are of high-grade large B cell type and diagnosis is usually straightforward (cytological atypia/destructive monomorphous infiltrate), with confirmatory immunohistochemistry for lymphoid markers and negative epithelial markers. Distinction between low-grade malignant lymphoma and lymphoid hyperplasia, as in *Helicobacter pylorii* gastritis or peptic ulcer, can be problematic and diagnosis depends on the density and atypia of the lymphoid infiltrate and degree of gland distortion and loss. *Immunoglobulin gene rearrangements* provide supportive evidence although monoclonality does not always correlate with potential for progression to malignancy and can be seen in a minority of cases of chronic gastritis. Sometimes designation of low-grade malignant lymphoma is only attained after several biopsy episodes and when there is a lack of response of the lymphoid infiltrate to eradication of *Helicobacter pylorii*. Persistence of monoclonality over time may be helpful. Various scoring systems exist for making a diagnosis of low-grade MALToma and assessing its response to HP eradication. Minimal residual disease shows persistent basal lymphoid aggregates whereas response gives a diminished lymphoid infiltrate and fine fibrosis in the lamina propria.

Overall prognosis is reasonably good (*40–60% 5 year survival*), low-grade malignant lymphomas following an indolent course (65–95 % 5 year survival). However, about 50 % of high-grade malignant lymphomas are aggressive with spread beyond the stomach (40–55 % 5 year survival). *Prognosis* relates to both *grade* and *stage* of disease at the time of presentation. Treatment of extensive low-grade and high-grade disease is with *chemotherapy* and/or *surgery*, the latter particularly if there are anatomical considerations e.g. multifocality, bulky ulcerated luminal disease, anaemia or gastric outlet obstruction. Initial full clinical staging is carried out (CT scan, bone marrow biopsy).

Other forms of malignant lymphoma are unusual in the stomach e.g. follicle centre cell lymphoma, mantle cell lymphoma, Burkitt's lymphoma, anaplastic large cell lymphoma and T cell lymphoma. Hodgkin's lymphoma is rare.

Leukaemia

- Stomach can be involved in up to 25 % of cases.
- CD34, CD43, CD 68, CD117/chloroacetate esterase/myeloperoxidase positive cells (myeloid/granulocytic sarcoma).

Miscellaneous Rare Malignancy

- Kaposi's sarcoma: visceral involvement can be present in 30–60 % of AIDS patients.
- Angiosarcoma, rhabdomyosarcoma, alveolar soft part sarcoma, teratoma, choriocarcinoma, yolk sac tumour.
- Metastatic malignant melanoma in the stomach is now seen with increasingly powerful chemo-/immunosuppressive therapies leading to unusual patterns of metastatic disease.

Bibliography

Allen DC. Histopathology reporting: guidelines for surgical cancer. 2nd ed. London: Springer; 2006.

Allum WH, Blazeby JM, Griffin SM, Cunningham D, Jankowski JA, Wong R, On behalf of the Association of Upper Gastrointestinal Surgeons of Great Britain and Northern Ireland, the British Society of Gastroenterology and the British Association of Surgical Oncology. Guidelines for the management of oesophageal and gastric cancer. Gut. 2011;60: 1449–72.

Bacon CM, Du M-Q, Dogan A. Mucosa-associated lymphoid tissue (MALT) lymphoma: a practical guide for pathologists. J Clin Pathol. 2007;60: 361–72.

Banks PM. Gastrointestinal lymphoproliferative disorders. Histopathology. 2007;50:42–54.

Bosman FT, Carneiro F. WHO classification of tumours of the digestive system. 4th ed. Lyon: IARC press; 2010.

Chandrasama P, Wickramasinghe K, Ma Y, DeMeester T. Adenocarcinomas of the distal esophagus and "gastric cardia" are predominantly esophageal carcinomas. Am J Surg Pathol. 2007;31:569–75.

Chetty R. Gastrointestinal cancers accompanied by a dense lymphoid component: an overview with special reference to gastric and colonic medullary and lymphoepithelioma-like carcinomas. J Clin Pathol. 2012;65:1062–5.

Copie-Bergman C, Gaulard P, Lavergne-Slove A, et al. Proposal for a new histological grading system for post treatment evaluation of gastric MALT lymphoma. Gut. 2003;52:1656.

Cotton P, Williams C. Practical gastrointestinal endoscopy. 4th ed. London: Blackwell Science; 1996.

Day DW, Jass JR, Price AB, Shepherd NA, Sloan JM, Talbot IC, Warren BF, Williams GT. Morson and Dawson's gastrointestinal pathology. 4th ed. Oxford: Blackwell Sciences; 2003.

Dixon MF, Martin IG, Sue-Ling HM, Wyatt JI, Quirke P, Johnston D. Goseki grading in gastric cancer: comparison with existing systems of grading and its reproducibility. Histopathology. 1994;25:309–16.

Goddard AF, Badreldin R, Pritchard DM, Walker MM, Warren B. The management of gastric polyps. Gut. 2010;59:1270–6.

Hull MJ, Mino-Kenudson M, Nishioka NS, Ban S, Sepehr A, Puricelli W, Nakatsuka L, Ota S, Shimizu M, Brugge WR, Lauwers GY. Endoscopic mucosal resection. An improved diagnostic procedure for early gastroesophageal epithelial neoplasms. Am J Surg Pathol. 2006;30:114–8.

Isaacson P. Biopsy appearances easily mistaken for malignancy in gastrointestinal endoscopy. Histopathology. 1982;6:377–89.

Joensuu H. Risk stratification of patients diagnosed with gastrointestinal stromal tumor. Hum Pathol. 2008;39: 1411–9.

Lauren P. The two histological main types of gastric carcinoma. Acta Pathol Microbiol Scand. 1965;64:31–49.

Lewin KJ, Appelman HD. Tumors of the esophagus and stomach. Atlas of tumor pathology. 3rd series. Fascicle 18. Washington: AFIP; 1996.

Logan RPH, Harris A, Misciewicz JJ, Baron JH, editors. ABC of the upper gastrointestinal tract. London: BMJ Books; 2002.

Miettinen M, Sobin LH, Lasota J. Gastrointestinal stromal tumours of the stomach. A clinicopathologic, immunohistochemical and molecular genetic study of 1765 cases with long-term follow-up. Am J Surg Pathol. 2005;29:52–68.

Morson BC, Sobin LH, Grundmann E, Johansen A, Nagayo T, Serck-Hanssen A. Precancerous conditions and epithelial dysplasia in the stomach. J Clin Pathol. 1980;33:711–21.

Odze RD, Goldblum JR. Surgical pathology of the GI tract, liver, biliary tract and pancreas. 2nd ed. Philadelphia: Saunders/Elsevier; 2009.

Plockinger U, Rindi G, Arnold R, Eriksson B, Krenning EP, de Herder WW, et al. Guidelines for the diagnosis and treatment of neuroendocrine gastrointestinal tumours. A consensus statement on behalf of the European Neuroendocrine Tumour Society (ENETS). Neuroendocrinology. 2004;80:394–424.

Pritchard SA. ACP best practice. Best practice in macroscopic examination of gastric resections. J Clin Pathol. 2008;61:172–8.

Schlemper RJ, Riddell RH, Kato Y, et al. The Vienna classification of gastrointestinal epithelial neoplasia. Gut. 2000;47:251–5.

Siewert JR, Stein HJ. Classification of adenocarcinoma of the oesophagogastric junction. Br J Surg. 1998;25: 1457–9.

The Royal College of Pathologists: Cancer Datasets (Oesophageal Carcinoma, Gastric Carcinoma, Carcinomas of the Pancreas, ampulla of Vater and Common Bile Duct, Colorectal Cancer, Gastrointestinal Stromal Tumours (GISTs), Liver Resection Specimens and Liver Biopsies for Primary and Metastatic Carcinoma, Endocrine Tumours of the Gastrointestinal Tract including Pancreas) and Tissue Pathways (Gastrointestinal and Pancreatobiliary Pathology, Liver Biopsies for the Investigation of Medical Disease and for Focal Liver Lesions). Accessed at http://www.rcpath.org/index. asp?PageID=254.

Ushiku T, Matsusaka K, Iwasaki Y, Tateishi Y, Funata N, Seto Y, Fukayama M. Gastric carcinoma with invasive micropapillary pattern and its association with lymph node metastasis. Histopathology. 2011; 59:1081–9.

Williams GT. Endocrine tumours of the gastrointestinal tract–selected topics. Histopathology. 2007;50: 30–41.

Wittekind CF, Greene FL, Hutter RVP, Klimpfinger M, Sobib LH. TNM atlas: illustrated guide to the TNM/ pTNM classification of malignant tumours. 5th ed. Berlin: Springer; 2005.

Yantis RK, Odze RD. Neoplastic precursor lesions of the upper gastrointestinal tract. Diagn Histopathol. 2008; 14:437–52.

Ampulla of Vater and Head of Pancreas Carcinomas

Ampullary adenocarcinoma represents 0.5 % of gastrointestinal malignancies and is strongly associated with mucosal adenoma(s), either sporadic in older patients or Familial Adenomatous Polyposis (FAP) in younger patients. Pancreatic cancer occurs mainly in patients 60–80 years of age and in the developed countries of Northern Europe and North America (particularly in African Americans). In the UK some 8,000 new cases are reported each year. Risk factors are hereditary (family history of pancreatic cancer or BRCA gene positivity), smoking, obesity, high intake of saturated fatty acids, low intake of fruit and vegetables, lack of exercise, diabetes, alcohol intake and a history of chronic pancreatitis (risk ×10). Males are affected 50 % more often than females.

Pancreatic and ampullary cancers classically present with anorexia, weight loss and dark urine with pale stools due to painless obstructive (cholestatic) jaundice. Investigation includes liver function tests (increased bilirubin, alkaline phosphatase) and serum CA19-9. Tissue diagnosis is obtained in a majority, but not all patients, using a combination of oesophagogastroduodenoscopy (OGD), endoscopic retrograde cholangiopancreatography (ERCP) and endoluminal ultrasound (ELUS) providing a range of biopsy, brush and aspiration cytology samples. Ultrasound can confirm extrahepatic duct obstruction. Staging for local and distant disease also includes MR cholangiopancreatography (MRCP), MRI scan, CT scan chest, abdomen and pelvis, and PET scan. Radiological imaging is the most important diagnostic tool for pancreatic cancer and determines operability. Staging laparoscopy may also be done prior to consideration of radical surgery which is contraindicated by liver, peritoneal and distant metastases. The fitness of the patient and any comorbidity are also important factors.

Pancreatic neuroendocrine tumours more often present as a consequence of a functional hormonal syndrome due to elevated serum hormone levels. Localisation of the primary lesion and metastases is by octreotide isotope scan, ultrasound and CT scans. Treatment entails complete local excision of the primary tumour with a combination of surgery and medical treatment for metastatic disease.

3.1 Gross Description

Specimen

- Endoscopic brushings or biopsy/transduodenal or percutaneous fine needle aspirate cytology (FNAC) or needle core biopsy.
- Whipple's procedure (partial gastrectomy, duodenectomy and partial pancreatectomy). A pylorus preserving pancreaticoduodectomy may be used for small periampullary tumours thus maintaining the storage and release functions of the distal stomach and proximal 3 cm of duodenum.
- Total pancreatectomy (partial gastrectomy, duodenectomy, total pancreatectomy and splenectomy).
- Weight (g) and size/length (cm) of component parts, number of fragments, core lengths (mm).

Carcinomas of the ampulla and head of pancreas are considered together because of their anatomical juxtaposition, overlap and common potentially operative resection (Whipple's procedure). *A majority of ampullary cancers are operable but only a minority of pancreatic carcinomas.*

Tumour

Site

- Non-ampullary duodenal mucosa/duodenal papilla/ampullary mucous membrane/muscularis/pancreatic head (60–70 % of pancreatic carcinomas)/terminal common bile duct/multifocal.

Size

- Length × width × depth (cm) or maximum dimension (cm).
- Ampullary cancers >2.5 cm diameter have a decreased 5 year survival. Pancreatic exocrine cancers >3 cm are often inoperable. Pancreatic neuroendocrine tumours >2–3 cm show greater local and vascular invasion and metastatic potential.

Appearance

- Polypoid/nodular/diffuse/ulcerated: ampullary tumours.
- Scirrhous/mucoid/cystic: pancreatic exocrine tumours.
- Circumscribed/pale: pancreatic neuroendocrine tumours.

Edge

- Circumscribed/irregular.

3.2   Histological Type

Ampulla

- Comprise *6–20 % of peripancreatic tumours* and *10–50 % of cancers resected* by pancreaticoduodenectomy.
- *Premalignant lesions*: include intestinal type adenomas (commonest), non-invasive papillary neoplasms of pancreaticobiliary type, and flat

intraepithelial neoplasia (dysplasia) of the ampullary epithelium.

- *Adenocarcinoma*: 80 % of cases and usually of well to moderately differentiated *intestinal* pattern arising from adenomatous dysplasia in the peri-/intraampullary mucosa. A minority are of *pancreaticobiliary* type and a subset of these have a more aggressive *micropapillary* pattern. Endoscopic biopsy underestimates the nature and extent of disease yielding a positive diagnosis of malignancy in only about 40 % of cases. It samples the surface dysplasia but not the underlying adenocarcinoma which is better demonstrated as a mass lesion on imaging studies (ELUS, CT scan). A useful clue in biopsies of the periampullary region and duodenal papilla is the presence of tumor microemboli in lamina propria lymphovascular channels or dysplasia of the ampullary duct epithelium.
- *Papillary adenocarcinoma*: intraluminal, exophytic, well differentiated of better prognosis and can be multifocal in the extrahepatic biliary tree.
- *Mucinous adenocarcinoma*: mucin in >50 % of the tumour. It may co-exist with usual ampullary cancer subtypes.
- *Signet ring cell adenocarcinoma*: 2 % of cases.
- *Others*: adenosquamous, clear cell, small cell, hepatoid, squamous cell and undifferentiated carcinomas.
- *Metastatic carcinoma*: usually by direct spread e.g. stomach, pancreas, terminal common bile duct, renal carcinoma. Some 10–15 % of ampullary adenocarcinomas arise from the terminal portion of either the main pancreatic or common bile ducts, and therefore, have a biliary phenotype making distinction from invasion by pancreatic adenocarcinoma difficult.

Pancreas

Classification is based on the *gross appearance* of the tumour (solid/cystic/intraductal), and the *line of cellular differentiation* which is either exocrine (ductal/acinar) or neuroendocrine.

Solid tumours: ductal adenocarcinoma, acinar cell carcinoma, pancreaticoblastoma, and neuroendocrine (including solid-pseudopapil-lary) tumours.

Cystic tumours: serous cystadenoma (30 %), mucinous cystic neoplasm (MCN 40 %), intra-ductal papillary mucinous neoplasm (IPMN 30 %), and degenerative forms of all the above types.

(a) **Exocrine**

- *Ductal adenocarcinoma*:
  80–90 % of cases comprising a tubuloaci-nar pattern of malignant ductal epithelium in a desmoplastic stroma. There is often perineural invasion and dysplasia of the adjacent duct epithelium (20–30 %). *Pancreatic Intraepithelial Neoplasia (PanIN)* is a microscopic papillary or flat, non-invasive epithelial neoplasm (dys-plasia) comprising cubocolumnar epithe-lial cells with variable degrees of cytoarchitectural atypia. It usually arises in pancreatic ducts <5 mm diameter, is multifocal and seen adjacent to existing adenocarcinoma being regarded as a pre-cursor to it. High-grade PanIN is equiva-lent to severe dysplasia or carcinoma in situ. PanIN in a needle biopsy in the con-text of a clinical or radiological mass lesion may be considered justification for radical surgery. Note that PanIN can be mimicked by florid reactive atypia or cancerisation of ducts by invasive ductal carcinoma.
  Multifocality 15–40 %.
  Male preponderance.

- *Ductal adenocarcinoma variants*:
  Well differentiated large duct pattern: look for perineural, lymphovascular or fat invasion, or a proliferation of irregu-larly shaped glandular structures.
  Mucinous non-cystic colloid carcinoma: *1–3 % of cases* and mucin in >80 % of the tumour.
  Adenosquamous: at least 30 % is the squa-mous cell component – poor prognosis.
  Microglandular/signet ring cell: poor prognosis. Exclude a gastric carcinoma secondary deposit.
  Others: oncocytic, clear cell, hepatoid, medullary (sporadic or HNPCC).

- *Undifferentiated carcinoma*:
  2–7 % of cases and variably termed pleomorphic/anaplastic/giant cell/sarco-matoid carcinoma. It shows spindle cells, pleomorphic cells, mitoses and lymphovascular invasion. There is a variant with osteoclast-like giant cells (CD68 positive – poor prognosis).

- *Intraductal papillary or mucinous neo-plasm (IPMN)*:
  IPMN (*3–5 % of cases*) is a clinically detectable grossly visible, non-invasive, mucin producing papillary epithelial neoplasm of gastric, intestinal, pancreati-cobiliary or oncocytic types. It arises from the main pancreatic duct or branch ducts (better prognosis) with varying duct dilatation (>1 cm) and cytoarchitec-tural atypia. It is benign/borderline or malignant according to the degree of dys-plasia±invasion. About *20–30 % are associated with colloid or ductal adeno-carcinoma*, 80 % are in the head of pan-creas and multifocal within the duct system. It shows *indolent behaviour* marked by MUC 2 phenotype in distinc-tion from the MUC 1 aggressive ductal phenotype of usual pancreatic cancer. *Intraductal tubulopapillary neoplasm (ITPN)* is a more recently described and rare lesion with relatively indolent behavior.

- *Serous cystic tumours*:
  Elderly patients in the body or tail (50–75 %) and *mostly benign* (macro/micro-cystic /oligocystic serous adenoma) but rarely malignant. It comprises glycogen-rich, clear cuboidal epithelium lining fluid filled microcysts with a central scar. Diagnosis can be aided by analysis of aspi-rated cyst fluid which, in distinction from mucinous cystic tumours and pseudocysts, has low viscosity and zero levels of leuco-cyte esterase. *Surgical excision is curative*. It is also seen in 35–75 % of patients with Von – Hippel Lindau syndrome.

- *Mucinous cystic neoplasm (MCN)*:
  Benign/borderline/malignant spectrum of appearance and behaviour tending to

malignancy. Prognosis relates to the degree of invasion (which can be focal within a lesion) into the pancreatic and extrapancreatic tissues. The carcinoma is usually ductal in character, occasionally adenosquamous, pleomorphic/giant cell or with sarcomatous stroma. In general MCN shows *indolent growth* with spread to the abdominal cavity occurring in middle-aged women, but with *90–95% 5 year survival if completely excised*. Surgical resection is potentially curative for non-invasive MCN. Those with an invasive component have 50 % 5 year survival figures. It can be either unilocular or multilocular, in the body or tail of pancreas (95 %). There is characteristic ovarian type stroma in the wall (helpful to distinguish from pancreatic pseudocyst where the epithelial lining is lost) and has no connection to the duct system.

- *Solid pseudopapillary tumour (syn. solid-cystic-papillary tumour)*:
  Adolescent girls/young women and of *low malignant potential* (10 % metastasise to liver and peritoneum) but *usually benign*. It comprises pseudopapillae covered by several layers of uniform, endocrine like epithelial cells and a vascularised, hyalinised stroma with necrosis and mucinous cystic change. Alpha-1-antitrypsin/vimentin/CD10/βcatenin/E-cadherin/progesterone positive, ± neuroendocrine markers (chromogranin/CD56/synaptophysin), and cytokeratin negative.
- *Acinar cell carcinoma*:
  1–2% of cases in the head of pancreas and uniform cells with cytoplasmic granules resembling normal pancreas. It is enzyme antibody positive, e.g. lipase, amylase, trypsin. Lymph node and liver metastases can be present in 50 % of cases at diagnosis with *aggressive behaviour*.
- *Mixed differentiation carcinoma*:
  Acinar/neuroendocrine or ductal/neuroendocrine are rare and behave as for ductal carcinoma. The endocrine component must be at least 30 % of the tumour.

- *Small cell carcinoma*:
  A poorly differentiated/high-grade neuroendocrine carcinoma it presents at a late stage with *poor prognosis*. It can be associated with ectopic ACTH secretion and hypercalcaemia.
- *Pancreaticoblastoma*:
  Malignant in children and favourable prognosis if resected before metastases occur (nodal/hepatic in 35 % of cases). It is also chemoresponsive, and consists of epithelial (acini, squamous nests) and mesenchymal (spindle cell) components.

(b) **Neuroendocrine/endocrine tumours**
- Also termed islet cell tumours, and they arise from pluripotential ductal cells showing neuroendocrine differentiation.
- They form a *minority of pancreatic neoplasms (1–5%)* usually occurring in adults. Functional tumours are usually <2 cm and non-functional 2–5 cm due to later presentation. Circumscribed, pale and solid/trabecular/gyriform/glandular cell patterns with hyaline (± amyloid) stroma. The cells have a salt and pepper nuclear chromatin pattern. The tumour cells are positive for general neuroendocrine (chromogranin/synaptophysin) and specific markers e.g. gastrin, insulin. The majority are *benign insulinomas (80–90%)*. *Prognosis depends on the functional subtype, tumour size and grade, adequacy of surgical excision and the extent of disease*.
  1. Functional   hormonal   syndrome (60–70 %)
     Gastrinoma: pancreatic head, duodenum, gastric antrum, Zollinger-Ellison syndrome (multiple gastroduodenal ulcers, endocrine (carcinoid) tumourlets or microadenomas(<5 mm)).
     Insulinoma: body and tail – psychiatric/neurological   symptoms/hypoglycaemia.
     Vipoma: body and tail – watery diarrhoea, hypocalcaemia and achlorhydria.
     Glucagonoma: body and tail – diabetes mellitus/skin rash/stomatitis.

2. Non-functional

Somatostatinoma: also in the duodenum with a glandular pattern and psammoma bodies, and must be distinguished from well differentiated adenocarcinoma. It is positive for synaptophysin, chromogranin A (50 %) and somatostatin, and can be associated with neurofibromatosis and MEN syndromes.

Others: ppoma, neurotensinoma, calcitoninoma.

Indicators of malignancy: cellular density, atypia, necrosis, CK19/CD117 positivity, and a grading system based on proliferative rate (mitoses/10 HPFs, Ki-67 index) are a guide to malignant potential. See Sect. 3.3. Other indicators are

- *Tumour type*: insulinoma 85–90 % benign; gastrinoma 60–85 % malignant with 5 and 10 year survivals of 65 and 45 % respectively.
- *Tumour size* (>2–3 cm), *site* (e.g. duodenal) and *invasion of vessels*.
- *Unequivocal evidence of malignancy* is gross invasion of adjacent organs, and metastases to regional lymph nodes, liver and other distant sites. *Tumour growth is indolent* and even patients with metastases can survive several years with response to chemotherapy, e.g. streptozotocin. Occasional cases are of poorly differentiated (G3) high-grade small cell or large cell type. *Over 50 % of patients with pancreatic neuroendocrine tumours present with liver metastases at diagnosis*. It is important on a needle core biopsy of a liver metastasis to not only demonstrate the neuroendocrine nature of the tumour, as opposed to the more commonly occurring diagnoses of metastatic colorectal or pancreatic ductal carcinomas, but also to provide its grading for prognosis and tailored oncological management.

Association with multiple endocrine neoplasia (MEN) syndrome: the pancreas is involved in 80–100 % of type 1 MEN syndrome, gastrinoma being the commonest (50 %) lesion. Associated abnormalities are hyperplasia or tumours of parathyroid, pituitary and adrenal glands. Also seen in Von-Hippel Lindau syndrome.

(c) **Mixed exocrine/neuroendocrine carcinoma**
- *<1 % of cases* comprising bivalent amphicrine cells or adjacent foci of mixed differentiation (the neuroendocrine component being at least 30 % of the tumour).

(d) **Metastatic carcinoma**
- *Direct spread*: stomach, colorectum, biliary tract, kidney, abdominal mesothelioma/malignant lymphoma.
- *Distant spread*: pleomorphic carcinoma of the pancreas has to be distinguished from metastatic malignant melanoma, sarcoma, choriocarcinoma and large cell lung carcinoma. Small cell lung carcinoma and renal carcinoma can also involve the pancreas.

Site of origin: it can be difficult to distinguish adenocarcinoma of the pancreas and adenocarcinoma of the terminal common bile duct from adenocarcinoma of the ampulla of Vater as they can share similar histological features of biliary phenotype. Careful examination of the exact *anatomical location of the tumour epicentre* is required and circumstantial evidence for a point of origin, e.g. an adenomatous lesion in the ampullary mucosa or dysplasia in the pancreatic/bile duct epithelium. Ampullary cancers tend to an intestinal phenotype and immunoprofile (CK20/CDX-2 positive and CK7 negative) and pancreatic cancers a ductal appearance and corresponding profile (CK7/MUC1/CK20 positive). In up to 20 % of cases the only conclusion can be adenocarcinoma of the peripancreatic or pancreatico-ampullary-biliary region.

3.3 Differentiation

Well/moderate/poor/undifferentiated, or, Grade 1/2/3/4.

Pancreatic ductal and ampullary adenocarcinoma can be graded according to the percentage tumour gland formation (well/G1 >95 %: moderate/G2 50–95 %: poor/G3 <50 %) and mitotic activity (<5, 5–10, >10/10 hpfs).

By convention and definition signet ring cell adenocarcinoma and undifferentiated carcinoma (no glandular differentiation) are grade 3 and grade 4, respectively. Well differentiated pancreatic adenocarcinoma can be difficult to distinguish from non-neoplastic ducts. Malignant glands are of variable size, shape and angularity with atypical nuclear and nucleolar features. Cell cytoplasm is tall and pale to clear in character. *Perineural, lymphovascular and fat invasion are diagnostically helpful.*

Intraduct papillary lesions are:

Low-grade	Mild nuclear atypia
	No mitoses
Intermediate	Moderate nuclear atypia
	<5 mitoses/10 high-power fields
High-grade	Severe cellular atypia
	Mitoses >5/10 high-power fields

In general, gastrointestinal neuroendocrine tumours are graded based on their proliferative activity: *low-grade or well differentiated tumour* (G1: 0–1 mitoses/10hpfs, Ki-67 index 0–2 %; G2: 2–20 mitoses/10 hpfs, Ki-67 index 3–20 %[1]), or *High-grade/poorly differentiated carcinoma* (G3: >20 mitoses/10hpfs, Ki-67 index >20 %). There can be inconsistent correlation of cytological features and growth pattern with biological behaviour, but grading is broadly indicative in that G1, G2 and G3 tumours tend to show benign, uncertain/low-grade malignant, and high-grade malignant outcomes, respectively. Each case needs detailed clinicopathological discussion at a specialist multidisciplinary meeting.

3.4 Extent of Local Tumour Spread

Border: pushing/infiltrative.

Lymphocytic reaction: prominent/sparse.

The TNM7 classification applies to carcinomas of the Ampulla of Vater, exocrine pancreas and pancreatic neuroendocrine tumours[2].

Ampulla

pTis	Carcinoma in situ
pT1	Tumour limited to the ampulla or sphincter of Oddi
pT2	Tumour invades duodenal wall
pT3	Tumour invades pancreas
pT4	Tumour invades peripancreatic soft tissues or other adjacent organs or structures (Figs. 3.1, 3.2, 3.3, and 3.4)

Pancreas

pTis	Carcinoma in situ
pT1	Tumour limited to the pancreas, ≤2 cm maximum dimension
pT2	Tumour limited to the pancreas, >2 cm dimension
pT3	Tumour extends beyond pancreas[a], but without involvement of coeliac axis or superior mesenteric artery.
pT4	Tumour involves coeliac axis or superior mesenteric artery.

[a]Beyond pancreas includes the retroperitoneal fat and space, mesenteric fat, mesocolon, greater and lesser omenta and peritoneum. Direct invasion to bile ducts and duodenum includes involvement of the Ampulla of Vater. *Peripancreatic soft tissue involvement is an adverse prognostic indicator* Figs. 3.5 and 3.6

3.5 Lymphovascular Invasion

Present/absent.

Intra-/extratumoural.

Perineural space involvement is common in pancreatic carcinoma and *lymphovascular invasion* is present in up to 50 % of cases with spread to local regional lymph nodes at the time of diagnosis. *Invasion of portal vein* has *adverse independent prognostic significance*. Therefore, assessment of any segmental resection of portal/

---

[1]A 5 % prognostic threshold is also recognized for pancreatic neuroendocrine tumours.

[2]The European Neuroendocrine Tumour Society designates pancreatic neuroendocrine tumours as: pT2 >2 cm and ≤4 cm, pT3 >4 cm, pT4 invading adjacent large vessels or stomach, spleen, colon or adrenal gland.

Fig. 3.1 Ampulla of Vater carcinoma (Reproduced, with permission, from Wittekind et al. (2005), © 2005)

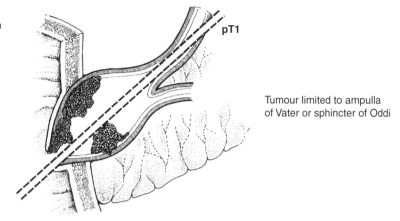

Tumour limited to ampulla of Vater or sphincter of Oddi

Fig. 3.2 Ampulla of Vater carcinoma (Reproduced, with permission, from Wittekind et al. (2005), © 2005)

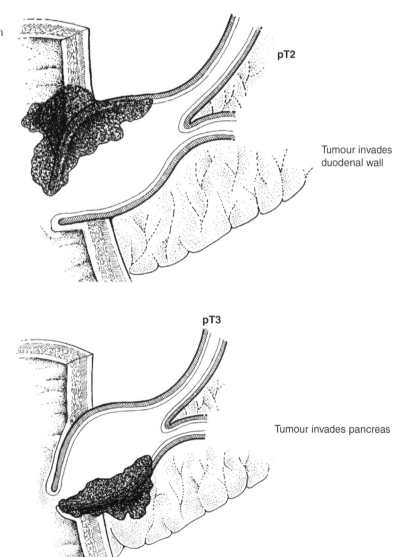

Tumour invades duodenal wall

Tumour invades pancreas

Fig. 3.3 Ampulla of Vater carcinoma (Reproduced, with permission, from Wittekind et al. (2005), © 2005)

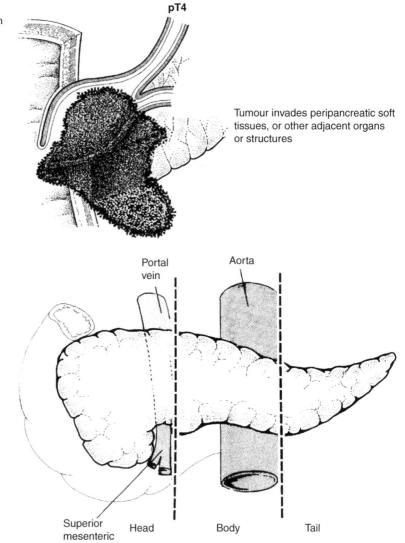

Fig. 3.4 Ampulla of Vater carcinoma (Reproduced, with permission, from Wittekind et al. (2005), © 2005)

pT4

Tumour invades peripancreatic soft tissues, or other adjacent organs or structures

Fig. 3.5 Pancreas (Reproduced, with permission, from Wittekind et al. (2005), © 2005)

Portal vein

Aorta

Superior mesenteric   Head   Body   Tail

superior mesenteric vein removed en bloc with the pancreaticoduodenectomy (5–10 % of cases) is important for prognosis and staging. Sites of *distant metastases* are the liver, peritoneum, lung, adrenal, bone, skin and central nervous system. Metastases to ovary can mimic primary ovarian mucinous neoplasms. Regional lymph node involvement is also present in 35–50 % of ampullary carcinomas.

3.6 Lymph Nodes

Site/number/size/number involved/limit node/extracapsular spread.

Regional nodes: peripancreatic, pancreaticoduodenal, common bile duct, pyloric and proximal mesenteric. A regional lymphadenectomy will ordinarily include a minimum of ten lymph nodes.

Fig. 3.6 Pancreatic carcinoma (Reproduced, with permission, from Allen (2006), © 2006)

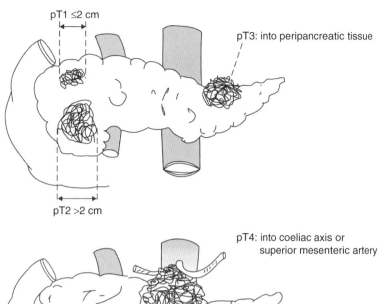

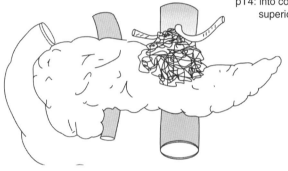

pN0	No regional lymph node metastasis
pN1	Metastasis in regional lymph node(s).

Up to 50 % of patients have involved regional lymph nodes at presentation.

3.7 Excision Margins

Distances (mm) to the following transected or dissected margins

Transected: proximal (gastric/duodenal), distal (duodenal), common bile duct, distal pancreatic

Dissected: posterior pancreatic surface (deep radial) and uncinate (medial).

Tumour <1 mm from the margin is reported as *positive (R1) in up to 35 % of cases*. Due to the dispersed tumour growth pattern at the periphery of pancreatic cancer assessment of complete excision is more problematic than for other gastrointestinal cancers.

The commonest site for *local recurrence of invasive carcinoma (occurs in 60–80 % of cases)* after a Whipple's procedure is the *posterior pancreatic surface margin*. This should be inked accordingly and the distance of tumour to it measured. Similarly for the *non-peritonealised medial margin of the uncinate process* which is identified by the superior mesenteric vein groove and the superior mesentery artery bare area. Local recurrence from intraductal tumour is more likely at a ductal resection margin.

3.8 Other Pathology

Ampulla

- *Duodenal adenoma(s)*, *Familial Adenomatous Polyposis*: periampullary carcinoma is one of the commonest causes of death in FAP.

Pancreas

- 3–10 % of pancreatic carcinomas are *hereditary*: either a positive family history of pancreatic carcinoma, BRCA2 gene positivity, or in the setting of HNPCC.
- *Disseminated intravascular coagulation (DIC)*, *thrombophlebitis migrans*: clinically present in 25 % of cases, particularly with mucin secreting tumours.
- *Gastrointestinal neuroendocrine syndromes*: e.g. Zollinger-Ellison syndrome (diarrhoea, gastric hyperacidity with gastric/duodenal/jejunal ulcers), Werner-Morrison syndrome/WDHA syndrome (watery diarrhoea, hypokalaemia, achlorhydria).
- *Chronic pancreatitis and autoimmune (IgG4) sclerosing pancreatitis*: can mimic pancreatic cancer clinically, on imaging and at operative inspection and palpation.
- *Chronic pancreatitis*: shows acinar atrophy, distortion and regenerative changes with stromal fibrosis and clusters of residual islet tissue that can *mimic pancreatic carcinoma*. Similar changes are also seen upstream and adjacent to pancreatic carcinoma due to duct obstruction indicating that interpretation and sampling can be problematic. Duct structures in chronic pancreatitis tend to retain their rounded contour and lobular architecture, lack significant malignant cytological change, show no invasion of nerve sheaths or peripancreatic fat, or juxtaposition to thick walled muscular vessels.
- *Pancreatic cancer*: jaundice of short duration in a patient older than 60 years is suspicious of malignancy. Other indicators are elevated serum CA19-9 (usually in cancers >3 cm diameter), duct stricture at ERCP, or a mass lesion on CT scan/ELUS. *Radiological imaging* is important in establishing *contraindications to surgery* (distant lymph node or major vessel involvement), or *other potentially operable diagnoses* e.g. serous or mucinous cystic tumours. A tissue diagnosis may be obtained by positive duct cytology brushings or transduodenal/percutaneous FNAC or needle core biopsy. This is particularly important to direct appropriate *palliative chemotherapy* in patients with *non-resectable disease*, and to exclude *other treatable malignancies* e.g. malignant lymphoma in peripancreatic nodes. In a proportion of cases (15–20 %) a firm diagnosis will not be obtained and must be assumed on the basis of clinical probability allowing radical surgery to proceed in a medically fit patient with resectable disease on imaging. As a result of these diagnostic difficulties there is inevitably a low risk (1–5 %) of a *false positive clinical diagnosis of cancer*, and it not being present in the resection specimen.

Immunophenotype

- *Neuroendocrine*: chromogranin, synaptophysin, CD56. A high Ki-67 index and CK19 positivity are a guide to metastatic potential. Poorly differentiated/high-grade (G3) neuroendocrine carcinoma shows reduced staining intensity for chromogranin A, and well differentiated/low-grade tumours for CD56.
- *Hormonal*: specific peptides – insulin, glucagon, gastrin, pancreatic polypeptide, VIP, ACTH, somatostatin.
- *Exocrine carcinoma*: cytokeratins (including CK7, CK8, CK18, CK19, ±CK20), CEA, CA19-9, CA-125, MUC I – expressed in >80 % of ductal lesions, ± CDX-2, p53, loss of SMAD4/DPC4.

Prognosis

Prognosis in pancreatic ductal carcinoma is poor with a majority of patients dead within several months of diagnosis. It relates to *tumour site* (body and tail are worse than head, as the latter may present early with obstructive jaundice), *size* (>4.5 cm is adverse), *histological grade* and *stage*. Overall 5 year survival is 5–10 %, resectable disease confined to the pancreas only achieving 15 % and with a median survival of 12–18 months. There is *limited suitability for resection in 10–20% of cases*, namely, lymph node negative tumours of the pancreatic head <3 cm diameter with no major vessel (superior mesenteric or portal vein) invasion. These patients may also receive benefit from *neoadjuvant* and *postoperative adjuvant chemotherapy*. Serum CA19-9 levels can be of use in monitoring response to therapy and as a surveillance tool during follow up to detect recurrent disease. The majority of patients present late with symptoms due to advanced disease in lymph node and retroperitoneal tissues. *Treatment is often palliative* with relief of ductal biliary obstruction by open or laparoscopic bypass, or endoscopic stent insertion, and, chemotherapy for select patients. *Non-invasive MCN and IPMN are potentially curable* by complete surgical resection. Those with an invasive component have 27–65 % 5 year survivals depending on the extent and histological type of the invasive component. *Pancreatic neuroendocrine tumours* may present with their associated metabolic or gastrointestinal syndrome and have an *indolent time course* being of low to intermediate-grade malignancy. *Ampullary carcinoma is more favourable* than pancreatic or bile duct carcinoma with a 5 year survival of 25–50 %. This can improve to 80–85 % if the tumour is at an early stage and confined to the sphincter of Oddi (pT1). Transduodenal wide local excision may be adequate for carefully selected ampullary tumours e.g. adenoma, but only after careful staging and exclusion of an underlying mass lesion requiring radical surgery.

3.9 Other Malignancy

Leukaemia

Malignant Lymphoma

- Usually spread from paraaortic/peripancreatic nodal lymphoma.
- Extramedullary plasmacytoma.

Sarcoma

- Rare
- Leiomyosarcoma, liposarcoma, fibrosarcoma, osteosarcoma.
- Exclude secondary from gastrointestinal tract (spindle cell carcinoma/GIST/sarcoma) or retroperitoneum.

Bibliography

Albores-Saavedra J, Henson DE, Klimstra DS. Tumors of the gallbladder, extrahepatic bile ducts and ampulla of vater. Atlas of tumor pathology. 3rd series. Fascicle 27. Washington: AFIP; 2000.

Allen DC. Histopathology reporting: guidelines for surgical cancer. 2nd ed. London: Springer; 2006.

Alsaad K, Chetty R. Serous cystic neoplasms of the pancreas. Curr Diagn Pathol. 2005;11:102–9.

Beckingham IJ, editor. ABC of liver, pancreas and gall bladder diseases. London: BMJ Books; 2001.

Bond-Smith G, Banga N, Hammond TM, Imber CJ. Pancreatic adenocarcinoma. BMJ. 2012;344:45–50.

Bosman FT, Carneiro F. WHO classification of tumours of the digestive system. 4th ed. Lyon: IARC press; 2010.

British Society of Gastroenterology. Guidelines for the management of patients with pancreatic cancer, periampullary and ampullary carcinomas. Gut. 2005;54:v1–15.

Campbell F, Azadeh B. Cystic neoplasms of the exocrine pancreas. Histopathology. 2008;52:539–51.

Carter D, Russell RCG, Pitt HA, Bismuth H, editors. Rob and Smith's operative surgery: hepatobiliary and pancreatic surgery. 5th ed. London: Chapman and Hall; 1996.

Chetty R. Pancreatic endocrine neoplasia: familial syndromes. Diagn Histopathol. 2009;15:95–8.

Day DW, Jass JR, Price AB, Shepherd NA, Sloan JM, Talbot IC, Warren BF, Williams GT. Morson and Dawson's gastrointestinal pathology. 4th ed. Oxford: Blackwell Sciences; 2003.

Ghaneh P, Costello E, Neoptolemos JP. Biology and management of pancreatic cancer. Gut. 2007;56: 1134–52.

Govender G. Mucinous cystic neoplasms of the pancreas. Curr Diagn Pathol. 2005;11:110–6.

Haugk B. Pancreatic intraepithelial neoplasia – can we detect early pancreatic cancer? Histopathology. 2010;57:503–14.

Hruban RH, Takaori K, Klimstra DS, Adsay NV, et al. An illustrated consensus on the classification of pancreatic intraepithelial neoplasia and intraductal papillary mucinous neoplasms. Am J Surg Pathol. 2004;28: 977–87.

Hruban RH, Pitman MB, Klimstra DS. Tumors of the pancreas. Atlas of tumor pathology. 4th Series. Fascicle 6. Washington: AFIP; 2007.

Katabi N, Klimstra DS. Intraductal papillary mucinous neoplasms of the pancreas: clinical and pathological features and diagnostic approach. J Clin Pathol. 2008;61:1303–13.

Odze RD, Goldblum JR. Surgical pathology of the GI tract, liver, biliary tract and pancreas. 2nd ed. Philadelphia: Saunders/Elsevier; 2009.

Plockinger U, Rindi G, Arnold R, Eriksson B, Krenning EP, de Herder WW, et al. Guidelines for the diagnosis and treatment of neuroendocrine gastrointestinal tumours. A consensus statement on behalf of the European Neuroendocrine Tumour Society (ENETS). Neuroendocrinology. 2004;80:394–424.

Ramage JK, Davies AHG, Ardill F, et al. Guidelines for the management of gastroenteropancreatic neuroendocrine (including carcinoid) tumours. Gut. 2005;54: iv1–16.

Serra S, Chetty R. Revision 2: an immunohistochemical approach and evaluation of solid pseudopapillary tumour of the pancreas. J Clin Pathol. 2008;61:1153–9.

Stephenson TJ. Prognostic and predictive factors in endocrine tumours. Histopathology. 2006;48:629–43.

Takhar AS, Palaniappan P, Dhingse R, Lobo DN. Recent development in diagnosis of pancreatic cancer. BMJ. 2004;329:668–73.

The Royal College of Pathologists: Cancer Datasets (Oesophageal Carcinoma, Gastric Carcinoma, Carcinomas of the Pancreas, ampulla of Vater and Common Bile Duct, Colorectal Cancer, Gastrointestinal Stromal Tumours (GISTs), Liver Resection Specimens and Liver Biopsies for Primary and Metastatic Carcinoma, Endocrine Tumours of the Gastrointestinal Tract including Pancreas) and Tissue Pathways (Gastrointestinal and Pancreatobiliary Pathology, Liver Biopsies for the Investigation of Medical Disease and for Focal Liver Lesions). Accessed at http://www.rcpath.org/index.asp?PageID=254

Verbeke CS. Resection margins and R1 rates in pancreatic cancer – are we there yet? Histopathology. 2008;52: 787–96.

Verbeke CS. Endocrine tumours of the pancreas. Histopathology. 2010;56:669–82.

Verbeke CS, Knapp J, Gladhaug IP. Tumour growth is more dispersed in pancreatic head cancers than in rectal cancer: implications for resection margin assessment. Histopathology. 2011;59:1111–21.

Wittekind CF, Greene FL, Hutter RVP, Klimpfinger M, Sobib LH. TNM atlas: illustrated guide to the TNM/pTNM classification of malignant tumours. 5th ed. Berlin: Springer; 2005.

Small Intestinal Carcinoma

Small intestinal carcinoma is uncommon with more arising in the duodenum than in the jejunum and ileum combined. African Americans are a high risk group. Other risk factors are smoking, alcohol, chronic inflammation (Crohn's disease, coeliac disease) and Familial Adenomatous Polyposis (FAP). Presentation can vary with poorly localized central abdominal pain, obstruction with vomiting, colicky pain, constipation and distension. There may be a palpable mass or gastrointestinal bleeding.

Up to 60 % of duodenal polyp/mass lesions are benign viz Brunner's gland hyperplasia/adenoma, nodular gastric heterotopia (first part duodenum – D1) and duodenal adenoma. Malignant lesions are relatively uncommon, usually in D2, and occurring in patients 60–79 years of age. About 16 % of these represent metastases from other sites e.g. lung, breast, colon and pancreas, and they have a poor prognosis despite surgical resection. Radical surgery is considered for a primary lesion in the absence of widespread metastases. Assessment is by upper gastrointestinal endoscopy and CT scan. Palliative treatment may be considered as a first line approach including duodenal stenting to overcome bowel obstruction by a compressing extrinsic tumour mass. Tissue diagnosis is important to exclude other treatable malignancies e.g. malignant melanoma, or malignant lymphoma in adjacent paraduodenal lymph nodes.

Localised jejunal and distal ileal mass lesions require a segmental resection and right hemicolectomy respectively, with en-bloc resection of the relevant mesenteric pedicle. Distal ileal lesions may be seen and biopsied at colonoscopy. More proximal small intestinal lesions may be characterized by push endoscopy, barium follow through studies or CT scan. Serosal disease e.g. seedlings of metastatic carcinoma can be visualized and biopsied at laparoscopy or exploratory laparotomy.

4.1 Gross Description

Specimen

- Endoscopic/laparoscopic or open biopsy/resection.
  Whipples pancreaticoduodenectomy, segmental bowel resection, right hemicolectomy: depending on the tumour site in the proximal/mid-/distal small bowel, respectively. Needle core biopsy of a small intestinal or mesenteric mass is usually avoided due to the risk of capsule rupture and tumour seeding jeopardising complete primary resection, suitability for which is assessed by CT scan.
- Weight (g) and size/length (cm), number of fragments.

Tumour

Site

- Duodenum (particularly periampullary) 70 %: see Chap. 3.
- Jejunum/ileum 30 %.
- Mucous membrane/muscularis/extra-mural.
- Serosal/mesenteric/nodal/single/multifocal.
- Mesenteric/anti-mesenteric border.
- Meckel's diverticulum.

Size

- Length × width × depth (cm) or maximum dimension (cm).

Appearance

- Polypoid/sessile/ulcerated/diffusely infiltrative/fleshy/pigmented/yellow/ stricture/intussusception ± secondary ischaemic necrosis of the tumour tip/intussusceptum or receiving segment (intussuscipiens).

Duodenal carcinomas tend to be papillary or polypoid, *ileojejunal carcinomas* ulcerated and annular with constriction of the bowel wall (napkin ring like). Presentation can be non-specific e.g. anaemia or weight loss, with poorly defined central abdominal pain or signs of subacute obstruction. There may be a detectable mass either on abdominal examination or CT scan. *Well differentiated endocrine (carcinoid) tumour* is nodular, yellow, solitary or multifocal, causing bowel obstruction due to fibrosis or acting as the apex of an intussusception. On CT scan it forms a characteristic dense spiculate mesenteric mass associated with coarse flecks of calcification. *Malignant lymphoma* can be subtle in the edge of a perforated jejunitis, unicentric or multifocal, and a fungating, fleshy mural or mesenteric mass. There may or may not be a preceding history of coeliac disease. *Metastatic carcinoma* variably forms serosal seedlings, nodules or plaques. *Gastrointestinal stromal tumours (GISTs)* are mural lesions which can be dumbbell shaped with luminal and extramural components. They can also be separate from the bowel wall and mesenteric in location. Deposits of *malignant melanoma* may be darkly pigmented, and *choriocarcinoma* haemorrhagic.

Edge

- Circumscribed/irregular.

4.2 Histological Type

Adenocarcinoma

- *Enteric pattern*: the usual type and well or moderately differentiated.
- *Anaplastic*: poorly differentiated forms occur more frequently than in colorectal cancer.
- *Mucinous carcinoma*: mucin forms >50 % of the tumour area.
- *Signet ring cell carcinoma*: mucin in >50 % of the tumour cells.

Diagnosis of primary small intestinal adenocarcinoma is by *exclusion of spread from more common sites* e.g. colorectum and stomach. As in the large intestine there is some evidence for a dysplasia (adenoma) – carcinoma sequence in the adjacent mucosa. *Prognosis is poor* due to late presentation at an advanced stage.

Carcinoid (Neuroendocrine) Tumour

- Yellow/nodular/solitary or multifocal (25 %).
- A well differentiated/low-grade neuroendocrine tumour which is positive for chromogranin/synaptophysin/CD56±/CDX-2. Mitoses are usually <2 per 10 high power fields and Ki-67 index ≤2 % (i.e. a G1 tumour).
- Typically an insular pattern of uniform cells in a dense fibrous stroma with vascular thickening.
- 20 % have *carcinoid syndrome* implying liver metastases. It is characterized by facial flushing, asthma and thickening of cardiac valves due to release of vasoactive peptides (e.g. serotonin) into the systemic circulation.
- *Tumour grade* is based on cell type, atypia, necrosis and proliferative activity: mitoses/10hpfs, Ki-67 index (see Chap. 3. Differentiation).
- *Low-grade malignancy*: any functioning well differentiated tumour; any tumour with angio-invasion; non-functioning tumour ≥2 cm or with invasion beyond the submucosa.

- *High-grade malignancy*: tumour with a high mitotic rate, cellular atypia or necrosis and poorly differentiated neuroendocrine large cell/small cell carcinomas. Chromogranin±, synaptophysin/CD56/Ki-67 positive.

Prognosis: well differentiated neuroendocrine (carcinoid) tumour has an overall *50–65 % 5 year survival rate*. It is better for small lesions (metastatic rate: <1 cm (2 %), 1–2 cm (50 %), >2 cm (80 %)) confined to the wall (85 % 5 year survival) than those invading the serosa or beyond (5 % 5 year survival). Metastases are to *regional lymph nodes and liver* (multiple, solid/cystic), and also bone, skin and thyroid. The above comments relate mostly to classical EC (enterochromaffin) cell ileojejunal well differentiated neuroendocrine (carcinoid) tumours. Duodenal lesions (5–8 % of cases) are sporadic or arise in association with MEN or neurofibromatosis syndromes. They have a better prognosis, occur mainly in D1/D2 and include *non-functioning G cell tumours*, *gastrinomas* (Zollinger Ellison/MEN syndromes), *somatostatinoma* (look for psammoma bodies) and *gangliocytic paraganglioma*.

Others

- Rare: adenosquamous, sarcomatoid carcinoma; aggressive.

Metastatic Carcinoma

- *Direct spread*: colorectum, ovary, stomach, pancreas.
- *Distant spread*: lung, breast, malignant melanoma and choriocarcinoma.

The bulk of disease is *extramural* but tumour can invade muscularis and mucous membrane causing obstruction or perforation, and *mimicking a primary lesion* on macroscopic and microscopic examination. Adjacent mucosal dysplasia is a useful pointer and adenoma is present in 24 % of primary lesions. Small bowel is a common site of metastatic malignancy with formation of peritoneal seedlings, multiple nodules, plaques and strictures causing obstruction.

Metastatic Malignant Melanoma

- Pigmented/multifocal.
- Amelanotic/oligomelanotic.
- Malignant melanoma requires confirmation with S100, HMB-45, melan-A.

4.3   Differentiation

Adenocarcinoma: well/moderate/poor/undifferentiated, or, Grade 1/2/3/4 based on the percentage tumour gland formation (well/G1 >95 %: moderate/G2 50–95 %: poor/G3 <50 %). Signet ring cell carcinoma is grade 3, small cell and undifferentiated carcinoma (no gland formation) grade 4.

Well differentiated neuroendocrine (carcinoid) tumour/ high-grade neuroendocrine carcinoma: see Chap. 3. Differentiation.

Malignant lymphoma: low-/high-grade based on the number of blast cells present.

Sarcoma: low-/high-grade based on the degree of cellularity, atypia, necrosis and mitoses.

4.4   Extent of Local Tumour Spread

Border: pushing/infiltrative.
Lymphocytic reaction: prominent/sparse.
TMN7 classification for carcinoma.

pTis	Carcinoma in situ
pT1	Tumour invades:
pT1a	Lamina propria or muscularis mucosae
pT1b	Submucosa
pT2	Tumour invades muscularis propria
pT3	Tumour invades through muscularis propria into subserosa or into non-peritonealised perimuscular tissue (mesentery or retroperitoneum) with extension ≤2 cm
pT4	Tumour perforates visceral peritoneum or directly invades other organs/structures (including loops of small intestine, mesentery, retroperitoneum >2 cm and abdominal wall via serosa; also for duodenum – invasion of pancreas) (Figs. 4.1 and 4.2).

The non-peritonealised perimuscular tissue is, for jejunum and ileum, part of the mesentery and,

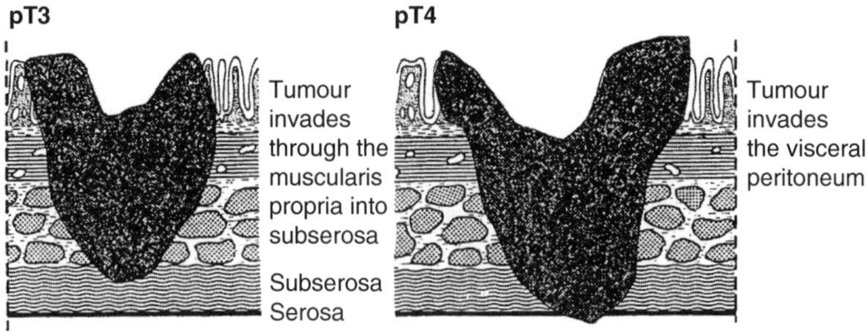

Fig. 4.1 Small intestinal carcinoma (Reproduced, with permission, from Wittekind et al. (2005), © 2005)

Fig. 4.2 Small intestinal carcinoma (Reproduced, with permission, from Wittekind et al. (2005), © 2005)

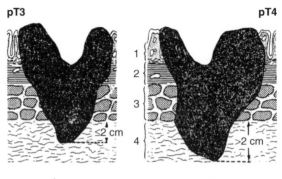

for duodenum in areas where serosa is lacking, part of the retroperitoneum.

TNM7 classification for well differentiated neuroendocrine (carcinoid) tumour.

pT1	Tumour invades lamina propria or submucosa, and is ≤1 cm in size
pT2	Tumour invades muscularis propria or is >1 cm in size
pT3	Tumour invades subserosa (jejunal/ileal), or, pancreas or retroperitoneum (ampullary/duodenal)
pT4	Tumour invades serosa or adjacent organs.

4.5 Lymphovascular Invasion

Present/absent.

Intra-/extratumoural.

Vessel wall fibrosis/stenosis in well differentiated neuroendocrine (carcinoid) tumour.

Metastatic carcinoma often shows quite extensive lymphovascular invasion in the various layers of the bowel wall.

4.6 Lymph Nodes

Site/number/size/number involved/limit node/extracapsular spread.

Regional nodes: duodenum – gastroduodenal, pancreaticoduodenal, pyloric, hepatic, superior mesenteric; ileum/jejunum – mesenteric; terminal ileum – ileocolic, posterior caecal. A regional lymphadenectomy will ordinarily include a minimum of 6 lymph nodes.

pN0	No regional lymph node metastasis
pN1	Metastasis in 1–3 regional lymph node(s)
pN2	Metastasis in ≥4 regional lymph nodes.

4.7 Excision Margins

Distances (mm) to the nearest longitudinal limit of resection and the painted deep radial (non-peritonealised soft tissue) mesenteric margin. In a segmental bowel resection it is usual to clear a 5 cm length of intestine on either side of the tumour with en bloc resection of a wedge of mesentery.

4.8   Other Pathology

There is increased incidence of adenocarcinoma in:

- *Familial Adenomatous Polyposis*: particularly periampullary related to duodenal adenomas. It is a significant cause of mortality in FAP.
- *Hereditary non-polyposis colon cancer (HNPCC)*.
- *Peutz-Jegher's polyposis*: beware of epithelial misplacement/pseudo-invasion mimicking carcinoma; rare.
- *Crohn's disease*.
- *Coeliac disease*.
- *Ileostomy, ileal conduits*.
- *Meckel's diverticulum's*: rare, but can also be a site for well differentiated neuroendocrine (carcinoid) tumour, GIST, or leiomyosarcoma.
- *Coeliac disease/ulcerative jejunitis/gluten induced intestinal or enteropathy associated T cell lymphoma (EATCL)*: change in or lack of responsiveness to a gluten free diet in a previously well maintained patient, or presentation as an ulcerative/perforated jejunitis, or an abdominal mass in an older patient can indicate onset of EATCL.

  Stricture – carcinoid, metastases.

  Intussusception – carcinoid, malignant lymphoma.

  Multifocal – carcinoid, malignant lymphoma, malignant melanoma, metastases.

  Meckel's diverticulum – carcinoid, adenocarcinoma, leiomyomatous tumours.

Immunophenotype

Small bowel adenocarcinoma is CAM 5.2, AE1/AE3, CEA, CK20 (40 %), CDX-2 positive. About 50 % are also CK7 positive.

Prognosis

Small bowel adenocarcinoma is unusual, being 50 times less common than large bowel carcinoma. Some 70 % occur in the duodenum, particularly the periampullary region. *Presentation is late* due to the fluid content of the bowel. Many patients already have transmural spread and lymph node metastases and the majority subsequently dies from their disease. *Five year survival rates are approximately 10–30 %* with the most important prognostic indicator being *depth of spread* or *stage* of disease. Localised, regional and metastatic disease have 5 year survival rates of 57, 34 and 3 % respectively. Duodenum is less favourable than ileum and jejunum. *Surgical resection* is the curative intent treatment of choice.

4.9   Other Malignancy

Malignant Lymphoma

- Comprises *30–50 % of small bowel malignancy*. Single or multifocal, primary or secondary to lymph node/systemic disease. Primary disease centres on the bowel with or without spread to regional lymph nodes.
- *MALToma*:

  Low/high-grade.

  B cell (70–90 % of bowel lymphomas are of B cell lineage).

  Centrocyte like cells with variable numbers of blasts (>20 %=high-grade).

  Lymphoepithelial lesions.

  Monotypic immunoglobulin expression.

  ± Eosinophilia.

  High-grade lesions are on a spectrum with *diffuse large B cell lymphoma* which forms *40–60 % of small intestinal lymphoma cases*, with or without a component of MALT lymphoma.
- *Burkitt's type/B lymphoblastic*:

  Children, or adults with HIV (non-endemic/non-EBV related).

  Terminal ileum/ileocaecal valve – a high-grade lymphoma.

  CD20, CD10, CD79a, tdt positive (lymphoblastic lymphoma). High Ki67 index (>90 %) and a starry sky appearance.

- *Multiple lymphomatous polyposis*:
  Centrocytic lymphoma or mantle cell lymphoma – splenic, small and large bowel disease with numerous intestinal polyps.
  An intermediate-grade lymphoma – *aggressive disease* with advanced stage at presentation. CD20, CD5, cyclin D1 positive.
- *EATCL*:
  Aggressive forming *5 % of GI lymphomas* usually in the proximal jejunum. Pleomorphic medium to large cell infiltrate (CD3 positive) and adjacent *enteropathic mucosa* (villous atrophy/increased surface intraepithelial lymphocytes) showing '*pre-lymphomatous*' *changes* or type 2 refractory coeliac disease viz clonal intraepithelial lymphocytes with T cell receptor gene rearrangements and an aberrant immunophenotype (loss of CD4/CD8 expression) .
- *Follicle centre cell (follicular) lymphoma*:
  More usually spread from lymph node disease rather than primary.
- *Immunoproliferative small intestinal disease (IPSID)*:
  Mediterranean countries.
  Alpha chain disease.
- *Post-transplant lymphoproliferative disorders*:
  Polyclonal/monclonal/disparate morphology and behaviour.
  Some regress on decreasing immunosuppression therapy e.g. cyclosporin (see Chap. 35).
  Prognosis: is better for low-grade B cell lymphomas (44–75 % 5 year survival) than high-grade B or T cell lymphomas (25–37 % 5 year survival). Adverse prognostic indicators are *perforation, high-grade histology, T cell phenotype, multiple tumours, large size, serosal penetration and advanced stage* (Ann Arbor System: see Chap. 35).

Gastrointestinal Mesenchymal or Stromal Tumours (GISTs)

- Spindle cells, epithelioid cells, skeinoid collagen fibres. Note also that extra-intestinal mesenteric or retroperitoneal lesions can occur.
- Ileum 50 %, jejunum 40 %, duodenum 10 %.

Myogenic: 10 % of cases are desmin/h-caldesmon/smooth muscle actin positive and DOG-1/c-kit(CD117) negative, representing true leiomyoma or leiomyosarcoma.

Neural: 10 % of cases are S100/synaptophysin positive and DOG-1/c-kit(CD117) negative, representing neurilemmoma (Schwannoma: characteristic peritumoural lymphoid infiltrate) or neurofibroma (can be associated with von Recklinghausen's disease/MEN syndrome and GISTs elsewhere in the gut).

Stromal: *DOG-1/c-kit(CD117*: tyrosine kinase receptor)/CD34 positive, with absent or incomplete myogenic/neural differentiation. Putative precursors are the interstitial cells of Cajal, which are gut pacemaker cells located in the deep submucosa and myenteric plexus. In general antigen positivity is DOG-1 and CD117 (95 %), CD34 (70–85 %), smooth muscle actin (20–40 %), h-caldesmon (60–80 %) and nestin (90–100 %). DOG-1/CD117 negative GISTs may be identified by positive protein kinase c theta and PDGFR mutation analysis. *C-kit mutation analysis* (exon 11 in 60–70 % of cases) is helpful in confirming the *diagnosis* and in prediction of *prognosis* and *response to drug treatment*. Exon 11 changes are more responsive than tumours with alterations in exon 9. Mutation analysis is generally recommended if immunohistochemistry is equivocal, and in cases of borderline/malignant GISTs. Note that other malignant tumours can also be CD117 positive e.g. seminoma, malignant melanoma and some metastatic carcinomas e.g. breast, ovary, colorectal, small cell carcinoma. DOG-1 (transmembrane protein <u>D</u>iscovered <u>O</u>n GIST<u>1</u>) is a highly sensitive and specific marker for GIST but may also show weak to moderate expression in some other tumours e.g. colorectal, endometrioid and acinic cell carcinomas, spindle cell malignant melanoma and malignant peripheral nerve sheath tumours. GANT (gastrointestinal autonomic nerve tumour) is now regarded as a variant of GIST and assessed accordingly. A small minority of patients with GISTs may have any of: a positive family history of GISTs, Carney triad (gastric GIST, pulmonary chondroma, extra-adrenal paraganglioma) or type 1 neurofibromatosis.

Table 4.1 Risk factors in ileojejunal GISTs – risk of progressive disease, metastases or tumour related death

	Tumour dia (cm)	Mitoses/ 50hpfs	Percentage risk
No risk	≤2	<5	0
Low risk	>2–5	<5	4.3
Moderate risk	>5–10	<5	24
High risk	>10	<5	52
	Any size	>5	73–90

Malignancy relates to: size (>2–5 cm), cellularity, atypia, cell type (epithelioid is worse than spindle cell), necrosis, margins and mitoses. *Prognosis* (approximately *50 % 5 year survival*) is also stage dependent. DNA ploidy, Ki-67 proliferation indices, over expression of p53, loss of DOG-1/CD117 immunoexpression and morphometry also correlate with these parameters.

Clinical risk: small intestinal GISTs are categorised as being no risk, low, moderate or high *metastatic risk* on the basis of size and mitoses (see Table 4.1).

Prognosis: in GISTs is dependent on *patient age, tumour size* (>5 cm), *tumour site* and *mitotic activity*. A robust criterion in stomach tumours is >5 *mitoses/50 high-power fields*, but *mid- and hindgut lesions are more aggressive* (even if <5 cm diameter and with low mitotic counts) *than foregut tumours*. Behaviour can also be unpredictable, with clinicopathological factors at best being only broadly indicative. The old terminology "gastrointestinal stromal tumour of uncertain malignant potential" has been replaced by clinical risk stratification. With an established diagnosis of *sarcoma* histological grading is not a reliable index of metastatic potential and *tumour size* is a better indicator. So much so that the TNM7 staging system is size based: pT1 ≤2 cm dia, pT2 >2–5 cm dia, pT3 >5–10 cm dia and pT4 >10 cm dia.

Metastases: *are commonly to peritoneum, liver, pancreas, retroperitoneum* and *lungs*. Lymph node metastases can occur but are rare. Metastases are CT/PET scan positive but become negative on treatment. Metastatic disease responds well to *targeted tyrosine kinase inhibitor therapy* (*Glivec* (*imatinib*)) resulting in tumour shrinkage, myxoid, hyaline and cystic degeneration. It gives several disease free years,

or tumour down staging that can facilitate operative resection, but usually therapeutic escape occurs with *recurrent peritoneal disease or size progression of liver metastases*. This may relate to new acquired genetic mutations in the tumour cells. About 13 % of patients are resistant to therapy with disease progression within 6 months.

Kaposi's Sarcoma

- HIV: 50 % of high risk patients have visceral involvement.

Leukaemia

- 14.8–25 % of cases.
- Granulocytic sarcoma (CD34/CD43/CD 68/ CD117/chloroacetate esterase and myleoperoxidase positive).

Bibliography

Banks PM. Gastrointestinal lymphoproliferative disorders. Histopathology. 2007;50:42–54.

Bosman FT, Carneiro F. WHO classification of tumours of the digestive system. 4th ed. Lyon: IARC press; 2010.

Day DW, Jass JR, Price AB, Shepherd NA, Sloan JM, Talbot IC, Warren BF, Williams GT. Morson and Dawson's gastrointestinal pathology. 4th ed. Oxford: Blackwell Sciences; 2003.

Domizio P, Owen RA, Shepherd NA, Talbot IC, Norton AJ. Primary lymphoma of the small intestine. A clinicopathological study of 119 cases. Am J Surg Pathol. 1993;17:429–42.

Dudley H, Pories W, Carter D, editors. Rob and Smith's operative surgery: alimentary tract and abdominal wall. 4th ed. London: Butterworths; 1993.

Hemminger J, Iwenofu OH. Discovered on gastrointestinal stromal tumours 1 (DOG1) expression in non-gastrointestinal stromal tumour (GIST) neoplasms. Histopathology. 2012;61:170–7.

Ho-Yen C, Chang F, van der Walt J, Mitchell T, Ciclitira P. Recent advances in refractory coeliac disease: a review. Histopathology. 2009;54:783–95.

Joensuu H. Risk stratification of patients diagnosed with gastrointestinal stromal tumor. Hum Pathol. 2008;39: 1411–9.

Kanthan R, Gomez D, Senger J-L, Kantan SC. Endoscopic biopsies of duodenal polyp/mass lesions: a surgical pathology review. J Clin Pathol. 2010; 63:921–5.

Lioe TF, Biggart JD. Primary adenocarcinoma of the jeju-
    num and ileum: clinicopathological review of 25
    cases. J Clin Pathol. 1990;43:533–6.
Miettinen M, Makhlouf H, Sobin LH, Lasota J.
    Gastrointestinal stromal tumors of the jejunum and
    ileum. A clinicopathologic, immunohistochemical,
    and molecular genetic study of 906 cases before ima-
    tinib with long-term follow-up. Am J Surg Pathol.
    2006;30:477–89.
Novelli M, Rossi S, Rodriguez-Justo M, Taniere P, Seddon
    B, Toffolatti L, Sartor C, Hogendoorn PCW, Sciot R,
    van Glabbeke M, Verweij J, Blay JY, Hohenberger P,
    Flanagan A, Tos APD. DOG1 and CD117 are the anti-
    bodies of choice in the diagnosis of gastrointestinal
    stromal tumours. Histopathology. 2010;57:259–70.
Odze RD, Goldblum JR. Surgical pathology of the GI
    tract, liver, biliary tract and pancreas. 2nd ed.
    Philadelphia: Saunders/Elsevier; 2009.
Pauwels P, Debiec-Rychter M, Stul M, de Wever I,
    van Oosterom AT, Sciot R. Changing phenotype
    of gastrointestinal stromal tumours under imatinib
    mesylate treatment: a potential diagnostic pitfall.
    Histopathology. 2005;47:41–7.
Riddell RH, Petras RE, Williams GT, Sobin LH. Tumors
    of the intestines. Atlas of tumor pathology. 3rd Series.
    Fascicle 32. Washington: AFIP; 2003.
The Royal College of Pathologists: Cancer Datasets
    (Oesophageal Carcinoma, Gastric Carcinoma, Carci-
    nomas of the Pancreas, ampulla of Vater and Common
Bile Duct, Colorectal Cancer, Gastrointestinal Stromal
    Tumours (GISTs), Liver Resection Specimens and
    Liver Biopsies for Primary and Metastatic Carcinoma,
    Endocrine Tumours of the Gastrointestinal Tract includ-
    ing Pancreas) and Tissue Pathways (Gastrointestinal
    and Pancreatobiliary Pathology, Liver Biopsies for the
    Investigation of Medical Disease and for Focal Liver
    Lesions). Accessed at http://www.rcpath.org/index.
    asp?PageID=254.
Walker MM, Murray JA. An update in the diagnosis of
    coeliac disease. Histopathology. 2011;59:166–79.
Williams GT. Endocrine tumours of the gastrointestinal
    tract – selected topics. Histopathology. 2007;50:
    30–41.
Wittekind CF, Greene FL, Hutter RVP, Klimpfinger M,
    Sobib LH. TNM atlas: illustrated guide to the TNM/
    pTNM classification of malignant tumours. 5th ed.
    Berlin: Springer; 2005.
Wong NACS. Gastrointestinal stromal tumours – an
    update for histopathologists. Histopathology. 2011;59:
    807–21.
Wong NACS, Deans ZC, Ramsden SC. The UK NEQUAS
    for molecular genetics scheme for gastrointestinal
    stromal tumour: findings and recommendations fol-
    lowing four rounds of circulation. J Clin Pathol.
    2012;65:786–90.
Yantis RK, Odze RD. Neoplastic precursor lesions of the
    upper gastrointestinal tract. Diagn Histopathol. 2008;
    14:437–52.

Colorectal Carcinoma

Colorectal cancer accounts for about 10 % of all new cancers worldwide and is the fourth commonest in men (after lung, prostate, stomach) and the third in women (after breast and cervix). Its geographical incidence varies greatly and is high but stabilizing in the industrialized countries of Europe, Australia, North America and Japan. Risk factors are: obesity with a diet of highly calorific food rich in animal fats, low fruit and fibre and high red meat intake, lack of exercise, smoking, alcohol and chronic inflammation e.g. inflammatory bowel disease. It is estimated that some 10–35 % of colorectal cancers can be attributed to inherited susceptibility, with 5 % on the basis of specific predisposing syndromes such as Familial Adenomatous Polyposis (FAP) and hereditary non-polyposis colorectal cancer (HNPCC).

Presentation of colorectal cancer is variable depending on the tumour site and growth pattern e.g. bright red bleeding per rectum, abdominal pain or mass, change in bowel habit, tenesmus (feeling of incomplete faecal evacuation), or, as an iron deficiency anaemia due to chronic blood loss from the ulcerated surface of the lesion. A significant minority (10–15 %) present as a surgical emergency due to intestinal obstruction, or perforation either directly through the tumour itself, or of the dilated bowel proximal to the stenotic tumour. National bowel screening programmes are based on detection of faecal blood loss and targeted at asymptomatic late middle aged patients with the aim of identifying precursor lesions and early stage cancers.

Investigation of colorectal cancer is by endoscopy and biopsy with staging of biopsy proven cancers by CT scan of chest, abdomen and pelvis for local and distant spread. MRI scan of rectal cancers complements this and clinical examination by imparting information about lymph node disease, possible vascular invasion, and the status of the tumour edge in relation to the mesorectal envelope and its fascial plane. These influence neoadjuvant and operative management decisions and rates of local recurrence.

Ideally, endoscopy is colonoscopy to visualize the entirety of the colorectum to assess for synchronous lesions. Any or a combination of CT colonogram, sigmoidoscopy and barium enema can be of use in a medically unfit patient or where there is a distal stricture not passable by the colonoscope or amenable to biopsy. A tight stricture may be negotiated by a gastroscope which is of a narrower diameter.

Curative colorectal cancer surgery excises the primary lesion with adequate longitudinal and deep radial margins and en bloc resection of the relevant colonic mesenteric lymphovascular pedicle, or, the mesorectum. The type of resection is determined by the site, distribution and any multiplicity of lesions detected at preoperative colonoscopy. Planned elective laparoscopic surgery is the preferred option. Open abdominal surgery (laparotomy) may be necessary for extensive disease, or if the presentation is as an acute emergency. Palliative intent surgery delivers a more limited resection. Some patients with obstructing cancers undergo piecemeal

D.C. Allen, *Histopathology Reporting*,
DOI 10.1007/978-1-4471-5263-7_5, © Springer-Verlag London 2013

resection, partial laser ablation, or stenting to restore intestinal continuity and avoid the risk of perforation. This may allow elective resection to be planned for a later date. Stenting is contraindicated in low rectal tumours and right sided colonic obstruction due to difficulties in stent placement and migration. Clinical follow up of colorectal cancer is by CT scan and serum CEA levels which can be elevated in recurrent or metastatic disease. Assay of serum CEA is not recommended for making a diagnosis of primary colorectal cancer. CT/PET scan can be of use in detecting extrahepatic metastases which would be a contraindication to consideration of hepatic metastasectomy, or treatment with cetuximab following surgical clearance of the colorectal primary.

5.1 Gross Description

Specimen

- Rectal/sigmoidoscopic/colonoscopic biopsy, local resection (EMR(endoscopic mucosal resection)/ESD(endoscopic submucosal dissection)/TEMS(transanal endoscopic microsurgery)), right or left hemi-/transverse/ sigmoid/ subtotal or total colectomy/anterior (AR) or abdominoperineal (APER) resection/ panproctocolectomy.
- Weight (g) and size/length (cm), number of fragments.

Tumour

Site
- Caecum/ascending colon/hepatic flexure/ transverse colon/splenic flexure/descending or sigmoid colon/ rectum/multifocal (10 % – synchronous or metachronous). *Rectosigmoid (50 % of cases)* are the commonest sites. *Tumour site strongly influences clinical presentation* e.g. caecal carcinoma – anaemia, right iliac fossa mass; sigmoid colon carcinoma – alteration in bowel habit; rectal cancer - bright red blood per rectum, tenesmus.

- *For rectum*: *above/at/below the peritoneal reflection*. Tumours below the reflection have a *higher rate of local recurrence* and tumours above/at the reflection anteriorly may *involve peritoneum*. The lateral angled descent of the peritoneum results in variation of the anatomical relationships with the upper rectum orientated to mesorectum posteriorly and laterally and peritoneum anteriorly. The mid rectum is surrounded by mesorectum, whereas the lower rectum is below the level of the mesorectum encircled by pelvic sphincteric and levator ani muscle. Elsewhere in the colon the bowel is orientated to serosa and a mesentery but the ascending and descending colons have a posterior non-peritonealised retroperitoneal bare area. As in the mesorectum this constitutes a deep radial soft tissue resection margin although this can be difficult to identify in individual cases. Sigmoid colon ends where the external longitudinal muscle bands (taeniae coli) blend with the rectal muscularis propria (Fig. 5.1).
- Distances (cm) to the dentate line and nearest longitudinal resection limit. These figures can audit the rates of *AR versus APER*, with the former being the operation of choice (*with total mesorectal excision*: *TME*) for mid- and upper rectal cancers. Low rectal cancers also have higher local recurrence rates. Clinical (endoscopic/radiological: MRI scan) and anatomical definition of the rectum varies, but in general, distances from the anal verge are: lower rectum 0–5 cm, mid rectum 5–10 cm, and upper rectum 10–15 cm. *Tumour site within the rectum* not only *influences the choice of operative procedure* but also *neoadjuvant therapy* e.g. low rectal cancers are given long course as opposed to short course preoperative radiotherapy. A further important audit factor is the *integrity or completeness of the mesorectal envelope in the postoperative specimen*. Deficiencies indicate a suboptimal operation and greater potential for local pelvic recurrence. A suggested grading classification is Quirke 1 (incomplete), 2 (nearly complete) and 3 (complete). Categories 1 and 2 show variable mesorectal bulk and deficiencies or cuts into the mesorectal capsule, but it is

smooth and intact in category 3. In low rectal cancers the need to achieve a clear radial margin has led to increased use of *extended (cylindrical/extralevator) APER* in order to give as wide a soft tissue clearance as possible. High risk factors for local recurrence are a threatened (<1 mm) or breached radial fascial envelope, tumour encroaching onto the intersphincteric plane or with levator ani muscle involvement.

Size

- Length × width × depth (cm) or maximum luminal dimension (cm).

Not shown to be an independent prognostic indicator but allows correlation with preoperative CT and MRI imaging and can be a gauge as to the effect of neoadjuvant therapy.

Appearance

- Polypoid/annular/ulcerated/mucoid/linitis plastica/stricture/plaque.
- No independent influence on prognosis except linitis plastica (signet ring cell carcinoma). Proximal cancers tend to be exophytic masses, other sites ulcerated, endophytic and annular.
- Expanding metallic mesh stent in situ: suitable for lesions from the distal transverse colon to the upper rectum. Outside of these locations there can be complications due to inadequate placement of the stent and its subsequent migration.

Edge

- Circumscribed/irregular (adverse prognostic indicator).

Perforation

- Present/absent. *Perforation has a higher incidence of local recurrence and poorer prognosis*. Perforation through the tumour is TNM7 stage pT4 because of the potential contact with peritoneum. This does not include proximal ischaemic back pressure perforation (e.g. caecum) due to an obstructing distal cancer. In this case the pT stage is determined by the degree of local spread of the distal cancer. Perforation localized to the mesocolic or mesorectal fat is in theory pT3 disease but it is often categorized as pT4 due to the higher recurrence rates that ensue.

5.2 Histological Type

Adenocarcinoma

- *85 % of cases are colorectal adenocarcinoma of usual type.*
- *Diagnostic criteria are*: (a) neoplastic epithelial changes, in (b) a desmoplastic stroma, with (c) invasion beneath the muscularis mucosae. In practice a combination of (a) and (b) is the most useful indicating a biopsy derived from the ulcerated surface of the tumour. (c) is seen in material derived from the tumour edge. Neoplastic epithelial changes are both architectural (angular tubules/ cribriform nests/segmental or garland necrosis with dirty lumenal debris/ single cells) and cytological (nuclear/nucleolar enlargement, overlap and stratification). Some 5–10 % of biopsies will show high-grade dysplasia suspicious for, but not totally diagnostic of malignancy. A significant proportion of these cases will not require further biopsy as surgical resection will be merited on the basis of finding glandular neoplasia in the context of appropriate clinical and imaging features e.g. an ulcerated mass lesion or irregular stricture.

Mucinous Carcinoma

- *10 % of cases.*
- Tumour area is >50 % mucinous component.
- *Potentially of worse prognosis* often presenting at a more advanced stage and with a 2–8 % increased hazard of death compared with an equivalent stage adenocarcinoma of usual type. Mucinous adenocarcinomas are regarded as either *low-grade* (a minority) or *high-grade* with 5 year survival decreased by 10–15 % on average. High-grade tumours are either microsatellite stable (MSS) or have a low level of microsatellite instability (MSI-L), and low-grade tumours a high level of microsatellite instability (MSI-H). For further discussion see HNPCC.

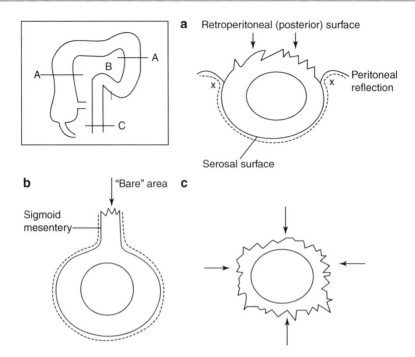

Fig. 5.1 Extent of serosal covering of the large intestine. *Arrows* indicate the "bare" non-peritonealized areas of different levels. (**a**) The ascending and descending colon are devoid of peritoneum on their posterior surface. (**b**) The sigmoid colon is completely covered with peritoneum, which extends over the mesentery. (**c**) The lower rectum lies beneath the pelvic peritoneal reflection. The *asterisks* in (a) indicate the sites where serosal involvement by tumour is likely to occur (Reproduced with permission from Burroughs and Williams (2000), BMJ Publishing Group)

Signet Ring Cell Adenocarcinoma

- >50 % signet ring cells.
- *Poor prognosis* in the rectosigmoid of young or elderly people with a linitis plastica pattern of annular thickening and stenosis.
- Distinguish from secondary carcinoma e.g. gastric signet ring cell carcinoma in young females, prostate carcinoma (PSA positive) in older males.

Others

- *Adenosquamous carcinoma*:
  Caecum. Requires glandular and squamous cell (keratinisation/intercellular bridges) features. *Aggressive*.
- *Squamous cell carcinoma*:
  Rectal: can be seen in ulcerative colitis/schistosomiasis/amoebiasis. Exclude spread from an anal carcinoma or cervical carcinoma.

Need intercellular bridges ± keratinisation with no gland/mucin formation.
- *Undifferentiated carcinoma*:
  (a) Good prognosis – medullary carcinoma. Circumscribed and expansile margin with solid sheets of tumour cells, intratumoural infiltrating lymphocytes (TILs) and a prominent peritumoural lymphocytic reaction. Sporadic or in HNPCC and strongly associated with MSI-H.
  (b) Poor prognosis – pleomorphic and diffusely infiltrative.
- *Neuroendocrine tumours*:
  Either well differentiated/low-grade neuroendocrine (carcinoid) tumour, or rarely, poorly differentiated/high-grade neuroendocrine (small cell/large cell) carcinoma. See Sect. 5.9.
- *Mixed differentiation*:
  MANEC – mixed adenoneuroendocrine carcinoma e.g. usual adenocarcinoma with small cell carcinoma or carcinoid tumour.

- *Metastatic carcinoma*:
  Transcoelomic spread: stomach, ovary, endometrium, gastrointestinal tract, pancreas.
  Direct spread: prostate, anus, cervix, kidney, stomach.
  Distant spread: breast (infiltrating lobular), malignant melanoma, lung cancer.
  Metastatic disease can infiltrate bowel wall and protrude into the mucosa *mimicking a primary lesion endoscopically and macroscopically* – a relevant previous history, extrinsic or mural disposition of the tumour, and a lack of mucosal tumour origin are crucial to the diagnosis.

5.3 Differentiation

Well/moderate/poor/undifferentiated, or, Grade 1/2/3/4 based on the percentage tumour gland formation (well/G1 > 95 %: moderate/G2 50–95 %: poor/G3 < 50 %). Undifferentiated carcinoma (grade 4) shows no gland formation.

Low-grade or *high-grade*: due to the difference in prognosis a two tier grading system is recommended with low-grade (well/moderately differentiated) and high-grade (poor/undifferentiated). Signet ring cell (grade 3), small cell and undifferentiated carcinomas (both grade 4) are high-grade cancers.

- *70–80 % of cases are low-grade or well/moderately differentiated.*
- Tumour grade is based on the *predominant area* and not the tumour margins, which can often show poorly differentiated microscopic foci. If there is a substantial component of poor differentiation this should be commented upon. Some studies indicate that a poorly differentiated invasive margin (with *tumour budding*, microacini and undifferentiated cells) in an otherwise moderately differentiated tumour is predictive of lymph node metastases and adverse prognosis. There are similar implications for adenocarcinoma with a *micropapillary* pattern as in other organ sites e.g. breast, bladder, lung i.e. a propensity for lymphovascular and lymph node spread.

5.4 Extent of Local Tumour Spread

Border: pushing/infiltrative.

Lymphocytic reaction: prominent/sparse.

An expanding growth pattern/margin with a Crohn's like inflammatory response is an indicator of better prognosis than an infiltrating, irregular margin with no inflammation.

Degree of mesorectal/mesocolic spread measured from the outer border of the muscularis propria (>5 mm) seems to influence prognosis but is not well established. It also facilitates audit of preoperative radiological staging of extramural spread.

When the mesocolic or mesorectal circumferential radial margin (CRM) is involved the degree of tumour spread is an indicator of either advanced disease or alternatively inadequate surgery.

The TNM classification applies only to carcinomas (Figs. 5.2, 5.3 and 5.4).

pTis	Carcinoma in situ: intraepithelial (within basement membrane) or invasion of lamina propria (intramucosal) with no extension through muscularis mucosae into submucosa
pT1	Tumour invades submucosa
pT2	Tumour invades muscularis propria
pT3	Tumour invades beyond muscularis propria into subserosa or non-peritonealised pericolic/perirectal tissues
pT4	Tumour invades the serosal surface or adjacent organs and/or perforation of visceral peritoneum[a]

[a]Other descriptors: pT4a (other organs/structures), pT4b (visceral peritoneum). In the UK the Royal College of Pathologists recommends ongoing use of TNM5 whereas TNM7 designates involvement of serosa pT4a and adjacent organs/structures pT4b

Serosal involvement is tumour either at or ulcerating the serosal surface as this is prognostically worse than tumour in a subserosal inflammatory reaction. About 10 % of patients develop peritoneal or ovarian (Krükenberg) deposits and there is a higher rate of distant metastases than in direct invasion of adjacent organs or structures alone. Serosal pT4 disease may include direct involvement of other segments of colon e.g. sigmoid colon by a caecal carcinoma. If no tumour is present in adhesions to other structures e.g. bladder, classify as pT3. Separate *mesenteric, omental or distant peritoneal deposits are metastatic (M1) disease.*

In low rectal cancer involvement of internal sphincteric muscle is pT3 and external voluntary sphincteric levator ani muscle is pT4.

Intramural extension to adjacent bowel e.g. caecal carcinoma to ileum does not affect the pT stage.

A *minimum of four blocks of tumour and bowel wall* is necessary to assess the pT stage adequately and to find extramural vascular invasion. The specimen is cut into serial transverse slices 4–5 mm thick, laid out in order and relevant slices selected for blocking.

Multiple carcinomas should be assessed and staged individually.

Direct implantation spread can be seen at anastomoses, peritoneal and abdominal wall wounds. Anastomotic site recurrence is unusual if the longitudinal margin clearance in the primary specimen is >5 cm.

5.5 Lymphovascular Invasion

Present/absent.

Intra-/extratumoural.

Extramural venous invasion is an adverse prognostic factor: 35 % 5 year survival. Often it comprises a sausage like tumour filled longitudinal structure orientated perpendicularly to the muscularis propria which can be quite distinctive in appearance on MRI scan and at the pathology cut up bench. At microscopy, the "protruding tongue" sign with smooth muscle fibres in its wall, adjacent "widowed" or "orphaned" small arteries and an elastin stain can help identification. The significance of mural "small vessel" lymphovascular invasion (LVI) is uncertain but should be reported as distinction between lymphatics and small venules can be difficult and oncologists regard LVI as an indicator for consideration of post-operative chemotherapy.

Neural invasion (epineural/perineural/endoneural/myenteric plexus) is also identified and commented upon.

5.6 Lymph Nodes

Lymph nodes and liver are the commonest sites of metastases. Other sites include *peritoneum, lung,* and, *ovaries, vagina* and *bladder* where the *metastases can mimic primary adenocarcinoma of those organs.* Immunophenotypical profiles may aid distinction e.g. ovarian cancer is CK7 positive, CK20/CDX-2 variable and weak for CEA, whereas intestinal cancer is strongly CEA/CK20/CDX-2 positive and CK7 negative. Occasional colorectal cancers express CK7 and a minority are CK20 negative, particularly those with a high level of microsatellite instability e.g. HNPCC. Some metastatic deposits can also lose their immunogenicity. Note that enteric differentiation and immunophenotype adenocarcinomas do arise as primary lesions in various organ sites e.g. urinary bladder – exclusion of a colorectal metastasis then largely rests on a *relevant prior history, clinical investigation* and *radiological imaging.*

Site/number/size/number involved/limit node/extracapsular spread.

Regional nodes: pericolic, perirectal, those located along the ileocolic, colic, inferior mesenteric, superior rectal and internal iliac arteries. A regional lymphadenectomy will ordinarily include a minimum of 12 lymph nodes. *Lymph node yield varies greatly even after careful dissection.* It is related to variation in individual anatomy, site (mesorectum yields fewer lymph nodes/ileocaecal angle mesentery more), the extent of resection performed, and history of preoperative neoadjuvant therapy. The latter leads to lymph node shrinkage and hyalinization. External iliac, common iliac and superior mesenteric artery nodes are distant metastases (pM disease).

pN0	No regional lymph node metastasis
pN1	1–3 involved regional lymph nodes
pN2	4 or more involved regional lymph nodes

Dukes'	C1 nodes involved but apical node negative
Dukes'	C2 suture tie limit apical node positive.

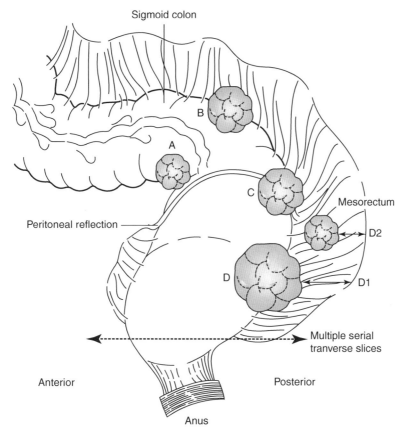

Sigmoid colon

B

A

C

Mesorectum

Peritoneal reflection

D2

D

D1

Multiple serial
tranverse slices

Anterior

Posterior

Anus

The upper anterior rectum is invested in peritoneum
The anterior mesorectum is thinner (0.75 – 1 cm) than the posterior mesorectum (1.5 – 3cm)
Cut the resection specimen into multiple serial transverse slices about 5 mm thick
Blocks for histology are:

Above the reflection	A	Tumour,rectal wall and serosa
	B	Tumour,rectal wall and serosa
		Tumour,rectal wall and mesentery
At the reflection	C	Tumour,rectal wall and serosa
		Tumour,rectal wall and mesorectum
Below the reflection	D	Tumour,rectal wall and mesorectum
	D1	Distance (mm) of the deepest point of continuous tumour extension to the nearest point of the painted CRM
	D2	Distance (mm) of the deepest point of discontinuous tumour extension(or in a lymphatic,node or vessel) to the nearest point of the painted CRM

Fig. 5.2   Rectal carcinoma (Reproduced, with permission, from Allen (2006), © 2006)

ALL *regional lymph nodes should be sampled for histology*:

- A minimum target of 10 will identify the vast majority of Dukes' C lesions. Finding more than 15 does not confer additional benefit although this is not universally accepted.

Essentially ALL fatty tissue should be carefully examined and ALL available lymph nodes harvested with a *departmental median count of 12 lymph nodes per specimen* achieved. Techniques such as fat clearance and methylene blue staining can increase

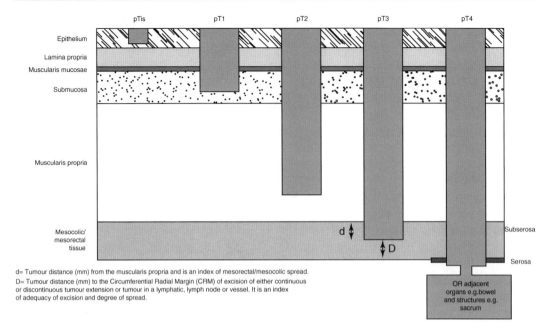

Fig. 5.3 Colorectal carcinoma (Reproduced, with permission, from Allen (2006), © 2006)

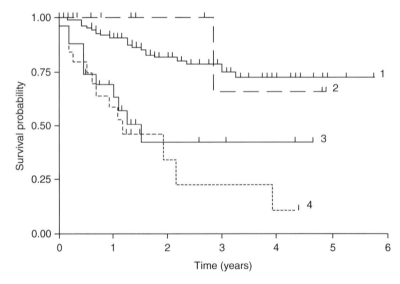

Fig. 5.4 Kaplan-Meier cumulative survival curve for peritoneal involvement (Shepherd et al. (1995). Reproduced with permission from the BMJ Publishing Group) *Group 1*, tumour well clear of the closest peritoneal surface; *group 2*, mesothelial inflammatory/ hyperplastic reaction with tumour close to but not actually at the peritoneal surface; *group 3*, tumour present at the peritoneal surface with inflammatory reaction/mesothelial hyperplasia/"ulceration"; *group 4*, tumour cells free in peritoneum and adjacent "ulceration"

lymph node yield but there is as yet no clear evidence that it increases numbers of positive lymph nodes or upstages the tumour. Lymph node mapping in rectal TME specimens shows differences from cadaveric studies. Lymph nodes are increased in number and *randomly distributed in the anterior, bilateral, posterior and distal mesorectal compartments* emphasizing the need for a complete surgical TME and comprehensive sampling in the laboratory. In addition in up to *48 % of cases metastases are present within small (<0.5 cm) lymph nodes* which should not be overlooked on macroscopic or microscopic examination. It also highlights some of the difficulties in determining an accurate clinical N stage on pre-treatment MRI scans. Mesorectal lymph node metastases also do not follow a predictable sentinel lymph node pathway.

- Remember to assess the small lymph nodes seen on histology adjacent to the tumour margin. The biological significance of nodal micrometastases (≤0.2 cm) is uncertain. Processing the lymph nodes in their *entirety versus a representative mid slice* can upstage 1 % of cases although usually there are other accompanying adverse prognostic factors e.g. pT4b disease that would in any case lead to consideration of adjuvant therapy for the patient.

- Comment if an involved lymph node lies adjacent to (≤1 mm) the mesorectal CRM (circumferential radial margin) or mesocolic margin as under TNM this equates to involvement of that margin. In the latter it raises the possibility of other involved lymph nodes left in place in any residual mesenteric pedicle. The biological significance of proximity to an intact mesorectal fascia where there is no residual soft tissue external to it in the bony pelvis is less certain (and a point of frustration for colorectal surgeons!).

- Direct invasion into a lymph node is regarded as a lymph node metastasis.

- A tumour nodule >3 mm in diameter in the perirectal/pericolic fat without evidence of residual lymph node is classified as a replaced nodal metastasis. If ≤3 mm diameter classify as discontinuous extension, i.e. pT3. It is important to note that this is a TNM5 rule. The TNM6 rule which probably more accurately reflects biological events is: a tumour nodule in the pericolic/perirectal adipose tissue without histological evidence of residual lymph node in the nodule is a lymph node metastasis if the nodule has the form and smooth contour of a lymph node. If of irregular contour it is classified as discontinuous pT3 spread and also as microscopic (V1) or macroscopic (V2) venous invasion as this is its likely origin. The TNM7 classification also defines these *prognostically adverse fatty tissue deposits* as satellites (pN1c) if the primary lesion is otherwise pT1 or pT2. Furthermore nodal involvement is stratified as: pN1a (1 involved node), pN1b (2–3 nodes), pN2a (4–6 nodes) and pN2b (≥7 nodes). In the UK the Royal College of Pathologists has recommended ongoing use of TMN5 rather than TMN6/TNM7 due to concerns over the validity of ongoing clinical trials and the observer reproducibility in applying TNM6/7 rules for defining a lymph node metastasis. The resolution of this issue awaits further studies. In either case it should be ensured that the nodule does not represent tumour in an identifiable extramural vein, and in practice pathologists often use a combination of these staging approaches.

- More than one vascular pedicle suture tie may mean more than one apical node needs to be identified as such.

5.7 Excision Margins

Doughnuts/anastomotic rings/staple gun transections – involved/not involved.

Distances to the nearest longitudinal resection limit (mm), mesorectal CRM (circumferential radial margin, mm), and mesocolic resection margin (mm).

Longitudinal spread beyond the gross edge of a colorectal carcinoma is unusual (<5 % of cases) and anterior resection of rectal carcinoma is generally considered satisfactory if a macroscopic clearance of 2–3 cm beyond the lesion edge is feasible. Block the nearest longitudinal surgical margin if ≤3 cm from the tumour edge, or if >3 cm but with any of: an unusually infiltrative tumour margin, extensive lymphovascular or mesorectal invasion, or morphology such as signet ring cell, small cell, undifferentiated carcinoma.

CRM involvement = direct or discontinuous tumour spread, or tumour within a lymphatic, lymph node or vessel ≤1 mm from the painted margin. Distances to this margin are best assessed using transverse serial slices of the resection specimen. At the multidisciplinary meeting they are correlated with the pretreatment MRI scan images as radiological demonstration of *rectal cancer threatening the integrity of the CRM investing fascia is an indicator for long course rather than short neoadjuvant radio-/chemotherapy*. Note that a non-peritonealised CRM exists not only in the mesorectum but also in relation to the posterolateral aspect of the ascending colon.

The prognostic significance of mesocolic margin involvement (7–10 % of cases) has not been fully clarified but is clearly an index of spread of disease and/or adequacy of surgery again emphasizing the need for complete resection of the mesocolic pedicle.

5.8 Other Pathology

Predisposing Conditions

Inflammatory: ulcerative colitis/Crohn's disease (1 % of colorectal carcinoma), schistosomiasis, juvenile polyposis syndrome (10 % risk). Carcinoma in ulcerative colitis occurs in patients with quiescent *disease of pancolic distribution* (>50 % colorectal involvement → 15 % lifetime risk of cancer) and *long duration* (>10–20 years). It may be associated with preceding or concurrent *mucosal dysplasia* above, adjacent to or distant from the tumour. A rectosigmoid biopsy positive for mucosal dysplasia is an indicator of the possible presence of a neoplasm elsewhere in the colorectum. Carcinomas may be multiple, right sided and in up to one third of cases difficult to define on endoscopic and gross examination. This is due to aberrant growth patterns with tumour arising in polypoid, villous or flat mucosal dysplasia in a background of mucosa already distorted by the effects of chronic inflammation, e.g. inflammatory polyps and strictures. Therefore *colonoscopic interval biopsy of flat mucosa and target biopsy of possible DALMs (dysplasia associated lesion or mass)* is employed to detect dysplasia as a marker of potential carcinoma which may be occult and submucosal in location. Due to variation in observer reproducibility mucosal dysplasia should be assessed by two experienced pathologists according to Riddell and/or the Vienna classification (Table 2.1). In the absence of a DALM *low-grade dysplasia may be followed up by colonoscopy* whereas *persistent low-grade dysplasia, DALM associated dysplasia, or, high-grade dysplasia should be considered for either local endoscopic resection or colectomy*. Surface over expression of Ki-67/AMACR and p53 is usual in a high-grade dysplasia and may help to distinguish from florid regenerative changes. Distinction from a sporadic adenoma in a patient with colitis can be difficult and is usually made by a combination of the dysplasia morphology ('top-down' in adenoma, 'bottom-up' with dystrophic goblet cells in colitis), and the absence of dysplasia or colitis in the flat mucosa adjacent to and away from an adenoma. Prognosis of colorectal cancer in ulcerative colitis is variable as some lesions present late masked by the symptoms of ulcerative colitis. Conversely, others are found early at regular (annual/biennial after 5–10 years disease duration) surveillance colonoscopy. Patients at high risk of developing colorectal cancer are those with: extensive ulcerative colitis or Crohn's disease with moderate or severe inflammation, a colonic stricture or mucosal dysplasia in the last 5 years, primary sclerosing cholangitis, or a family history of colorectal cancer in a first degree relative aged under 50 years. Early colonoscopy with chromoscopy is the recommended method of surveillance.

Neoplastic: aberrant crypt foci (hyperplasia (serration) or dysplasia), adenoma(s), Familial Adenomatous Polyposis (and the related Gardner's syndrome), previous or synchronous carcinoma(s), HNPCC (see below), hyperplastic polyposis (rare).

The dysplasia – carcinoma sequence indicates that development of adenocarcinoma increases with the *size of adenoma, its degree of villous architecture and grade of dysplasia, multiplicity of lesions and age of the patient*. High risk factors for developing colorectal cancer are 5 or more adenomas and lesion size >1 cm. A maximum diameter >2 cm and villous morphology confer approximate cancer risks of 50 % and 40 % respectively. These risk factors in a rectal adenoma are also good indicators in individual patients for full colonoscopic survey and follow up to detect right sided colonic neoplasms.

In the UK *severe or high-grade dysplasia is applied to epithelial proliferation of any degree of complexity that is mucosa based, i.e. above the muscularis mucosae. Adenocarcinoma is reserved for those lesions that show invasion below the muscularis mucosae*. Terms such as carcinoma in situ tend to be avoided due to the relative lack of mucosal lymphatics, the rarity of lymph node metastases with such lesions and the fear of over treatment with unnecessary radical resection. However, it is not always possible to demonstrate invasion through the muscularis mucosae in biopsy specimens and neoplastic epithelial changes with a desmoplastic stromal response in an appropriate clinical, endoscopic and radiological context are sufficient for a designation of adenocarcinoma. *Sampling error* must always be borne in mind in that a dysplastic fragment may not show the adjacent invasive component. Undoubtedly there are also malignant polyps for which terminology such as carcinoma in situ or intramucosal carcinoma is appropriate. In these circumstances there should be active discussion with the surgeon, emphasising that the process is "mucosa confined", and comments made on the *adequacy of local excision* and *absence of lymphovascular invasion*. It should also be checked with the endoscopist that the specimen is a complete polypectomy and not simply a diagnostic biopsy from the adenomatous edge of an established carcinoma.

Malignant Polyps

Therapeutic polypectomy is achieved if the adenocarcinoma is:
(a) Well or moderately differentiated,
(b) Clear of the stalk base,
(c) Without lymphovascular invasion.

Resection is considered if the adenocarcinoma is:
(a) Poorly differentiated
(b) At (≤1 mm) the stalk base
(c) Shows lymphovascular invasion

Resection is more likely if the patient is young and medically fit to obviate the risk of lymph node metastases which can occur with pT1 lesions, potentially varying from 3 to 8 % and 15 % in the right colon, left colon and rectum, respectively. In an older patient with comorbidity the polypectomy site may be revisited, tattooed and reviewed at a later date. The polyp may recur and be amenable to mucosal resection, or, adenocarcinoma may ensue requiring further consideration of surgery depending on the fitness of the patient. A not uncommon finding, particularly in sigmoid lesions, is stalked adenomas that twist and prolapse resulting in *mucosal misplacement* or glandular herniation into submucosa *mimicking invasive carcinoma*. The presence of haemosiderin, lack of stromal desmoplasia, surrounding lamina propria and cytoarchitectural abnormalities similar to those of the overlying adenoma are helpful pointers to a benign lesion. In the rectum of a younger patient mucosal prolapse or solitary rectal ulcer syndrome must be considered if reactive glands are present within muscle and a misdiagnosis of adenocarcinoma avoided.

Sessile adenomas with invasion: resection is indicated as this represents invasion of actual mural submucosa (Haggitt level 4) rather than just stalk submucosa (Haggitt levels 1, 2 and 3). Local transanal resection is considered for the very elderly and medically unfit. It can be either mucosal and piecemeal (e.g. tubulovillous adenoma), or full depth mucous membrane or wall thickness (cancer). It is geared towards either a large adenoma not amenable to saline lift excision or snaring, or, "early" pT1 sm1 (superficial third of the submucosa) invasive disease. *Indications for more radical surgery are*: a lesion >3 cm diameter, incomplete tumour excision, deep submucosal (sm3) or muscularis propria invasion, lymphovascular invasion or the presence of a poorly differentiated invasive component (Fig. 5.5).

Flat adenomas: uncommon with a different genetic basis from usual adenomas and difficult

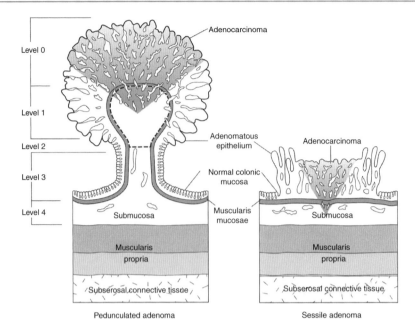

Fig. 5.5 Malignant colorectal polyp. Levels of invasion in a pedunculated adenoma (*left*) and a sessile adenoma (*right*). The *stippled areas* represent zones of carcinoma. Note that any invasion below the muscularis mucosae in a sessile lesion represents level 4 invasion, i.e. invasion into the submucosa of the bowel wall. In contrast, invasive carcinoma in a pedunculated adenoma (*left*) must traverse a considerable distance before it reaches the submucosa of the underlying bowel wall. The *dotted line* in the head of the pedunculated adenoma represents the zone of level 1 invasion (Haggit et al. (1985). ©1985 Reproduced, with permission, from American Gastroenterological Association)

to identify endoscopically on gross examination without magnification and dye spray techniques. Defined as up to twice the height of the adjacent mucosa with a height usually less than half its diameter (<10 mm across). These lesions have proportionately (×10 risk) *higher grades of dysplasia and frequency of carcinoma*. Depressed variants harbour carcinoma in up to 25 % of cases, overexpress p53 and the DNA aneuploidy rate is increased. They may account for a proportion of the 30 % of colorectal cancers with no identifiable adenoma at the tumour edge.

Hereditary non-polyposis colorectal cancer (HNPCC, syn. hereditary mismatch repair deficiency syndrome): hMLH1 and hMSH2 are the two most frequently mutated genes. *Autosomal dominant with 90 % penetrance* and a *70 % risk of developing cancer by the age of 70 years*. HNPCC forms *2 % of colorectal cancer cases* requiring three affected family members across two generations with at least one <50 years of age at presentation (*Amsterdam criteria*). HNPCC is found in about 20 % of patients with mismatch repair defi-

cient colorectal cancers. The latter can also show BRAF mutations although this is rare in HNPCC – a helpful finding in distinguishing between sporadic and HNPCC related MSI-H colorectal cancers. In HNPCC numbers of adenomas are low but they can progress more quickly, forming carcinomas tending to be right sided and multiple with an *18 % incidence of synchronous or metachronous tumours*. They are mucinous or poorly/ undifferentiated (medullary like) in character and less responsive to usual 5FU(fluorouracil)/oxaliplatin colorectal cancer chemotherapy. However they are more sensitive to topoisomerase II inhibitors e.g. irinotecan, and are of *better prognosis (66 % versus 44 % 5 year survival)*. They have expanding or circumscribed margins, peritumoural and intratumoural lymphocytes (TILs), show paired loss of mismatch repair antibody nuclear expression (usually MLH1/PMS2, or, MSH2/MSH6), and are less likely to show distant spread. There is often a *family history of cancer in other viscera*, e.g. stomach, small intestine, pancreas, endometrium, breast, ovary, ureter and renal pelvis, and the risk of colonic cancer in a first degree relative of an affected individual is about 50 %. The tumours have a *high level of microsatellite instability (MSI-H)* but this applies to only a small minority of sporadic colorectal cancers most of which show more extensive chromosomal abnormalities and are microsatellite stable. Most sporadic colorectal cancers arise on the basis of the p53/APC pathway (70 %) but 30 % (MSI-H and microsatellite stable cancers) are associated with the *serrated pathway* viz sessile serrated adenoma/traditional serrated adenoma/serrated cated cancer. Therefore, although the vast majority of serrated lesions are age related, left sided, small and innocuous hyperplastic polyps, larger sessile right sided lesions in a younger patient may be instrumental in the development of a minority of cancers. These sessile serrated adenomas/polyps are recognized by persistence of serrated epithelium down into distorted crypt bases which have a bulbous, L shape, inverted T or anchor shaped architecture, and variably equivocal to low-grade cytological dysplasia. Onset of dysplasia is regarded as an important indicator of potential progression to carcinoma.

Familial Adenomatous Polyposis (FAP): sporadic in 30–50 % of cases or *familial and autosomal dominant* with a high degree of penetrance (chromosome 5q21). The site of gene mutation can determine the phenotype and type of surgery required. A minimum of 100 colorectal polyps is required for a morphological diagnosis and these can vary from unicryptal dysplasia to macroscopic lesions. Usually thousands of polyps are present and, if left untreated, one or more cancers occur on average *20 years earlier (90 % by 50 years of age) than usual colorectal carcinomas* and more often in the left colon than the right. *Prophylactic colectomy with surveillance of the rectal stump or panproctocolectomy are undertaken.* FAP is also associated with adenomas and periampullary carcinoma in the duodenum (5 % risk of cancer and a significant cause of mortality), gastric fundic gland cyst polyps, and desmoid tumours (fibromatosis) as part of Gardner's syndrome (including epidermoid cysts and bone osteomas). Attenuated FAP has fewer lesions (30 polyps) that are more often right sided with rectal sparing.

National Bowel Cancer Screening Programme: in the UK this tests *50–70 year olds* with *2 yearly faecal occult bloods (FOBs)*, and if positive, follow up *colonoscopy* geared to detecting a higher percentage of Dukes' A cancers and increasing 5 year survival rates. Results to date indicate that 2 % of these asymptomatic patients have positive FOBs and in 50 % of these colonoscopy or CT colonography shows a detectable abnormality. This is either adenoma or carcinoma (80 % of cases) or other pathology (20 % of cases e.g. chronic inflammatory bowel disease) with a demonstrable shift to "earlier" lesions viz polyp cancers and Dukes' A cancers. Future plans for the programme include age extension to 75 years and one off sigmoidoscopy at age 55 years.

In sporadic colorectal cancer rates for *synchronous* and *metachronous carcinomas* range from 5 to 15 %.

Associated Conditions

Presentation with *obstruction is adverse* leading either to direct tumour perforation (pT4), proximal dilatation with ischaemic perforation of the caecum, and obstructive enterocolitis. The latter can mimic inflammatory bowel disease with continuous and skip lesions of transmural inflammation either adjacent to or distant from the distal carcinoma.

Immunophenotype

CK20 positive/CK7 negative, βcatenin, CEA, CA19-9, sialomucin/sulphomucin, large intestinal mucus antigen (LIMA)/MUC-2, tumour associated glycoprotein (TAG-72: antibody B72.3) positive. Serum CA125 and CA19-9 may also be elevated. Some 60 % of cases are p53 positive but this does not appear to be an independent prognostic variable. Note that some rectal, right sided colonic and HNPCC cancers may also lose CK20 positivity and 10 % of cases can be CK7 positive – a complicating factor in typing metastatic adenocarcinoma of unknown origin or in biopsy diagnosis of colorectal cancer with aberrant morphology. CDX-2 homeobox gene expression is positive in a majority of primary and secondary colorectal cancers. EGFR (epidermal growth factor receptor) – see below.

Adjuvant Therapy

Postoperative adjuvant therapy is used for *Dukes' C carcinomas and "bad" Bs*, i.e. Dukes' B carcinomas with any of: perforation, involved serosa, involved deep margin or extramural venous spread. These parameters score 2, 1, 1 and 1 respectively with a total of ≥2 necessitating postoperative chemotherapy.

In rectal cancer international trials are examining whether treatment should be chemotherapy or radiotherapy in isolation or combination, and also preoperative or postoperative. Prior to definitive surgery with curative intent, rectal cancer is assessed for evidence of local (MRI scan) and distant (CT scan) spread. *Low, or clinically fixed high risk rectal cancer*, with MRI scan evidence of significant direct mesorectal or lymph node spread with or without proximity to the mesorectal fascia, receives *long course (6 weeks) preoperative radio-/chemotherapy*. *Short course (5 days) radiotherapy* is given to *intermediate risk rectal cancers* i.e. mid-rectal lesions with early cT3 and/or equivocal N disease. *Low risk tumours* (cT1/cT2/N0) are treated by surgery alone. *Neoadjuvant therapy* can induce in a significant number of cases (30–50 %) marked changes of tumour regression: cell vacuolation, mucinous degeneration, apoptosis, necrosis, inflammation, and fibrosis leaving only microscopic residual tumour foci. The *degree of tumour response can be graded* as complete/moderate/no response based on the amount of residual tumour, and must be assessed in the context of the pretreatment clinical and MRI scan measurements. When significant it has implications for assessing the pathological stage in the resection specimen – the pT stage being determined by the deepest focus of residual tumour and not the fibrous reaction where tumour may have been. Its role in reducing tumour bulk at the involved deep margin is uncertain but it does seem to *improve resectability*. Downstaging

of lymph node disease remains controversial although lymph nodes diminish in size and number making harvesting difficult. Prognosis of colorectal cancer and response to neoadjuvant therapy are patient dependent and can also partly relate to tumour genotype, as to whether the cancer is positive or negative for microsatellite instability (DNA mismatch repair deficient), KRAS or BRAF mutations, or other factors such as tumour tissue levels of thymidylate synthetase. Thus tumour characteristics allied to more sophisticated preoperative staging (e.g. MRI, ELUS) will allow selection of those patients who will benefit most from neoadjuvant therapy, with tailoring of the drug regime accordingly.

Recurrent or Metastatic Disease

Significantly elevated serum CEA levels correlate with either *recurrent* or *metastatic disease*. After adequate local resection of the colorectal primary liver metastases can be excised to good effect by wedge resection, *partial hepatectomy* or subjected to *targeted radiofrequency or microwave ablation*. With widespread liver metastases *palliative chemotherapy* has a role to play – the primary may also be reduced in bulk by *laser*, or a *stent* inserted across it to avoid obstruction and potential perforation with peritonitis. Due to difficulties in stent placement and subsequent migration this procedure is only suitable for lesions in the distal transverse to sigmoid colons.

Novel targeted medical therapy in irinotecan resistant metastatic cancer is *cetuximab (Erbitux)*, an antibody against tumour cell expression of *epidermal growth factor receptor (EGFR)*. EGFR positivity can be demonstrated by immunohistochemistry although levels of tissue expression do not consistently correlate with tumour response. Importantly about *50 % of colorectal cancers show KRAS mutation by genetic analysis – this confers reduced survival and resistance to EGFR monoclonal antibody therapy with cetuximab*. This analysis is carried out either on the diagnostic biopsy or resection specimen prior to commencing inappropriate and expensive treatment. Cetuximab therapy is broadly indicated where there is

- A resected or potentially resectable colorectal primary
- The colorectal primary is KRAS mutation negative i.e. wild type with retention of potential sensitivity to cetuximab
- The metastases are liver confined and irresectable, or the patient is fit enough for liver resection should the metastases respond to the cetuximab treatment.

Patients with MSI-H BRAF mutated tumours have intermediate disease free progression and overall survival.

Stage

TNM: see above.

Dukes'	A	Tumour limited to the wall, nodes negative
	B	Tumour beyond the muscularis propria, nodes negative
	C1	Nodes positive, apical node negative
	C2	Apical node positive
	D	Non-regional metastatic disease.

For routine practice a combination of Dukes' and pTNM are recommended.

Resection

RO	Tumour completely excised locally
R1	Microscopic involvement of margin by tumour (to within 1 mm)
R2	Macroscopic tumour left behind or gross involvement of margin.

RO clear proximal, distal and radial margins irrespective of serosal involvement

Prognosis

Adverse Prognosis

Tumour perforation (pT4) and obstruction.

Mucinous tumour (>50 % of the tumour area) possibly due to presentation at a more advanced stage with less host immune response.

Poor differentiation.
Splenic flexure lesion.
Male sex.
Young and old age due to delay in presentation and greater numbers of mucinous and signet ring tumours.

Prognosis relates mainly to tumour stage (particularly peritoneal and lymph node spread), differentiation and adequacy of local excision with overall 5 year survival 35–40%.

Stage	Dukes'	5 year survival (%)	Incidence (%)
	A	95	15
	B	75	35
	C	35	25
	D	25	25

Differentiation	Well/moderate	75 %
	Poor	25 %

Local excision	CRM positive 25 % with 85 % risk of local recurrence
	CRM negative 75 % with 10 % risk of local recurrence.

Not infrequently there is poor correlation between surgical and histological assessment of *margin clearance*. A *positive resection margin* (usually the CRM) has strong prognostic significance for *local recurrence* (×12 risk) and *death* (×3 risk). It is one of the most important causes of morbidity in rectal cancer. Low rectal cancers also have higher recurrence rates than mid- or upper rectal tumours. For every 100 patients with colorectal cancer it is estimated that 50 will be cured, 10 will die from pelvic recurrence, 5 from lymphatic spread and 35 from haematogenous spread. Sites of spread are *regional lymph nodes, liver (75%), lung (15%), bone and brain (5% each)*. Patients with bone marrow micrometastases are reported by some to have shorter disease-free survival, but the clinical significance of the immunohistochemical and molecular detection of minimal residual disease in lymph nodes and marrow samples which are tumour negative on routine examination awaits results from large international trials.

5.9 Other Malignancy

Gastrointestinal Mesenchymal or Stromal Tumours

- GISTs are rare in the colorectum. See also Chaps. 2 and 4.

Colon

- Benign appearing lesions are rare.
- Usually *aggressive* with metastases and death related to: mitoses >6/50 high-power fields, infiltrative growth pattern into the muscularis propria, mucosal invasion, cellularity, and coagulative necrosis.

Anorectal

- Lesions arising from the muscularis mucosae (i.e. *mucosal leiomyomatous polyp*) are usually treatable by local excision or polypectomy.
- Lesions arising from the muscularis mucosae are considered malignant if: cellular, >5 cm diameter, infiltrative into the muscularis propria. However, if originating in the muscularis propria even bland lesions (low cellularity, 0–1 mitoses/50 high-power fields) need long term follow up as there is a tendency for local recurrence and even potential metastases.

Carcinoid Tumour and Small Cell Carcinoma

- Well differentiated/low-grade neuroendocrine (carcinoid) tumour and variably positive for chromogranin, synaptophysin and CD56(±) with a low Ki-67(≤2 %) index and mitotic rate (<2 per 10 high power fields). Presentation is most often as an incidental rectal polyp.
  - (a) Chronic ulcerative colitis→enteroendocrine cell hyperplasia→microcarcinoids.
  - (b) Carcinoid polyp <1 cm diameter (pT1a). (a) and (b) are benign and managed by *endoscopic surveillance* and *biopsy with snare polypectomy*, usually with no further clinical consequences.
  - (c) Ulcerated tumour: malignancy relates to; size ≥2 cm diameter or invasion beyond submucosa (both pT2), or angioinvasion, with these features necessitating *resection*.
- Lesions 1–2 cm diameter (pT1b) are also potentially malignant and require *wide local excision*.
- Right colonic carcinoids tend to be large and ulcerated with adverse prognosis but the commoner rectal carcinoid is usually solitary and <1 cm in diameter. The latter are of L cell origin and show variable expression of neuroendocrine markers (chromogranin negative, synaptophysin positive). Many are prostatic acid phosphatase positive which can cause diagnostic confusion with the differential diagnosis of secondary prostatic adenocarcinoma (PSA positive).

Neuroendocrine differentiation can be present in up to 50 % of usual type colorectal adenocarcinomas and is not prognostically significant. However a poorly differentiated high-grade endocrine (small cell) carcinoma component is adverse. Pure *small cell carcinoma* does occasionally occur as a large locally advanced primary tumour in the rectum. Metastasis from a lung cancer must be excluded by negative radiological imaging, and CDX-2 expression by a rectal small cell carcinoma can be of help.

Malignant Lymphoma

- Predisposing conditions are chronic ulcerative colitis and AIDS (which can also result in Kaposi's sarcoma).
- Solitary or multifocal.
- Of probable mucosa associated lymphoid tissue (MALT) origin (>70 %) with a heterogeneous, polymorphous cell population: *low-grade* <20 % blasts, *high-grade* >20 % blasts and on a spectrum with *diffuse large B cell lymphoma*.
- B (>90 %) or T cell±high content of eosinophils.
- Prognosis relates to the grade and stage of disease.

Others (see Chap. 4): centrocytic or mantle cell lymphoma (multiple lymphomatous polyposis) which is of intermediate-grade and aggressive. Rarely follicle centre (follicular) lymphoma spreading from systemic nodal disease. Burkitt's type/B lymphoblastic in children or adults (with AIDS) in the terminal ileum/ileocaecal valve are high-grade lymphomas.

Leukaemia

- 50 % of children with acute leukaemia who die in relapse.
- Chronic lymphocytic leukaemia in the elderly and usually found incidentally in a resection done for other reasons e.g. diverticular disease or colorectal cancer.
- Myeloid/granulocytic sarcoma (CD34,CD43, CD 68,CD117/chloroacetate esterase/ myeloperoidase positive).
- Single/multiple deposits.

Malignant Melanoma

- Primary or secondary; metastases are commoner.

Kaposi's Sarcoma

- AIDS/inflammatory bowel disease/human herpes virus 8 (HHV 8).
- 50 % show visceral involvement, 8 % in the hindgut.

Teratoma

- Rare; primary in caecum, sigmoid and rectum but exclude spread from ovary or sacrococcygeal area. Choriocarcinoma must be distinguished from adenocarcinoma with trophoblastic differentiation.

Bibliography

Allen DC. Histopathology reporting: guidelines for surgical cancer. 2nd ed. London: Springer; 2006.

Association of Directors of Anatomic and Surgical Pathology. Recommendations for the reporting of surgically resected specimens of colorectal carcinoma. Am J Surg Pathol. 2008; 129:13–23.

Bateman AC, Carr NJ, Warren BF. The retroperitoneal surface in distal caecal and proximal ascending colon carcinoma: the Cinderella surgical margin? J Clin Pathol. 2005;58:426–8.

Bettington M, Walker N, Clouston A, Brown I, Leggett B, Whitehall V. The serrated pathway to colorectal carcinoma: current concepts and challenges. Histopathology. 2013;62:376–86.

Bosman FT, Carneiro F. WHO classification of tumours of the digestive system. 4th ed. Lyon: IARC press; 2010.

Bull AD, Biffin AHB, Mella J, Radcliffe AG, Stamatakis JD, Steele RJC, Williams GT. Colorectal cancer pathology reporting: a regional audit. J Clin Pathol. 1997;50:138–42.

Burroughs SH, William GT. Examination of large intestine resection specimens. J Clin Pathol. 2000;50: 344–9.

Burroughs SH, Williams GT. ACP best practice no. 159. Examination of large-intestine resection specimens. J Clin Pathol. 2000;53:345.

Cairns SR, Scholefield JH, Steele RJ, British Society of Gastroenterology, et al. Guidelines for colorectal cancer screening and surveillance in moderate and high risk groups (update from 2002). Gut. 2010;59: 666–89.

Chetty R. Gastrointestinal cancers accompanied by a dense lymphoid component: an overview with special reference to gastric and colonic medullary and lymphoepithelioma-like carcinomas. J Clin Pathol. 2012;65:1062–5.

Cooper HS. Pathology of the endoscopically removed malignant colorectal polyp. Curr Diagn Pathol. 2007;13:423–37.

Cooper HS, Deppisch LM, Kahn EI, Lev R, Manley PN, Pascal RR, Qizilbash AH, Rickert RR, Silverman JF, Wirman JA. Pathology of the malignant colorectal polyp. Hum Pathol. 1998;29:15–26.

Cotton P, Williams C. Practical gastrointestinal endoscopy. 4th ed. London: Blackwell Science; 1996.

Cserni G, Bori R, Sejben I. Limited lymph-node recovery based on lymph-node localisation is sufficient for accurate staging. J Clin Pathol. 2011; 64:13–5.

Day DW, Jass JR, Price AB, Shepherd NA, Sloan JM, Talbot IC, Warren BF, Williams GT. Morson and Dawson's gastrointestinal pathology. 4th ed. Oxford: Blackwell Sciences; 2003.

Dirschmid K, Sterlacci W, Oellig F, Edlinger M, Jasarevic Z, Rhomberg M, Dirschmid H, Offner F. Absence of extramural venous invasion is an excellent predictor of metastasis-free survival in colorectal carcinoma stage II – a study using tangential tissue sectioning. J Clin Pathol. 2012;65:619–23.

Doyle VJ, Bateman AC. Colorectal cancer staging using TNM7: is it time to use this new staging system? J Clin Pathol. 2012;65:372–4.

Dudley H, Pories W, Carter D, editors. Rob and Smith's operative surgery: alimentary tract and abdominal wall. 4th ed. London: Butterworths; 1993.

Dukes CE, Bussey HJR. The spread of rectal cancer and its effect on prognosis. Br J Cancer. 1958; 12:309–20.

Ensari A, Bosman FT, Offerhaus GJA. The serrated polyp: getting it right! J Clin Pathol. 2010;63:665–8.

Ervine A, Houghton J, Park R. Should lymph nodes from colorectal cancer resection specimens be processed in their entirety? J Clin Pathol. 2012;65:114–6.

Fielding LP, Goldberg SM, editors. Rob and Smith's operative surgery: surgery of the colon, rectum and anus. Oxford: Elsevier Science Ltd; 2002.

Finlay I. Preoperative staging for rectal cancer. Magnetic resonance imaging can accurately predict the success of surgical resection. BMJ. 2006;333:766–7.

Goldstein NS. Lymph node recoveries from 2427 pT3 colorectal resection specimens spanning 454 cases. Recommendations for a minimum number of recovered lymph nodes based on predictive probabilities. Am J Surg Pathol. 2002;26:179–89.

Guidelines from the Bowel Cancer Screening Programme Pathology Group. Reporting lesions in the NHS Bowel Cancer Screening Programme; NHS BCSP Publication No 1. 2007.

Haggitt RC, Glotzbach RE, Soffer EE, Wruble LD. Prognostic factors in colorectal carcinomas arising in adenomas: implications for lesions removed by endoscopic polypectomy. Gastroenterology. 1985;89:328–36.

Hurlstone DP, Brown S, Cross SS. The role of flat and depressed colorectal lesions in colorectal carcinogenesis: new insights for clinicopathological findings in high-magnification chromoscopic colonoscopy. Histopathology. 2003;43:413–26.

Jass JR. Classification of colorectal cancer based on correlation of clinical, morphological and molecular features. Histopathology. 2007;50:113–30.

Jones DJ, editor. ABC of colorectal diseases. 2nd ed. London: BMJ Books; 1999.

Konishi F, Morson BC. Pathology of colorectal adenomas: a colonoscopic survey. J Clin Pathol. 1982;35: 830–41.

Littleford SE, Baird A, Rotimi O, Verbeke CS, Scott S. Interobserver variation in the reporting of local peritoneal involvement and extramural venous invasion in colonic cancer. Histopathology. 2009; 55:407–13.

Ludeman L, Shepherd NA. Macroscopic assessment and dissection of colorectal cancer resection specimens. Curr Diagn Pathol. 2006;12:220–30.

MacGregor TP, Maughan TS, Sharma RA. Pathological grading of regression following neoadjuvant chemoradiation therapy: the clinical need is now. J Clin Pathol. 2012;65:867–71.

Makinen MJ. Colorectal serrated adenocarcinoma. Histopathology. 2007;50:131–50.

Mann CV, Russell RCG, Williams NS, editors. Bailey & Love's short practice of surgery. 22nd ed. London: Chapman and Hall Medical; 1995.

McGregor DK, Wu TT, Rashid A, Luthra R, Hamilton SR. Reduced expression of cytokeratin 20 in colorectal carcinomas with high levels of microsatellite instability. Am J Surg Pathol. 2004;28:712–8.

Mekenkamp LJM, van Krieken JHJM, Marijnen CAM, van de Velde CJH, Nagtegaal ID. Lymph node retrieval in rectal cancer is dependent on many factors – the role of the tumor, the patient, the surgeon, the radiotherapist, and the pathologist. Am J Surg Pathol. 2009;33: 1547–53.

Mitchard JR, Love SB, Baxter KJ, Shepherd NA. How important is peritoneal involvement in rectal cancer? A prospective study of 331 cases. Histopathology. 2010;57:671–9.

Morson BC, Whiteway JE, Jones EA, Macrac FA, Williams CB. Histopathology and prognosis of malignant colorectal polyps treated by endoscopic polypectomy. Gut. 1984;25:437–44.

Odze RD, Goldblum JR. Surgical pathology of the GI tract, liver, biliary tract and pancreas. 2nd ed. Philadelphia: Saunders/Elsevier; 2009.

Pheby DFH, Levine DF, Pitcher RW, Shepherd NA. Lymph node harvests directly influence the staging of colorectal cancer: evidence from a regional audit. J Clin Pathol. 2004;57:43–7.

Poston GJ, Tait D, O'Connell S, Bennett A, Berendse S, Guideline Development Group. Diagnosis and management of colorectal cancer: summary of NICE guidance. BMJ. 2011;343:1010–2.

Prall F. Tumour budding in colorectal carcinoma. Histopathology. 2007;50:151–62.

Pritchard CC, Grady WM. Colorectal cancer molecular biology moves into clinical practice. Gut. 2011;60: 116–29.

Puppa G, Senore C, Sheahan K, et al. Diagnostic reproducibility of tumour budding in colorectal cancer: a multicentre, multinational study using virtual microscopy. Histopathology. 2012;61:562–75.

Quirke P. Training and quality assurance for rectal cancer: 20 years of data is enough. Lancet. 2004;4:695–701.

Quirke P, Morris E. Reporting colorectal cancer. Histopathology. 2007;50:103–12.

Quirke P, Durdey P, Dixon MF, Williams NS. Local recurrence of rectal adenocarcinoma due to inadequate surgical resection. Histopathological study of lateral tumour spread and surgical excision. Lancet. 1986;2:996–8.

Quirke P, Williams GT, Ectors N, Ensari A, Piard F, Nagtegaal I. The future of the TNM staging system in colorectal cancer: time for a debate? Lancet Oncol. 2007;8:651–7.

Riddell RH, Goldman H, Ransonoff DF, Appelman HD, Fenoglio CM, Haggitt RC, Ahren C, Correa P, Hamilton SK, Morson BC, Sommers SC, Yardley JH. Dysplasia in inflammatory bowel disease: standardised classification with provisional clinical applications. Hum Pathol. 1983;14:931–68.

Riddell RH, Petras RE, Williams GT, Sobin LH. Tumors of the intestines. Atlas of tumor pathology. 3rd Series. Fascicle 32. Washington: AFIP; 2003.

Ryan R, Gibbons D, Hyland JMP, Treanor D, White A, Mulcahy HE, O'Donoghue DP, Moriarty M, Fennelly

D, Sheahan K. Pathological response following long-course neoadjuvant chemoradiotherapy for locally advanced rectal cancer. Histopathology. 2005;47: 141–6.

Schlemper RJ, Riddell RH, Kato Y, et al. The Vienna classification of gastrointestinal epithelial neoplasia. Gut. 2000;47:251–5.

Shepherd NA. Pathological mimics of chronic inflammatory bowel disease. J Clin Pathol. 1991;44:726–33.

Shepherd NA, Baxter KJ, Love SB. Influence of local peritoneal involvement on pelvic recurrence and prognosis in rectal cancer. J Clin Pathol. 1995;48:849–55.

Snover DC, Jass JR, Fenoglio-Preiser C, Batts KP. Serrated polyps of the large intestine. A morphologic and molecular review of an evolving concept. Am J Clin Pathol. 2005;124:380–91.

Stewart CJR, Morris M, de Boer B, Iacopetta B. Identification of serosal invasion and extramural venous invasion on review of Dukes' stage B colonic carcinomas and correlation with survival. Histopathology. 2007;51:372–8.

Swamy R. Histopathological reporting of pT4 tumour stage in colorectal carcinomas: dotting 'i's and crossing 't's. J Clin Pathol. 2010;63:110–5.

Talbot IC, Ritchie S, Leighton M, Hughes AO, Bussey HJR, Morson BC. Invasion of veins by carcinoma of rectum: method of detection, histological features and significance. Histopathology. 1981;5:141–63.

Talbot I, Price A, Salto-Tellez M. Biopsy pathology – colorectal disease. 2nd ed. London: Hodder Arnold; 2007.

The Royal College of Pathologists: Cancer Datasets (Oesophageal Carcinoma, Gastric Carcinoma, Carcinomas of the Pancreas, ampulla of Vater and Common Bile Duct, Colorectal Cancer, Gastrointestinal Stromal Tumours (GISTs), Liver Resection Specimens and Liver Biopsies for Primary and Metastatic Carcinoma, Endocrine Tumours of the Gastrointestinal Tract including Pancreas) and Tissue Pathways (Gastrointestinal and Pancreatobiliary Pathology, Liver Biopsies for the Investigation of Medical Disease and for Focal Liver Lesions). Accessed at http://www.rcpath.org/index. asp?PageID=254.

Verhulst J, Ferdinande L, Demetter P, Ceelen W. Mucinous subtype as prognostic factor in colorectal cancer: a systematic review and meta-analysis. J Clin Pathol. 2012;65:381–8.

Wheeler JM, Warren BF, Mortensen NJ. Quantification of histologic regression of rectal cancer after irradiation: a proposal for a modified staging system. Dis Colon Rectum. 2002;45:1051–6.

Williams GT. Endocrine tumours of the gastrointestinal tract – selected topics. Histopathology. 2007;50:30–41.

Xu F, Xu J, Lou Z, Di M, Wang F, Hu H, Lai M. Micropapillary component in colorectal carcinoma is associated with lymph node metastasis in T1 and T2 stages and decreased survivial time in TNM stages I and II. Am J Surg Pathol. 2009;33:1287–92.

Yantiss RK. Serrated colorectal polyps and the serrated neoplastic pathway: emerging concepts in colorectal carcinongenesis. Curr Diagn Pathol. 2007; 13:456–66.

Yao Y-F, Wang L, Liu Y-Q, Li J-Y, Gu J. Lymph node distribution and pattern of metastases in the mesorectum following total mesorectal excision using the modified fat clearing technique. J Clin Pathol. 2011;64:1073–7.

Potentially malignant and malignant appendiceal tumours include well differentiated neuroendocrine (carcinoid) tumour (85 % of cases), low-grade appendiceal mucinous neoplasm (LAMN), and adenocarcinoma. The latter two categories and serrated mucosal hyperplasia may be associated with polyps or contiguous tumour in the caecal pouch or elsewhere in the colorectum. Colonoscopy or CT colonogram is therefore required to assess the status of the entire colorectum. Goblet cell carcinoid is more appropriately designated crypt cell adenocarcinoma and has particular propensity to involve the appendiceal base or result in transcoelomic peritoneal spread.

Appendiceal tumours are usually encountered because of symptomatic acute appendicitis, an inflammatory appendix mass, or as part of a colectomy for other reasons e.g. colonic tumour. They are also seen in the context of the CT scan investigation of lower abdominopelvic symptoms or mass lesions e.g. ovarian cystic tumours. Related to this the patient may present with abdominal distension due to widespread pseudomyxoma peritonei associated with a ruptured appendiceal LAMN, or, ascitic fluid or peritoneal seedlings secondary to carcinomatosis peritonei. Planned elective laparoscopic surgery is the preferred option for appendicectomy. Open abdominal surgery may be required: either a classical right iliac fossa gridiron approach, or an extended midline incision, if there has been perforation with extensive inflammatory peritoneal contamination, or malignancy is suspected.

6.1 Gross Description

Specimen

- Appendicectomy/right hemicolectomy.
- Length and diameter (cm).
- Mucocoele/perforation/diverticulum/appendicitis/appendicular mass.

Tumour

Site

- Tip/base/diverticulum/body.

Size

- Length × width × depth (cm) or maximum dimension (cm).

Appearance

- Polypoid/sessile/plaque/ulcerated/infiltrative/ mucoid/yellow/serosal mucin.

Edge

- Circumscribed/irregular.

6.2 Histological Type

Carcinoid Tumour

- 0.5–1.5 % of appendicectomy specimens.
- *85 % of appendiceal tumours.*
- Usually a coincidental finding of yellow pale

tumour at the tip although it may contribute to appendicitis when at the appendix base (10 %).

- A well differentiated/low-grade neuroendocrine tumour and variably chromogranin, synaptophysin, CD56(±) positive depending on EC (usual enterochromaffin) or L cell origin. Low Ki-67 index (≤2 %) and mitotic count (<2 per 10 high power fields).

Usual type: 70 % of cases and at the appendiceal tip. Solid nests/cords/ribbons/acini of uniform cells often with invasion of the muscularis±serosa and lymphatics. *Benign behaviour* with *appendicectomy the treatment of choice*.

Rarely cases spread to abdominopelvic peritoneum, regional nodes and liver with 75–85 and 35 % 5 year survival figures, respectively. These are usually >2 cm diameter with *size the main factor predictive of outcome*. Radical surgery should be considered in these circumstances. *Extensive invasion of the mesoappendix (>3 mm)* and the *appendiceal base* are also adverse indicators.

Goblet cell carcinoid (mucinous/adenocarcinoid/crypt cell carcinoma) type: clusters, strands or glandular collections of mucus secreting epithelial cells with a goblet cell or signet ring morphology. There is a range of appearances with the degree of cytological atypia, stromal desmoplastic reaction, and extent of infiltration impacting on prognosis. Usually only a minor population of endocrine cells is present demonstrated by immunohistochemistry. More correctly *designated crypt cell adenocarcinoma to reflect its biological behaviour*, it is an example of a MANEC (mixed adenoneuroendocrine carcinoma). It has potential for extra-appendiceal spread (20 % of cases) and occasionally involvement of regional lymph nodes and liver. It shows a propensity for *transperitoneal spread* to involve the ovaries and direct spread through the appendix base and into the caecum. Localised, regional and distant disease have 5 year survival rates of 86, 74 and 18 % respectively.

Right hemicolectomy should be considered if there is extensive spread with an infiltrative growth pattern, involvement of the appendix base or tumour pleomorphism and mitoses. The term MANEC may also be used if there is a mix of endocrine tumour with an infiltrating component

of usual colorectal type adenocarcinoma, and again radical surgery should be considered.

Distinguish from: (1) secondary colorectal carcinoma involving the appendix either directly (e.g. from caecal pouch) or via the peritoneum (signet ring cell carcinoma of rectosigmoid area), and, (2) primary colonic type mucinous adenocarcinoma of the appendix which is aggressive in behaviour and requires radical surgery. A pre-existing mucosal adenoma/LAMN in an adenocarcinoma can help to confirm a primary origin.

Adenoma

- Rare (<1 % of appendicectomies).
- Localised (polypoid) or diffuse.
- Tubular/tubulovillous/villous[1] with variable grades of dysplasia.
- The adenomatous mucosa can be flattened and simplified.
- In up to *20–40% of cases* there are *polyps or adenocarcinoma elsewhere in the colorectum*.

Adenocarcinoma

- 0.1 % of appendicectomy specimens.
- Requires invasion through the muscularis mucosae by malignant glands (sometimes but often not with a desmoplastic reaction) and/or the presence of epithelium in extra-appendiceal mucus (cytokeratins and CEA can be useful in demonstrating this). The latter can be difficult to distinguish from a LAMN with mural dissection and peritoneal spillage of mucin containing epithelium (see below).
- Identified as primary by a mucosal adenoma/LAMN lesion.
- Histologically of usual colorectal type, but often cystic and well differentiated mucinous in character.
- Rarely signet ring cell carcinoma: distinguish from goblet cell carcinoid (focally chromogranin/synaptophysin positive) and

---

[1]See section "Mucocoele" (Appendiceal Mucinous Neoplasms).

metastatic gastric/breast carcinoma (infiltrating lobular type). In this respect it is necessary to know of previous operations to the stomach and breast and these sites may have to be investigated. Breast carcinoma may also be ER/PR positive and CK7 positive/CK20 negative whereas gastrointestinal cancers are usually CEA positive and CK20 positive/CK7 negative. The intracytoplasmic vacuoles of lobular carcinoma are PAS-AB positive.

- *Treatment is right hemicolectomy* with regional lymphadenectomy. Prognosis reflects the histological grade of tumour and TNM stage/Dukes' classification. There is an overall 5 year survival rate of 60–65 % for hemicolectomy, but this falls to 20 % for appendicectomy alone.

Metastatic Carcinoma

- *Peritoneal spread*: colorectum, ovary, stomach.
- *Distant spread*: lung, breast.

6.3 Differentiation

Well/moderate/poor/undifferentiated, or, Grade 1/2/3/4 based on the percentage tumour gland formation (well/G1 >95 %: moderate/G2 50–90 %: poor/G3 <50 %) for adenocarcinoma.

Undifferentiated carcinoma (grade 4) shows no gland formation.

In MANECs the behaviour and prognosis is determined by that of the individual components. Neuroendocrine tumours are graded according to their subtype, and proliferative activity (mitoses, Ki-67 index: see Sect. 3.3).

6.4 Extent of Local Tumour Spread

Border: pushing/infiltrative.

Lymphocytic reaction: prominent/sparse.

Limited to the appendix, into mesoappendix, appendiceal base and caecum.

As in colorectal carcinoma prognosis relates to Dukes' stage:

A	Tumour confined to the appendix wall, nodes negative
B	Tumour through the appendix wall, nodes negative
C	Tumour in regional lymph nodes irrespective of the depth of wall invasion.

In the TNM5/6 classifications appendix is an anatomical subsite of colorectum and it applies only to carcinoma.

pTis	Carcinoma in situ: intraepithelial (within basement membrane) or invasion of the lamina propria (intramucosal) with no extension through muscularis mucosae into submucosa
pT1	Tumour invades submucosa
pT2	Tumour invades muscularis propria
pT3	Tumour invades beyond muscularis propria into subserosa or mesoappendix
pT4	Tumour invades the serosal surface or adjacent organs and/or perforation of visceral peritoneum.

In addition in the TNM7 classification distinction is made between *non-mucinous* and *mucinous carcinoma*. The latter is categorized as *low-grade* (well differentiated) or *high-grade* mucinous carcinoma, and due to the differences in prognosis staged as tumour either confined to (pT4a) or beyond (pM1a) the right lower quadrant. Non-peritoneal metastasis is pM1b disease. This staging classification also applies to *goblet cell carcinoid* (*crypt cell adenocarcinoma*).

Well differentiated neuroendocrine (usual carcinoid) tumours are classified separately

pT1	Tumour 2 cm or less
pT1a	≤1 cm
pT1b	>1–2 cm
pT2	Tumour >2–4 cm, or with extension to caecum
pT3	Tumour >4 cm, or with extension to ileum
pT4	Tumour perforates peritoneum, or invades other organs or structures e.g. abdominal wall or skeletal muscle.

The European Neuroendocrine Tumour Society designates: pT1 ≤1 cm, pT2 ≤2 cm and/or mesoappendix/subserosa invasion ≤3 mm, pT3 >2 cm and/or invasion into mesoappendix/subserosa >3 mm.

6.5   Lymphovascular Invasion

Present/absent.
    Intra-/extratumoural.
    Serosa/mesoappendix.
    Lymphovascular invasion in adenocarcinoma is more significant than in a usual appendiceal tip carcinoid tumour where it is not infrequently present with no adverse prognostic effect.

6.6   Lymph Nodes

Site/number/size/number involved/limit node/extracapsular spread.
    Regional nodes: ileocolic. A regional lymphadenectomy will ordinarily include a minimum of 12 lymph nodes.
    Dukes' C: metastasis in regional lymph nodes.

pN0	No regional lymph node metastasis
pN1	1–3 involved regional lymph nodes
pN2	4 or more involved regional lymph nodes.

    Well differentiated neuroendocrine (carcinoid) tumour is limited to pN0 (not involved) or pN1 (involved) categories.

6.7   Excision Margins

Distances (mm) to the caecal base/proximal limit of excision and edge of the mesoappendix.

6.8   Other Pathology

Carcinoid syndrome: rarely occurs due to the scarcity of appendiceal carcinoid tumours metastatic to the liver.

Mucocoele

Mucocoeles of obstructed or non-obstructed types: both result in marked distension of the lumen by abundant mucus. Obstructed mucocoele is usually <1–2 cm diameter and effectively a retention cyst lined by variably attenuated, non-dysplastic atrophic mucosa. The much commoner non-obstructed mucocoeles are generally >1–2 cm diameter and due to an abnormality of the underlying mucosa caused either by *serrated epithelial change* (diffuse hyperplasia or serrated polyp/adenoma), *mucinous cystadenoma*, or *mucinous adenocarcinoma*. The latter two lesions comprise the group of *Appendiceal Mucinous Neoplasms* which can be either *low-grade* (*LAMN/ mucinous cystadenoma*) *or high-grade* (*MACA/mucinous adenocarcinoma*). LAMNs are of particular relevance to formation of *pseudomyxoma peritonei* and *ovarian mucinous cystic tumours*. They often have a bland attenuated epithelial lining which can be confined to the mucosa or dissect through the appendiceal wall. MACAs tend to invade adjacent tissues with potential for lymphatic and haematogenous metastases.

Pseudomyxoma Peritonei

Mucocoeles can be associated with rupture or perforation resulting in *pseudomyxoma peritonei* which is either localised or diffuse. Obstructed mucocoeles and those due to serrated hyperplastic change and mucosa confined adenoma usually remain localized. Diffuse pseudomyxoma peritonei is due to *spillage of mucin containing either variably atypical, or unequivocally malignant epithelium* associated with a LAMN or MACA, respectively. *Clinical behaviour and prognosis relates to the extent of extra-appendiceal mucus and the cellularity and atypia of the neoplastic cells within it.* However, generalised abdomino-pelvic disease can result even when the epithelial component is cytologically bland and relatively scanty. Anatomical distribution tends to spare some of the peritoneal surfaces with preferential location in the greater omentum, pelvis, left paracolic gutter and subdiaphragmatic space. There can be superficial invasion with a pushing border into various organs including omentum, spleen, ovary, myometrium and bowel. TNM7 distinguishes between disease localized to (pT4a) or beyond (pM1a) the right lower quadrant. Diffuse pseudomyxoma peritonei may be helped by *cytoreductive debulking procedures* such as peritoneal stripping and removal of involved organs (Sugarbaker technique), with *hyperthermic intraperitoneal chemotherapy*. However, it is largely *refractory to treatment, slowly but relentlessly progressive* and causes death by bowel obstruction (*45 % 10 year survival*). The outlook also varies according to whether the epithelial content is of *low-grade* or *high-grade* morphology, with 5 year survival rates of 63 and 23 %, respectively. Where compete cytoreduction is achieved the corresponding figures can improve to 84 and 48 %.

In this condition there is also a strong association with cystic intestinal type ovarian mucinous borderline tumours which are now regarded as being an implantation deposit from the appendix. Comparative immunophenotyping can help determine the relationship between the tumours. In this respect it should be noted that up to 5 % of appendiceal mucinous tumours express CK7 as well as the usual CK20. Ovarian mucinous tumours are also CK7/CK20 positive indicating either an ovarian primary or possible spread from appendix. If CK20 positive alone it is most likely a deposit from an appendiceal or other colorectal lesion. Ovarian tumours of mucinous type can show a wide spectrum of intestinal differentiation and it is possible that a number of these represent deposits from appendiceal, colonic, gastric or pancreatic sites. In addition the appendiceal lesion may not be grossly evident and it is recommended that appendicectomy be carried out, particularly if the ovarian tumours are bilateral and mucinous peritoneal disease is present. Occasionally pseudomyxoma peritonei may be due to mucinous carcinomas from other sites e.g. colorectal, urachus, stomach, gall bladder, breast or lung. However, it is in the vast majority of cases (94 %) appendiceal in origin, either from a LAMN (80 %) or a MACA (20 %).

Synchronous/metachronous colorectal lesions: the presence of serrated, adenomatous or cystadenocarcinomatous epithelium in the appendix is a marker of concurrent or subsequent epithelial neoplasms elsewhere in the colorectum. The patient should have postoperative colonoscopy or CT colonogram to visualise the entirety of the colorectum. Acquired *appendiceal diverticulum* has also been reported to have an increased incidence of appendiceal mucosal precursor and neoplastic lesions and concurrent locoregional colorectal carcinoma.

Appendicitis: can form an inflammatory appendix mass in the right iliac fossa that mimics colorectal cancer clinically and radiologically. Appendiceal tumours may also present in this fashion.

6.9 Other Malignancy

Malignant Lymphoma

- Primary (rare) or secondary to systemic/lymph node disease.
- Burkitt's lymphoma: ileocaecal angle in childhood and *aggressive highngrade* disease.

Kaposi's Sarcoma

- AIDS.

Bibliography

Bosman FT, Carneiro F. WHO classification of tumours of the digestive system. 4th ed. Lyon: IARC press; 2010.

Bradley RF, Cortina G, Geisinger KR. Pseudomyxoma peritonei: review of the controversy. Curr Diagn Pathol. 2007;13:410–6.

Carr NJ, Finch J, Ilesley IC, Chandrakumaran K, Mohamed F, Mirnezami A, Cecil T, Moran B. Pathology and prognosis in pseudomyxoma peritonei: a review of 274 cases. J Clin Pathol. 2012;65:919–23.

Day DW, Jass JR, Price AB, Shepherd NA, Sloan JM, Talbot IC, Warren BF, Williams GT. Morson and Dawson's gastrointestinal pathology. 4th ed. Oxford: Blackwell Sciences; 2003.

Misdraji J. Epithelial neoplasms and other epithelial lesions of the appendix (excluding carcinoid tumours). Curr Diagn Pathol. 2005a;11:60–71.

Misdraji J. Neuroendocrine tumours of the appendix. Curr Diagn Pathol. 2005b;11:180–93.

Misdraji J, Yantiss RK, Graeme-Cook FM, Baliss UJ, Young RH. Appendiceal mucinous neoplasm: a clinicopathologic analysis of 107 cases. Am J Surg Pathol. 2003;27:1089–103.

Odze RD, Goldblum JR. Surgical pathology of the GI tract, liver, biliary tract and pancreas. 2nd ed. Philadelphia: Saunders/Elsevier; 2009.

Plockinger U, Rindi G, Arnold R, Eriksson B, Krenning EP, de Herder WW, et al. Guidelines for the diagnosis and treatment of neuroendocrine gastrointestinal tumours. A consensus statement on behalf of the European Neuroendocrine Tumour Society (ENETS). Neuroendocrinology. 2004;80:394–424.

Riddell RH, Petras RE, Williams GT, Sobin LH. Tumors of the intestines. Atlas of tumor pathology. 3rd Series. Fascicle 32. Washington: AFIP; 2003.

Ronnett BM, Kurman RJ, Shmookler BM, Sugarbaker PH, Young RH. The morphologic spectrum of ovarian metastases of appendiceal adenocarcinomas. Am J Surg Pathol. 1997;21:1144–55.

Tang LH, Shia J, Soslow RA, Dhall D, Wong WD, O'Reilly E, et al. Pathologic classification and clinical behaviour of the spectrum of goblet cell carcinoid tumors of the appendix. Am J Surg Pathol. 2008;32:1429–43.

The Royal College of Pathologists: Cancer Datasets (Oesophageal Carcinoma, Gastric Carcinoma, Carcinomas of the Pancreas, ampulla of Vater and Common Bile Duct, Colorectal Cancer, Gastrointestinal Stromal Tumours (GISTs), Liver Resection Specimens and Liver Biopsies for Primary and Metastatic Carcinoma, Endocrine Tumours of the Gastrointestinal Tract including Pancreas) and Tissue Pathways (Gastrointestinal and Pancreatobiliary Pathology, Liver Biopsies for the Investigation of Medical Disease and for Focal Liver Lesions). Accessed at http://www.rcpath.org/index.asp?PageID=254.

Van Eeden S, Offerhaus GJA, Hart AAM, Boerrigter L, Nederlof PM, Porter E, van Velthuysen MLF. Goblet cell carcinoid of the appendix: a specific type of carcinoma. Histopathology. 2007;51:763–73.

Younes M, Katikaneni PR, Lechago J. Association between mucosal hyperplasia of the appendix and adenocarcinoma of the colon. Histopathology. 1995; 26:33–7.

Anal Canal Carcinoma (with Comments on Pelvic Exenteration)

The incidence of anal carcinoma is increasing in the Western hemisphere (2.5–5 fold in recent decades) due to cigarette smoking, Human Papilloma Virus (HPV) infection and immunosuppression e.g. HIV. Females are more frequently affected than males. Squamous cell carcinoma outnumbers adenocarcinoma by a ratio of 10–20:1. The 5 year survival figures for localised and extensive disease are 65–80 % and 15 % respectively.

Anal tumours present as a mass or feeling of fullness. Symptoms can be non-specific and develop late in the disease course. Patients are often reluctant to consult their doctors for investigation. Anal Intraepithelial Neoplasia (AIN) is often an incidental microscopic finding in minor surgical excision specimens or adjacent to carcinoma in local excisions.

For therapeutic reasons clear clinicopathological distinctions must be made

- Rectal type adenocarcinoma arising from the distal rectum or the colorectal zone of the upper anal canal can spread downwards and present as an anal tumour. Treatment is surgical (APER) preceeded by neoadjuvant therapy (see Chap. 5).
- Anal canal squamous cell carcinoma can spread upwards or downwards presenting as low rectal or perianal/anal margin tumour, respectively. Treatment is primarily radio-/chemotherapy with surgery reserved for non-responsive or recurrent disease.
- Perianal/anal margin squamous cell carcinoma can be confined to the skin or spread to involve the distal anus. Treatment is local surgical excision

for the former. Extended local excision or more radical surgery, or radiotherapy alone or in combination are indicated for the latter.
- Anal canal adenocarcinoma, malignant melanoma or sarcoma are surgically resected.
- Investigation of anal tumours is by anoproctoscopy and biopsy with endoanal ultrasound, MRI and CT scans to stage biopsy proven disease.

7.1 Gross Description

Specimen

- Biopsy/resection (wide local excision or abdominoperineal(APER)).
- Weight (g) and size/length (cm), number of fragments.

Tumour

Site
- Mucous membrane/muscularis/extra-mural.
- Low rectal/anal canal/perianal margin or skin.
- Anatomy:
  1. Upper zone: colorectal mucosa
  2. Transitional/cloacal zone: stratified cuboidal epithelium with surface umbrella cells + anal glands in submucosa dentate (pectinate) line
  3. Lower zone: stratified squamous epithelium continuous with appendage bearing perianal skin (Fig. 7.1).

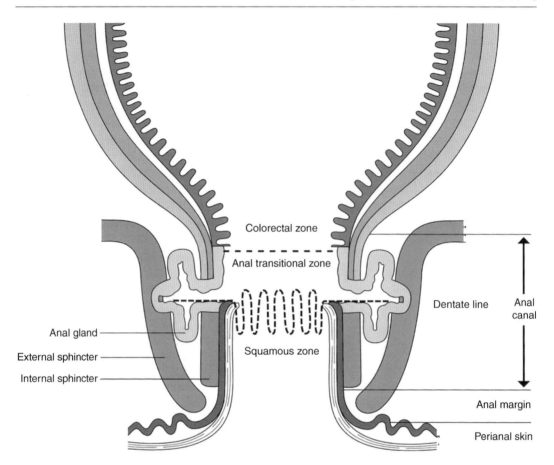

Fig. 7.1 The anatomy of the anal canal (Williams and Talbot (1994). Reproduced with permission from Blackwell Publishing Ltd)

Size

- Length × width × depth (cm) or maximum dimension (cm).

Appearance

- Polypoid/sessile/ulcerated/stricture/pigmented/fleshy/mucoid.

Edge

- Circumscribed/irregular.

7.2   Histological Type

Anal Margin/Perianal Skin

As for non-melanocytic skin carcinoma (Chap. 20), in particular well differentiated keratinising squamous cell carcinoma and variants including verrucous carcinoma. Also basal cell carcinoma, Bowen's disease, Paget's disease.

Anal Canal

Carcinoma of the anal canal is regarded as being a *squamous cell carcinoma* showing variable degrees of *squamous cell* (>90 % of cases), *basaloid* (65 % of cases) and *ductular* (26 % of cases) *differentiation*. Distal canal and anal margin cancers tend to show more overt well differentiated keratinising squamous cell differentiation – proximal tumours are generally non-keratinising and basaloid in character (Fig. 7.2).

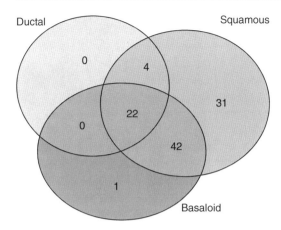

Fig. 7.2 Anal canal carcinoma: overlap in histological subtypes (Williams and Talbot (1994). Reproduced with permission from Blackwell Publishing Ltd)

Squamous Cell Carcinoma

- Keratinising/non-keratinising large cell or basaloid in character.

Basaloid Carcinoma

- (syn. cloacogenic/non-keratinising small cell squamous carcinoma).
- Palisading nests of basophilic cells with surrounding retraction artifact, central eosinophilic necrosis ± ductular differentiation.
- *Comprises 50% of anal carcinomas.*
- Mixed basaloid/squamous cell types.
- Increased incidence in Crohn's disease, smoking, immunosuppression and sexually transmitted disease.
- Association with HPV 16/18 and AIN.

Others

Squamous cell carcinoma variants: verrucous carcinoma, spindle cell carcinoma (rare), squamous carcinoma with microcysts (worse prognosis).

Mucinous (colloid) adenocarcinoma: in anal fistula which may be associated with Crohn's disease or hindgut duplication.

Anal gland adenocarcinoma: rare. In contrast to anorectal adenocarcinoma it is CK7 positive/CK20 negative. Late diagnosis and poor prognosis.

Extra-mammary Paget's disease: in 20% an underlying adnexal or rectal adenocarcinoma is found. The *majority of cases are primary* and remain *confined to the epithelium.*

Well differentiated neuroendocrine (carcinoid) tumour: carcinoid <2 cm is treated by local excision, if ≥2 cm consider more radical surgery.

Poorly differentiated/high-grade neuroendocrine carcinoma: small cell or large cell – both rare.

Malignant melanoma: primary mucosal origin with adjacent junctional atypia that can be destroyed by surface ulceration. Spindle cell or epithelioid cell types. *1.5% of anal malignancy* – aggressive with early spread and death in months from liver and lung metastases. *Five year survival is <20%, median survival 19 months.* No significant survival advantages for radical surgery over local palliative excision.

Metastatic carcinoma: direct spread – adenocarcinoma of rectal type arising from the colorectal mucosa of the upper anal zone cannot be distinguished from usual low rectal carcinoma and is grouped with it. Other possibilities are prostatic adenocarcinoma (PSA/PSAP positive) and cervical carcinoma.

7.3 Differentiation

Well/moderate/poor/undifferentiated or Grade 1/2/3/4.

For squamous cell cancers differentiation features are keratinisation and intercellular bridges, and, for adenocarcinomas the percentage tumour gland formation (well/G1 >95 %: moderate/G2 50–95 %: poor/G3 <50 %). Undifferentiated carcinomas (no gland formation) are classified as grade 4.

Sarcoma: low-grade/high-grade based on necrosis, cellular atypia and mitotic counts.

7.4 Extent of Local Tumour Spread

Border: pushing/infiltrative.

Lymphocytic reaction: prominent/sparse.

Depth of spread: submucosa, muscularis of rectum or anal sphincters, extrarectal and extraanal tissue including ischiorectal fossae and pelvic structures. Clinical assessment is by MRI

Fig. 7.3 Anal canal carcinoma (Reproduced, with permission, from Wittekind et al. (2005), © 2005)

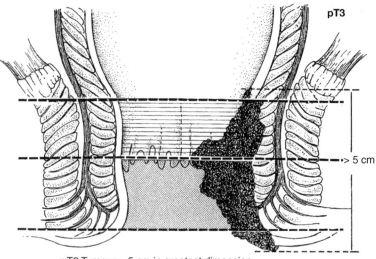

pT3 Tumour > 5 cm in greatest dimension

Fig. 7.4 Anal canal carcinoma (Reproduced, with permission, from Wittekind et al. (2005), © 2005)

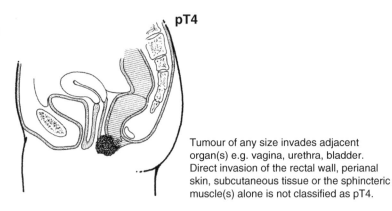

Tumour of any size invades adjacent organ(s) e.g. vagina, urethra, bladder. Direct invasion of the rectal wall, perianal skin, subcutaneous tissue or the sphincteric muscle(s) alone is not classified as pT4.

scan and endoanal ultrasound for local spread, and CT scan for distant disease.

At diagnosis a majority have spread through sphincteric muscle into adjacent soft tissues.

The TMN7 classification applies only to carcinomas (Figs. 7.3 and 7.4).

pTis	Carcinoma in situ
pT1	Tumour ≤2 cm in greatest dimension
pT2	2 cm< tumour ≤5 cm in greatest dimension
pT3	Tumour >5 cm in greatest dimension
pT4	Tumour of any size invading adjacent organ(s) e.g. vagina, urethra, bladder.

7.5 Lymphovascular Invasion

Present/absent.
  Intra-/extratumoural.
  Perineural spread.

Distant metastases are present in 5–10 % of cases at the time of diagnosis. Haematogenous spread is to liver, lung and skin.

7.6 Lymph Nodes

Site/number/size/number involved/limit node/extracapsular spread.

Regional nodes: perirectal, internal iliac, inguinal. Anal margin tumours go initially to inguinal nodes → iliac nodes. Anal canal tumours go initially to haemorrhoidal nodes → perirectal and inguinal nodes. A regional perirectal/pelvic lymphadenectomy will ordinarily include a minimum of 12 lymph nodes, an inguinal lymphadenectomy 6 or more lymph nodes.

pN0	No regional lymph node metastasis
pN1	Metastasis in perirectal lymph node(s)
pN2	Metastasis in unilateral internal iliac and/or inguinal lymph node(s)
pN3	Metastasis in perirectal and inguinal lymph nodes and/or bilateral internal iliac and/or inguinal lymph nodes.

Lymph node involvement is present in 10–50 % of cases at presentation.

7.7   Excision Margins

Distances (mm) to the nearest longitudinal (rectal or perianal) resection limit and deep circumferential radial margin.

7.8   Other Pathology

Carcinoma of the anal canal: (F:M 3:2) is commoner (3:1) than carcinoma of the anal margin (M:F 4:1).

HPV infection: a common aetiological agent associated with a spectrum of anal viral lesions, preneoplasia and carcinoma. *Preneoplasia* is variably site designated as *AIN*, *SIL* (squamous intraepithelial lesion) and *PSIN* (perianal squamous intraepithelial neoplasia). HPV subtypes 16 and 18 are particularly neoplasia progressive. Infection with HIV and other sexually transmitted viruses also contributes.

Traditionally used clinical terms: that are no longer preferred include condyloma accuminatum, giant condyloma of Buschke-Löwenstein, and Bowen's disease of anal skin. Some authors equate giant condyloma to verrucous carcinoma (indolent growth, exophytic, deep bulbous processes with bland cytology, more aggressive after radiotherapy). Bowenoid papulosis (perineal brown patches in younger patients, histology of Bowen's disease) has no significant malignant potential.

Multifocal anogenital neoplasia: there is potential for concurrent cervical intraepithelial neoplasia (CIN) and AIN associated with anal canal carcinoma. A premalignant phase or model of progression in AIN is not as well established

as in CIN although cancer risk appears to be greatest for high-grade AIN III. As with vulval intraepithelial neoplasia (VIN) *AIN is either classical or differentiated/simplex in character*. The former is commoner, occurs in younger patients with HPV infection, shows Bowenoid morphology and is p16 positive/p53 negative. The latter is in older patients and p53 positive/p16 negative. Diagnosis of AIN can be facilitated by use of p16, p53 and Ki-67 positive immunohistochemistry. It can be treated by local excision if small (<50 % of the anal circumference), ablation (laser, photodynamic) or immunomodulation therapy (Imiquimod).

Differential diagnoses: a significant proportion of anal canal carcinomas arise in the vicinity of the dentate line from the transitional/cloacal zone and spread preferentially upwards in the submucosal plane thereby presenting as ulcerating tumour of the lower rectum. Due to the differential options of primary neoadjuvant therapy versus primary resection, anal canal carcinoma must be distinguished by biopsy from both rectal adenocarcinoma superiorly and basal cell carcinoma or squamous cell carcinoma of the perianal margin/skin inferiorly.

Anal Paget's disease: must be distinguished from AIN/SIL/PSIN and Pagetoid spread of malignant melanoma. Mucin stains and immunohistochemistry are necessary (mucicarmine, PAS±diastase, cytokeratins, melanoma markers: pigment, S100, HMB-45, melan-A). It may be associated with concurrent or subsequent low rectal adenocarcinoma with the Paget's cells showing intestinal type gland formation and CK20 positivity. More often it is a primary epithelial lesion lacking intestinal glandular differentiation and CK20 positivity but is CK7/GCDFP-15 positive. Other associations are with bladder and cervical carcinoma. It may progress to submucosal invasion with a tendency for local recurrence. However, a *majority remain as intraepithelial malignancy*. A further differential diagnosis is Pagetoid spread from a primary anorectal signet ring cell carcinoma.

Immunohistochemistry: also important in the differential diagnosis of anal basaloid squamous cell carcinoma (CK5/6, p63, p16, EMA, CEA positive), malignant melanoma, malignant lymphoma (CD 45 positive), spindle cell carcinoma (cytokeratin positive), and leiomyosarcoma (desmin, h-caldesmon, smooth muscle actin positive). Distinction between anal canal basaloid squamous cell carcinoma and basal cell carcinoma of the anal margin is by the anatomical location as well as histological characteristics.

Radiotherapy necrosis.

Leukoplakia: clinically a white plaque with or without AIN is occasionally seen and it requires biopsy to establish the presence of dysplasia.

Prognosis

Carcinoma of the anal margin/perianal skin is treated primarily by *surgery ± radiotherapy*. Well differentiated tumours <2 cm diameter or occupying <50 % of the anal circumference can initially be locally excised and followed up surgically. An oncoplastic surgical procedure with flap rotation may be required to give skin coverage. *Anal canal squamous carcinoma* responds well to *primary radio-/chemotherapy* and abdominoperineal resection is reserved for locally extensive, recurrent or non-responsive tumours, or other lesions such as malignant melanoma and leiomyosarcoma. *Perianal carcinoma: 5 year survival 85%; anal canal carcinoma: 5 year survival 65–80%*. Adverse prognostic indicators are advanced stage or depth of spread, tumour in inguinal lymph nodes (10–50 %) and post-treatment recurrence in the pelvic and perianal regions, e.g. pT1 carcinoma has a 5 year survival of 91 %, pT3 16 %. Histological grade is not a strong indicator but may be helpful in poorly differentiated squamous cell carcinoma of large cell type. Ductal differentiation in basaloid squamous cell carcinoma is an adverse factor. Recurrence in men is pelvic and perineal, in women pelvic and vaginal.

7.9 Other Malignancy

Malignant Lymphoma/Leukaemia

- Secondary to systemic/nodal disease.
- HIV: also Kaposi's sarcoma.

Leiomyosarcoma

- Low-grade/high-grade based on cellularity, atypia, necrosis, infiltrative margins and mitoses. Desmin, h-caldesmon positive.

Presacral Tumours

- Teratoma, peripheral neuroectodermal tumours (including Ewing's sarcoma), multiple myeloma, metastatic carcinoma.

Rhabdomyosarcoma

- Childhood, embryonal (desmin/myo D1/myogenin positive).

7.10 Comments on Pelvic Exenteration

In general pelvic exenteration is considered for locally advanced or recurrent pelvic malignancy in the absence of extra-pelvic metastases.

- *Degree of disease spread*: assessed by
  - CT scan – pelvic and retroperitoneal lymphadenopathy, extra-pelvic metastases.
  - MRI scan – local cancer spread into adjacent tissues.
  - CT/PET scan – detects metabolic activity in malignant tumours and is useful in localising recurrent or distant metastatic disease, and distinguishing neoplasia from radiotherapy induced fibrosis.
- *Relevant malignancies*: cervical carcinoma, rectal carcinoma, anal carcinoma, soft tissue lesions (e.g. malignant fibrous histiocytoma, aggressive angiomyxoma), aggressive muscle invasive bladder cancer, and occasionally advanced high-grade endometrial, vaginal or vulval cancers. Exenteration is not recommended in ovarian malignancy as high stage disease shows peritoneal involvement outside the pelvis.
- *Contraindications*: significant comorbidity, distant metastases (except resectable liver metastases from a rectal carcinoma) and

Fig. 7.5 Pelvic exenterations (Reproduced, with
permission, from Allen
(2006), © 2006)

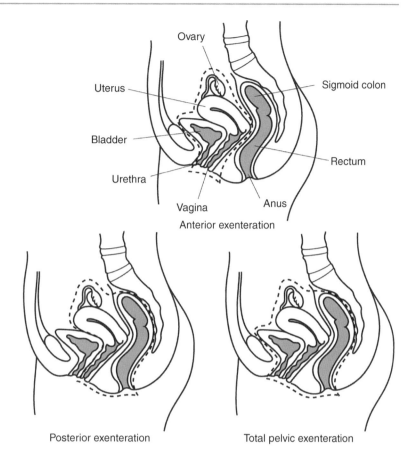

involvement of major pelvic vessels, nerves,
pelvic side walls or sacrum, although the latter
can be resected en-bloc in rectal cancer.

- *Preoperative adjuvant therapy*: may result in
  significant tumour regression so that it can be
  difficult to find residual disease and lymph
  nodes which shrink and hyalinise. Deep
  spread and margins fibrose making accurate
  assessment of pT stage and resection status
  problematic.
- *Surgery*: may be with curative intent or palliative to obviate complex and debilitating pelvic
  symptoms due either to spread of malignancy
  or as a consequence of adjuvant therapy e.g.
  pain, fistulae. The latter can produce unusual
  symptoms e.g. pneumaturia or faecaluria.
- *Pelvic exenterations* (Fig. 7.5)
  - *Anterior*: bladder, lower ureters, reproduc-
    tive organs, draining lymph nodes and pel-
    vic peritoneum.

  - *Posterior*: rectum, distal colon, internal
    reproductive organs, draining lymph nodes
    and pelvic peritoneum.
  - *Total*: anterior and posterior.
- *Principles of specimen reporting*
  - Identify the specimen type and component
    organs.
  - Block longitudinal transection limits i.e. ure-
    ters, urethra, vagina and proximal/distal bowel.
  - Paint circumferential radial fascial or soft
    tissue margins, comment on the uterine/
    bladder dome/colonic/upper anterior rectal
    peritoneum, and integrity of the mesorec-
    tum and its fascia.
  - *Sagittal hemisection* can be very useful in
    demonstrating the relationships between
    the tumour and the constituent organs.
    Fistulae can be cut along the line of an
    exploring probe. Also document the status
    of circumferential radial margins.

- Report as per individual cancers noting in particular the degree of locoregional spread, margin status and effects of preoperative adjuvant therapy.
- The diagnosis and organ of origin will have been previously established by clinical and radiological investigation and diagnostic biopsy. In an exenteration specimen good macroscopic description, orientation, fixation and blocking are paramount to establish that a *complete (R0) resection* has been achieved. Microscopy further identifies lymphovascular and microscopic margin involvement that determines adjuvant treatment. It also documents the effects of neoadjuvant therapy.

Bibliography

Allen DC. Histopathology reporting: guidelines for surgical cancer. 2nd ed. London: Springer; 2006.

Balachandra B, Marcus V, Jass JR. Poorly differentiated tumours of the anal canal: a diagnostic strategy for the surgical pathologist. Histopathology. 2007;50:163–74.

Bosman FT, Carneiro F. WHO classification of tumours of the digestive system. 4th ed. Lyon: IARC press; 2010.

Day DW, Jass JR, Price AB, Shepherd NA, Sloan JM, Talbot IC, Warren BF, Williams GT. Morson and Dawson's gastrointestinal pathology. 4th ed. Oxford: Blackwell Sciences; 2003.

Fielding LP, Goldberg SM, editors. Rob and Smith's operative surgery: surgery of the colon, rectum and anus. 5th ed. London: Butterworth-Heinemann; 1993.

Goldblum JR, Hart WR. Perianal Paget's disease. A histologic and immunohistochemical study of 11 cases

with and without associated rectal adenocarcinoma. Am J Surg Pathol. 1998;22:170–9.

Mitchell KA, Owens SR. Anal carcinoma and its differential diagnosis. Diagn Histopathol. 2008;14:61–7.

Odze RD, Goldblum JR. Surgical pathology of the GI tract, liver, biliary tract and pancreas. 2nd ed. Philadelphia: Saunders/Elsevier; 2009.

Riddell RH, Petras RE, Williams GT, Sobin LH. Tumors of the intestines. Atlas of tumor pathology. 3rd series. Fascicle 32. AFIP: Washington; 2003.

Serra A, Chetty R. Tumours of the anal canal. Curr Diagn Pathol. 2006;12:136–51.

Simpson JAD, Scholefield JH. Diagnosis and management of anal intraepithelial neoplasia and anal cancer. BMJ. 2011;343:1004–9.

Williams GR, Sheffield JP, Love SB, Talbot IC. Morphology of anal carcinoma: a reappraisal. Curr Diagn Pathol. 1995;2:32–7.

Williams GR, Talbot IC. Anal carcinoma: a histological review. Histopathology. 1994;25:507–16.

Wittekind CF, Greene FL, Hutter RVP, Klimpfinger M, Sobib LH. TNM atlas: illustrated guide to the TNM/pTNM classification of malignant tumours. 5th ed. Berlin: Springer; 2005.

Pelvic Exenteration

Ferenschild FTJ, Vermaas M, Verhoef C, Ansink AC, Kirkels WJ, Eggermont AMM, de Wilt JHW. Total pelvic exenteration for primary and recurrent malignancies. World J Surg. 2009;33:1502–8.

Rodrigues-Bigas MA, Petrelli NJ. Pelvic exenteration and its modifications. Am J Surg. 1996;171:293–8.

Temple WJ, Saettler EB. Locally recurrent rectal cancer: role of composite resection of extensive pelvic tumors with strategies for minimizing risk of recurrence. J Surg Oncol. 2000;73:47–58.

Gall Bladder Carcinoma

Gall bladder cancer accounts for 28 and 51 % of cancers of the biliary tree in males and females respectively. A positive genetic background, calculi (80 % of cases) and an abnormally functioning choledochopancreatic junction are the main risk factors. Gall bladder disease generally presents in middle-aged to elderly females with dyspepsia, bloating and right hypochondrial pain. Investigation includes liver function tests and abdominal ultrasound scan looking for calculi, luminal/mural lesions, cystic duct or extrahepatic large duct obstruction. If abnormal, CT scan and cholangiography (percutaneous or endoscopic) are of use in demonstrating and staging a tumour mass. Although usually asymptomatic or masked by the inflammatory changes of cholelithiasis, gall bladder cancer can cause weight loss and jaundice, the latter due to metastatic disease compressing bile ducts. About 50 % of gall bladder cancers are an incidental finding after routine cholecystectomy. Some 10 % of calcified porcelain gall bladders contain carcinoma.

The presence of extensive adhesions may require intraoperative conversion from the usual laparoscopic technique to an open cholecystectomy procedure. An elective staged resection is indicated for pT1b and higher stage cancers although clinical suitability for this is established on an individual patient basis. Alternatively gall bladder cancer is diagnosed on clinical imaging and submitted as part of an elective extended cholecystectomy. After determination of the extent of local spread by operative ultrasound the hepatic gall bladder bed and regional nodes are resected. A deeper tumour may require hepatic segmental resection. However, pT4 disease involving main portal vein, hepatic artery or two or more extrahepatic organs/structures is considered inoperable. Adjuvant therapy has a role to play. With extensive locally infiltrative disease palliation may involve stenting or bypass surgery of the biliary tree or other local structures, to relieve jaundice or gastric outlet obstruction.

8.1 Gross Description

Specimen

- Size (cm) and weight (g).
- Open/intact.
- Contents: bile/calculi (number, size, shape, colour).
- Lymph nodes: site/size/number.

Tumour

Site
- Fundus (50 %)/body/cystic duct.

Size
- Length × width × depth (cm) or maximum dimension (cm).

Appearance
- Grossly apparent/inapparent.
- Diffuse (65 %)/polypoid (30 % – including papillary)/ulcerated.

Edge

- Circumscribed/irregular.

8.2 Histological Type

More than 95% of gall bladder cancers are adenocarcinoma.

Adenocarcinoma

- *Tubular/acinar*: usual type and a well to moderately differentiated biliary pattern of low cuboidal to tall columnar cells.
- *Papillary*: polypoid/well differentiated/better prognosis. An exophytic luminal lesion with invasion often restricted to the superficial aspect of the mucosa. It can be difficult to distinguish between papillary adenoma (usually of intestinal phenotype), intracystic papillary neoplasm (usually of biliary phenotype), and well differentiated adenocarcinoma.
- *Gastric foveolar/intestinal/mucinous/signet ring cell/clear cell*: all unusual. Distinguish from metastatic stomach or bowel cancer by adjacent mucosal dysplasia. Mucinous/signet ring cell adenocarcinomas require >50 % of the tumour to be composed of this pattern.

Adenosquamous Carcinoma

- Moderately differentiated with mucin secretion and keratin pearl formation.

Squamous Cell Carcinoma

- Most represent adenosquamous carcinoma with a focal glandular component.

Neuroendocrine Tumour/Carcinoma

- Low-grade/high-grade gastrointestinal neuroendocrine tumours e.g. well differentiated neuroendocrine (carcinoid) tumour, or, poorly differentiated/high-grade (small cell/large cell) neuroendocrine carcinomas including composite tumours (MANECs – mixed adenoneuroendocrine carcinomas).
- Small cell carcinoma is *aggressive* and may be a component of usual adenocarcinoma. It occurs more frequently in the gall bladder than at other gastrointestinal sites. Synaptophysin/CD56 positive, high Ki-67 index.
- About 50 % of carcinoid tumours are confined to the gall bladder at diagnosis. Chromogranin/synaptophysin positive, CD56±, low Ki-67 index (≤2 %).

Spindle Cell Carcinoma/ Carcinosarcoma

- Biphasic carcinoma/sarcoma like components ± specific mesenchymal differentiation. These represent carcinomas with variable homologous or heterologous stromal differentiation and overlap with undifferentiated carcinoma.
- Elderly patients, poor prognosis.

Undifferentiated Carcinoma

- Nodular and solid/spindle cell/giant cell/osteoclast-like giant cell variants. Also non-neuroendocrine small cell pattern.

Malignant Melanoma

- Secondary (15 % of disseminated melanoma at autopsy), or rarely, primary (nodular, adjacent mucosal junctional change).

Metastatic Carcinoma

- *Direct spread*: stomach, colon, pancreas, cholangiocarcinoma.
- *Distant spread*: breast, lung, kidney.

8.3 Differentiation

Well/moderate/poor/undifferentiated, or, Grade 1/2/3/4 based on the percentage tumour gland formation (well/G1 >95 %: moderate/G2 50–95 %: poor/G3 <50 %).

- Usually well to moderately differentiated arising from mucosal dysplasia (BilIN: <u>Bil</u>iary <u>I</u>ntraepithelial <u>N</u>eoplasia), or mucosal intestinal metaplasia and dysplasia.
- Signet ring cell carcinoma is grade 3, small cell and undifferentiated carcinoma (no gland formation) grade 4.

8.4 Extent of Local Tumour Spread

Border: pushing/infiltrative.

Lymphocytic reaction: prominent/sparse.

Characteristic perineural spread (25 % of cases).

The TNM7 classification applies only to carcinomas of the gall bladder and cystic duct.

pTis	Carcinoma in situ
pT1	Tumour limited to gall bladder or cystic duct wall
pT1a	Invades lamina propria
pT1b	Invades muscularis
pT2	Tumour invades perimuscular connective tissue, no extension beyond serosa or into liver.

pT3	Tumour perforates serosa and/or directly invades the liver and/or directly invades one adjacent organ e.g. stomach, duodenum, colon, pancreas, omentum, extrahepatic bile ducts.
pT4	Tumour invades main portal vein or hepatic artery, or invades two or more extrahepatic organs or structures.

Note that carcinoma in situ and adenocarcinoma may extend into Rokitansky-Aschoff sinuses or gall bladder bed Lushka's ducts, and this must be distinguished from deeply invasive tumour which shows a lack of low power lobular organisation, deficient basement membrane and stromal desmoplasia (Figs. 8.1, 8.2 and 8.3).

8.5 Lymphovascular Invasion

Present/absent.

Intra-/extratumoural.

Perineural invasion is a helpful diagnostic clue to adenocarcinoma but is also an adverse prognostic factor.

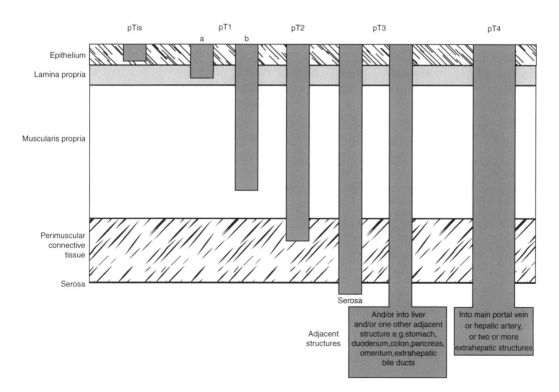

Fig. 8.1 Gall bladder carcinoma (Reproduced, with permission, from Allen (2006), © 2006)

Fig. 8.2 Gall bladder carcinoma (Reproduced, with permission, from Wittekind et al. (2005), © 2005)

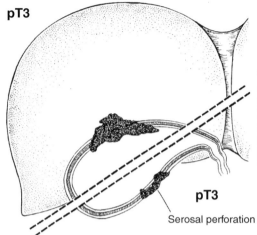

pT3

Tumour perforates serosa (visceral peritoneum) and/or directly invades the liver and/or one other adjacent organ or structure, e.g., stomach,duodenum,colon, pancreas,omentum, extrahepatic bile ducts

pT3

Serosal perforation

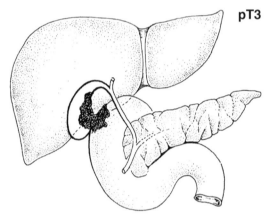

pT3

| pN0 | No regional lymph node metastasis |
| pN1 | Metastasis in regional lymph node (s). |

The most commonly involved lymph nodes are the pericholedochal (Fig. 8.4).

Fig. 8.3 Gall bladder carcinoma (Reproduced, with permission, from Wittekind et al. (2005), © 2005)

8.6 Lymph Nodes

Site/number/size/number involved/limit node/extracapsular spread.

Regional nodes: hepatic hilus nodes (along the common bile duct, common hepatic artery, portal vein and cystic duct). Coeliac, periduodenal, peripancreatic and superior mesenteric artery nodes are considered metastatic (pM1) disease. A regional lymphadenectomy will ordinarily include a minimum of three lymph nodes.

8.7 Excision Margins

Distances (mm) of tumour to the proximal limit of the cystic duct and adventitial or liver bed margin. Microscopic involvement (R1) is generally regarded as tumour clearance <1 mm.

Mucosal dysplasia (BilIN) in adjacent gall bladder mucosa, the cystic duct and its limit. Histological detection of mucosal dysplasia in a routine cholecystectomy block should prompt extra blocks to look for an occult invasive cancer.

8.8 Other Pathology

Adenoma: rare (0.5 % cholecystectomies) and exclude *Familial Adenomatous Polyposis (FAP)*. As in the colorectum the risk of malignancy in an adenoma increases with size, villousity and degree of dysplasia. Histologically there are

Fig. 8.4 Gall bladder: regional lymph nodes (Reproduced, with permission, from Wittekind et al. (2005), © 2005)

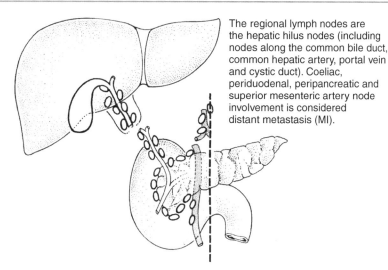

The regional lymph nodes are the hepatic hilus nodes (including nodes along the common bile duct, common hepatic artery, portal vein and cystic duct). Coeliac, periduodenal, peripancreatic and superior mesenteric artery node involvement is considered distant metastasis (MI).

pyloric gland (commonest), intestinal, and biliary subtypes. A true adenoma should not be confused with the commoner fundal cholecystitis glandularis proliferans – a reactive mucosal hyperplasia and herniation associated with smooth muscle proliferation.

Immunophenotype

Gall bladder carcinoma is cytokeratin (CAM 5.2, AE1/AE3, CK7, CK19), CA19-9 and CEA positive.

Prognosis

Calculi, and anomalous choledochopancreatic duct anatomy are *risk factors*, with *calculi* present in 80–90 % of cases in female patients (F:M 3:1). A majority of gall bladder carcinomas are *clinically inapparent* and found incidentally as diffuse thickening of the wall at cholecystectomy for gall stones. *Prognosis* is strongly related to *cancer type, grade and stage*. It is better if lesions are of papillary type, low histological grade and confined to the mucous membrane, when resection is potentially curative (90 % 5 year survival). *Full wall thickess infiltration has a 10 year survival rate of*

52 %. A significant number of carcinomas are grossly inapparent and a microscopic finding only. However, curative resection is unusual and up to 50–70 % present with regional lymph node metastases and involvement of the gall bladder bed liver. In these patients 5 year survival rates are 5–10 %.

8.9 Other Malignancy

Malignant Lymphoma/Leukaemia

- MALToma or more usually secondary to systemic nodal disease.

Sarcoma (Rare)

- Embryonal rhabdomyosarcoma (children: desmin/myo D1/myogenin positive), leiomyosarcoma, angiosarcoma.

Bibliography

Albores-Saavedra J, Henson DE, Klimstra DS. Tumors of the gallbladder, extrahepatic bile ducts and ampulla of vater. Atlas of tumor pathology. 3rd series. Fascicle 27. Washington: AFIP; 2000.

Allen DC. Histopathology reporting: guidelines for surgical cancer. 2nd ed. London: Springer; 2006.

Beckingham IJ, editor. ABC of liver, pancreas and gall bladder diseases. London: BMJ Books; 2001.

Bosman FT, Carneiro F. WHO classification of tumours of the digestive system. 4th ed. Lyon: IARC press; 2010.

Carter D, Russell RCG, Pitt HA, Bismuth H, editors. Rob and Smith's operative surgery: hepatobiliary and pancreatic surgery. 5th ed. London: Chapman and Hall; 1996.

Day DW, Jass JR, Price AB, Shepherd NA, Sloan JM, Talbot IC, Warren BF, Williams GT. Morson and Dawson's gastrointestinal pathology. 4th ed. Oxford: Blackwell Sciences; 2003.

Goldin RD, Roa JC. Gallbladder cancer: a morphological and molecular update. Histopathology. 2009;55:218–29.

Mann CV, Russell RCG, Williams NS, editors. Bailey & Love's short practice of surgery. 22nd ed. London: Chapman and Hall Medical; 1995.

Odze RD, Goldblum JR. Surgical pathology of the GI tract, liver, biliary tract and pancreas. 2nd ed. Philadelphia: Saunders/Elsevier; 2009.

Wittekind CF, Greene FL, Hutter RVP, Klimpfinger M, Sobib LH. TNM atlas: illustrated guide to the TNM/pTNM classification of malignant tumours. 5th ed. Berlin: Springer; 2005.

Predisposing conditions to extrahepatic bile duct carcinoma include chronic ulcerative colitis, primary sclerosing cholangitis, gall stones and choledochal cysts.

Extrahepatic bile duct cancer presents with obstructive jaundice, right upper quadrant pain, weight loss and malaise. Pyrexia can result from ascending cholangitis and the gall bladder may be distended depending on the anatomical site of the tumour. Investigations include: serum CA19-9 levels, liver function tests, ultrasound scan and cholangiography (either percutaneous, at MRI scan or ERCP(endoscopic retrograde cholangiopancreatography)) to detect large duct obstruction and strictures, and, CT/MRI scans for tumour staging of local and distant disease. Cytology material is obtained at ERCP which is used either for diagnostic or therapeutic purposes (stone retrieval, stent insertion). Diagnostic yields for malignancy are at best 30–40 % and a presumptive working diagnosis may have to be based on clinical grounds.

Radical resection is usually for a distal bile duct or ampullary mass (Whipple's pancreaticoduodenectomy) causing obstructive jaundice. This may or may not have been proven by ERCP brushings or endoscopic biopsy of the ampulla or duodenal papilla. Sometimes a segmental resection for a mid bile duct tumour is carried out, or occasionally combined with hepatic segmental resection for a proximal or peri-/infrahilar tumour. Intraoperative frozen section may be required for assessment of bile duct resection margins, enlarged suspicious lymph nodes or a subcapsular liver nodule. This is augmented by diagnostic and staging laparoscopy with biopsy of suspected lymph node, peritoneal and subcapsular liver deposits that would preclude radical surgery.

9.1 Gross Description

Specimen

- Cytological brushings and washings/biopsy/resection.
- Weight (g) and size/length (cm), number of fragments.

Tumour

Site

- Tumours of the extrahepatic ducts are outside the liver and above the level of the ampulla of Vater. Choledochal cyst tumours are included but cystic duct tumours are grouped with gall bladder cancer (Fig. 9.1).
- Perihilar tumour/proximal third (50–60 %: equally between the right/left/common hepatic, and upper common bile ducts), intermediate third (25 %), distal third (10 %), multifocal/diffuse (15 %).

Size

- Length × width × depth (cm) or maximum dimension (cm).
- Tumour size may be deceptive as there can be extensive fibrosis due to cholangitis or stenting.

Fig. 9.1 Extrahepatic bile
ducts (Reproduced, with
permission, from Wittekind
et al. (2005), © 2005)

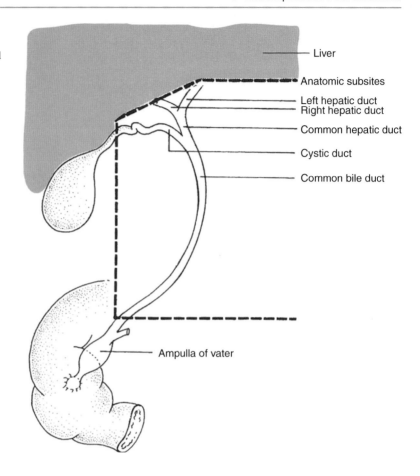

Liver

Anatomic subsites

Left hepatic duct
Right hepatic duct

Common hepatic duct

Cystic duct

Common bile duct

Ampulla of vater

In contrast to this there can be microscopic
infiltration of tumour beyond its macroscopic
edge.

• Localised (a majority), the entire common bile
  duct or multifocal throughout the extrahepatic
  biliary system.

Appearance
• Papillary/polypoid: distal third.
• Nodular: intermediate third.
• Ulcerated/sclerotic/scirrhous: proximal third.
  The majority are nodular or sclerosing with
deep penetration of the wall, although the macro-
scopic appearances overlap considerably. A small
minority have a cystic component.

Edge
• Circumscribed/irregular.

9.2   Histological Type

Adenocarcinoma

• *Tubular/acinar:* usual type and a well to moderately differentiated biliary pattern of low
  cuboidal to tall columnar cells.
• *Papillary:* polypoid and well differentiated in
  the distal third with a better prognosis. It is of
  biliary or intestinal phenotype.
• *Intestinal:* well to moderate differentia-
  tion±mucin secretion in a fibrous stroma.
• *Sclerosing:* perihilar tumour. Well to moderately differentiated tubular adenocarcinoma
  and rarely mucinous or signet ring cell. Fibrous
  nodule, short or long segmental stenosis with a
  periductal infiltrative pattern, or papillary.
  Indolent growth with potentially prolonged

survival and ultimately *death is from liver failure rather than tumour dissemination.* Includes the classical Klatskin tumour at the confluence of the right and left hepatic ducts and which also often shows intrahepatic extension. Arises in a field of mucosal dysplasia and resection limits should be checked for this.

- *Others:* mucinous carcinoma/signet ring cell carcinoma (>50 % of the tumour area), clear cell carcinoma are unusual.
- *Cystadenocarcinoma:* a small number are the malignant counterpart of bile duct cystadenoma with variable benign, borderline and focal malignant change. Middle aged females, resectable, good prognosis.

Adenosquamous Carcinoma

- Moderately differentiated with mucin secretion and keratin pearl formation.

Squamous Cell Carcinoma

- Most represent adenosquamous carcinoma with a minor glandular component.

Neuroendocrine Tumour/Carcinoma

- Gastrointestinal neuroendocrine tumours e.g. well differentiated/low-grade neuroendocrine (carcinoid) tumour, or poorly differentiated/high-grade (small cell/large cell) neuroendocrine carcinoma. Variably chromogranin, synaptophysin, CD56, Ki-67 positive.

Carcinosarcoma/Spindle Cell Carcinoma

- Cytokeratin positive spindle cells and varying degrees of homologous or heterologous stromal mesenchymal differentiation.

Undifferentiated Carcinoma

- Nodular or solid/spindle cell/giant cell variants.

Malignant Melanoma

- Metastatic or primary (rare). Comprises up to 50 % of metastatic cancers to the gall bladder and biliary tree.

Metastatic Carcinoma

- Stomach, breast (infiltrating lobular), colorectum, kidney.

9.3   Differentiation

Well/moderate/poor/undifferentiated, or, Grade 1/2/3/4 based on the percentage tumour gland formation (well/G1 >95 %: moderate/G2 50–95 %: poor/G3 <50 %). Signet ring cell carcinoma is grade 3, small cell and undifferentiated carcinoma (no gland formation) grade 4 – these are prognostically adverse cancers.

9.4   Extent of Local Tumour Spread

Border: pushing/infiltrative.
    Lymphocytic reaction: prominent/sparse.
    Perineural spread is a characteristic and may be *present beyond the resection line causing surgical failure.*
    The TNM7 classification distinguishes between carcinomas of the extrahepatic bile ducts by their location. Either distal (distal to the insertion of the cystic duct) or perihilar (proximal to the cystic duct origin up to and including the second branches of the left and right hepatic ducts) (Fig. 9.2).

Distal

pTis	Carcinoma in situ
pT1	Tumour confined to the bile duct[a] histologically
pT2	Tumour invades beyond the wall of the bile duct[a]
pT3	Tumour invades adjacent structures: liver, pancreas, gall bladder, duodenum or other adjacent organs
pT4	Tumour invades the coeliac axis or superior mesenteric artery

[a]The wall of the bile duct comprises the subepithelial connective tissues and underlying fibromuscular layer

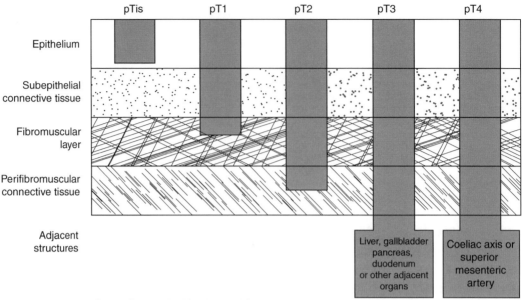

pT1: confined to the bile duct wall (mucous membrane plus muscularis)
pT2: beyond the bile duct wall

Fig. 9.2 Distal extrahepatic bile duct carcinoma (Reproduced, with permission, from Allen (2006), © 2006)

Perihilar

pT1	Tumour confined to the bile duct wall
pT2	Tumour invades beyond the bile duct wall into either
pT2a	Periductal adipose tissue or
pT2b	Adjacent hepatic parenchyma
pT3	Tumour invades unilateral branches of portal vein or hepatic artery
pT4	Tumour invades main portal vein, bilateral branches, common hepatic artery, second order biliary radicles bilaterally (or, unilateral with contralateral portal vein or hepatic artery involvement).

9.5   Lymphovascular Invasion

Present/absent.

Intra-/extratumoural.

An adverse prognostic indicator.

9.6   Lymph Nodes

Site/number/size/number involved/limit node/extracapsular spread.

Regional nodes: distal – common bile duct, common hepatic artery, coeliac trunk,

pancreaticoduodenal, superior mesenteric vein and artery (right lateral wall). Perihilar – hilar, pericholodochal. A regional lymphadenectomy will ordinarily include a minimum of 12 and 15 lymph nodes for distal and perihilar lesions, respectively.

pN0	No regional lymph node metastasis
pN1	Metastasis in regional lymph node (s).

Lymph node metastases are usually present at the time of diagnosis with subsequent spread to local structures (liver, pancreas, gall bladder, duodenum), lungs and peritoneal cavity.

9.7   Excision Margins

Distances (mm) to the nearest longitudinal and circumferential resection margins of carcinoma and presence of mucosal dysplasia at the longitudinal limits.

Local recurrence usually relates to longitudinal or soft tissue radial margin involvement by adenocarcinoma and is commonest in proximal tumours. Microscopic involvement (R1) is generally regarded as tumour clearance <1 mm.

9.8 Other Pathology

Diagnostic presentation: 90 % of patients (>60 years, F:M 1:1) present with jaundice and diagnosis is by cholangiography (retrograde endoscopic or percutaneous transhepatic) supplemented by fine needle aspiration/brushings/washings cytology and/or biopsy.

Frozen section diagnosis: of bile duct carcinoma can be difficult due to the presence of ductulo-glandular structures in normal bile duct submucosa and the distortion that can occur in inflammatory strictures.

Dysplasia (BilIN): of adjacent bile duct mucosa can have a flat or micropapillary epithelial pattern and must be noted at the resection limits. Intraductal papillary neoplasia or biliary papillomatosis is a relatively uncommon precancerous lesion which can develop an associated invasive component.

Predisposing conditions: chronic inflammatory bowel disease (ulcerative colitis), primary sclerosing cholangitis, gall stones and choledochal cysts all show an increased incidence. Radiologically it can be difficult to distinguish between primary sclerosing cholangitis and a stenotic carcinoma.

Immunophenotype

Markers (e.g. cytokeratins, CEA) may be helpful in identifying poorly differentiated single cell infiltration on biopsy. Other markers of bile duct carcinoma are cytokeratins 7 and 19, EMA and CA19-9. There is also over expression of p53 in contradistinction to normal duct structures. Perineural invasion can point to a diagnosis of malignancy.

Prognosis

Prognosis is worse for carcinoma of the upper third and hilum which is diffuse and/or multifocal. Distal lesions which are polypoid or nodular are potentially resectable with better prognosis. Despite being sclerotic and diffuse, perihilar Klatskin tumours have a well differentiated morphology and indolent time course. *Prognosis of bile duct carcinoma is poor* with most patients dead within 2–3 years. It relates to *tumour location, stage, histological type and grade. Overall survival is 10 %* with 25 % for lesions of the distal third and resectable lesions with negative margins. This can improve to 50–80 % 5 year survival if the tumour is ampullary and of early stage (pT1: limited to the sphincter of Oddi). Treatment for proximal lesions is resection (± hepatic lobectomy) with hepatojejunostomy. A Whipple's procedure is indicated for distal lesions. *Bile duct cancer is treated conservatively in 80–90 % of cases* and *resection is only considered in tumours that are localised to the wall without metastatic spread (21 % 5 year survival).* Palliative treatment can involve biliary drainage, stenting or radiotherapy.

9.9 Other Malignancy

Malignant Lymphoma/Leukaemia

- Secondary to systemic/nodal disease.

Sarcoma

- Embryonal (botryoid) rhabdomyosarcoma in children with direct invasion of abdominal structures, metastases to bone and lungs and poor prognosis. Desmin/myo D1/myogenin positive small cells, subepithelial cellular cambium layer, deeper myxoid zone.
- Leiomyosarcoma, angiosarcoma.

Bibliography

Albores-Saavedra J, Henson DE, Klimstra DS. Tumors of the gallbladder, extrahepatic bile ducts and ampulla of vater. Atlas of tumor pathology. 3rd series. Fascicle 27. Washington: AFIP; 2000.

Allen DC. Histopathology reporting: guidelines for surgical cancer. 2nd ed. London: Springer; 2006.

Beckingham IJ, editor. ABC of liver, pancreas and gall bladder diseases. London: BMJ Books; 2001.

Bosman FT, Carneiro F. WHO classification of tumours of the digestive system. 4th ed. Lyon: IARC press; 2010.

Carter D, Russell RCG, Pitt HA, Bismuth H, editors. Rob and Smith's operative surgery: hepatobiliary and pancreatic surgery. 5th ed. London: Chapman and Hall; 1996.

Day DW, Jass JR, Price AB, Shepherd NA, Sloan JM, Talbot IC, Warren BF, Williams GT. Morson and Dawson's gastrointestinal pathology. 4th ed. Oxford: Blackwell Sciences; 2003.

Kakar S, Burgart LJ. Tumours of the biliary system. Curr Diagn Pathol. 2005;11:34–43.

Mann CV, Russell RCG, Williams NS, editors. Bailey & Love's short practice of surgery. 22nd ed. London: Chapman and Hall Medical; 1995.

Odze RD, Goldblum JR. Surgical pathology of the GI tract, liver, biliary tract and pancreas. 2nd ed. Philadelphia: Saunders/Elsevier; 2009.

Wittekind CF, Greene FL, Hutter RVP, Klimpfinger M, Sobib LH. TNM atlas: illustrated guide to the TNM/ pTNM classification of malignant tumours. 5th ed. Berlin: Springer; 2005.

Liver Carcinoma

Primary liver cancer is the sixth commonest cause of cancer worldwide and second commonest cancer in Asia and the fourth in Africa. Hepatocellular carcinoma is the most frequent subtype (90 %). Risk factors are chronic viral infection (hepatitis B(HBV), hepatitis C(HCV)), alcohol, tobacco, aflatoxin ingestion, and in Western society cirrhosis due to various causes e.g. alcohol, alpha-1-antitrypsin deficiency, and haemochromatosis. There is a rising incidence of hepatocellular carcinoma in Europe and the USA due to the increasing prevalence of chronic liver disease e.g. HCV, non-alcoholic fatty liver disease. Some 50–90 % of cases arise in a background of cirrhosis, the presence of cirrhosis or advanced fibrosis being an indicator of an "unstable liver" and a contraindication to resection as it is a predictor of local recurrence.

Intrahepatic cholangiocarcinoma forms a minority of primary liver cancers and risk factors include long standing ulcerative colitis, particularly when associated with primary sclerosing cholangitis.

Liver disease can be asymptomatic until relatively late in the disease course. Otherwise presentation of hepatic malignancy may be with jaundice, weight loss, anaemia and anorexia. There can be right upper quadrant pain or a palpable mass and investigations include serum alpha-fetoprotein (AFP) and CA19-9, liver function tests and imaging studies. Diagnosis of hepatocellular carcinoma is usually based on a combination of elevated (>400 ng/ml) or continuously rising serum AFP levels and appropriate radiological features obviating the need for biopsy. Cholangiocarcinoma is diagnosed by demonstration of obstruction and distortion of the intrahepatic bile duct system usually by magnetic resonance cholangiography (MRC). Suspected metastatic colorectal or pancreatic cancer may have an appropriate past history and raised serum CEA and CA19-9 tumour markers. CT/PET scan is of use in distinguishing metabolically active tumour from benign or necrotic mass lesions. Where metastases or a primary hepatocellular carcinoma are potentially resectable, or transplant is considered, there is a reluctance to carry out fine needle aspiration (FNA)/needle biopsy for fear of upstaging the tumour e.g. needle tract implantation (1–2 % of cases). However in the absence of a significantly elevated serum AFP or other obvious primary site targeted needle biopsy (percutaneous or transjugular) under USS/CT scan guidance may be needed for a firm tissue diagnosis and to exclude other treatable tumours e.g. malignant lymphoma. Needle biopsy yields either a positive diagnosis or the changes adjacent to a mass lesion i.e. liver plate atrophy, prominent sinusoids and focal inflammation.

Transjugular cores are very fine and require careful handling in the laboratory. However they can produce useful morphological and immunohistochemical results if the tumour is in a suitably accessible location. Some of the potential upstaging risks are also obviated if a percutaneous route is avoided.

Hepatic resection in malignant disease is dependent on careful patient selection and is potentially considered for

Fig. 10.1 Liver and regional lymph nodes (Reproduced, with permission, from Wittekind et al. (2005), © 2005)

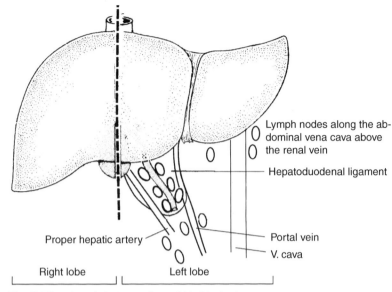

Lymph nodes along the ab-dominal vena cava above the renal vein

Hepatoduodenal ligament

Proper hepatic artery

Portal vein

V. cava

Right lobe   Left lobe

The dividing plane is between the gall bladder bed and inferior vena cava

The regional lymph nodes are the hilar, hepatic (along the proper hepatic artery), periportal (along the portal vein) nodes and those along the abdominal inferior vena cava above the renal vein (except the inferior phrenic nodes).

- Primary liver tumour involving a single lobe with no invasion of portal vein or inferior vena cava and no significant background cirrhosis. Also one lesion <5 cm or up to three lesions <3 cm.
- Isolated metastases (e.g. well differentiated neuroendocrine (carcinoid) tumour, colorectal carcinoma) localised to a single lobe with no metastatic spread elsewhere, and adequate excision of the primary lesion. More recently this criterion has been extended to include multiple hepatic metastases provided resection is technically feasible leaving sufficient functioning hepatic remnant. Use of neoadjuvant chemotherapy, intravascular chemoembolisation or radiofrequency ablation can facilitate operative resection or be used in a palliative setting by down sizing the tumour deposits. Patient fitness must also be taken into account, but in patients with colorectal cancer and low volume metastatic disease 40 % 5 year survival can be achieved by metastasectomy. Diagnostic and staging assessment of patients for liver resection of primary and metastatic cancer is performed by regional or network specialist teams.

Depending on the anatomical extent of disease as determined by MRI/CT/ultrasound scans the resection can be major (partial hepatectomy, lobectomy) or segmental, the latter excised with its supplying lymphovascular pedicle. Note that the surgical definition of lobes and their constituent segments differs from the classical anatomical lobes. Small subcapsular metastases of carcinoma can be removed by open or laparoscopic non-anatomical wedge resection, or erroneously diagnosed as such at frozen section during radical cancer surgery due to mimicry by a bile duct adenoma or Von Meyenberg complex (Fig. 10.1).

10.1 Gross Description

Specimen

- FNAC (fine needle aspiration cytology)/core biopsy/wedge excision/segmentectomy/partial hepatectomy/R/L lobectomy.
- Size (cm) and weight (g).

Tumour

Site

- Subcapsular/parenchymal/ductocentric/vasculocentric/lobe/multifocal (particularly when cirrhosis is present).

Size

- Length × width × depth (cm) or maximum dimension (cm).
- In a cirrhotic liver a solid irregular lesion >5 cm diameter is probably a hepatocellular carcinoma.
- The diffuse, periductal pattern of cholangiocarcinoma often shows microscopic infiltration beyond its clinical macroscopic extent.

Appearance

- Hepatocellular carcinoma: solitary/nodular/diffuse/multifocal (particularly in cirrhosis)/bile stained/venous spread/pedunculated/encapsulated/background cirrhosis/haemochromatosis. The cancer often shows a mosaic of macroscopic patterns.
- Cholangiocarcinoma: papillary/nodular/stenotic/scirrhous/ductocentric/multifocal.
- Metastatic carcinoma:single/multiple/necrotic/umbilicated/calcification/diffuse/mucoid/subcapsular.

Edge

- Circumscribed/irregular.

10.2 Histological Type

Hepatocellular Carcinoma

- *Trabecular*, *plate like or sinusoidal*.
- *Pseudoglandular* (*acinar*).
- These are the *usual types* comprising hepatoid cells, bile cytoplasmic staining and canalicular plugging, eosinophilic intranuclear pseudoinclusions, and a sinusoidal vascular pattern with a CD34 positive endothelial lining (capillarisation).
- *Solid* (*compact*): inconspicuous sinusoids.
- *Scirrhous*: fibrotic. Distinguish from cholangiocarcinoma and post chemo-/radiotherapy changes.

- *Rarely*: pleomorphic, clear cell, spindle cell, lymphoepithelial (EBV positive) or osteoclast like.
- *Variants with good prognosis*: fibrolamellar carcinoma (90 % <25 years old); pedunculated carcinoma; minute, small or encapsulated carcinoma (see Sect. 10.8.).

Intrahepatic Cholangiocarcinoma

- *5–15 % of primary liver cancers*. Usually *mass forming* (single/multifocal/peripheral), *periductal infiltrative* (perihilar tumours/scirrhous) or *intraductal* (papillary: rare in the West).
- *Ductulo-acinar pattern* of heterogeneous cuboidal to columnar mucin secreting cells in a fibrous stroma with a hyalinised sclerotic hypocellular centre and more cellular periphery. Sometimes papillary.
- *Portal expansion/periportal sleeve like* and *parenchymal sinusoidal* distributions.
- Few survive longer than 2–3 years due to late presentation and limited resectability.
- *Rarely*: mucinous; signet ring cell; adenosquamous; clear cell; pleomorphic; osteoclast like; spindle cell (sarcomatoid). These are prognostically adverse variants.

Combined Hepatocellular/ Cholangiocarcinoma

- *1 % of cases*. Mixed phenotypes of usual morphology and immunohistochemical expression, with foci of intermediate character.

Hepatoblastoma

- 50–60 % of childhood liver cancers, 90 % are <5 years of age.
- Usually a large solitary mass and raised serum AFP. Epithelial component of two cell types (fetal/embryonal hepatocytes or small cell anaplastic) and fibrous mesenchyme (25 % of cases: osteoid or undifferentiated spindle cells). Treatment is neoadjuvant chemotherapy to shrink the tumour and then surgery with a 50–70 % long term survival. Age <1 year, large size and a significant small cell component are adverse factors.

Metastatic Carcinoma

- *In order of frequency*: secondary carcinoma (breast, colorectum, pancreas, stomach, lung), neuroendocrine tumour (pancreas) and malignant melanoma. Malignant lymphoma and sarcoma (except metastatic GIST) are uncommon although diffuse large B cell malignant lymphoma and granulocytic sarcoma (myeloid leukaemia) can form single or multiple mass lesions mimicking metastatic carcinoma.
- *Direct spread*: stomach, colorectum, pancreas, gall bladder and biliary tree.
- *Distant spread*: stomach, oesophagus, colorectum, lung, breast, malignant melanoma, kidney, urinary bladder, ovary, teratoma.

The *tumour distribution* and *appearance* may reflect its origin e.g.

- Colorectum: multiple, large nodules with central necrosis and umbilication, ± mucin, ± calcification. As in renal cell carcinoma can be solitary and massive.
- Gall bladder: the bulk of disease is centred on the gall bladder bed.
- Lung: medium sized nodules and fleshy appearance (small cell carcinoma).
- Breast, stomach: medium sized nodules or diffuse cirrhotic like pattern of sinusoidal infiltration.
- Malignant melanoma: pigmented.
- Angiosarcoma, choriocarcinoma, leiomyosarcoma, renal/thyroid carcinoma, gastrointestinal neuroendocrine tumours, GIST: haemorrhagic/cystic.

Note that *carcinoma rarely metastasises to a cirrhotic liver*, i.e. the tumour is more likely to be a primary liver cancer. Histologically there can be considerable difficulty distinguishing hepatocellular carcinoma and its variants from other metastases e.g. neuroendocrine tumour, renal cell carcinoma, adrenal cortical carcinoma and malignant melanoma. Similarly cholangiocarcinoma (look for adjacent BilIN/mucosal dysplasia) from gastrointestinal secondaries. *Morphology allied to a panel of antibodies* should be used including:

Hepatocellular – Hep Par 1, AFP, canalicular polyclonal CEA/CD 10.

Adrenal – inhibin, melan-A, vimentin, synaptophysin.

Renal – EMA, vimentin, RCCab, CD10, pax8.

Colorectum – CK20, CDX-2.

Lung adenocarcinoma – CK7, TTF-1, napsin A.

Malignant melanoma – S100, HMB-45, melan-A.

GIST – DOG-1, CD117.

Neuroendocrine tumours – chromogranin A, synaptophysin, CD56(±), Ki-67, CDX-2 (from gastrointestinal tract), TTF-1 (from lung).

Resection of hepatic metastases: can be done to good effect e.g. well differentiated endocrine (carcinoid) tumour, colorectal carcinoma. Tumour macroscopic and microscopic appearances may be altered by preoperative ablative or neoadjuvant therapy. Extensive sampling is required to establish response which can be assessed as complete, incomplete or absent. *Tumour regression* is often accompanied by a histiocytic and fibrous reaction with mucin lakes. The *number of metastatic deposits and clearance of metastasectomy surgical margins are prognostically significant* although equivocal margins are often obliterated by operative diathermy and haemostasis techniques.

Hepatic mass lesions at clinical follow up: a common issue at specialty multidisciplinary team meetings is the finding of a solitary (or several) liver lesion(s) on CT scan staging or post treatment follow up of a cancer originating from various primary sites. A circumscribed hypodense, or, characteristic appearance may allow the radiologist to designate simple cysts or specific entities such as haemangioma with confidence. *Indeterminate lesions can be monitored for size and contour change with time.* Irregularity of edge or content signal is more worrying for a metastatic deposit and *further characterisation* can be sought with *MRI* and *CT/PET scans*. This is correlated with *serum tumour marker levels* e.g. CEA, CA125, CA19-9. Ultimately, if radiologically accessible, a *tissue diagnosis* may be desirable either by FNAC or core biopsy, as a basis for proceeding to further surgical or medical oncological treatment. Importantly *new pathology* can also be excluded e.g. a patient with previously treated colorectal cancer developing metastatic pancreatic neuroendocrine tumour rather than colorectal metastases, or a mass forming diffuse large B cell malignant lymphoma.

10.3   Differentiation/Grade

For hepatocellular carcinoma well/moderate/poor, or, Edmonson/Steiner Grade I/II/III/IV.

This is based on the degree of *resemblance to hepatic tissue*. Well differentiated (GI/II)

Fig. 10.2 Hepatocellular carcinoma (Reproduced, with permission, from Wittekind et al. (2005), © 2005)

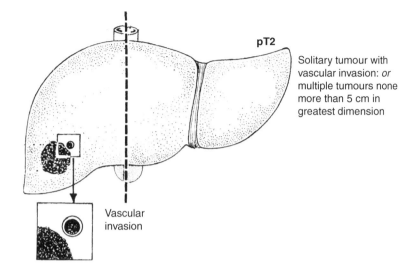

pT2

Solitary tumour with vascular invasion: *or* multiple tumours none more than 5 cm in greatest dimension

Vascular invasion

hepatocellular carcinomas resemble a dysplastic nodule in cirrhosis, or an adenoma in non-cirrhotics. Poorly differentiated (GIV) cancers are not recognisably hepatic in character, requiring more usual foci, appropriate immunophenotype and raised serum AFP. Well to moderately differentiated lesions show trabecular (plate like) or pseudoglandular patterns seen in tumours <2–3 cm diameter. Larger lesions (>3 cm) usually only have a well differentiated periphery, with a less differentiated centre characterised by greater cytoarchitectural atypia and no discernable sinusoids. This nodule within nodule appearance is diagnostically useful and highlights the heterogeneity and active evolution of hepatocellular carcinoma. Tumour grade in a preoperative biopsy can predict patient survival.

For cholangiocarcinoma based on the percentage tumour gland formation: well/G1 >95 %: moderate/G2 50–95 %: poor/G3 <50 %: undifferentiated/G4 no glands.

It is recognised that hepatocellular carcinoma and cholangiocarcinoma form a morphological spectrum with origin from a common progenitor stem cell. Mixed cancers can therefore occur.

10.4   Extent of Local Tumour Spread

Border: pushing/infiltrative.
Lymphocytic reaction: prominent/sparse.
Invasion through the hepatic (Glisson's) capsule.

The TNM7 classification distinguishes between hepatocellular carcinoma and intrahepatic cholangiocarcinoma.

Hepatocellular Carcinoma

pT1	Solitary tumour with no vascular invasion
pT2	Solitary tumour with vascular invasion or multiple tumours, none >5 cm
pT3	Multiple tumours >5 cm (pT3a) or tumour involving a major branch of the portal or hepatic vein(s) (pT3b)
pT4	Tumour with direct invasion of adjacent organs other than the gall bladder or with perforation of visceral peritoneum

Vascular invasion is diagnosed by clinical imaging. The pathological classification includes gross and histological involvement. Criteria are: location within a portal tract appropriate to the site of a portal vein, an identifiable lumen and endothelial lining.

Multiple tumours includes multiple independent primaries or intrahepatic metastases from a single hepatic carcinoma. A *multicentric distribution* is associated with a *poor prognosis* (Figs. 10.2, 10.3, 10.4, 10.5 and 10.6).

Intrahepatic Cholangiocarcinoma

pT1	Solitary tumour without vascular invasion
pT2	Solitary tumour with vascular invasion (pT2a) or multiple tumour deposits with or without vascular invasion (pT2b)

Fig. 10.3 Hepatocellular
carcinoma (Reproduced,
with permission, from
Wittekind et al. (2005),
© 2005)

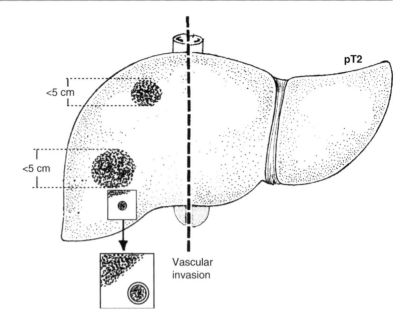

Fig. 10.4 Hepatocellular
carcinoma (Reproduced,
with permission, from
Wittekind et al. (2005),
© 2005)

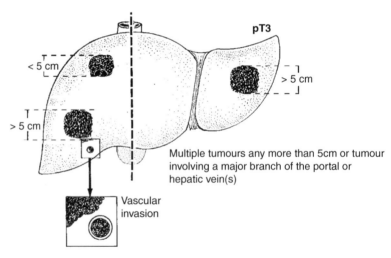

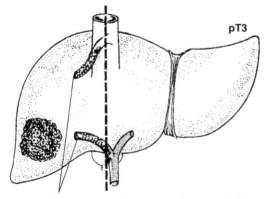

Major branch of the portal or hepatic vein(s)

Fig. 10.5 Hepatocellular carcinoma (Reproduced, with
permission, from Wittekind et al. (2005), © 2005)

Fig. 10.6 Hepatocellular carcinoma (Reproduced, with permission, from Wittekind et al. (2005), © 2005)

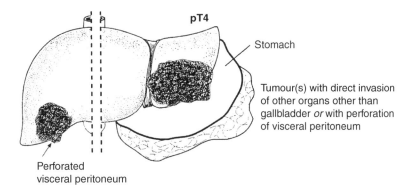

pT4

Stomach

Tumour(s) with direct invasion of other organs other than gallbladder *or* with perforation of visceral peritoneum

Perforated visceral peritoneum

pT3	Tumour perforates the visceral peritoneum or directly invades adjacent extrahepatic structures
pT4	Tumour with periductal invasion (periductal growth pattern).

Cholangiocarcinoma can be *mass forming* directly invading the adjacent liver parenchyma, *periductal* infiltrating along portal pedicles, or, rarely shows *ductal intraluminal spread*.

10.5   Lymphovascular Invasion

Present/absent.

Intra-/ extratumoural.

Note the particular propensity for *vascular invasion by hepatocellular carcinoma* to involve portal tract veins, major branches of portal and hepatic veins and inferior vena cava, ultimately with metastases to lung (47 %), adrenal gland (12 %) and bone (37 %).

Cholangiocarcinoma typically shows *lymphovascular and perineural invasion* with spread to regional lymph nodes, lungs, bone, adrenal gland, kidney, pancreas and peritoneum.

10.6   Lymph Nodes

Site/number/size/number involved/limit node/extracapsular spread.

Regional nodes: hilar (hepatoduodenal ligament), hepatic (along the hepatic artery), periportal (along portal vein) and those along the inferior vena cava above the renal veins. For cholangiocarcinoma also the periduodenal, peripancreatic and gastrohepatic lymph nodes whereas periaortic,

pericaval, superior mesenteric and coeliac lymph nodes are distant metastases (pM1). For primary liver cancers a regional lymphadenectomy will ordinarily include three or more lymph nodes. In cholangiocarcinoma lymph node metastases are often microscopic and subcapsular requiring careful scrutiny of serial slices of the lymph nodes.

pN0	No regional lymph node metastasis
pN1	Metastasis in regional lymph node(s).

10.7   Excision Margins

Distances (mm) to the limits of excision of parenchyma, bile ducts and veins. Microscopic involvement (R1) is generally regarded as tumour clearance <1 mm.

Mucosal dysplasia (BilIN) at the bile duct excision limits.

10.8   Other Pathology

Budd Chiari Syndrome

Veno-occlusion or small/large calibre hepatic venular obstruction secondary to malignant infiltration and thrombosis. It leads to hepatic ischaemia.

Hepatocellular Carcinoma

Risk factors: *Hepatitis B and C*: in 50–70 and 20–30 % of cases respectively, world-wide. Seropositive hepatitis B patients have ×*100 risk* of developing hepatocellular carcinoma.

Cirrhosis: its extent is assessed clinically by the Child-Pugh score and it is present in *60–80 %* of cases in the West secondary to viral hepatitis, alcohol, congenital bile duct atresia, alpha-1-antitrypsin deficiency or haemochromatosis.

Small/large cell liver cell change or dysplasia: a microscopic finding and usually <1 mm, there is a strong association between large cell change and hepatitis B surface antigen. *Small cell change* (enlarged nucleus, decreased volume of cytoplasm, nuclear crowding) is regarded as being *premalignant* and a more important risk factor for the development of carcinoma. Liver nodules can be macroregenerative, focal nodular hyperplasia like, or dysplastic.

Dysplastic nodules: arise in a background of cirrhosis and range from 1 mm to 2–3 cm diameter (usually 5–15 mm), ± a fibrous rim, and variable cytoarchitectural atypia (plates 3 cells thick, irregular edges, loss of reticulin, ± cellular dysplasia, arterialisation, increased Ki-67 proliferation index). They show a spectrum of changes towards hepatocellular carcinoma with *type 2* (*high-grade dysplastic*) *nodules* particularly significant. Increasingly sophisticated radiological imaging is leading to greater detection of these premalignant dysplastic nodules and small, early hepatocellular carcinomas. Nodules <1 cm require reassessment by 3–6 month interval ultrasound. Nodules 1–2 cm in size are treated as hepatocellular carcinoma if there is typical hypervascularity and portal venous phase wash out on dynamic imaging (CT/MRI scan or contrast enhanced US). If the radiological investigations are inconsistent biopsy may be required. Nodules >2 cm in size with characteristic imaging findings do not require biopsy as a presumptive diagnosis of malignancy can be made.

Immunophenotype: hepatocellular carcinoma is positive for Hep Par 1 (86 %), AFP (37 %: high specificity but low sensitivity) and polyclonal CEA/CD 10 in bile canaliculi. Also CAM 5.2 (but not AE1/AE3), cytokeratins 8, 18 (but not 7,19), ER/PR. PAS positive cytoplasmic glycogen, intracellular PAS positive globular inclusions, loss of pericellular reticulin. EMA, Ber EP4 negative. Also positive for glypican 3, HSP70, glutamine synthetase one protein and nuclear Ki-67.

Cholangiocarcinoma

Risk factors: *hepatolithiasis/primary sclerosing cholangitis/ulcerative colitis/liver fluke/biliary tree anomaly.* Arises from flat mucosal dysplasia or BilIN – rarely from an intraductal papillary neoplasm (previously designated as biliary papillomatosis). *Treatment is surgical* (partial/total hepatic resection ± liver transplantation) but often *palliative* with stenting to relieve obstructive jaundice as prognosis is poor and overall *mean survival is <2 years.*

Immunophenotype: cytokeratins (7,19), EMA, CEA, CA19-9, mucin positive. Also CAM 5.2 (low molecular weight cytokeratins, as for hepatocellular carcinoma) and AE1/AE3 (including high molecular weight cytokeratins, negative in hepatocellular carcinoma).

Differential Diagnosis of Hepatic Mass Lesions

Focal nodular hyperplasia: the commonest benign liver nodule after cavernous haemangioma. It occurs in young to middle aged women, is usually solitary, <5 cm diameter and asymptomatic. It has a radiological and gross central scar devoid of bile ducts with thick walled vessels, marginal ductular proliferation, plates 2 or 3 cells thick, and is a cirrhosis like nodule with adjacent normal parenchyma. It is a vascular anomaly representing an area of hyperplastic liver due to hyperperfusion by an anomalous artery.

Hepatocellular adenoma: 5–15 cm diameter in middle aged women sometimes with an acute haemorrhagic abdominal presentation and history of oral contraception (60 %), obesity or diabetes mellitus (both 30 %). It has no portal tracts or central veins, shows unaccompanied arteries, liver cell plates ≥2 cells thick with retention of reticulin pattern and sinusoidal Kupffer cells (CD 68 positive). It comprises steatotic, inflammatory and unclassified variants.

Hepatocellular carcinoma: there is often evidence of risk factors e.g. cirrhosis. Plates are >2–3 cells thick, show loss of reticulin pattern and Kupffer cells, sinusoid capillarisation

(CD34), cellular atypia, and look for stromal, capsular and vascular invasion. Serum AFP is markedly elevated in 40 % of cases. CT/MRI scan shows the location of the lesion, its extent of invasion and multicentric distribution.

Poorly differentiated metastatic carcinoma: specific histological appearance (e.g. small cell carcinoma lung), immunogenicity (e.g. PSA positive) or histochemical feature (e.g. mucin positive – this cannot distinguish secondary adenocarcinoma from primary cholangiocarcinoma).

Problematic cases: sometimes the distinction between a regenerative nodule, adenoma and well differentiated hepatocellular carcinoma is not possible and the subsequent *clinical course* establishes the diagnosis. FNAC of hepatic mass lesions is useful for simple cysts, abscesses and some metastatic cancers (e.g. small cell lung carcinoma). Secondary adenocarcinoma cannot always be distinguished from cholangiocarcinoma and previous history is important e.g. resection for colorectal carcinoma. Differential cytokeratin expression may help: colorectal cancer (CK20+/CK7−), cholangiocarcinoma (CK7, 19+/CK20 ±). FNAC is reasonably robust for moderately differentiated hepatocellular carcinoma but needs to be supplemented by core/open biopsy in poorly differentiated carcinomas (to exclude metastatic cancers) and well differentiated lesions (to exclude adenoma, focal nodular hyperplasia, cirrhosis).

Diagnostic features for hepatocellular carcinoma: hepatoid cells (polygonal with central nucleus), nuclear/nucleolar enlargement, a trabecular pattern with sinusoidal capillarisation, nuclear pseudoinclusions, bile secretion and an absence of bile duct epithelial and inflammatory cells. Immunostaining may also be helpful e.g. AFP/polyclonal CEA/CD10/CD34/glypican 3 positive and CK7/19 negative for hepatocellular carcinoma.

Prognosis

Treatment of hepatocellular carcinoma depends on *surgical resection ± liver transplantation* the latter treating the underlying causative disease. *Local resection of carefully selected patients has a* *50 % 5 year survival rate but a 70 % recurrence rate*. Small tumours may also be successfully treated by *high radiofrequency ablation (RFA)*. *Chemotherapy* is used for recurrent or inoperable tumours with new agents emerging combined with adjuvant radiotherapy. Prognosis relates to tumour size (>5 cm), cell type or differentiation, encapsulation, multifocality, high serum AFP levels (>100 ng/ml at diagnosis), vascular invasion and the presence or absence of a background cirrhosis (an adverse indicator). *Five year survival is at most 10–15 % and more usually about 3 %*. The majority die within several months of presentation with liver failure, haemorrhage and infection. Small tumours (<3–5 cm) and variants such as fibrolamellar and pedunculated carcinoma are potentially curable (see below). In cases that are resected tumour stage and resection margin status are important prognostic indicators. *Hepatic arterial chemoembolisation*, *percutaneous alcohol injection* and *radiofrequency ablation* also have roles to play with potential survival benefit and easing of pain in non-operable disease. These modalities can also be applicable to metastatic deposits in the liver e.g. colorectal carcinoma. *Cholangiocarcinoma* is an *aggressive disease* with early invasion, widespread metastases, late presentation and ineffectual treatment modalities. A mass forming tumour has a more favourable outlook (39 % 5 year survivial) than a periductal infiltrating type lesion with few patients surviving beyond 2–3 years.

Fibrolamellar Carcinoma

- Large eosinophilic cells in a fibrous stroma, potentially resectable.
- 50 % cure rate.
- Serum AFP is not raised, and there is no cirrhosis. May also have areas of usual liver cell carcinoma and cholangiocarcinoma.
- Can express CK7,19.

Pedunculated Carcinoma

- Inferoanterior aspect right lobe, up to 1 kg weight.

Minute, Small Encapsulated Carcinoma

- 2–5 cm, encapsulated by fibrous tissue.
- 90–100 % 5 year survival if no angio-invasion.

10.9   Other Malignancy

Malignant Lymphoma/Leukaemia

- Secondary involvement by *Hodgkin's/non-Hodgkin's malignant lymphoma* (50–60 % of cases) or *leukaemia* (80 % of CLL cases). *Malignant lymphoma is mainly portal* and *leukaemia sinusoidal* but mixed patterns of distribution are common.
- Primary malignant lymphoma is rare but of more favourable prognosis. Solitary/multiple masses or diffuse and *high-grade large B cell* in type. Associated with hepatitis C infection, HIV and primary biliary cirrhosis.

Angiosarcoma

- Cirrhosis, PVC, thorotrast exposure, the *commonest liver sarcoma*.
- Exclude peliosis (well-differentiated angiosarcoma) and primary and secondary carcinoma (poorly differentiated angiosarcoma).
- Growth is typically along vascular structures (sinusoids, vessels) and the liver cell plates. The endothelial cells are atypical and CD31/34 positive.

Epithelioid Haemangioendothelioma

- Multinodular fibrous masses with a zoned periphery of cords and tube like structures of spindle and epithelioid cells in myxoid stroma and a central hyalinised scar. *Paranuclear cytoplasmic vacuoles, CD31 positive.*
- Associated with Budd Chiari syndrome.
- Of *low to intermediate-grade malignancy*: also seen in *skin, lung and bone*.

Kaposi's Sarcoma

- AIDS (15–20 % of fatal cases).

Embryonal Sarcoma

- 15 % 5 year survival in patients of 6–10 years of age.Spindle/stellate/pleomorphic/rounded cells.

Embryonal Rhabdomyosarcoma

- <5 years of age, poor prognosis although changing with emerging neoadjuvant therapies and aggressive surgery. Desmin/myo D1/myogenin positive small cells in a cellular subepithelial cambium layer.
- Arises from major bile ducts near the porta hepatis.

Leiomyosarcoma, Fibrosarcoma

- Rare. More often represents spread from a retroperitoneal primary.
- Exclude sarcomatoid liver carcinoma, and, more commonly secondary sarcoma e.g. GIST.

Well Differentiated Neuroendocrine (Carcinoid) Tumour

- Usually represents metastases from gastrointestinal tract or pancreas. Associated with carcinoid syndrome. Detected clinically by octreotide or CT scans.

Mimics of Malignancy

- *Abscess* secondary to ascending cholangitis, portal pyaemia or septicaemia, *cavernous haemangioma*, *sclerosed haemangioma*, *inflammatory myofibroblastic or pseudotumour* (spindle cells in a storiform pattern, plasma cells), *PEComa/angiomyolipoma* (fat, dystrophic vessels, HMB 45 positive spindle cells, coexisting renal lesion(s)), *solitary fibrous tumour* (storiform spindle cells, CD34 positive).

Bibliography

Anthony PP. Hepatocellular carcinoma: an overview. Histopathology. 2001;39:109–18.

Beckingham IJ, editor. ABC of liver, pancreas and gall bladder diseases. London: BMJ Books; 2001.

Bellamy COC, Maxwell RS, Prost S, Azodo IA, Powell JJ, Manning JR. The value of immunophenotyping hepatocellular adenomas: consecutive resections at one UK centre. Histopathology. 2013;62:431–45.

Burt AD, Portmann BC, Ferrell LD. MacSween's pathology of the liver. 5th ed. Edinburgh/New York: Churchill Livingstone; 2007.

Carter D, Russell RCG, Pitt HA, Bismuth H, editors. Rob and Smith's operative surgery: hepatobiliary and pancreatic surgery. 5th ed. London: Chapman and Hall; 1996.

Ishak KG, Goodman ZD, Stocker JT. Tumors of the liver and intrahepatic bile ducts. Atlas of tumor pathology. 3rd series. Fascicle 31. Washington: AFIP; 2001.

Kumagi T, Hiasa Y, Hirschfield GM. Hepatocellular carcinoma for the non-specialist. BMJ. 2009;339:1366–70.

Leong TYM, Wannakrairot P, Lee ES, Leong ASY. Pathology of cholangiocarcinoma. Curr Diagn Pathol. 2007;13:54–64.

Paterson AC, Cooper K. Tumours and tumour-like lesions of the hepatic parenchyma. Curr Diagn Pathol. 2005;11:19–53.

Quaglia A, Battacharjya S, Dhillon P. Limitations of the histopathological diagnosis and prognostic assessment of hepatocellular carcinoma. Histopathology. 2001; 38:167–74.

Ryder S. Predicting survival in early hepatocellular carcinoma. Gut. 2005;54:328–9.

Scheuer PJ, Lefkowitch JH. Liver biopsy interpretation. 8th ed. London: Saunders/Elsevier; 2010.

The Royal College of Pathologists: Cancer Datasets (Oesophageal Carcinoma, Gastric Carcinoma, Carcinomas of the Pancreas, ampulla of Vater and Common Bile Duct, Colorectal Cancer, Gastrointestinal Stromal Tumours (GISTs), Liver Resection Specimens and Liver Biopsies for Primary and Metastatic Carcinoma, Endocrine Tumours of the Gastrointestinal Tract including Pancreas) and Tissue Pathways (Gastrointestinal and Pancreatobiliary Pathology, Liver Biopsies for the Investigation of Medical Disease and for Focal Liver Lesions). Accessed at http://www.rcpath.org/index.asp?PageID=254.

Wittekind CF, Greene FL, Hutter RVP, Klimpfinger M, Sobib LH. TNM atlas: illustrated guide to the TNM/pTNM classification of malignant tumours. 5th ed. Berlin: Springer; 2005.

- Lip and Oral Cavity Carcinomas
- Oropharyngeal Carcinoma (with Comments on Nasopharynx and Hypopharynx)
- Nasal Cavity and Paranasal Sinus Carcinomas
- Laryngeal Carcinoma
- Salivary Gland Tumours
- Thyroid Gland Tumours (with Comments on Parathyroid)

1.1 General Comments

See: Royal College of Pathologists. Datasets for histopathology reporting of mucosal malignancies of: oral cavity, pharynx, larynx, nasal cavities and paranasal sinuses, salivary neoplasms, nodal excisions and neck dissection specimens associated with head and neck carcinomas, thyroid gland and parathyroid gland. Accessed at http://www.rcpath.org/publications-media/publications/datasets/datasets-TP.htm

Basic rules are applied to carcinomas arising at various sites in the upper aerodigestive tract (lip, oral cavity, pharynx, nasal cavity, paranasal sinuses and larynx), 95 % of which are squamous cell carcinoma.

The surgeon should mark clinically relevant resection margins in the primary specimen and lymph node territories in neck dissections.

Prognosis

Prognosis and prediction of response to adjuvant radiation and/or chemo-therapy relate to carcinoma:

Type

- e.g. Keratinising squamous cell carcinoma versus undifferentiated naso-pharyngeal carcinoma. This also influences treatment modality e.g. surgery in the former, chemo-/radiotherapy in the latter.

Grade

- The majority are moderately differentiated but identify well and poorly differentiated lesions. Base the tumour grade on the most aggressive area (medium magnification field).

Size

- Maximum diameter (mm): macroscopic or microscopic, whichever is greater.

Depth

- Maximum depth of invasion (mm) below the luminal aspect of the surface measured from the extrapolated level of the adjacent mucosa. At least one block per cm diameter of the tumour is required and the whole lesion is submitted if less than 1 cm in maximum dimension. For large tumours an estimate of depth may be an approximation.

Invasive Edge

- A cohesive versus non-cohesive pattern of infiltration. The latter equates to single cells, small groups or multiple thin (<15 cells across) strands of cells at the deep aspect of the tumour. It is of worse prognosis than an invasive border comprising broad cohesive sheets of tumour cells.

Margins of Excision

>5 mm	Clear
1–5 mm	Close to; also a high risk of recurrence if the invasive edge is non-cohesive or shows vascular invasion
<1 mm	Involved.

Incomplete excision is associated with a significantly increased risk of local recurrence. Note also the presence of severe dysplasia at the resection edge – if present to within 5 mm it can also predict likelihood of local recurrence.

Lymphovascular and Perineural Spread

- Vascular invasion is a relatively weak predictor of cervical lymph node metastases. Perineural invasion is an indicator of more aggressive disease, local recurrence and lymph node metastases.

Bone Invasion

- Distinguish erosion of the cortex from infiltration of the medulla. Bone involvement is important for accurate staging.

Lymph Node Status

- The number identified and *number involved* at each anatomical level of the neck dissection (Fig. 1). The number of involved nodes affects TNM staging – the pattern of involvement influences postoperative treatment. A typical radial neck dissection without previous chemotherapy or radiotherapy should yield an average of 20 lymph nodes. Isolated tumour nodules in the connective tissue are regarded as lymph node metastases unless within 10 mm of the main tumour where they may represent discontinuous extension.
- An important prognostic factor is involvement of the *lower cervical lymph nodes*, that is level IV (lower jugular chain deep to the lower one-third of sternocleidomastoid muscle) and level V (posterior triangle of neck behind the posterior border of sternocleidomastoid).
- The *maximum dimension* of the largest nodal deposit is a determinant in TNM staging.
- *Extracapsular spread:* if present prompts the use of adjuvant radiotherapy.
- The significance of *micrometastases* is uncertain but should be counted as involved.
- *Persistent cervical lymph node enlargement* in an older patient is commonly malignant due to either malignant lymphoma or metastases. The latter are generally due to head and neck tumours particularly mucosal squamous cell carcinomas, malignant melanoma of skin and thyroid gland carcinoma. Pharyngeal and laryngeal lesions should also be considered and once a tissue diagnosis has been obtained by fine needle aspiration cytology (FNAC), panendoscopy of the upper aerodigestive tract is undertaken to establish and biopsy the primary site, and, to exclude the possibility (10 % of cases) of a synchronous cancer e.g. oesophagus. CT, MRI, and CT/PET scans and thyroid ultrasound are also used for investigation and staging. A small minority (10 %) can be due to metastatic spread of non-head and neck cancers e.g. lung, stomach, prostate or testis. Patients can present with their metastatic disease the occult primary being in the nasopharynx, posterior one third of tongue, tonsil or hypopharynx. Positivity of the lymph node metastasis for p16 and HPV in situ hybridisation may indicate an oropharyngeal origin, and EBER positivity a nasopharyngeal primary.

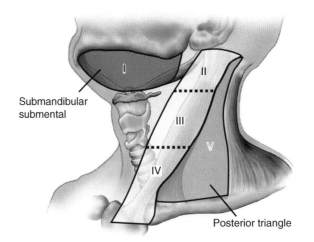

Fig. 1 Lymph node groups in block dissection of the neck (Reproduced, with permission, from Histopathology reporting: guidelines for surgical reporting, 2nd ed., © 2006, Springer)

- *Neck dissection* is either *therapeutic* (to remove metastases) or *elective* in a clinically negative neck to avoid the 20 % risk of this future possibility. Alternatively a *'watch and wait' policy* is followed or elective *irradiation* of the neck. This decision will depend on the risk factors present, age, and fitness of the patient. *Extent of resection* relates to the tumour type, site and expected pattern of spread and is usually more limited (selective neck dissection e.g. levels I–II or II–IV) in elective cases. Oral and oropharyngeal cancers tend to spread to levels I–IV lymph nodes, laryngeal and hypopharyngeal to levels II and III. Therapeutic dissection (comprehensive/radical or modified radical, levels I–V ± sternomastoid, internal jugular vein, spinal accessory nerve and submandibular gland) aims to give maximum disease clearance where there are large (>6 cm) and/or multiple deposits, extranodal spread or recurrent disease. Positive lymph nodes (≥2) and/or the presence of extracapsular spread in the resection warrant *postoperative radiotherapy*. Head and neck cancer specimens should also be interpreted in the light of any previous radiotherapy or chemotherapy due to potential morphological alterations and tumour regression that may make accurate staging more difficult. The role of sentinel lymph node dissection as a means to avoiding the morbidity associated with neck dissection is currently being evaluated.

Lip and Oral Cavity Carcinomas

Oral cancers comprise 1–2 % of malignancies and are increasing in incidence with ageing populations. Tobacco and alcohol use are multiplicative risk factors for oral cancer which usually occurs in patients between 40 and 60 years of age. Lower socioeconomic classes are also disproportionately affected, and males more often than females.

Pathological lesions present either as a lump, ulcer, or white/red mucosal patches that require biopsy to determine their nature. White/red patches are assessed histologically for the presence of dysplasia – a potentially precancerous lesion. If no carcinoma is present these lesions may be locally excised or ablated by laser or photodynamic therapy. FNAC (fine needle aspiration cytology) may be of help for submucosal masses and to determine if cervical lymphadenopathy is due to metastatic disease. Preoperative investigation of a mass will include direct biopsy, plain x-ray, MRI and CT scans to assess local spread, bone destruction and for the presence of cervical lymph node metastases.

Local wedge excision (± shave excision of the adjacent mucosa) is used for small tumours of the lip and tip/lateral border of the tongue. Hemiglossectomy is indicated for deeply infiltrative cancers, and (sub)total glossectomy for large tumours crossing the midline or involving the posterior one third that have recurred following front line chemoradiotherapy. Sublingual gland is submitted with anterior floor of mouth lesions and superficial gingival tumours require mucosal excision only. Periosteum acts as a barrier to bone spread but where it is demonstrated radiologically rim or hemimandibulectomy may be required. Previous irradiation can disrupt the periosteum increasing bone spread. Adequate demonstration will require decalcification with the overlying soft tissues in place. Where there is proven or likely lymph node metastases an en bloc neck dissection is performed. Thus treatment of the patient is determined by the tumour site, local spread, lymph node metastases, presence of any other synchronous primary lesion and patient fitness. Lip cancer can present early with relatively good prognosis but oral cancer is often late in its presentation with 5 year survival of 50 %.

11.1 Gross Description

Specimen

- FNAC/diagnostic (punch/incisional) or (wedge) excision biopsy/transoral laser resection/resection e.g. glossectomy (hemi-/partial/total)/mandibulectomy/maxillectomy/neck dissection. Specimen orientation by the surgeon is crucial in assessing clearance of resection margins.
- Size (cm) and weight (g).

Tumour

Site
- Lip:
  External upper.
  External lower.
  Commissures.

When the skin is involved if >50 % of the tumour is within the vermillion border the tumour is designated as lip in origin. Otherwise it is a cutaneous lesion associated with longstanding sun exposure.

- Oral cavity:
  Buccal mucosa – lips/cheek/retromolar areas/ bucco-alveolar sulci.
  Upper alveolus and gingiva (upper gum).
  Lower alveolus and gingiva (lower gum).
  Hard palate.
  Tongue – dorsal surface and lateral borders (anterior two thirds); inferior (ventral) surface.
  Floor of mouth.

The *commonest sites* are, in order of decreasing frequency: lip (90 % lower), lateral borders of tongue (35 %), anterior floor of mouth (20 %) and the soft palate complex (soft palate, anterior pillar of fauces and retromolar areas).

Multifocal lesions are not uncommon (*10%*), both synchronous and metachronous, also at other upper aerodigestive sites e.g. oesophagus. Upper aerodigestive tract panendoscopy is performed prior to surgery to identify any occult second primary neoplasm.

Size

- Length × width × depth (cm) or maximum dimension (cm).
- Depth of invasion >4–5 mm is predictive of cervical lymph node metastases for oral pT1/ pT2 carcinomas.
- Large size at presentation is associated with greater local recurrence, lymph node metastases and reduced survival.

Appearance

- Verrucous/warty/nodular/sessile/plaque/ ulcerated.

Edge

- Circumscribed/irregular.

11.2   Histological Type

Squamous Cell Carcinoma

- *90% of cases.*
- Keratinising/non-keratinising.

- Variants:
- *Verrucous*: elderly, tobacco usage, broad based exophytic and "church spire" hyperkeratosis with a pushing deep margin of cytologically bland bulbous processes. Locally invasive (75 % 5 year survival) but may become aggressive after radiotherapy although this association is anecdotal.
- *Papillary*: >70 % exophytic or papillary malignant epithelial fronds with focal invasion at the base (70 % 5 year survival).
- *Spindle cell*: polypoid and pleomorphic, cytokeratin (AE1/AE3, CK5/6) and p63 positive, distinguish from sarcoma. A more obvious in situ or invasive squamous component may be seen and lymph node metastases can show a spectrum of epithelial and spindle cell changes. Prognosis (80 % 5 year survival) relates to the depth of invasion.
- *Basaloid*: poor prognosis, nests of palisaded basaloid cells with central comedonecrosis, hyalinised stroma. More radiosensitive than other squamous cell carcinoma subtypes.
- *Adenoid squamous*: usual prognosis, acantholytic (pseudoglandular) pattern.
- *Adenosquamous*: poor prognosis, mixed differentiation squamous cell carcinoma and adenocarcinoma (either obvious glands or solid with mucin positive cells).
- *Undifferentiated carcinoma.*
- Note that the above variants can coexist in any one lesion.

Salivary Gland Tumours

- There is a higher frequency in the oral cavity (particularly palate and floor of mouth) of carcinoma of minor salivary gland origin e.g. polymorphous low-grade adenocarcinoma (cytological uniformity with architectural diversity), adenoid cystic carcinoma, mucoepidermoid carcinoma, acinic cell carcinoma, carcinoma ex pleomorphic adenoma.

Small Cell Carcinoma

- A poorly differentiated/high-grade neuroendocrine carcinoma. *Aggressive*: pure or with a squamous cell component. Chromogranin±/synaptophysin/CD56/TTF-1/paranuclear dot CAM 5.2 positive, and a high Ki-67 index.

Malignant Melanoma

- Represents 25 % of mucosal malignant melanomas. Japanese/Africans, palate and gingiva, ± adjacent junctional activity. *Prognosis is poor* (<25 % 5 year survival) with local recurrence, lymph node and distant metastases common. This aggressive behavior is recognised in TNM7 by designating malignant melanoma as moderately advanced (pT3: mucosal) or very advanced (pT4: beyond the mucosa) disease.
- Lip: desmoplastic melanoma. Shows S100 positivity to distinguish it from fibrous tissue; ± neurotropism. Can be negative for HMB-45 and melan-A.

Metastatic Carcinoma

- *Direct spread*: nasal cavity/maxillary sinus.
- *Distant spread*: lung, breast, kidney, gastrointestinal tract, malignant melanoma.

11.3 Differentiation

Well/moderate/poor/undifferentiated, or, Grade 1/2/3/4.
- For squamous cell carcinoma based on cellular atypia, keratinisation and intercellular bridges.
- Usually moderately differentiated whereas carcinomas at the base of the tongue can be poorly differentiated/undifferentiated. Immunohistochemistry for cytokeratins is needed to distinguish from malignant lymphoma.
- Undifferentiated carcinoma is grade 4. Where differentiation varies prognosis related to the worst area.
- Most *salivary gland tumours* are *graded according to type* e.g. acinic cell carcinoma

and polymorphous low grade adenocarcinoma are low-grade but salivary duct and undifferentiated carcinoma are high-grade. Mucoepidermoid carcinoma has a specific grading system.

11.4 Extent of Local Tumour Spread

Border: pushing/infiltrative. An infiltrative pattern of invasion at the deep aspect of the carcinoma is of proven adverse prognostic value.

Lymphocytic reaction: prominent/sparse. Lack of host immune response at the tumour edge is adverse.

The TNM7 classification applies to carcinomas of the lip and oral cavity including those of minor glands.

pTis	Carcinoma in situ
pT1	Tumour ≤2 cm in greatest dimension
pT2	Tumour >2 cm but ≤4 cm in greatest dimension
pT3	Tumour >4 cm in greatest dimension
pT4a	Moderately advanced local disease
	Lip: tumour invades adjacent structures, e.g. through cortical bone, inferior alveolar nerve, floor of mouth, skin (chin or nose).
	Oral cavity: tumour invades adjacent structures, e.g. through cortical bone, into deep (extrinsic) muscle of tongue, maxillary sinus, skin of face
pT4b	Very advanced local disease
	Lip and oral cavity: tumour invades masticator space, pterygoid plates, or skull base, or encases internal carotid artery

(Figs. 11.1, 11.2, 11.3, 11.4 and 11.5)

Cancers of the lip and lateral borders of the tongue may remain localised for considerable periods of time prior to invasion of local adjacent structures.

Distinguish tumour extending to or overlying bone from gross erosion or radiographic destruction of bone – the periosteum can act as a spatial and temporal barrier to local invasion.

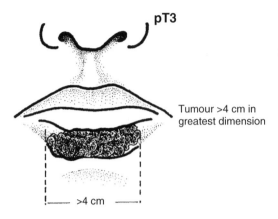

Fig. 11.1 Lip and oral cavity carcinoma (Reproduced, with permission, from Wittekind et al. (2005), © 2005)

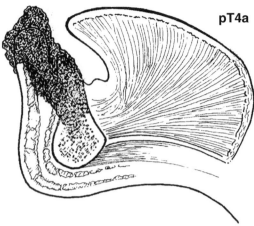

Fig. 11.3 Lip and oral cavity carcinoma (Reproduced, with permission, from Wittekind et al. (2005), © 2005)

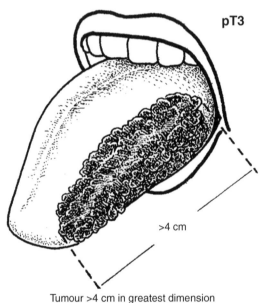

Fig. 11.2 Lip and oral cavity carcinoma (Reproduced, with permission, from Wittekind et al. (2005), © 2005)

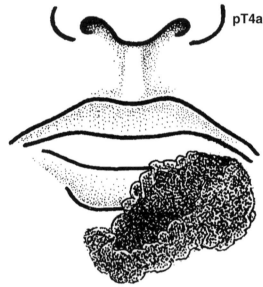

Fig. 11.4 Lip and oral cavity carcinoma (Reproduced, with permission, from Wittekind et al. (2005), © 2005)

11.5 Lymphovascular Invasion

Present/absent.

Intra-/extratumoural.

Perineural spread: a predictor of *local recurrence* and more *aggressive disease*. Vascular invasion is a relatively weak predictor of cervical lymph node metastases.

11.6 Lymph Nodes

Metastases are mainly lymphatic with the more anterior the tumour the lower the position of the cervical nodes involved. Lymph node metastases may also undergo cystic degeneration with central straw coloured fluid and viable cells at the tumour margin only. Residual paucicellular masses of keratin with

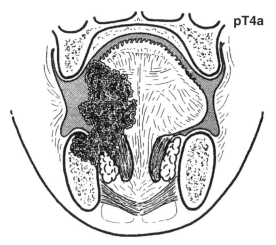

pT4a

Fig. 11.5 Lip and oral cavity carcinoma (Reproduced, with permission, from Wittekind et al. (2005), © 2005)

a foreign body reaction may result from radiation therapy. These features should be borne in mind on FNAC of cervical lymph nodes and a careful search made for malignant cells, which may be very well differentiated and difficult to distinguish from mature squames. A positive result is of considerable use in determining the nature of a bulky oral lesion. A common differential diagnosis of a neck mass in a younger to middle aged patient is branchial cyst.

Site/number/size/number involved/limit node/ extracapsular spread.

Regional nodes: cervical.

Level I	Submental, submandibular
Level II	Upper jugular
Level III	Middle jugular
Level IV	Lower jugular
Level V	Posterior triangle

A selective neck dissection will ordinarily include a minimum of six lymph nodes, a (modified) radical dissection ten lymph nodes.

pN0	No regional lymph node metastasis
pN1	Metastasis in a single ipsilateral node ≤3 cm
pN2	Metastasis in:
	(a) Ipsilateral single node >3–6 cm
	(b) Ipsilateral multiple nodes ≤6 cm
	(c) Bilateral, contralateral nodes ≤6 cm
pN3	Metastasis in a lymph node >6 cm

Extracapsular lymph node extension increases the risk of local recurrence and distant (4–26 %) spread. Metastasis is usually to *ipsilateral lymph nodes* but lesions of the tip of the tongue, those that cross the midline or the posterior one third can cause contralateral lymph node involvement. Up to *30 % of patients* with excision of the tongue and floor of mouth will have *clinically occult cervical lymph node metastases*.

11.7   Excision Margins

Distances (mm) of tumour to the nearest painted excision margins.

Epithelial dysplasia/carcinoma in situ present at excision margins. Tumour or mucosal dysplasia at or near (<5 mm) a margin is a *predictor of local recurrence*. Proximity of the surgical margin is often determined by the site, size and pattern of spread of the carcinoma.

An ideal therapeutic margin is 10 mm but often resections only afford 2–3 mm which is compounded by a peritumoural zone of dysplastic or hypertrophic mucosa.

11.8   Other Pathology

Predisposing Factors

Gender (M : F 2 : 1), smoking and alcohol are the main risk factors.

Clinical

Leukoplakia	Thin, smooth	
	Thick, fissured	
	Granular, verruciform	↓ Increasing risk trend
	Erythroleukoplakia 25–33 % risk	
Erythroplakia	50 % cancer risk	

Histological: Dysplasia

- Mild/moderate/severe. Most clinical examples of leukoplakia do not show histological dysplasia although if present it indicates a greater predisposition to carcinoma: *low-grade (mild/moderate) dysplasia – 5%, high-grade (severe) dysplasia – 50%*. Note that carcinoma can also arise from lesions with no dysplasia.

Others

- *Smokeless tobacco keratosis.*
- *Chronic hyperplastic candidosis*: this may also mimic squamous cell carcinoma histologically and treatment of infection is advised prior to any designation of malignancy.
- *HPV16,18*: aetiological factor contributing to verrucous and squamous cell carcinomas.
- *Smoking, alcohol, post-transplant immunosuppression.*
  Squamous cell carcinoma is positive for p63 and a range of cytokeratins including AE1/AE3, CK5/6, and 34βE12, but excluding CK 20 and CAM 5.2. This is of use in the distinction of spindle cell carcinoma from sarcoma. Routine p16 staining as a surrogate marker of HPV infection is not currently done in oral cavity and lip carcinoma.

Prognosis

Prognosis relates to tumour site, size, stage and histological grade. Histological type of squamous cell carcinoma can also influence prognosis: *better* (verrucous, papillary), *usual* (spindle cell, adenoid squamous) and *worse* (basaloid, adenosquamous).

Lip	90 % 5 year survival
Anterior tongue	60 % 5 year survival (20 % with large tumours and positive lymph nodes)
Posterior tongue, floor of mouth	40 % 5 year survival

Treatment is by surgery and/or radiotherapy supplemented by chemotherapy depending on the site and stage of disease.

11.9 Other Malignancy

Malignant Lymphoma

- Waldeyer's ring is the commonest site of oropharyngeal *non-Hodgkin's malignant lymphoma (NHL)* but it can arise in gingiva, buccal mucosa and palate. Most are *B cell and diffuse* although others e.g. T cell NHL and anaplastic large cell lymphoma do occur. Some are MALT derived and associated with extranodal malignant lymphomas elsewhere e.g. stomach, whereas others are of nodal type e.g. mantle cell. Prognosis relates to histological type and grade and stage of disease. There is an increasing incidence with HIV.

Leukaemia

- Direct infiltration or ulceration with opportunistic infection e.g. herpes simplex virus, cytomegalovirus. Gingival involvement is seen in *4% of acute myeloid leukaemia*. Rarely in granulocytic sarcoma (CD34/CD43/CD68/CD117/chloroacetate esterase/myeloperoxidase positive) an oral lesion is the first presentation of disease.

Plasmacytoma/Myeloma

κ, λ light chain restriction. Look for evidence of systemic disease e.g. serum immune paresis and monoclonal gammopathy, Bence-Jones proteinuria, radiological lytic bone lesions.

Odontogenic/Osseous Cancers by Direct Spread

Sarcoma

- Kaposi's sarcoma: HIV, palate.
- Leiomyosarcoma: cheek.
- Rhabdomyosarcoma: embryonal – children soft palate, desmin/myo D1/myogenin positive.
- Synovial sarcoma: young adults, cheek, tongue, palate.

Granular Cell Tumour

- A benign nerve sheath tumour composed of S100 positive granular cells. Commonly, overlying pseudoepitheliomatous hyperplasia can mimic squamous cell carcinoma and a careful search for granular cells in the biopsy subepithelial connective tissues must be made.

Bibliography

Barnest L, Eveson J, Reichart P, Sidransky D. WHO classification of tumours. Pathology and genetics. Tumours of the head and neck. Lyon: IARC Press; 2005.

Bouquot JE, Speight PM, Farthing PM. Epithelial dysplasia of the oral mucosa – diagnostic problems and prognostic features. Curr Diagn Pathol. 2006;12:11–21.

British Association of Otorhinolaryngologists – Head and Neck Surgeons. Effective head and neck cancer management. Second consensus document. London: Royal College of Surgeons; 2000.

Gnepp DR, editor. Diagnostic surgical pathology of the head and neck. 2nd ed. Philadelphia: WB Saunders; 2009.

Mehanna H, Paleri V, West CML, Nutting C. Head and neck cancer – part 1: epidemiology, presentation, and prevention. BMJ. 2010a;341:663–6.

Mehanna H, West CML, Nutting C, Paleri V. Head and neck cancer – part 2: treatment and prognostic factors. BMJ. 2010b;431:721–5.

Shah JP, Patel SG. Head and neck surgery and oncology. 3rd ed. Edinburgh: Mosby; 2003.

Slootweg PJ. Complex head and neck specimens and neck dissections. How to handle them. ACP best practice no 182. J Clin Pathol. 2005;58:243–8.

Speight PM, Farthing PM, Bouquot JE. The pathology of oral cancer and precancer. Curr Diagn Pathol. 1996;3: 165–76.

Thariat J, Badoual C, Faure C, Butori C, Marcy PY, Righini CA. Basaloid squamous cell carcinoma of the head and neck: role of HPV and implication in treatment and prognosis. J Clin Pathol. 2010;63: 857–66.

The Royal College of Pathologists. Head and Neck Tissues – Cancer Datasets (Head and Neck Carcinomas and Salivary Neoplasms, Parathyroid Cancer, Thyroid Cancer) and Tissue Pathways (Head and Neck Pathology, Endocrine Pathology). Accessed at http://www.rcpath.org/index.asp?PageID=254.

Thomas GJ, Barrett AW. Papillary and verrucous lesions of the oral mucosa. Diagn Histopathol. 2009;15: 279–85.

Van Heerden WFP, van Zyl AW. Surgical pathology of oral cancer. Diagn Histopathol. 2009;15:296–302.

Wittekind CF, Greene FL, Hutter RVP, Klimpfinger M, Sobib LH. TNM atlas: illustrated guide to the TNM/ pTNM classification of malignant tumours. 5th ed. Berlin: Springer; 2005.

Oropharyngeal Carcinoma (with Comments on Nasopharynx and Hypopharynx)

12

Tobacco and alcohol are the major risk factors and usually in male patients aged 40–60 years. Post cricoid carcinoma is associated with Plummer-Vinson syndrome in older females (iron deficiency anaemia, achlorhydria, upper oesophageal web). Human Papilloma Virus (HPV) infection has a role in the aetiology of a significant proportion of tonsillar and oropharyngeal carcinomas in non-smokers. It can be identified by in situ hybridisation or over expression of the surrogate marker tumour suppressor gene protein product p16.

Depending on the anatomical site of the lesion patients can present with dysphagia, hoarseness, deafness, cranial nerve palsy or cervical lymphadenopathy. Investigation is by endoscopy with biopsy, and ultrasound with cervical lymph node fine needle aspiration cytology (FNAC) to obtain a diagnosis. Biopsies can be superficial and miss submucosal invasive cancer. CT and MRI scans are used to assess local tumour spread and metastasis to the neck and elsewhere. Chest x-ray can detect concurrent lung cancer.

Extent of resection depends on the tumour site, stage, lymph node spread, fitness of the patient and any concurrent tumour that is detected at upper aerodigestive tract endoscopy. Tonsil is submitted when there is asymmetrical enlargement or as a possible site of an occult primary in FNAC proven cervical lymph node metastases. Carcinoma in the post nasal space is a not infrequent source. Serology for Epstein-Barr virus (EBV) may help in the diagnosis of nasopharyngeal carcinoma, and in assessing efficacy of its treatment and subsequent local recurrence.

12.1 Gross Description

Specimen

- FNAC/biopsy (punch, incisional)/tonsillectomy/adenoidectomy/transoral laser resection/pharyngectomy/pharyngooesophagectomy ± laryngectomy/neck dissection.
- Weight (g) and size (cm), number of fragments.

Tumour

Site

Oropharynx: lies between the soft palate and tip of the epiglottis. Most tumours arise in the posterior third of tongue and the tonsil.

Boundaries:

1. Anterior wall	Posterior third tongue, vallecula
2. Lateral wall	Tonsil, tonsillar fossa and pillars
3. Posterior wall	
4. Superior	Wall inferior surface soft palate, uvula.

Nasopharynx (post nasal space): superiorly from the skull base and delineated inferiorly by the superior surface of the soft palate.

Hypopharynx: demarcated anteriorly by the larynx and aryepiglottic folds, laterally the piriform sinus and superiorly the oropharynx at the level of the hyoid bone. It lies below the tip of the epiglottis down to the start of the oesophagus at the postcricoid area. The majority (75 %) of tumours arise in the piriform fossa (Fig. 12.1).

D.C. Allen, *Histopathology Reporting*,
DOI 10.1007/978-1-4471-5263-7_12, © Springer-Verlag London 2013

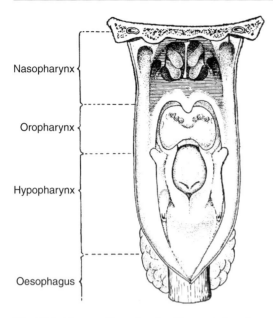

Nasopharynx

Oropharynx

Hypopharynx

Oesophagus

Fig. 12.1 Pharynx (Reproduced, with permission, from Wittekind et al. (2005), © 2005)

Size

- Length × width × depth (cm) or maximum dimension (cm).
- Depth of invasion >4 mm is predictive of cervical lymph node metastases. Tumour of the posterior tongue tends to be large at presentation. Tonsillar tumour is more often occult presenting with cervical lymph node metastases.

Appearance

- Polypoid/sessile/ulcerated/fleshy.

Edge

- Circumscribed/irregular.

12.2 Histological Type

Squamous Cell Carcinoma

- *85 % of cases* and predominantly well differentiated keratinising.
- Keratinising/non-keratinising.
- Prognosis is *better* (verrucous/papillary/HPV related), *usual* (spindle cell/adenoid squamous) or *worse* (basaloid/adenosquamous).
- *HPV related cancers* are usually submucosal, lobulated and non-keratinising with minimal

stromal reaction in contrast to usual squamous cell carcinoma with irregular nests of keratinising malignant squamous epithelium and a desmoplastic stroma.

- Variants:
- *Verrucous:* elderly, tobacco usage, broad based exophytic and "church spire" hyperkeratosis with a pushing deep margin of cytologically bland bulbous processes. Locally invasive (75 % 5 year survival) but may become aggressive after radiotherapy although this association is anecdotal.
- *Papillary:* >70 % exophytic or papillary malignant epithelial fronds with focal invasion at the base (70 % 5 year survival).
- *Spindle cell:* polypoid and pleomorphic, cytokeratin (AE1/AE3, CK5/6) and p63 positive, distinguish from sarcoma. A more obvious in situ or invasive squamous cell component may be seen and lymph node metastases can show a spectrum of epithelial and spindle cell changes. Prognosis (80 % 5 year survival) relates to the depth of invasion.
- *Basaloid:* poor prognosis, nests of palisaded basaloid cells with central comedonecrosis. More radiosensitive than other squamous cell carcinoma subtypes.
- *Adenoid squamous:* usual prognosis, acantholytic (pseudoglandular) pattern.
- *Adenosquamous:* poor prognosis, mixed differentiation squamous cell carcinoma and adenocarcinoma (either obvious glands or solid with mucin positive cells).
- *Sinonasal "transitional type":* a descriptive term and morphological features are intermediate between squamous cell and transitional cell carcinoma with variable keratinisation and differentiation.

Undifferentiated Carcinoma

- *15 % of cases.*
- Absence of squamous cell or glandular differentiation.
- Particularly *nasopharynx* where it is *EBV related* and associated with a prominent lymphocytic component (lymphoepithelioma) of tumour infiltrating lymphocytes (TILs). Asian/oriental males 40–60 years of age, CK5/6, p63, EBER positive.

Salivary Gland Tumours

- Adenoid cystic carcinoma.
- Acinic cell carcinoma.
- Mucoepidermoid carcinoma.
- Polymorphous low-grade adenocarcinoma.

Malignant Melanoma

- Primary or secondary, *poor prognosis*. This *aggressive behaviour* is recognised in TNM7 by designating malignant melanoma as moderately advanced (pT3: mucosal) or very advanced (pT4: beyond mucosa) disease.

Neuroendocrine Tumour/Carcinoma

- Well to moderately differentiated/low-grade neuroendocrine (carcinoid/atypical carcinoid) tumour, or poorly differentiated/high-grade neuroendocrine (small cell/large cell) carcinoma. Small cell and large cell mucosal neuroendocrine carcinomas of the head and neck region have relatively *poor prognosis*. They are variably chromogranin, synaptophysin, CD56, Ki-67 positive.

Metastatic Carcinoma

- Renal cell carcinoma, breast, lung, gut.

12.3 Differentiation

Well/moderate/poor/undifferentiated, or, Grade 1/2/3/4.
- For squamous carcinoma based on cellular atypia, keratinisation and intercellular bridges.
- Undifferentiated carcinoma is grade 4.
- Mainly well-differentiated keratinising but varies according to tumour site e.g. nasopharyngeal carcinoma is of undifferentiated type. *Carcinoma of the tonsil and base of the tongue also tend to be poorly differentiated*. When differentiation varies prognosis relates to the worst area.
- Most *salivary gland tumours* are *graded according to type* e.g. acinic cell carcinoma and

polymorphous low-grade adenocarcinoma are low-grade but salivary duct and undifferentiated carcinoma are high-grade. Mucoepidermoid carcinoma has a specific grading system.

12.4 Extent of Local Tumour Spread

Border: pushing/infiltrative. An infiltrative pattern of invasion at the deep aspect of the carcinoma is of adverse prognostic value.

Lymphocytic reaction: prominent/sparse.

The TNM7 classification applies only to carcinomas.

Oro-(Hypopharynx)

pT1	Tumour ≤2 cm in greatest dimension (hypopharynx – and limited to one subsite)	
pT2	2 cm < tumour ≤4 cm in greatest dimension (hypopharynx – and more than one subsite or adjacent site, without fixation of hemilarynx)	
pT3	Tumour >4 cm in greatest dimension or extension to lingual surface of epiglottis (hypopharynx – or with fixation of hemilarynx[a] or extension to oesophagus)	
pT4	Tumour invades any of	
	Oropharynx	4a: larynx, deep/extrinsic muscle of tongue[b], medial pterygoid, hard palate, and mandible
		4b: lateral pterygoid muscle, pterygoid plates, lateral nasopharynx, skull base, or encases carotid artery.
	Hypopharynx	4a: thyroid/cricoid cartilage, hyoid bone, thyroid gland, oesophagus, central compartment soft tissue (including prelaryngeal strap muscles and subcutaneous fat)
		4b: prevertebral fasia, encases carotid artery, or invades mediastinal structures.

pT4a and pT4b represent moderately advanced and very advanced local disease, respectively (Figs. 12.2 and 12.3)

[a]Fixation of hemilarynx is diagnosed endoscopically by immobility of the arytenoid or vocal cord

[b]Invasion of deep muscle of tongue is usually associated with restriction of tongue mobility clinically

Nasopharynx

pT1	Tumour confined to nasopharynx or extends to oropharynx and/or nasal cavity
pT2	Tumour with posterolateral parapharyngeal extension
pT3	Tumour into bone of skull base and/or nasal sinuses
pT4	Intracranial extension and/or into cranial nerves, hypopharynx, orbit, infratemporal fossa, or masticator space (Figs. 12.4 and 12.5).

12.5   Lymphovascular Invasion

Present/absent.

Intra-/extratumoural.

Perineural spread: predictor of *local recurrence* and more *aggressive disease.* Vascular invasion is a relatively weak indicator for cervical lymph node metastases.

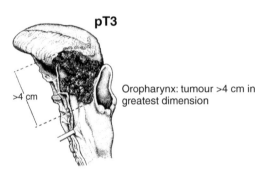

pT3

>4 cm

Oropharynx: tumour >4 cm in greatest dimension

Fig. 12.2 Oropharyngeal carcinoma (Reproduced, with permission, from Wittekind et al. (2005), © 2005)

12.6   Lymph Nodes

Site/number/size/number involved/limit node/extracapsular spread.

Regional nodes: cervical

Level I	Submental, submandibular
Level II	Upper jugular
Level III	Middle jugular
Level IV	Lower jugular
Level V	Posterior triangle

A selective neck dissection will ordinarily include a minimum of six lymph nodes, a (modified) radical dissection ten lymph nodes.

Oro- and Hypopharynx

pN0	No regional lymph node metastasis
pN1	Metastasis in a single ipsilateral node ≤3 cm
pN2	Metastasis in
	(a) Ipsilateral single node >3–6 cm
	(b) Ipsilateral multiple nodes ≤6 cm
	(c) Bilateral, contralateral nodes ≤6 cm
pN3	Metastasis in a lymph node >6 cm.

Nasopharynx

pN0	No regional lymph node metastasis
pN1	Unilateral cervical nodal metastasis ≤6 cm, above supraclavicular fossa, and/or uni-/bilateral retropharyngeal nodal metastasis
pN2	Bilateral cervical nodal metastasis ≤6 cm, above supraclavicular fossa
pN3	Cervical metastasis in (a) nodes >6 cm or (b) in supraclavicular fossa.

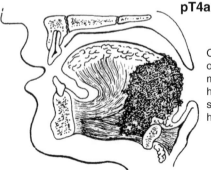

pT4a

Oropharynx: tumour invades any of the following: larynx, deep/extrinsic muscle of tongue (genioglossus, hyoglossus, palatoglossus, and styloglossus), medial pterygoid, hard palate, and mandible

Fig. 12.3 Oropharyngeal carcinoma (Reproduced, with permission, from Wittekind et al. (2005), © 2005)

Fig. 12.4 Nasopharyngeal carcinoma (Reproduced, with permission, from Wittekind et al. (2005), © 2005)

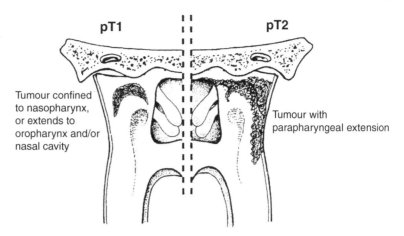

Fig. 12.5 Nasopharyngeal carcinoma (Reproduced, with permission, from Wittekind et al. (2005), © 2005)

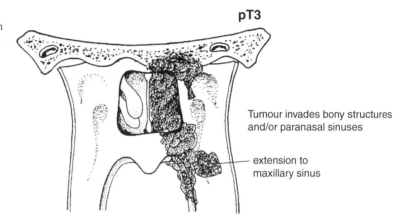

Presentation in up to 10 % of cases is with *upper cervical lymph node metastases* mimicking malignant lymphoma. Cervical metastases of nasopharyngeal carcinoma may also show a necrotising granulomatous nodal reaction. Carcinomas of the base of the tongue and oropharynx tend to metastasise to the retropharyngeal nodes and rarely (6 %) the posterior triangle of neck.

12.7   Excision Margins

Distances (mm) to the nearest longitudinal and circumferential excision margins. Tumour or mucosal dysplasia at or near (<5 mm) a lateral resection margin may predict local recurrence.

Due to anatomical limitations on resection, margins are usually only several millimetres.

12.8   Other Pathology

Concurrent carcinoma bronchus, oropharyngo-laryngeal ring: 10–15 % of cases. Bronchoscopic assessment may be required further to any indicators on CT staging scan.

HPV associated oropharyngeal carcinomas: usually non-keratinising, arise in the tonsils or base of the tongue, and are of better prognosis than non-HPV associated carcinomas. There is overexpression of p16 on immunohistochemistry and if positive confirm by in situ hybridization for HPV 16.

Primary treatment of oropharyngeal and hypopharyngeal carcinoma: surgical ± neoadjuvant chemoradiotherapy, with the majority of lesions being well to moderately differentiated keratinising squamous cell carcinoma. Small oropharyngeal lesions can be locally excised (80 % 5 year survival) but larger lesions are treated by primary chemoradiation with surgery reserved for recurrent disease. HPV related cases are particularly chemoradiation responsive.

Primary treatment of nasopharyngeal carcinoma is radio-/chemotherapy: a majority of nasopharyngeal carcinomas are of undifferentiated type comprising a syncytial arrangement of enlarged tumour cells with a prominent nucleolus, and an accompanying lymphoid stroma characterized by prominent tumour infiltrating lymphocytes (TILs). The tumour is strongly associated with *EBV infection*, which can be shown by immunohistochemistry (EBV LMP (latent membrane protein)) or EBER (EBV encoded RNA) in situ hybridisation techniques. Strength of LMP expression has been associated with cervical lymph node metastases. *Serum EBV levels* are also useful for *monitoring the effects of treatment* and in *detecting recurrence*. Markers are helpful in distinguishing carcinoma (cytokeratins, p63, EMA) from high-grade malignant lymphoma (CD 45) and malignant melanoma (S100, HMB-45, melan-A). Nasopharyngeal carcinoma has a biphasic age presentation (15–25 years, 60–90 years) with the keratinising squamous cell variant (not EBV related) occurring in the older age group. Nasopharynx has separate pT and pN staging in the TNM7 system. Hypopharynx may also be submitted with a laryngectomy specimen due to spread from a laryngeal carcinoma.

Prognosis

Prognosis of oropharyngeal carcinoma varies and relates to tumour site, stage and histological grade. Small early lesions are adequately treated by curative local excision, but there are *20–40 % 5 year survival rates* for cancers of the posterior tongue, tonsil and palate. Undifferentiated carcinoma has a very poor prognosis. However, the *chemo-/radiosensitivity of nasopharyngeal carcinoma* results in complete remission in 80 % of cases and 10 year survival rates of 40–70 %. The keratinising squamous cell variant in the older age group is of worse prognosis as are cancers

with lower cervical rather than upper cervical lymph node metastases.

12.9 Other Malignancy

Leukaemia

Malignant Lymphoma
- Diffuse large B cell non-Hodgkin's malignant lymphoma.
- Mantle cell lymphoma: intermediate-grade and aggressive.
- MALToma with recurrence in other MALT sites e.g. stomach, Waldeyer's ring.
- Angiocentric T cell lymphoma: aggressive.

Plasmacytoma/Myeloma
κ, λ light chain restriction. Look for evidence of systemic disease e.g. serum immune paresis and monoclonal gammopathy, Bence-Jones proteinuria, radiological lytic bone lesions.

Sarcoma
- Children: embryonal rhabdomyosarcoma (subepithelial cellular cambium layer; deeper myxoid zone; desmin/myo D1/myogenin positive).
- Young adults: synovial sarcoma; pharynx, palate.
- Kaposi's sarcoma: AIDS.

Nasopharyngeal Chordoma (Locally Destructive), Olfactory Neuroblastoma, Primitive Neuroectodermal Tumour.
- See Chap. 13.

Bibliography

Barnest L, Eveson J, Reichart P, Sidransky D. WHO classification of tumours. Pathology and genetics. Tumours of the head and neck. Lyon: IARC Press; 2005.

British Association of Otorhinolaryngologists – Head and Neck Surgeons. Effective head and neck cancer management. Second consensus document. London: Royal College of Surgeons; 2000.

Gnepp DR, editor. Diagnostic surgical pathology of the head and neck. 2nd ed. Philadelphia: WB Saunders; 2009.

Kusafuka K, Abe M, Iida Y, Onitsuka T, Fuke T, Asano R, Kamijo T, Nakajima T. Mucosal large cell neuroendocrine carcinoma of the head and neck regions in Japanese patients: a distinct clinicopathological entity. J Clin Pathol. 2012;65:704–9.

Mehanna H, Paleri V, West CML, Nutting C. Head and neck cancer – part 1: epidemiology, presentation, and prevention. BMJ. 2010a;341:663–6.

Mehanna H, West CML, Nutting C, Paleri V. Head and neck cancer – part 2: treatment and prognostic factors. BMJ. 2010b;431:721–5.

Perez-Odonez B. Hamartomas, papillomas and adenocarcinomas of the sinonasal tract and nasopharynx. J Clin Pathol. 2009;62:1085–95.

Shah JP, Patel SG. Head and neck surgery and oncology. 3rd ed. Edinburgh: Mosby; 2003.

Slootweg PJ. Complex head and neck specimens and neck dissections. How to handle them. ACP best practice no 182. J Clin Pathol. 2005;58:243–8.

Thariat J, Badoual C, Faure C, Butori C, Marcy PY, Righini CA. Basaloid squamous cell carcinoma of the head and neck: role of HPV and implication in treatment and prognosis. J Clin Pathol. 2010;63: 857–66.

The Royal College of Pathologists. Head and Neck Tissues – Cancer Datasets (Head and Neck Carcinomas and Salivary Neoplasms, Parathyroid Cancer, Thyroid Cancer) and Tissue Pathways (Head and Neck Pathology, Endocrine Pathology). Accessed at http://www.rcpath.org/index.asp?PageID=254.

Wittekind CF, Greene FL, Hutter RVP, Klimpfinger M, Sobib LH. TNM atlas: illustrated guide to the TNM/pTNM classification of malignant tumours. 5th ed. Berlin: Springer; 2005.

Nasal Cavity and Paranasal Sinus Carcinomas

13

Sinonasal cancer accounts for about 3 % of head and neck malignancies and in general affects patients aged 55–65 years. About two thirds are of epithelial origin, with others including malignant melanoma and malignant lymphoma. Some also represent direct spread from adjacent local sites e.g. primary tumours in the oral cavity or nasopharynx.

Clinical presentation is with nasal obstruction, rhinorrhoea, epistaxis, deafness, ocular proptosis or facial pain. Investigation is by endonasal endoscopy with biopsy. Plain x-ray, CT and MRI scans can demonstrate and stage a soft tissue mass and any bone destruction that is present. Spread intracranially or into the orbit and relationship to the optic nerve and carotid artery can also be determined. A majority of cancers arise in the maxillary sinus.

Tumour can be removed piece-meal by functional endoscopic sinus surgery (FESS) or more formal resection. Nasal septal lesions are excised via a lateral rhinotomy. Medial maxillectomy is the commonest procedure for low-grade tumours of the lateral nasal cavity, or maxillary, ethmoid and frontal sinuses e.g. transitional papilloma or olfactory neuroblastoma. Craniofacial resection is for aggressive tumours or those of the frontal or ethmoid sinus that extend into the anterior cranial fossa. Orbital exenteration may be required if there is involvement of its bony wall. Neck dissection is carried out when there are proven cervical lymph node metastases. These are complex specimens and they require careful marking by and liaison with the surgeon.

13.1 Gross Description

Specimen

- FNAC (fine needle aspirate cytology)/biopsy/resection e.g. piece-meal, rhinectomy, maxillectomy, ethmoidectomy, craniofacial resection/neck dissection.
- Weight (g) and size (cm), number of fragments.

Tumour

Site

- Nasal cavity, maxillary sinus, ethmoid sinus, sphenoid/frontal sinuses (Figs. 13.1 and 13.2).
- Maxillary and ethmoid sinuses are the commonest tumour sites.
- Mucosal/osseous/extrinsic.

Size

- Length × width × depth (cm) or maximum dimension (cm).
- An indicator of disease extent and also allows correlation with clinical imaging studies. Not used for TNM staging.

Appearance

- Exophytic/papillary/mucoid/sclerotic/chondroid/osseous.

D.C. Allen, *Histopathology Reporting*,
DOI 10.1007/978-1-4471-5263-7_13, © Springer-Verlag London 2013

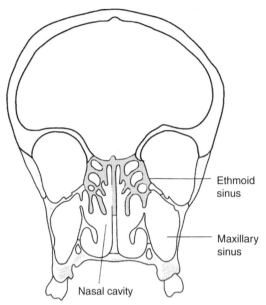

Fig. 13.1 Paranasal sinuses (Reproduced, with permission, from Wittekind et al. (2005), © 2005)

Edge

• Circumscribed/irregular.

13.2 Histological Type

Squamous Cell Carcinoma

• *85 % of cases* of sinonasal carcinoma.
• Keratinising/non-keratinising.
• Usually moderately differentiated keratinising.
• CK5/6, 34βE12, p63 positive.
• variants:
• *Verrucous*: elderly, tobacco usage, broad based exophytic and "church spire" hyperkeratosis with a pushing deep margin of cytologically bland bulbous processes. Locally invasive (75 % 5 year survival) but may become aggressive after radiotherapy although this association is anecdotal.
• *Papillary*: >70 % exophytic or papillary malignant epithelial fronds with focal invasion at the base, 70 % 5 year survival.
• *Spindle cell*: polypoid and pleomorphic, cytokeratin (AE1/AE3, CK5/6) and p63 positive, distinguish from sarcoma. A more obvious in

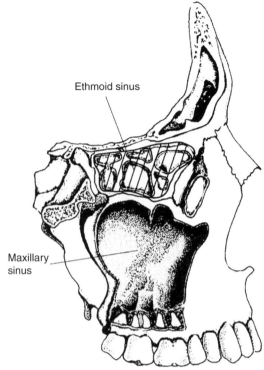

Fig. 13.2 Paranasal sinuses (Reproduced, with permission, from Wittekind et al. (2005), © 2005)

situ or invasive squamous cell component may be seen and lymph node metastases can show a spectrum of epithelial and spindle cell changes. Prognosis (80 % 5 year survival) relates to the depth of invasion.
• *Basaloid*: poor prognosis, nests of palisaded basaloid cells with central comedonecrosis. More radiosensitive than other squamous cell carcinoma subtypes.
• *Adenoid squamous*: usual prognosis, acantholytic (pseudoglandular) pattern.
• *Adenosquamous*: poor prognosis, mixed differentiation squamous cell carcinoma and adenocarcinoma (either obvious glands or solid with mucin positive cells).
• *Sinonasal "transitional type"*: a descriptive term with features intermediate between squamous cell and transitional cell carcinoma. Consider a possible origin in inverted transitional (Schneiderian) papilloma which is a benign, but in 20 % of cases, locally

recurrent sinonasal tumour. It is a papillary exophytic/endophytic neoplasm with features intermediate between transitional and squamous epithelia, and variably associated with HPV and EBV. Complicated by carcinoma in 3 % of cases which is either focal (good prognosis) or diffusely infiltrative (25 % survival rate), and of variable keratinisation and differentiation.

- *Lymphoepithelial carcinoma*: EBV related with prominent tumour infiltrating lymphocytes (TILs). Responds to radiotherapy.

Sinonasal Undifferentiated Carcinoma (SNUC)

- Absent or minimal squamous cell, glandular or neuroendocrine differentiation.
- Nests, lobules and sheets of cytologically atypical cells with prominent apoptotic and mitotic activity.
- Cytokeratin (CK8)/EMA positive but CK5/6 and p63 negative.
- *Primary sinonasal undifferentiated neoplasms* comprise a broad range of epithelial and non-epithelial lesions. The *epithelial group* includes: SNUC, nasopharyngeal type undifferentiated carcinoma, high-grade neuroendocrine small cell carcinoma, nuclear protein in testis (NUT) nasal midline carcinoma, squamous cell carcinoma and variants, and forms of adenocarcinoma. The *non-epithelial group* includes: malignant melanoma, neuroectodermal tumours (olfactory neuroblastoma, Ewing's sarcoma/PNET), haematopoietic tumours (malignant lymphoma, plasmacytoma/myeloma, granulocytic sarcoma), sarcoma (rhabdomyosarcoma, chondrosarcoma, synovial sarcoma) and malignant desmoplastic small round cell tumour.

Nasal Midline Carcinoma

- Rare, highly *aggressive* carcinoma of the midline axis in young adults with favourable response to chemoradiation.

- Undifferentiated basaloid cells with focal abrupt squamous cell differentiation.
- NUT antibody positive.

Neuroendocrine Tumour/Carcinoma

- Well to moderately differentiated neuroendocrine (carcinoid/atypical carcinoid) tumour, and poorly differentiated/high-grade neuroendocrine (small cell) carcinoma.
- Small cell carcinoma has a *poor prognosis*. An aggressive tumour which may follow radiation therapy for other head and neck malignancies.
- Paranuclear dot CAM5.2/synaptophysin/CD56/TTF-1 positive and a high Ki-67 index. Carcinoid tumour is chromogranin/synaptophysin positive, and variable for CD56/Ki-67.

Adenocarcinoma

- Salivary, intestinal or non-intestinal in type.
- *Salivary*: mucoepidermoid, acinic cell, adenoid cystic carcinomas.
- *Intestinal*: polypoid or solid/mucinous and a well-differentiated intestinal pattern. Occurs in woodworkers (wood dust exposure) in the middle turbinate or ethmoid sinus. It is locally aggressive and recurrent. Prognosis relates to the degree of glandular differentiation with 5 and 10 year survival rates of 36 and 25 % respectively.
- *Non-intestinal adenocarcinoma*: low-grade sinonasal and papillary adenocarcinoma, or, high-grade not otherwise specified. The latter is based on atypia, necrosis and mitotic rate with a poor prognosis and 20 % 3 year survival.

Malignant Melanoma

- Rare (commoner in nasal cavity), 2 % of malignant paranasal tumours, antrum, ethmoid, frontal sinuses.
- ± Adjacent mucosal junctional activity.

- *Poor prognosis* with 50 % developing distant metastases to lungs, brain, bone and liver (most dead within 5 years). This *aggressive behaviour* is recognised in TNM7 by designating malignant melanoma as moderately advanced (pT3: mucosal) or very advanced (pT4: beyond mucosa) disease, respectively.

Metastatic Carcinoma

- Renal, lung, breast, gastrointestinal tract carcinomas, malignant melanoma.

13.3 Differentiation

Well/moderate/poor/undifferentiated, or, Grade 1/2/3/4.
- For squamous cell carcinoma based on cellular atypia, keratinisation and intercellular bridges.
- The majority are moderately differentiated but this varies according to tumour site and type e.g. undifferentiated nasopharyngeal carcinoma (grade 4). Where differentiation varies prognosis relates to the worst area.
- For adenocarcinoma based on the percentage tumour gland formation (well/G1 >95 %: moderate/G2 50–95 %: poor/G3 <50 %: undifferentiated/G4 no glands).

13.4 Extent of Local Tumour Spread

Border: pushing/infiltrative. The microscopic pattern of invasion does not have a consistent prognostic value.

Lymphocytic reaction: prominent/sparse and the desmoplastic stromal response.

The TNM7 classification applies only to carcinomas.

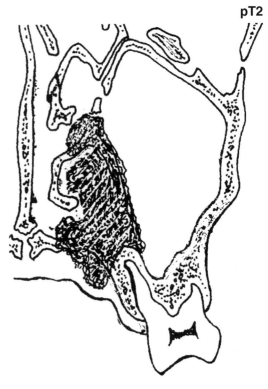

pT2

Fig. 13.3 Maxillary sinus carcinoma (Reproduced, with permission, from Wittekind et al. (2005), © 2005)

pTis	Carcinoma in situ.

Maxillary Sinus

pT1	Tumour limited to the antral mucosa
pT2	Tumour causes erosion or destruction of bone (including extension into hard palate and/or middle nasal meatus), except posterior antral wall and pterygoid plates
pT3	Tumour invades any of: posterior wall maxillary sinus, subcutaneous tissues, floor/medial wall orbit, pterygoid fossa, ethmoid sinus(es)
pT4	Tumour invades any of:
4a	Anterior orbital contents, skin of cheek, pterygoid plates, infratemporal fossa, cribriform plate, sphenoid or frontal sinuses.
4b	Orbital apex, dura, brain, middle cranial fossa, cranial nerves (other than maxillary division trigeminal nerve V2), nasopharynx, clivus (Figs. 13.3, 13.4, and 13.5).

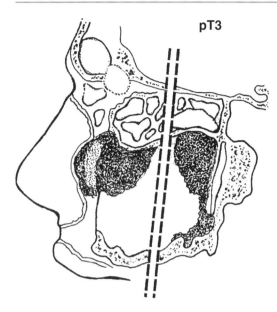

pT3

Fig. 13.4 Maxillary sinus carcinoma (Reproduced, with permission, from Wittekind et al. (2005), © 2005)

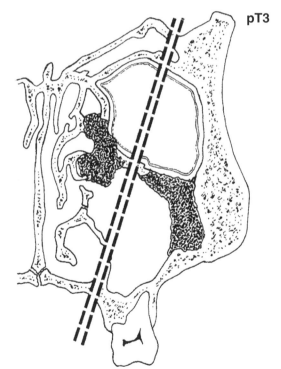

pT3

Fig. 13.5 Maxillary sinus carcinoma (Reproduced, with permission, from Wittekind et al. (2005), © 2005)

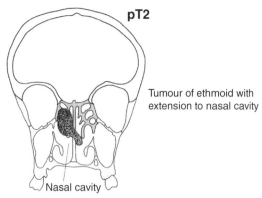

pT2

Tumour of ethmoid with extension to nasal cavity

Nasal cavity

Fig. 13.6 Ethmoid sinus carcinoma (Reproduced, with permission, from Wittekind et al. (2005), © 2005)

Nasal Cavity and Ethmoid Sinus

pT1	Tumour confined to one subsite of nasal cavity or ethmoid ± bone invasion
pT2	Tumour involves two subsites in a single site or extends to involve an adjacent site within the nasoethmoidal complex ± bone invasion.
pT3	Tumour extends to medial wall or floor of orbit, maxillary sinus, palate, or cribriform plate.
pT4	Tumour invades any of:
4a	Anterior orbital contents, skin of nose or cheek, minimal extension to anterior cranial fossa, pterygoid plates, sphenoid or frontal sinuses
4b	Orbital apex, dura, brain, middle cranial fossa, cranial nerves other than V2, nasopharynx, clivus.

Invasion of bone includes only involvement of the spongiosa, not the cortex.

Presentation is not infrequently late with bone destruction already present (Figs. 13.6 and 13.7).

13.5 Lymphovascular Invasion

Present/absent.

Intra-/extratumoural.

Vascular invasion is a relatively weak indicator for cervical lymph node metastases. *Perineural invasion* is an indicator of more *aggressive disease* with a

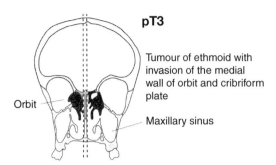

pT3

Tumour of ethmoid with invasion of the medial wall of orbit and cribriform plate

Orbit

Maxillary sinus

Fig. 13.7 Ethmoid sinus carcinoma (Reproduced, with permission, from Wittekind et al. (2005), © 2005)

greater likelihood of *local recurrence and metastases*. It may indicate the need for adjuvant therapy.

13.6 Lymph Nodes

Site/number/size/number involved/limit node/extracapsular spread.

Regional nodes: cervical. The external nose and anterior nasal cavity drain to the level I cervical lymph nodes, the rest of the nasal cavity and paranasal sinuses to the level II lymph nodes.

Level I	Submental, submandibular
Level II	Upper jugular
Level III	Middle jugular
Level IV	Lower jugular
Level V	Posterior triangle

A selective neck dissection will ordinarily include a minimum of 6 lymph nodes, a (modified) radical dissection 10 lymph nodes.

pN0	No regional lymph node metastasis
pN1	Metastasis in a single ipsilateral node ≤3 cm
pN2	Metastasis in
	(a) Ipsilateral single node >3 cm but ≤6 cm
	(b) Ipsilateral multiple nodes ≤6 cm
	(c) Bilateral, contralateral nodes ≤6 cm
pN3	Metastasis in a lymph node >6 cm

13.7 Excision Margins

Distance (mm) to the nearest painted excision margin.

Tumour at or close to (<5 mm) a margin is a predictor of *local recurrence* and may necessitate

adjuvant therapy. Dysplasia is uncommon except as part of the mucosa adjacent to an invasive carcinoma.

Due to anatomical limitations on resection, margins are usually only several millimetres.

13.8 Other Pathology

Relative incidence: malignant tumours are more common than benign in the paranasal sinuses with the reverse being the case in the nasal cavity. Equivalent nasal cavity tumours have a better prognosis. Immunohistochemical markers are of use in differentiating carcinoma from malignant melanoma and malignant lymphoma. About 55 % of sinonasal malignancies occur in the maxillary sinus, 35 % in the nasal cavity and 9 % in the ethmoid sinus. The majority of lesions (85 %) are squamous cell carcinoma and its variants with adenocarcinoma representing only 5–10 % of cases. Most cases are *locally advanced at presentation* and *local recurrence is common* despite surgery and radiotherapy. About 10 % of patients present with lymph node metastases.

Prognosis

Prognosis is strongly related to tumour stage. Treatment is by a combination of *surgery* and *radiotherapy* with on *average 20–60% 5 year survivals*. Undifferentiated carcinoma has a very poor prognosis and histologically squamous cell and glandular differentiation are precluded by definition. *Undifferentiated carcinoma of nasopharyngeal type is radiosensitive* with remission in 80 % and 10 year survival in 40 %. More recently cetuximab therapy targeted at human epidermal growth factor receptor (EGFR) has found a role to play in the treatment of metastatic squamous cell carcinoma of the head and neck region.

13.9 Other Malignancy

Malignant Lymphoma

- *Diffuse large B cell lymphoma* is commonest; CD 20 positive.
- *Angiocentric T cell lymphoma* (sinonasal NK (natural killer)/T cell lymphoma):

Destructive nasal/midline tumour with large areas of zonal necrosis and vasculocentric/destructive. It comprises polymorphic tumour cells (CD2/CD56/TIA-1 positive/CD 3 ±) which may be hard to recognise amongst the inflammatory infiltrate. EBV associated and of poor prognosis. It can show pseudoepitheliomatous hyperplasia mimicking squamous cell carcinoma. Serum cANCA levels help to distinguish it from Wegener's granulomatosis - another cause of sinonasal lethal midline granuloma.

Plasmacytoma/Myeloma

• Development of myeloma may take a number of years.
• κ, λ light chain restriction and clinical evidence of myeloma e.g. elevated ESR, serum immune paresis, and monoclonal gammopathy, Bence-Jones proteinuria, radiological lytic bone lesions.

Rhabdomyosarcoma (Embryonal – Children), Angiosarcoma, Fibrosarcoma, Malignant Fibrous Histiocytoma, Chondrosarcoma, Synovial Sarcoma, Osteosarcoma, Odontogenic Tumours by Direct Spread

• About 40 % of rhabdomyosarcomas occur in the head and neck and 20 % in the nasal cavity, nasopharynx and nasal sinuses. It is the commonest sarcoma in childhood and of embryonal type with a better prognosis (44–90 % 5 year survival) than the alveolar type seen in adults (<10 % 5 year survival). Desmin, myogenin, myo D1 positive.

Olfactory Neuroblastoma, Ewing's Sarcoma/Primitive Neuroectodermal Tumour (PNET)

• *Olfactory neuroblastoma* (*esthesioneuroblastoma*): an uncommon neuroectodermal malignancy arising in a broad age range from the olfactory membrane of the upper nasal cavity. It comprises small, round blue cell tumour aggregates (lobules/nests±rosettes) in a vascular

stroma with calcification. It is positive for neuroendocrine markers chromgranin, synaptophysin, NSE, neurofilament, GFAP and S100 sustentacular cells. Its *histological* (*Hyams*) *grade* is of *prognostic significance* and is based on the degree of lobular architecture, neurofibrillary stroma, cellular pleomorphism, necrosis and mitotic activity. Tumours confined to the nasal cavity have a reasonable prognosis while those in the nasal cavity and paranasal sinuses an intermediate outlook. Extranasal/paranasal and visceral lesions are of poor prognosis. Treatment is by a combination of *surgery* and *radiotherapy*. Overall *5 year survival is 50–60 % with a tendency for late recurrences*. Its immunophenotype aids in distinction from the differential diagnoses of malignant melanoma, malignant lymphoma, plasmacytoma/myeloma and embryonal/alveolar rhabdomyosarcoma.

• *Ewing's sarcoma/PNET tumour*: less differentiated than olfactory neuroblastoma, MIC 2 (CD99) positive and variably neuroendocrine marker positive (NSE, PGP 9.5, neurofilament) but potentially responsive to *high-dose irradiation* and *multi-drug chemotherapy* (*75 % 5 year survival*). There is overlap with cytokeratin positive sinonasal neuroendocrine carcinoma.

Pituitary Carcinoma

Chordoma
• A locally destructive midline low-grade malignancy derived from notochordal remnants with characteristic vacuolated physaliphorous cells positive for S100, cytokeratins (CAM 5.2, AE1/AE3, CK 8, CK 19), EMA and rarely CEA.

Malignant Meningioma

Malignant Teratoma
Desmoplastic Small Round Cell Tumour
• Polyphenotypic: positive for cytokeratins, EMA, vimentin, desmin, NSE, CD56, WT1.

Granulocytic Sarcoma

• Localised tumour of malignant myeloid cells presenting before, concurrently or following acute myeloid leukaemia. CD34/CD43/CD68/CD117/chloroacetate esterase/myeloperoxidase positive.

Bibliography

Barnest L, Eveson J, Reichart P, Sidransky D. WHO classification of tumours. Pathology and genetics. Tumours of the head and neck. Lyon: IARC Press; 2005.

British Association of Otorhinolaryngologists – Head and Neck Surgeons. Effective head and neck cancer management. Second consensus document. London: Royal College of Surgeons; 2000.

Franchi A, Palomba A, Cardesa A. Current diagnostic strategies for undifferentiated tumours of the nasal cavities and paranasal sinuses. Histopathology. 2011;59:1034–45.

Gnepp DR, editor. Diagnostic surgical pathology of the head and neck. 2nd ed. Philadelphia: WB Saunders; 2009.

Mehanna H, Paleri V, West CML, Nutting C. Head and neck cancer – part 1: epidemiology, presentation, and prevention. BMJ. 2010a;341:663–6.

Mehanna H, West CML, Nutting C, Paleri V. Head and neck cancer – part 2: treatment and prognostic factors. BMJ. 2010b;431:721–5.

Perez-Odonez B. Hamartomas, papillomas and adenocarcinomas of the sinonasal tract and nasopharynx. J Clin Pathol. 2009;62:1085–95.

Shah JP, Patel SG. Head and neck surgery and oncology. 3rd ed. Edinburgh: Mosby; 2003.

Slootweg PJ. Complex head and neck specimens and neck dissections. How to handle them. ACP best practice no 182. J Clin Pathol. 2005;58:243–8.

Thariat J, Badoual C, Faure C, Butori C, Marcy PY, Righini CA. Basaloid squamous cell carcinoma of the head and neck: role of HPV and implication in treatment and prognosis. J Clin Pathol. 2010;63:857–66.

The Royal College of Pathologists. Head and Neck Tissues – Cancer Datasets (Head and Neck Carcinomas and Salivary Neoplasms, Parathyroid Cancer, Thyroid Cancer) and Tissue Pathways (Head and Neck Pathology, Endocrine Pathology). Accessed at http://www.rcpath.org/index.asp?PageID=254.

Thompson LDR. Sinonasal carcinomas. Curr Diagn Pathol. 2006;12:40–53.

Wittekind CF, Greene FL, Hutter RVP, Klimpfinger M, Sobib LH. TNM atlas: illustrated guide to the TNM/pTNM classification of malignant tumours. 5th ed. Berlin: Springer; 2005.

Laryngeal Carcinoma

14

Typically presenting in 50–60 year old males with persistent hoarseness, tobacco and alcohol use are the usual risk factors. Investigation is by indirect larynoscopy with biopsy. Chest x-ray and endoscopy of the upper aerodigestive tract are done to exclude a concurrent cancer elsewhere. CT and MRI scans are used to stage the tumour and cervical lymph node enlargement necessitates ultrasound guided fine needle aspiration cytology (FNAC) to establish if there are metastases. Tumour stage and fitness of the patient determine the appropriate choice of treatment i.e. radiotherapy, laser resection, local excision, laryngectomy, or neck dissection. Laryngectomy may also accompany a pharyngectomy for cancer of the hypopharynx.

14.1 Gross Description

Specimen

- Biopsy/transoral laser resection/hemi-/partial or total laryngectomy/neck dissection.
- Size (cm) and weight (g).

Tumour

Site

Supraglottic	20 %
Glottic	70 %
Infraglottic	5 %
Transglottic	5 %

Supraglottis: from the tip of the epiglottis to the true cords including the aryepiglottic folds, false vocal cords and ventricles.

Glottis: true cords and anterior commissure.

Subglottis: from the lower border of the true cords to the first tracheal cartilage.

Anterior/posterior/lateral(right, left)/commissural/ventricles/false cords.

Anterior glottis is the commonest site (Fig. 14.1).

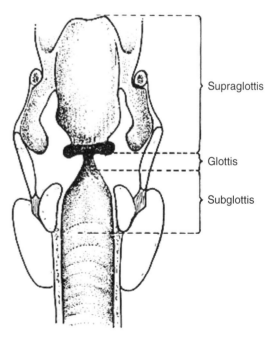

Fig. 14.1 Larynx (Reproduced, with permission, from Wittekind et al. (2005), © 2005)

D.C. Allen, *Histopathology Reporting*,
DOI 10.1007/978-1-4471-5263-7_14, © Springer-Verlag London 2013

Size

- Length × width × depth (cm) or maximum dimension (cm).
- Tumour size is the main contributor to pathological stage as it is an indicator of disease extent. The maximum depth of invasion is subordinate to the nature of the tissue planes involved. Invasion of thyroid or cricoid cartilage are important staging criteria.

Appearance

- Polypoid/verrucous/plaque/ulcerated/multifocal.
- Ulcerated endophytic cancers do less well than exophytic polypoid cancers.

Edge

- Circumscribed/irregular.

14.2 Histological Type

Squamous Cell Carcinoma

- *90 % of cases*.
- Keratinising/non-keratinising.
- Prognosis is *better* (verrucous/papillary), *usual* (spindle cell/adenoid squamous) or *worse* (basaloid/adenosquamous)
- variants:
- *Verrucous*: broad based exophytic and "church-spire" hyperkeratosis with a pushing deep margin of cytologically bland bulbous processes arising in the glottis. Locally invasive, rarely metastatic, radiation may result in anaplastic change although this association is anecdotal. Seventy percent 5 year survival.
- *Papillary*: >70 % papillary or exophytic fronds, covered by malignant type epithelium with focal invasion at the base. Better prognosis (70 % 5 year survival).
- *Spindle cell*: polypoid, glottic, elderly, ± history of irradiation for previous carcinoma. A minor squamous cell element is present (in situ or invasive) with a major variably monomorphic to pleomorphic fibrosarcoma like component. Diffuse or focal cytokeratin

(AE1/AE3, CK5/6) and p63 positivity suggests that it is a metaplastic form of squamous cell carcinoma. Prognosis is better if polypoid and superficial than infiltrative when the outlook is poor. Distinguish from sarcoma and bizarre post-irradiation granulation tissue.

- *Basaloid*: poor prognosis, nests of basaloid cells with peripheral palisading and central comedonecrosis. Presents with more extensive disease but is more radiosensitive than other squamous cell carcinoma subtypes.
- *Adenoid squamous*: usual prognosis, acantholytic (pseudoglandular) pattern.
- *Adenosquamous*: poor prognosis, mixed differentiation squamous cell carcinoma and adenocarcinoma (either obvious glands or solid with mucin positive cells).

Undifferentiated Carcinoma

- There is an absence of squamous cell or glandular differentiation.
- Includes lymphoepithelioma type which is aggressive with propensity for cervical lymph node and distant metastases.

Neuroendocrine Tumours/Carcinomas

- Chromogranin/synaptophysin positive ± CD56/CAM 5.2. Variable Ki-67 index and mitotic counts.
- Well differentiated/low-grade: *carcinoid tumour*. Low Ki-67 index (≤2 %) and mitotic count (<2/10hpfs).
- Moderately differentiated: *atypical carcinoid tumour* with characteristic spread to locoregional lymph nodes.
- Poorly differentiated/high-grade: *small cell/large cell carcinoma* 60–90 % of which present with distant metastases. High Ki–67 index and mitotic count.

Atypical carcinoid and large cell neuroendocrine carcinoma are commoner in the larynx than well differentiated neuroendocrine (carcinoid) tumour and they are *aggressive lesions with 50% mortality*.

Adenocarcinoma

- *Salivary type* e.g. adenoid cystic, mucoepidermoid carcinomas of mucosal gland origin.
- *Adenocarcinoma of no special type*.

Metastatic Carcinoma

- *Direct spread*: thyroid, oesophagus.
- *Distant spread*: malignant melanoma, kidney, breast, lung, pancreas, colon, ovary, and prostate carcinomas. Usually associated with disseminated disease.

14.3 Differentiation

Well/moderate/poor/undifferentiated, or, Grade 1/2/3/4.
- For squamous carcinoma based on cellular atypia, keratinisation and intercellular bridges.
- Undifferentiated carcinoma shows no squamous or glandular differentiation (grade 4). When differentiation varies prognosis relates to the worst area.

14.4 Extent of Local Tumour Spread

Border: pushing/infiltrative. An infiltrative pattern of invasion at the deep aspect of the tumour is of adverse prognostic value.

Lymphocytic reaction: prominent/sparse and desmoplastic stroma.

A glottic tumour is best sliced horizontally to demonstrate its anatomical relationships, a supraglottic tumour sagitally.

Anterior

- Mucous membrane, cricothyroid membrane, thyroid cartilage, thyroid gland, strap muscles, jugular vein.

Superior

- Base of epiglottis, vestibular folds, pyriform fossa and limits.

Inferior

- Trachea and limit.

The TNM7 classification applies only to carcinomas.

pTis	Carcinoma in situ

Supraglottis

pT1	One subsite, normal mobility
pT2	Mucosa of more than one adjacent subsite of supraglottis or glottis or adjacent region outside the supraglottis; without fixation
pT3	Cord fixation or invades post cricoid area, pre-epiglottic tissues, paraglottic space, thyroid cartilage erosion
pT4a	Through thyroid cartilage and/or into trachea, soft tissues of neck: deep/extrinsic muscle of tongue, strap muscles, thyroid, oesophagus
pT4b	Prevertebral space, mediastinal structures, carotid artery

Glottis

pT1	Limited to vocal cord (s), normal mobility (a) One cord (b) Both cords
pT2	Into supraglottis and/or subglottis and/or impaired cord mobility
pT3	Cord fixation and/or into paraglottic space and/or thyroid cartilage erosion

(continued)

| pT4a | Through thyroid cartilage or into trachea, soft tissues of neck: deep/extrinsic muscle of tongue, strap muscles, thyroid, oesophagus |
| pT4b | Prevertebral space, mediastinal structures, carotid artery (Fig. 14.2) |

Subglottis

pT1	Limited to subglottis
pT2	Extends to vocal cord(s) with normal/impaired mobility.
pT3	Cord fixation
pT4a	Through cricoid or thyroid cartilage and/or into trachea, deep/extrinsic muscle of tongue, strap muscles, thyroid, oesophagus
pT4b	Prevertebral space, mediastinal structures, carotid artery

14.5   Lymphovascular Invasion

Present/absent.
Intra-/extratumoural.
Vascular invasion is a relatively weak indicator for cervical lymph node metastasis. *Perineural invasion* indicates *more aggressive disease* with likelihood of local recurrence, cervical nodal metastasis and the need for adjuvant therapy.

14.6   Lymph Nodes

The *incidence of lymph node metastases at presentation* varies according to the site of the primary tumour from glottic (<10 %) to supra-/infraglottic (30–50 %). Well differentiated carcinomas are less likely to metastasise than poorly differentiated cancers.

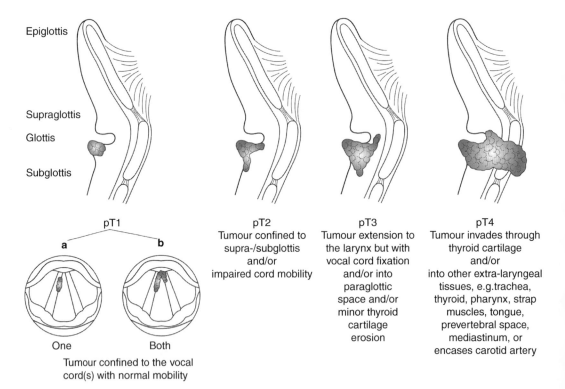

Epiglottis

Supraglottis
Glottis

Subglottis

pT1
a   b

One   Both
Tumour confined to the vocal cord(s) with normal mobility

pT2
Tumour confined to supra-/subglottis and/or impaired cord mobility

pT3
Tumour extension to the larynx but with vocal cord fixation and/or into paraglottic space and/or minor thyroid cartilage erosion

pT4
Tumour invades through thyroid cartilage and/or into other extra-laryngeal tissues, e.g.trachea, thyroid, pharynx, strap muscles, tongue, prevertebral space, mediastinum, or encases carotid artery

Fig. 14.2   Laryngeal carcinoma: glottis (Reproduced, with permission, from Allen (2006), © 2006)

Site/number/size/number involved/limit node/extracapsular spread.

Regional nodes: cervical.

Level I	Submental, submandibular
Level II	Upper jugular
Level III	Middle jugular
Level IV	Lower jugular
Level V	Posterior triangle

A selective neck dissection will ordinarily include a minimum of six lymph nodes, a (modified) radical dissection ten lymph nodes.

pN0	No regional lymph node metastasis
pN1	Metastasis in single ipsilateral node ≤3 cm
pN2	Metastasis in:
	(a) Single ipsilateral node >3 cm but ≤6 cm
	(b) Ipsilateral multiple nodes ≤6 cm
	(c) Bilateral, contralateral nodes ≤6 cm
pN3	Metastasis in lymph node >6 cm

Extracapsular lymph node spread is an adverse prognostic indicator with an increased risk of local recurrence and distant metastasis.

14.7   Excision Margins

Distances (mm) to the tracheal limit, aryepiglottic fold and pre-laryngeal anterior fascia of infiltrating carcinoma and any mucosal dysplasia or carcinoma in situ. Tumour or mucosal dysplasia at or near (<5 mm) a margin indicates a *greater likelihood of local recurrence* and requires consideration of adjuvant therapy. Intraoperative frozen section assessment of surgical margins may be required.

14.8   Other Pathology

Laryngeal carcinoma: predominantly (>95 %) in males who smoke and are 50–60 years of age. Smokers and heavy voice users can develop keratosis with hoarseness and thickened white cords on laryngoscopy. A proportion may be associated with dysplasia and progression to carcinoma in situ, and eventually over a period of years infiltrative squamous cell carcinoma. These premalignant changes can be treated by *local excision*, *laser* or *irradiation*. Carcinoma in situ may be leukoplakic, erythroplakic or inapparent and biopsy is necessary.

Radionecrosis: post-radiotherapy laryngeal dysfunction due to confluent necrosis which may lead to local airway obstruction ("crippled larynx") and necessitate laryngectomy.

Concurrent carcinoma bronchus/oropharynx: 10–15 % of cases. Can become apparent on CT staging scan of the primary laryngeal cancer and may require upper aerodigestive tract endoscopy and biopsy.

Verrucous squamous cell carcinoma: has to be distinguished from benign squamous epithelial papilloma (viral or non-viral) and hyperplasia by its pushing deep margin. It can also co-exist with squamous cell carcinoma of usual type. Beware granular cell tumour with overlying pseudoepitheliomatous hyperplasia – the granular cells (Schwann cell origin) are S100 protein positive.

Juvenile laryngeal papillomatosis: multiple HPV related squamous cell papillomas of the upper respiratory tract and a rare cause of squamous cell carcinoma, usually after erroneous application of radiotherapy. These papillomata often require *repeated endoscopic laser or microdebrider debulking* to avoid airway obstruction. A minority persist and can spread to trachea and bronchi.

Prognosis

Prognosis relates to tumour site, stage and histological grade. Early (pT1, pT2) glottic and supraglottic carcinomas may be treated by voice sparing *local excision*, *laser* or *radiotherapy*. *Partial laryngectomy* (supraglottic or vertical hemilaryngectomy) may be carried out for small volume T2 or T3 cancers. Advanced (T3/T4) carcinoma, infraglottic and transglottic tumours and cancers refractory to radiotherapy usually necessitate *laryngectomy supplemented by radiotherapy*.

Site-related 5 year survival:

Glottic	80 %
Supraglottic	65 %
Transglottic	50 %
Subglottic	40 %

Stage-related 5 year survival:

Glottic	I	90 %
	II	85 %
	III	60 %
	IV	<5 %

Most glottic carcinomas are well to moderately differentiated while non-glottic carcinomas are more frequently moderately to poorly differentiated.

14.9 Other Malignancy

Malignant lymphoma/leukaemia

- Primary MALToma or more commonly secondary to lymph node/systemic disease.
- Sinonasal (angiocentric) T/NK cell lymphoma.

Plasmacytoma/Myeloma

- Initially localised but generally becomes part of disseminated myeloma. Look for κ, λ light chain restriction and evidence of systemic disease (elevated ESR, serum immune paresis and monoclonal gammopathy, Bence-Jones proteinuria, radiological lytic bone lesions).

Sarcoma, Particularly low-Grade Chondrosarcoma and Rhabdomyosarcoma (Embryonal – Childhood), Occasionally Synovial Sarcoma, Angiosarcoma, Liposarcoma, Fibrosarcoma

Malignant Melanoma

- Primary or secondary (commoner). S100, HMB-45, melan-A positive.
- *Aggressive (20 % 5 year survival)* and recognised as such in TNM7 by designation as moderately advanced (pT3: mucosal) or very advanced (pT4: beyond mucosa) disease.

Kaposi's Sarcoma

- HIV.

Bibliography

Allen DC. Histopathology reporting: guidelines for surgical cancer. 2nd ed. London: Springer; 2006.

Barnest L, Eveson J, Reichart P, Sidransky D. WHO classification of tumours. Pathology and genetics. Tumours of the head and neck. Lyon: IARC Press; 2005.

British Association of Otorhinolaryngologists – Head and Neck Surgeons. Effective head and neck cancer management. Second consensus document. London: Royal College of Surgeons; 2000.

Gnepp DR, editor. Diagnostic surgical pathology of the head and neck. 2nd ed. Philadelphia: WB Saunders; 2009.

Gnepp DR, Barnes L, Crissman J, Zarbo R. Recommendations for the reporting of larynx specimens containing laryngeal neoplasms. Am J Clin Pathol. 1998;110:137–9.

Helliwell TR. Guidelines for the laboratory handling of laryngectomy specimens. ACP best practice no 157. J Clin Pathol. 2000;53:171–6.

Kusafuka K, Abe M, Iida Y, Onitsuka T, Fuke T, Asano R, Kamijo T, Nakajima T. Mucosal large cell neuroendocrine carcinoma of the head and neck regions in Japanese patients: a distinct clinicopathological entity. J Clin Pathol. 2012;65:704–9.

Mehanna H, Paleri V, West CML, Nutting C. Head and neck cancer – part 1: epidemiology, presentation, and prevention. BMJ. 2010a;341:663–6.

Mehanna H, West CML, Nutting C, Paleri V. Head and neck cancer – part 2: treatment and prognostic factors. BMJ. 2010b;431:721–5.

Shah JP, Patel SG. Head and neck surgery and oncology. 3rd ed. Edinburgh: Mosby; 2003.

Slootweg PJ. Complex head and neck specimens and neck dissections. How to handle them. ACP best practice no 182. J Clin Pathol. 2005;58:243–8.

Thariat J, Badoual C, Faure C, Butori C, Marcy PY, Righini CA. Basaloid squamous cell carcinoma of the head and neck: role of HPV and implication in treatment and prognosis. J Clin Pathol. 2010;63:857–66.

The Royal College of Pathologists. Head and Neck Tissues – Cancer Datasets (Head and Neck Carcinomas and Salivary Neoplasms, Parathyroid Cancer, Thyroid Cancer) and Tissue Pathways (Head and Neck Pathology, Endocrine Pathology). Accessed at http://www.rcpath.org/index.asp?PageID=254.

Wittekind CF, Greene FL, Hutter RVP, Klimpfinger M, Sobib LH. TNM atlas: illustrated guide to the TNM/pTNM classification of malignant tumours. 5th ed. Berlin: Springer; 2005.

Salivary Gland Tumours

Salivary gland swelling has diverse causes including calculus (sialolithiasis), infection secondary to duct obstruction by calculus, duct stenosis or mucous plugs, enlargement (sialadenosis) associated with systemic diseases e.g. diabetes, Sjögren's syndrome or HIV, and, primary or secondary neoplasms. Presentation can mimic cervical lymphadenopathy, and investigation is by ultrasonography with fine needle aspiration cytology (FNAC). Ultrasound can determine whether the swelling is focal or diffuse, cystic or non-cystic, salivary or non-salivary.

Comprising about 6 % of head and neck cancers salivary gland tumours present as persistent unilateral enlargement the majority of which are in the parotid gland and are benign. Facial pain is a worrying feature and suggestive of carcinoma involving branches of the facial (VIIth cranial) nerve. Other red flag symptoms suspicious of malignancy are a rapid increase in size, ulceration, induration or fixity of the buccal mucosa or overlying skin. A history of previous skin squamous cell cancer or malignant melanoma, Sjögren's syndrome or radiation to the head and neck area are relevant clues. There is a higher incidence of carcinoma arising in the submandibular glands (40 % of neoplasms at that site), sublingual (90 % of neoplasms at that site) and minor glands of the oral cavity i.e. the proportion of cancers increases with decreasing gland size. Tumours in the soft palate and upper lip are likely to be benign but malignant if sited in the tongue, floor of mouth and retromolar pad.

Assessment is by a specialist head and neck surgeon. Investigation is plain x-ray (for calculus), ultrasound scan, MRI and CT scans (for local and distant tumour stage, respectively). Free hand or ultrasound guided FNAC is the method of choice in obtaining a likely tissue diagnosis for the purposes of planning operative management. It effectively triages inflammatory, lymphoid and epithelial proliferations and can exclude the possibility of metastatic carcinoma. Salivary epithelial tumours can show considerable cytological overlap and findings must be interpreted in light of the patient's age, symptoms and clinical findings. Needle core and open biopsy are avoided due to the risk of nerve damage, salivary fistula and compromising complete local surgical clearance. Diagnostic biopsy of large minor gland lesions may assist in planning radical surgery.

Surgical treatment is by partial or total excision of the gland to include the tumour mass with a surround of either salivary gland tissue or soft tissues. Most specimens are a superficial parotidectomy. Total parotidectomy is indicated for tumours in the deep lobe, with or without facial nerve preservation, if there is tumour involvement of the nerve or local salivary gland extraparenchymal spread. Parotid tumours may also require excision of the skin and soft tissues of the side of the face and upper neck. Submandibular and sublingual glands are removed in their entirety if the site of tumour. Occult or clinically evident cervical lymph node metastases may require a therapeutic neck dissection. Post operative radiotherapy

D.C. Allen, *Histopathology Reporting*,
DOI 10.1007/978-1-4471-5263-7_15, © Springer-Verlag London 2013

is determined by the tumour size, grade and status of the surgical resection margins.

The most important prognostic features are tumour type (with grade influential in some malignancies), stage and adequacy of local excision.

15.1   Gross Description

Specimen

- Parotid/submandibular/sublingual/minor (oral).
- Incisional or excisional biopsy/surgical excision: conservative superficial/radical parotidectomy, submandibulectomy, excision of oral tumour (sublingual glands, or minor salivary glands of mucosal origin), neck dissection.
- Size (cm) and weight (g).

Tumour

Site
- Salivary gland/intrasalivary lymph node based.
- Parotid gland: superficial or deep lobe (subdivided by the plane of the facial nerve). Most arise in the superficial lobe.
- Bilateral: Warthin's tumour, pleomorphic adenoma, acinic cell carcinoma.

Size
- Length × width × depth (cm) or maximum dimension (cm).
- Size is part of TNM7 staging for carcinoma and a major factor in treatment outcome and survival.

Appearance
- Solid/cystic.
- Mucoid/chondroid/necrotic/fleshy/scirrhous.

Edge
- Circumscribed/irregular: presence of macroscopic extraglandular extension.

Gland
- Intrasalivary lymph nodes/nerves.

15.2   Histological Type

Adenomas

- Pleomorphic; 70 % of salivary gland tumours, 80 % in the parotid gland.
- Myoepithelioma.
- Basal cell.
- Warthin's tumour (adenolymphoma/papillary cystadenolymphomatosum).
- Oncocytoma.
- Canalicular.
- Sebaceous.
- Ductal papilloma (inverted/intra-ductal/sialadenoma papilliferum).
- Cystadenoma (papillary/mucinous).

Carcinomas

- Acinic cell.
- Mucoepidermoid: low-grade/well differentiated, high-grade/poorly differentiated.
- Adenoid cystic: cribriform/tubular/solid.
- Polymorphous low-grade.
- Epithelial/myoepithelial.
- Salivary duct.
- Basal cell.
- Sebaceous.
- Oncocytic.
- Papillary cystadenocarcinoma.
- Mucinous (colloid).
- Adenocarcinoma, not otherwise specified (NOS).
- Squamous cell.
- Carcinoma in pleomorphic adenoma (ex-PSA) usually adenocarcinoma, no special type.
- Myoepithelial: spindle/clear cell types.
- Lymphoepithelial.
- Small cell.
- Undifferentiated.
- Carcinosarcoma.

Malignant Lymphoma

- Extranodal lymphoma of salivary gland (MALToma).
- Malignant lymphoma of salivary gland lymph nodes (nodal lymphoma).

Metastatic Carcinoma

- Squamous cell carcinoma of head and neck region and upper aerodigestive tract, malignant melanoma from scalp or facial skin, renal cell carcinoma, lung, breast, prostate, and large bowel carcinomas. The metastasis is to adjacent or intra-salivary lymph nodes and the enlargement *mimics a primary lesion*. Note that secondary carcinoma of the sub-maxillary region is commoner than a primary neoplasm.

15.3   Differentiation

Well/moderate/poor/undifferentiated, or, Grade 1/2/3/4.

- *Grade* is related to the *risk of local recurrence*, *regional* and *distant metastasis* but is *less important than stage*. It is *type dependent* e.g. acinic cell, basal cell, myoepithelial and polymorphous low-grade adenocarcinomas are *low-grade*, but salivary duct, primary squamous cell, carcinoma ex-PSA, oncocytic and undifferentiated carcinomas are *high-grade*. Adenocarcinoma, NOS is graded according to the percentage tumour gland formation, and adenoid cystic carcinoma is grade 2 (intermediate) unless it is solid pattern (grade 3, high-grade). Mucoepidermoid carcinoma is assessed on the degree of cystic change, atypia, necrosis, perineural invasion and mitoses as low-, intermediate- or high-grade (grade 1/2/3). The latter tend to be solid and epidermoid in type with a scanty mucous component.
- A majority of salivary gland tumours are low-grade but *elderly patients* not infrequently present with high-grade tumours.

- Some carcinomas show a range of grade with *progression to high-grade or dedifferentiation*.
- *Ki-67 labelling index* may be of use in grading and a prognostic indicator in acinic cell, adenoid cystic and mucoepidermoid carcinomas. A *high Ki-67 index (>5%) correlates with poor survival*.

15.4   Extent of Local Tumour Spread

Border: pushing/infiltrative.

- *Infiltrative margins* are a useful diagnostic feature of malignancy in low-grade lesions e.g. polymorphous low-grade adenocarcinoma and adenoid cystic carcinoma.
- *Macroscopic extraparenchymal extension* of carcinoma to involve adjacent structures is a predictor of local recurrence and cervical lymph node metastasis for parotid carcinoma. Lymphocytic reaction: prominent/sparse.

Perineural space involvement particularly in adenoid cystic carcinoma resulting in intractable facial pain, and *predictive of lymph node metastases* and *poor outcome*. Perineural invasion is also *diagnostically useful* in adenoid cystic and polymorphous low-grade adenocarcinomas.

Skin, subcutis.

The TNM7 classification applies to major salivary glands: parotid, submandibular and sublingual. Minor salivary gland tumours (i.e. from the mucosa of the upper aerodigestive tract) are classified according to anatomical site, e.g. lip.

pT1	Tumour ≤2 cm, without extraparenchymal extension[a]
pT2	Tumour >2–4 cm, without extraparenchymal extension[a]
pT3	Tumour with extraparenchymal extension, and/or >4 cm
pT4	Tumour invades
	(a) Skin, mandible, ear canal, and/or facial nerve.
	(b) Base of skull, and/or pterygoid plates and/or encases carotid artery.

[a]Extraparenchymal extension is clinical or macroscopic evidence of invasion of skin, soft tissues, bone or nerve; microscopic evidence alone is not sufficient (Figs. 15.1, 15.2, 15.3 and 15.4)

Fig. 15.1 Salivary gland
carcinoma (Reproduced,
with permission,
from Wittekind et al.
2005, © 2005)

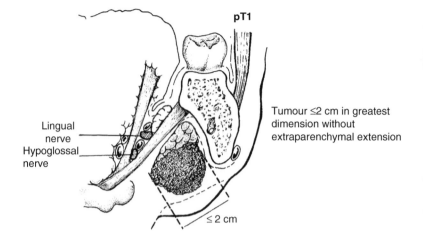

Fig. 15.2 Salivary gland
carcinoma (Reproduced, with
permission, from Wittekind
et al. 2005, © 2005)

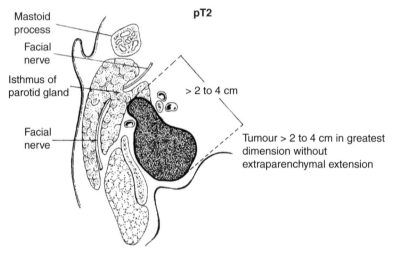

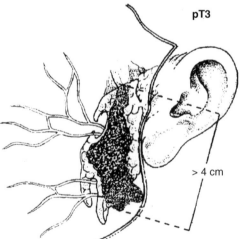

Fig. 15.3 Salivary gland
carcinoma (Reproduced,
with permission, from
Wittekind et al. 2005,
© 2005)

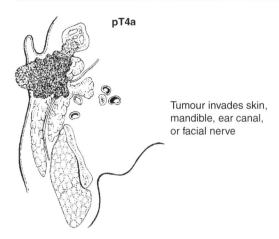

pT4a

Tumour invades skin, mandible, ear canal, or facial nerve

Fig. 15.4 Salivary gland carcinoma (Reproduced, with permission, from Wittekind et al. 2005, © 2005)

15.5   Lymphovascular Invasion

Present/absent.

Intra-/extratumoural.

Useful diagnostically in designation of a tumour as adenocarcinoma and predictive for local recurrence.

15.6   Lymph Nodes

Intra-/extraglandular: the parotid gland can contain up to 20–30 intraglandular lymph nodes.

Site/number/size/number involved/limit node/extracapsular spread.

Regional nodes: cervical.

Level I	Submental, submandibular
Level II	Upper jugular
Level III	Middle jugular
Level IV	Lower jugular
Level V	Posterior triangle

A selective neck dissection will ordinarily include a minimum of six lymph nodes, a (modified) radical dissection ten lymph nodes.

pN0	No regional lymph node metastasis
pN1	Metastasis in single ipsilateral node ≤3 cm
pN2	Metastasis in:
	(a) Single ipsilateral node >3 cm but ≤6 cm
	(b) Ipsilateral multiple nodes ≤6 cm
	(c) Bilateral or contralateral nodes ≤6 cm
pN3	Metastasis in lymph node >6 cm.

The *cervical regional lymph nodes* are the commonest site of *metastasis* followed by *lungs* and *bone*. The parotid gland drains to the superior deep cervical (level II) lymph nodes, the submandibular and sublingual glands to the submandibular, submental and level II lymph nodes. *Extracapsular lymph node spread* is an indicator of more *aggressive disease* and should prompt consideration of postoperative radiotherapy.

15.7   Excision Margins

Distance (mm) to the nearest painted excision margin. Tumour at or close to (<5 mm) the nearest excision margin is an important factor in *local control of disease* and *survival*.

Pleomorphic adenomas should not be surgically enucleated as the irregular lobulated margin with satellite nodules can lead to residual tumour and local recurrence.

15.8   Other Pathology

Fine needle aspiration cytology: has an important role to play in the primary diagnosis of salivary gland enlargement and is capable of designating *benignity* and *malignancy* in a majority of cases. It can indicate non-neoplastic disorders such as simple cysts, abscess and fatty infiltration. The separation of benign from malignant salivary tumours results in more *appropriate surgery* (superficial conservative versus radical parotidectomy) or *the avoidance of it* (malignant lymphoma, secondary carcinoma). The experienced cytopathologist can in many cases obtain sufficient material to stipulate the tumour subtype. Some *pitfalls* are *cystic lesions* (simple cyst versus cystic salivary tumour e.g. mucoepidermoid carcinoma, acinic cell carcinoma or metastatic squamous carcinoma), *clear cell lesions* (primary epithelial or myoepithelial tumour versus secondary renal, lung or thyroid carcinoma), *metastases* (primary squamous cell or mucoepidermoid carcinoma versus secondary squamous cell carcinoma), the onset of low-grade *malignant lymphoma* in lympho(myo-)epithelial sialadenitis and distinction from extranodal lymphoma and chronic sialadenitis. The technique is obviously reliant on *representative sampling* of the tumour and there can be a degree of cytological overlap between subtypes e.g. pleomorphic adenoma, adenoid cystic carcinoma and polymorphous low-grade adenocarcinoma.

Necrotising sialometaplasia: of minor salivary glands in the mouth and palate can *mimic carcinoma* e.g. mucoepidermoid carcinoma. It presents as an ulcerating lesion in middle aged men.

Site of carcinoma: there is a higher incidence of carcinoma in *minor salivary glands* e.g. mucoepidermoid adenocarcinoma or polymorphous low-grade adenocarcinoma of the palate or floor of mouth. The *relative site frequencies of salivary carcinomas* are: palate 44 %, submaxillary glands 38 %, parotid 17 %.

Salivary tumours with clear cells: tend to be *malignant*, and must also be distinguished from secondary renal cell carcinoma. A wide range of salivary tumours can show clear cell differentiation: acinic cell, mucoepidermoid, epithelial-myoepithelial, sebaceous, clear cell carcinomas and malignant myoepithelioma. Abdominal CT scan may be necessary to exclude metastatic renal cell carcinoma (EMA, CD10, vimentin, RCC ab); also S100, melan-A and HMB-45 (clear cell malignant melanoma), and thyroglobulin/TTF-1 (clear cell thyroid carcinoma). Primary clear cell carcinoma of low-grade arises in minor salivary glands, has uniform clear cells in a dense hyalinising stroma and is locally infiltrative.

Acinic cell carcinomas: occur in the parotid gland and have deceptively bland granular to clear or eosinophilic cells with a variably solid, papillary, follicular or microcystic pattern, but can still infiltrate and metastasise. More aggressive pleomorphic variants occur. Overall recurrence can be seen in 10–30 % and death in about 6 %. Peak incidence is in the third decade of life, but *like mucoepidermoid carcinoma, acinic cell carcinomas are seen in childhood and teenage years*. Gross invasion, cellular pleomorphism, a high Ki-67 index (>5 %) with mitoses >20/mm^2, and incomplete primary excision are adverse indicators.

Mucoepidermoid carcinoma: affects the palate and parotid gland and is *the commonest malignant salivary gland tumour (30 % of cases)*. It shows a spectrum of epidermoid and mucous cells in varying proportions (mucin stains may be necessary). Well differentiated lesions may be largely cystic with only mural tumour. Poorly differentiated (high-grade) lesions are more solid, squamoid and infiltrative. The mucin and keratin can be extruded into the interstitium causing an inflammatory reaction. *Tumour grade dictates prognosis* with multiple local recurrences dominating and lymph node metastases (10 % of cases) late.

Adenoid cystic carcinoma: forms 5 % of salivary gland neoplasms but *20 % of the carcinomas* with an equal distribution between the parotid and minor glands (palate). It shows *biphasic cell differentiation* (epithelial/myoepithelial: cytokeratins/S100, CK5/6, p63 and calponin), and *biphasic histochemical staining* of PAS positive luminal mucus and alcian blue positive matrix. It typically shows cribriform, hyaline and tubular patterns and indolent perineural spread with facial pain and late lymph node involvement. It is *slow growing* but *highly malignant* and *locally recurrent* with *10 year survival <50 %*. Prognosis relates adversely to a >30 % solid (basaloid) growth pattern, stage and incomplete primary excision, with *radical surgery* being the treatment of choice. Margins can be difficult to define as there is often spread beyond the identifiable clinical edge. Tumour cells may show oestrogen receptor positivity indicating potential use for anti-oestrogens and aromatase inhibitors for clinical control. It is also CD117 (c-kit) positive.

Polymorphous low-grade adenocarcinoma: is characterised by *cellular uniformity* and *architectural diversity* (solid/cribriform/single cell/cords/tubular/ductal/papillary) with abundant stroma. Typically in the *palate* (second commonest after adenoid cystic carcinoma) with local recurrence in 21 %, lymph node involvement in 6.5 % and distant metastases in 1.8 %. An infiltrative margin and perineural invasion can be helpful in making the diagnosis. A somewhat more aggressive tumour is the related low-grade papillary adenocarcinoma.

Epithelial/myoepithelial carcinoma: is a low-grade malignancy mainly of the parotid gland and recurs in one third of cases, comprising ductal cells and outer clear myoepithelial cells in a biphasic pattern. Myoepithelial differentiation can be demonstrated by CK5/6, S100, p63 and calponin. Although circumscribed it has an infiltrative margin with perineural invasion. Death can occur in 7 % and nuclear atypia in >20 % of cells is an adverse prognostic factor. Occasionally one element dedifferentiates resulting in carcinomatous or sarcomatous overgrowth.

Myoepithelial carcinoma: is a spindle cell lesion with mitotic activity, nuclear atypia, necrosis and invasion.

Ductal carcinoma: resembles high-grade ductal carcinoma in situ of the breast. It shows *aggressive behaviour* with poor prognosis and *70 % die within 3 years*. Patients are >50 years of age and the male to female ratio is 3:1 with parotid being the main site. Micropapillary and sarcomatoid variants are adverse. A low-grade variant also exists which probably represents intraductal carcinoma with or without microinvasion.

Primary squamous cell carcinoma: *5–10 % of cases*, mostly in the parotid gland and aggressive with 5 year survival rates of 40 %. Metastases to the parotid gland from other sites must be excluded, commonly upper aerodigestive tract or skin. Some primary lesions represent mucoepidermoid carcinoma or squamous cell carcinoma ex-PSA.

Carcinoma in pleomorphic adenoma (ex-PSA): *3–4 % of cases* and unusual manifesting as *symptomatic regrowth* or *facial pain in an existing lesion present for 15–30 years (9.5 % risk after 15 years)*. In descending order of frequency the malignancy is carcinoma (adenocarcinoma of no special type, poorly differentiated ductal and undifferentiated, squamous cell carcinoma), malignant myoepithelioma, carcinosarcoma and metastasising pleomorphic adenoma. The latter is usually due to previous surgery and vascular implantation. Prognosis of carcinoma ex-PSA which is adverse relates to the *proportion of carcinoma in the tumour* and strongly to the *degree of extracapsular extension* of the malignancy beyond that of the original benign tumour.

Basal cell carcinoma: is the malignant counterpart of basal cell adenoma (solid nests surrounded by basal hyaline lamina material) except that it shows infiltration, perineural and vascular invasion. It occurs in the patient's parotid gland, 50–60 years of age.

Carcinosarcoma, small cell carcinoma and undifferentiated carcinoma (some of which are lymphoepitheliomatous in character and EBV related similar to nasopharyngeal carcinoma) have poor prognosis.

Surgical treatment: most *low-grade carcinomas* of mucoepidermoid or acinic cell type can be treated by *superficial parotidectomy* whereas more *radical surgery* with sacrifice of the facial nerve is needed for *large (>4 cm), higher-grade or advanced carcinomas*. Submandibular and sublingual sited tumours are treated by total removal of the gland with a margin of normal tissue.

Immunohistochemistry: *diagnosis of salivary gland tumours is mainly morphological*. Immunohistochemistry can help to characterise neoplasms that contain myoepithelial cells (CK14, CK5/6, p63, calponin, caldesmon, S100) and luminal epithelial cells (cytokeratins 8, 18, 19). Adenoid cystic carcinoma is positive for CD117 (c-kit) and can be oestrogen receptor positive. Pleomorphic adenoma is GFAP positive. Ki-67 index is a gauge of grade and prognosis for some tumour types.

Prognosis

Prognosis relates to anatomical location, tumour histological type, grade, stage and adequacy of excision.

- Minor salivary gland tumours have a higher incidence of recurrence and metastases than equivalent parotid lesions.
- Examples of 5 year survival rates:
  Low-grade mucoepidermoid, 90–95 %
  High-grade mucoepidermoid, 50–60 %
  Squamous cell carcinoma, 40 %.
- Histological type:
  Better prognosis: low-grade mucoepidermoid/ acinic cell carcinomas
  Worse prognosis: high-grade mucoepidermoid/ acinic cell carcinomas; adenoid cystic carcinoma, malignant mixed tumour, salivary duct carcinoma, squamous cell carcinoma.

15.9   Other Malignancy

Rhabdomyosarcoma

- Children. Desmin/myo D1/myogenin positive. Note that mucoepidermoid and acinic cell carcinomas can also typically occur in childhood and young adults.

Malignant Fibrous Histiocytoma, Fibrosarcoma, Malignant Peripheral Nerve Sheath Tumour

- Adults

Malignant Lymphoma

- *2–5 % of salivary gland neoplasms.*
- 20 % have *Sjögren's syndrome* or *LESA* (lymphoepithelial or myoepithelial sialadenitis).
- One third are *diffuse large B cell lymphoma*, of lymph node or parenchymal origin.

- One third are *follicular lymphoma*, usually of lymph node origin.
- One third are *MALTomas* i.e. originating in mucosa associated lymphoid tissue. LESA has ×40 increased risk of developing low-grade malignant lymphoma and 15–20 % do so over a variable period of 5–20 years. MALToma is characterised by lymphoepithelial lesions surrounded by broad haloes or sheets of centrocyte like (marginal zone/ monocytoid) B cells. Other features include monotypic plasma cells and follicular colonisation. High-grade transformation to large cell lymphoma can occur. PCR demonstration of clonality does not always reliably predict those lymphoid lesions that will progress to clinical malignant lymphoma.

Bibliography

Cheuk W, Chan JKC. Advances in salivary gland pathology. Histopathology. 2007;51:1–20.

Ellis G, Auclair PL. Tumors of the salivary glands. Atlas of tumor pathology. 4th series. Fascicle 9. Washington: AFIP; 2006.

Gnepp DR, editor. Diagnostic surgical pathology of the head and neck. 2nd ed. Philadelphia: WB Saunders; 2009.

Mehanna H, McQueen A, Robinson M, Paleri V. Salivary gland swellings. BMJ. 2012;345:36–41.

Perez-Odonez B. Selected topics in salivary gland tumour pathology. Curr Diagn Pathol. 2004;9:355–65.

Shah JP, Patel SG. Head and neck surgery and oncology. 3rd ed. Edinburgh: Mosby; 2003.

Slootweg PJ. Complex head and neck specimens and neck dissections. How to handle them. ACP best practice no 182. J Clin Pathol. 2005;58:243–8.

Speight PM, Barrett AW. Diagnostic difficulties in lesions of the minor salivary glands. Diagn Histopathol. 2009; 15:311–7.

The Royal College of Pathologists. Head and Neck Tissues – Cancer Datasets (Head and Neck Carcinomas and Salivary Neoplasms, Parathyroid Cancer, Thyroid Cancer) and Tissue Pathways (Head and Neck Pathology, Endocrine Pathology). Accessed at http://www.rcpath.org/index.asp?PageID=254.

Wittekind CF, Greene FL, Hutter RVP, Klimpfinger M, Sobib LH. TNM atlas: illustrated guide to the TNM/ pTNM classification of malignant tumours. 5th ed. Berlin: Springer; 2005.

Thyroid Gland Tumours (with Comments on Parathyroid)

16

Thyroid cancer comprises about 1 % of human malignancies and is the commonest originating in the endocrine system. A majority are differentiated cancer, either papillary (60 %) or follicular (20 %) in type. They arise in young to middle aged adults, females more commonly than males, and are of indolent behaviour with 10 year survival rates in excess of 90 %. Clinical features and histology identify those undifferentiated cancers that show aggressive local and metastatic spread. Benign tumours are common and cancers relatively rare.

Thyroid gland tumours usually present with enlargement (goitre) due to a solitary "*cold*" *nodule* with euthyroid function. About 5 % of thyroid nodules are malignant. There is a range of thyroid function tests including serum levels of thyroxine, thyroid stimulating hormone (TSH), triiodothyronine, and autoantibodies to thyroglobulin, microsomal antigen and the TSH receptor. Iodine-123 radioactive scintiscan determines the functional status of the tissue. A functional "*hot*" *nodule* is very unlikely to be malignant. Differentiated cancer (papillary, follicular) may present with cervical lymph node or sclerotic bone metastases. Undifferentiated cancers are often of rapid onset with symptoms due to infiltration or compression of local structures e.g. hoarseness, dysphagia or respiratory stridor. Fine needle aspiration cytology (FNAC) is the investigation of choice either of a clinically palpable lesion or under ultrasound guidance, with clinical follow up for benign cytology and surgery for a suspicious or malignant aspirate. Needle core biopsy may be necessary to distinguish between anaplastic carcinoma and malignant lymphoma.

The extent of operative resection depends on the *patient's age*, *gender*, *tumour type* and *stage*. The latter is assessed by MRI and CT scans of the neck and chest respectively. Intraoperative frozen section is occasionally used to confirm a diagnosis of papillary, medullary or anaplastic carcinoma, or lymph node involvement. It is inappropriate for making the distinction between follicular adenoma and carcinoma as this requires full examination of the entirety of the tumour capsule in a well fixed specimen. High stage undifferentiated and anaplastic cancers are often treated non-surgically with radiotherapy.

16.1 Gross Description

Specimen

- FNAC/needle core biopsy/partial or (sub)total thyroidectomy/ left or right lobectomy/ hemithyroidectomy/isthmusectomy/parathyroidectomy/selective neck dissection.
- Size (cm) and weight (g).

Tumour

Site

- Left/right lobe, isthmus, multifocal.

Size

- Length × width × depth (cm) or maximum dimension (cm).
- Size is a criterion for TNM staging.

Appearance

- Solid/cystic/calcified/haemorrhagic/pale/tan/papillary.
- From small foci to tumour replacing the entire gland.

Edge

- Circumscribed/irregular   (encapsulated/non-encapsulated).

Gland

- Uniform, nodular, atrophic, pale in colour.

16.2   Histological Type

Follicular Adenoma

- *Usual type*: macrofollicular, microfollicular, embryonal/fetal, or mixed patterns.
- *Variants*: hyalinising trabecular (HTA); oxyphil (Hürthle). Most HTAs (organoid trabecular/nested pattern of spindle cells and collagen) are benign but a minority show overlap features with papillary carcinoma and/or capsular/vascular invasion and are regarded as hyalinising trabecular carcinoma. Thyroglobulin and NSE positive ± CK19.

Papillary Carcinoma

- *Usual type*: psammomatous.
- *Variants with better prognosis*:
  Encapsulated, including follicular variant
  Papillary microcarcinoma (≤1 cm).
- *Variants with usual prognosis*:
  Follicular
  Oxyphil (Hürthle cell).
- *Variants potentially more aggressive or with worse prognosis*:
  Diffuse sclerosing
  Diffuse follicular

Solid
Tall cell
Columnar cell

Follicular Carcinoma

- *Widely invasive*:
  Grossly apparent or extensive microscopic invasion of thyroid outside the lesion capsule and/or extrathyroidal soft tissue.
  Follicular/trabecular/solid patterns and vascular invasion.
  Cytological features of malignancy e.g. atypia/mitoses/necrosis.
  Mitotic counts >1–4/10 hpfs are adverse.
- *Minimally invasive*:
  Encapsulated – *angioinvasive* with potential for metastases, or, *capsular invasion* with equivocal potential for metastases.
  Note the number of foci of vascular and capsular invasion.
- *Variants*: oxyphil (Hürthle: >75 % of cells)/clear cell.

Undifferentiated (Anaplastic) Carcinoma

- Old age; *5–10 % of cases*. Clinically there is *rapid growth with involvement of vital neck structures and death in 6 months*. Treatment (decompressive surgery, external beam radiotherapy) is usually palliative.
- Spindle/squamoid/giant cells ± cartilage/osseous metaplasia ± a differentiated component i.e. evidence of origin from a more usual thyroid carcinoma e.g. papillary carcinoma. The tumour cells are cytokeratin positive/CD45 negative to distinguish from malignant lymphoma.

Poorly Differentiated Carcinoma

- "Insular" carcinoma: large solid nests or trabeculae of small to medium sized round uniform tumour cells (medullary like) and thyroglobulin/TTF-1   positive,   calcitonin negative. In older age and grossly invasive with *aggressive behaviour*.

- Also includes carcinomas of solid, scirrhous and trabecular patterns with necrosis and increased mitoses, and/or of tall cell or columnar type, either alone or as a dedifferentiated part of a carcinoma of more usual type. These tumours are intermediate between differentiated (papillary/follicular) and undifferentiated (anaplastic) thyroid cancers. More than 50 % of the tumour area requires to be poorly differentiated to be designated as such. Any focus of anaplastic change comprises undifferentiated/anaplastic carcinoma and is assigned pT4.

Small Cell Carcinoma

- A poorly differentiated/high-grade neuroendocrine carcinoma and synaptophysin/CD56/CAM5.2/TTF-1 positive with a high Ki-67 index.
- Exclude a metastasis from the lung.

Medullary Carcinoma

- *5–10 % of cases*, including mixed medullary/follicular. See Sect. 16.8.

Miscellaneous

- Signet ring cell carcinoma, squamous cell carcinoma, mucoepidermoid carcinoma, carcinoma showing thymus like differentiation (CASTLE).

Metastatic Carcinoma

- *Direct spread*: upper aerodigestive tract, metastases in cervical lymph nodes.
- *Distant spread*: malignant melanoma, breast, kidney, lung carcinomas. Renal cell carcinoma can mimic primary clear cell carcinoma (papillary or follicular) of the thyroid. Renal cell carcinoma may be multiple nodules, show

vascular invasion and thyroglobulin/TTF-1 negative, but positive for renal carcinoma markers (RCC antibody/vimentin/EMA/CD10).

16.3   Differentiation

Well/moderate/poor/undifferentiated, or, Grade 1/2/3/4.

Traditional cytoarchitectural features may be used but *grade* is often determined by the *nature of the tumour and its subtype* e.g. usual papillary carcinoma and minimally invasive follicular carcinoma are *low-grade*, whereas undifferentiated carcinoma is *high-grade*. Tumour heterogeneity and a *minor undifferentiated component* within an otherwise differentiated tumour should be noted as this is an *adverse indicator*.

16.4   Extent of Local Tumour Spread

Border: pushing/infiltrative.
Lymphocytic reaction: prominent/sparse.
Perineural space involvement.
Solitary/multifocal, one or two lobes.
Involvement of lesion capsule, *extracapsular spread*.
Involvement of thyroid capsule, *extrathyroid spread*.

Specimen blocking must be generous to detect tumour heterogeneity, multifocality, tumour capsule and thyroid capsule involvement, vascular invasion and status of the excision margins. One suggestion is to process all of the tumour up to 2–3 cm diameter, and upwards of ten blocks thereafter.

The TNM7 classification applies only to carcinomas.

pT1	Tumour ≤2 cm in greatest dimension, limited to thyroid
	(a) ≤1 cm
	(b) 1 cm < tumour ≤2 cm

(continued)

Fig. 16.1 Thyroid carcinoma (Reproduced, with permission, from Allen (2006), © 2006)

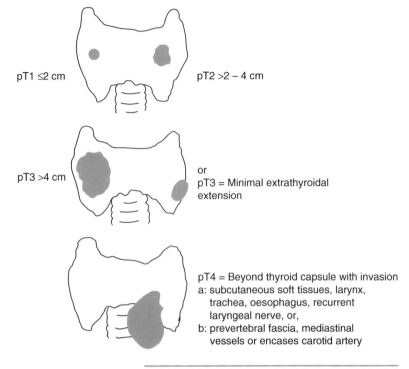

pT1 ≤2 cm

pT2 >2 – 4 cm

pT3 >4 cm

or
pT3 = Minimal extrathyroidal extension

pT4 = Beyond thyroid capsule with invasion
a: subcutaneous soft tissues, larynx,
    trachea, oesophagus, recurrent
    laryngeal nerve, or,
b: prevertebral fascia, mediastinal
    vessels or encases carotid artery

pT2	2 cm < tumour ≤4 cm in greatest dimension, limited to thyroid
pT3	(a) Tumour >4 cm in greatest dimension, limited to thyroid or
	(b) Any tumour with minimal extrathyroid extension (e.g. to sternothyroid muscles or perithyroid tissues)
pT4	(a) Tumour extends beyond capsule and involves any of: subcutaneous soft tissues, larynx, trachea, oesophagus, recurrent laryngeal nerve
	(b) Tumour invades prevertebral fascia, mediastinal vessels or encases carotid artery

See Fig. 16.1

All anaplastic/undifferentiated thyroid carcinomas are pT4 (pT4a: intrathyroidal and considered surgically resectable; pT4b: extrathyroidal spread and considered surgically non-resectable).

Other pathological descriptors:

- pT1, 2, 3:
  i. Grossly encapsulated tumour
  ii. Grossly non-encapsulated tumour

Separate *clinical stage groupings* are recommended for

1. Papillary or follicular carcinoma <45 year
2. Papillary or follicular carcinoma ≥45 year
3. Medullary carcinoma
4. Anaplastic/undifferentiated carcinoma (all stage IV).

16.5   Lymphovascular Invasion

Present/absent.

Intra-/extratumoural.

Papillary carcinoma tends to *lymphatic spread, follicular carcinoma* to *vascular spread.* Patient outcome also relates to the *number of foci (>4–5)* of vascular invasion in follicular carcinoma, and the encapsulated follicular variant of papillary carcinoma (also foci of capsular invasion).

16.6   Lymph Nodes

Site/number/size/number involved/limit node/extracapsular spread.

Regional nodes: cervical, upper/superior mediastinal

Level I	Submental, submandibular
Level II	Upper jugular
Level III	Middle jugular
Level IV	Lower jugular
Level V	Posterior triangle

A selective neck dissection will ordinarily include a minimum of six lymph nodes. Radical neck dissection is rarely performed for thyroid cancer.

pN0	No regional lymph nodes metastasis
pN1	Metastasis in regional lymph node(s)
	(a) Level VI (including pre-/paratracheal and prelaryngeal nodes)
	(b) Other unilateral, bilateral or contralateral cervical or upper/superior mediastinal nodes.

16.7   Excision Margins

Distances (mm) to the nearest painted capsule and surgical excision margins.

16.8   Other Pathology

Thyroid carcinoma: is commoner in females (2.5:1) with the most frequent subtypes being papillary carcinoma (60 %) and follicular carcinoma (20 %). Previous irradiation predisposes to papillary carcinoma.

Papillary carcinoma: occurs in younger patients (average age 40 years), is multifocal (intraglandular lymphatic metastases) in a significant proportion of cases (20 %), and shows a tendency to *lymphatic vessel* and *lymph node spread (40–50%)*. Despite this, *prognosis is excellent* with a *low disease-related mortality of about 5%*. Papillary carcinoma may undergo cystic change with only residual mural tumour – a potential pitfall on FNAC. Invasion is not necessary for its *diagnosis, which is mainly cytological*. Diagnostic features are a combination of optically clear (orphan Annie) ground glass, overlapping nuclei with longitudinal grooves and nuclear pseudoinclusions. Stromal (not intrafollicular) and tumour cell related calcified psammoma bodies are present (50 % of cases) and the stroma may be hyalinised, calcified or ossified. Architectural patterns are papillary, follicular or solid. The cells are thyroglobulin, TTF-1, cytokeratin 7, 19, galectin 3, HBME-1 and vimentin positive. Protooncogene product RET is variably positive and tumours positive for *BRAF mutation* can be *widely infiltrative and*

more *aggressive* presenting at a more advanced clinical stage of disease. Notably the papillae of Grave's disease and nodular hyperplasia are CK19 focal or negative helping in the differential diagnosis. Variants with an *excellent prognosis* are encapsulated carcinoma (totally surrounded by a capsule) and papillary microcarcinoma (≤1 cm diameter). *Potentially more locally aggressive* are diffuse sclerosing (sclerosing, numerous psammoma bodies, solid foci, squamous metaplasia, heavy lymphocytic infiltrate), diffuse follicular and solid types. There are *significantly worse outcomes* for tall cell (older patients, papillary, oncocytic cell with height two to three times the width) and columnar cell (nuclear stratification) variants with a high risk of lymph node and distant metastases, and *disease-related mortality of up to 25 %*.

Follicular carcinoma: tends to be in older patients (50–60 years) than papillary carcinoma, unifocal and spreads via the blood stream to lung and bone. *Minimally invasive carcinoma has an excellent prognosis* with lymph node metastases in <5 % of cases, whereas *widely invasive tumour has a mortality of 30–35%*. Multiple blocks (up to ten) of the lesion and its capsule are required for the distinction between follicular adenoma and minimally invasive follicular carcinoma. *Diagnostic criteria are invasion of the capsule and/or its vessels*. Cytological appearances of the epithelium are not particularly helpful as adenomas may be markedly atypical, although solid, trabecular and microfollicular growth patterns can be a low-power clue. Carcinoma often has a thick, partly desmoplastic fibrous capsule and its full width must be traversed to qualify as invasion. The invasive tumour front may then form a second fibrotic interface with the parenchyma giving a dumbbell type of distribution. *Vascular invasion, which is a more reliable indicator of malignancy*, requires vessels to be:

(a) Within or outside the capsule, i.e. extratumoural,

(b) Of venous rather than capillary calibre with a definite muscular wall and endothelial lining, and

(c) Partially or completely plugged by tumour in the lumen with a definite point of attachment to the vessel wall. A cluster of follicular cells found free floating in a vascular lumen may represent artifactual detachment and is therefore discounted. CD31/CD34 immunostains help to identify true vascular structures.

Note that capsular invasion needs to be distinguished from rupture following FNAC which often shows organising haemorrhage and a reparative response. It can also cause tumour infarction and entrapment of cells within the capsule.

Ultrasound and isotope scan examinations combined with FNAC: used in the investigation of a wide range of thyroid enlargement. Cytology can be diagnostic in

- *Inflammatory/autoimmune goitres*:
  Hashimoto's thyroiditis (lymphocytes, Askanazy epithelial cells, colloid poor).
  De Quervain's thyroiditis (lymphocytes, giant cells, degenerate follicular cells).
  Riedel's struma (spindle cells, scant aspirate).
  Abscess (polymorph rich).
- *Simple goitre*: multinodular colloid/adenomatous (characteristically *colloid rich/cell poor*) and forming the vast majority of thyroid nodules.
- *Simple thyroid cyst*: watery colloid and macrophages, scanty follicular cells.
- *Solitary, solid thyroid nodule*: adenoma, follicular carcinoma, papillary carcinoma and medullary carcinoma (see above and below).
  Adenoma and minimally invasive follicular carcinoma *cannot be distinguished on FNAC*. They are designated follicular lesion or neoplasm and are recognised by a variable *cell rich/colloid poor* pattern usually distinguishing them from simple goitres. *Surgical excision is necessary for the histological assessment of capsular and vascular invasion.*
- *Malignant goitre*:
  Widely invasive follicular carcinoma (cytological features of malignancy).
  Malignant lymphoma (dispersed atypical lymphoid cells, lymphoglandular bodies).
  Anaplastic carcinoma (spindle/giant cells with atypia).
  Metastatic carcinoma.
  Care must be taken to closely *correlate imaging and FNAC* results as well as in assessing *specimen adequacy* sufficient to constitute a

safe diagnosis e.g. 5–10 groups of follicular cells with 10–20 cells per group. Diagnostic categories (Thy 1–5) are: (1) insufficient, (2) benign (nodular goitre, hyperplastic nodule, thyroiditis), (3) follicular lesion, (4) suspicious of malignancy, and (5) malignant (papillary carcinoma, anaplastic carcinoma etc.).

Hürthle cell neoplasms: a higher proportion are malignant than follicular neoplasms of usual type. Once again capsular and vascular invasion are the hallmarks of malignancy. Hürthle cell carcinomas are *aggressive with 5 year mortality rates of 20–40%*. Follicular carcinomas are thyroglobulin, cytokeratin, TTF-1, EMA, galectin 3 and vimentin positive.

Medullary carcinoma: (C-cell differentiation – *5% of thyroid cancers*) is in *the majority of cases (80%) sporadic and unifocal*. The *hereditary forms* occur in *younger patients*, can be *multifocal and bilateral*, associated with diffuse C-cell hyperplasia (>50 C cells per low power field), C-cell tumourlets and the multiple endocrine neoplasia (MEN) syndromes types II and III. Its morphology is heterogeneous, but usually comprises polygonal or plump spindle cells with a nested, trabecular or solid pattern. The hyalinised stroma can be calcified and is typically positive for amyloid. The tumour cells are *CEA, calcitonin and chromogranin/synaptophysin positive*. Staining for TTF-1 and thyroglobulin is variable. Loss of calcitonin staining is adverse and in its absence CEA positivity acts as a surrogate marker. Lymph node metastases are seen in 30–60 % of cases but *5 year survival is 80%*. High serum calcitonin levels, soft tissue and regional lymph node involvement are associated with an adverse prognosis. Elevated serum calcitonin following ablative therapy can indicate recurrence or metastases. Family members should be *genetically screened* for the *RET mutation* to establish the hereditary cases (autosomal dominant), and *prophylactic thyroidectomy* can be offered to affected children. Serial blocking of the gland is often required to look for C cell hyperplasia and medullary microcarcinoma (≤1 cm). *Treatment is surgical* with radio-/chemotherapy of limited use.

Poorly differentiated carcinoma: 70 % 5 year survival with a prognosis intermediate between that of usual thyroid carcinoma (90–95 % 5 year survival) and anaplastic carcinoma. It is more frequently associated with old age, lymph node metastases and extrathyroid extension.

Anaplastic (syn. undifferentiated or sarcomatoid) carcinoma: requires immunohistochemistry to distinguish it from high-grade malignant lymphoma, malignant melanoma and angiosarcoma:

Immunophenotype

Carcinoma	Low molecular weight cytokeratin positive, thyroglobulin, CK19, TTF-1. Undifferentiated carcinoma may be negative for thyroglobulin and TTF-1 but cytokeratin and pax-8 positive.
Malignant lymphoma	CD 45, CD 20 (B) , CD 3 (T)
Malignant melanoma	S100, HMB-45, melan-A
Angiosarcoma	CD 31, CD 34, factor VIII positive.

Prognosis

Prognosis is worse in:
- Male patients.
- Patients >45 years of age.
- Large tumours: <1.5 cm, excellent; >3.5–5 cm, poor.
- Multicentric tumours.
- Unencapsulated tumours.
- Widely invasive tumours with extrathyroid extension.

Low-Grade Malignancy

- Minimally invasive follicular carcinoma.
- Papillary carcinoma.

Intermediate-Grade Malignancy

- Widely invasive follicular carcinoma.
- Medullary carcinoma.
- Poorly differentiated carcinoma.
- Malignant lymphoma.

High-Grade Malignancy

- Undifferentiated carcinoma.
- Angiosarcoma.

Thus, patients with differentiated cancer can be managed based on risk stratification according to gender, age, stage and histology (GASH):

Patient	Low-risk	F <45 year.
	High-risk	<16 year, F >45 year, all males.
Tumour	Low-risk	Papillary/minimally invasive follicular cancer <1 cm.
	High-risk	Papillary/follicular carcinoma >1 cm, multifocal or metastatic cancer.

Treatment: most solitary thyroid neoplasms are treated *surgically* by lobectomy with isthmusectomy, or, (sub)total thyroidectomy if a firm preoperative diagnosis of differentiated thyroid malignancy has been made. Total or completion thyroidectomy tends to be reserved for worse prognosis subtypes of papillary carcinoma, widely invasive follicular carcinoma, medullary carcinoma (particulary if familial) and undifferentiated carcinoma (if operable). Extensive differentiated thyroid cancer may also require laryngectomy, tracheal resection and pharyngectomy, and, neck dissection is performed for clinically palpable lymph node metastases. Alternative treatment modalities are tumour and TSH suppression by administration of *thyroxine or radioactive iodine* (papillary and follicular carcinoma), and *radiotherapy* (incompletely excised carcinomas or undifferentiated carcinoma). Treatment is therefore tailored to the patient's age, tumour type and stage.

16.9 Other Malignancy

Malignant Lymphoma

- Lymphocytic/Hashimoto's thyroiditis/MALToma (mucosa associated lymphoid tissue).
- Low-grade: centrocyte-like cells, lymphoepithelial lesions, follicle loss/ destruction.
- High-grade: blast cells.

The majority of lesions are *diffuse large B cell* and there is some evidence for progression from Hashimoto's thyroiditis through low-grade to high-grade MALToma/DLBCL. *Clinical onset can be rapid* with compression of neck structures and presentation is usually in elderly patients with an enlarging mass, stridor and dysphagia. *Overall 5 year survival is 50–80%* and spread can occur to other MALT sites, e.g. gastrointestinal tract. Advanced age, size (>10 cm), high-grade and stage of disease (particularly perithyroidal soft tissue extension) can decrease *5 year survival rates to 40%*. Malignant lymphoma responds to *chemoradiotherapy*.

Primary Hodgkin's lymphoma is extremely rare.

Plasmacytoma

- As part of systemic myeloma: elevated ESR, serum immune paresis and monoclonal gammopathy, Bence-Jones proteinuria, radiological lytic bone lesions.

Angiosarcoma

- Overlaps with undifferentiated carcinoma and is a pleomorphic tumour with vasoformative areas in elderly patients. Endothelial markers (CD31, CD 34) are required for confirmation.

16.10   Parathyroid

Hyperparathyroidism is due to over secretion of parathormone and results in *hypercalcaemia*. It arises in three main contexts

1. *Primary hyperparathyroidism* – over secretion by one or more parathyroid glands sometimes due to *diffuse hyperplasia* (10–25 % of cases 25 % of which are associated with MEN I and IIa syndromes) but more commonly (70–80 % of cases) an *adenoma*.

2. *Secondary hyperparathyroidism* – as a physiological response of all four glands to chronic hypocalcaemia due to renal failure, malabsorption or vitamin D deficiency.

3. *Tertiary hyperparathyroidism* – autonomous hypersecretion in long-standing secondary hyperparathyroidism after correction of the hypercalcaemia.

Investigation: is by serum calcium, phosphate, parathormone and alkaline phosphate levels. *Gland localisation* is by technetium labelled isotope scintigraphy (technetium 99 sestamibi) with CT scan and MRI scans.

Treatment: is by *surgical removal* of the adenoma (usually solitary, occasionally two) or hyperplastic glands, leaving a small amount (100 mg) of functioning tissue either in situ or implanted into the soft tissues of the arm. An alternative is total parathyroidectomy with replacement treatment (calcium/calcidiol). Recurrence >6 months after surgery can be due to inadequate neck exploration with removal of insufficient parathyroid tissue, or ectopic glands. Better preoperative localisation now allows minimally invasive procedures targeted at the single abnormal gland in primary hyperparathyroidism. However limitations in scan sensitivity can lead to missed multifocal disease and higher recurrence rates. Bilateral neck exploration is still more appropriate in 20–40 % of cases particularly in the context of secondary hyperparathyroidism or if more than one abnormal gland is suspected. There is histological overlap in the features of adenoma and nodular hyperplasia and designation is more appropriately decided by the number of enlarged glands (adenoma is usually solitary) and the clinical context. What is of crucial importance is that *the pathologist confirms by frozen section to the surgeon that parathyroid tissue has been excised at neck exploration and not lymph node, thymic remnant or thyroid nodule*. To this end each submitted specimen is finely weighed and its nature confirmed indicating whether there is any need for further surgical exploration.

Parathyroid carcinoma: is *rare (<2 % of cases)* and in elderly patients with high levels of parathormone. It may infiltrate adjacent soft tissues with *difficulty in surgical excision*. Suspicion is raised by an irregular, large and pale adherent gland. Histologically it has a solid or trabecular pattern with thick fibrous bands traversing it. Cytological atypia and mitoses are present but as these can be seen in an adenoma more reliable indicators are soft tissue, perineural and lymphovascular invasion. It may be resected in continuity with the ipsilateral lobe of thyroid gland, and neck dissection is considered for palpable metastases. Cervical and mediastinal lymph nodes, lungs, bone and liver are the commonest sites for metastatic spread. Parathyroid carcinoma is *slow growing* with a tendency for *multiple local recurrences* after a long disease free interval and *late metastases*. Cure is achieved in 50 % of cases, *death is due to the complications of hypercalcaemia*. Chemotherapy is not indicated but radiotherapy may have a role to play.

Bibliography

Allen DC. Histopathology reporting: guidelines for surgical cancer. 2nd ed. London: Springer; 2006.

Anderson CE, McLaren KM. Best practice in thyroid pathology. J Clin Pathol. 2004;56:401–5.

Asa SL. My approach to oncocytic tumours of the thyroid. J Clin Pathol. 2004;57:225–32.

Chetty R. Follicular patterned lesions of the thyroid gland: a practical algorithmic approach. J Clin Pathol. 2011;64:737–41.

De Matos PS. Thyroid epithelial tumours. Diagn Histopathol. 2008;14:236–46.

DeLellis RA, Lloyd RV, Heitz PU, Eng C. WHO classification of tumours. Pathology and genetics. Tumours of endocrine organs. Lyon: IARC Press; 2004.

Derringer GA, Thompson LDR, Frommett RA, Bijwaard KE, Hefess CS, Abbondanzo SL. Malignant lymphoma of the thyroid gland. A clinicopathologic study of 108 cases. Am J Surg Pathol. 2000;24:623–39.

Gnepp DR, editor. Diagnostic surgical pathology of the head and neck. 2nd ed. Philadelphia: WB Saunders; 2009.

Khonsari M, Scarsbrook AF, Bradley KM. Anatomical and functional imaging of the thyroid and parathyroid. CPD Cell Pathol. 2007;6:47–58.

LiVolsi VA, Baloch ZW. Familial thyroid carcinoma: the road less travelled in thyroid pathology. Diagn Histopathol. 2009;15:87–94.

McNichol AM. Criteria for diagnosis of follicular thyroid neoplasms and related conditions. In: Lowe DG, Underwood JCE, editors. Recent advances in histopathology, vol. 20. London: RSM Press; 2003. p. 1–16.

Rosai J, Carcangiu ML, DeLellis RA. Tumors of the thyroid gland. Atlas of tumor pathology. 3rd series. Fascicle 5. Washington: AFIP;. 1992.

Rosai J, Kuhn E, Carcanagiu ML. Pitfalls in thyroid tumour pathology. Histopathology. 2006;49:107–20.

Slootweg PJ. Complex head and neck specimens and neck dissections. How to handle them. ACP best practice no 182. J Clin Pathol. 2005;58:243–8.

Sneed DC. Protocol for the examination of specimens from patients with malignant tumors of the thyroid gland, exclusive of lymphomas. Arch Pathol Lab Med. 1999;123:45–9.

Sobrinho-Simóes M, Magalháes J, Fonseca E, Amendoeira I. Diagnostic pitfalls of thyroid pathology. Curr Diagn Pathol. 2005;11:52–61.

Stephenson TJ. Prognostic and predictive factors in endocrine tumours. Histopathology. 2006;48:629–43.

The Royal College of Pathologists. Head and Neck Tissues – Cancer Datasets (Head and Neck Carcinomas and Salivary Neoplasms, Parathyroid Cancer, Thyroid Cancer) and Tissue Pathways (Head and Neck Pathology, Endocrine Pathology). Accessed at http://www.rcpath.org/index.asp?PageID=254.

Thompson LDR. Endocrine pathology. Philadelphia: Elsevier; 2006.

Parathyroid

DeLellis RA. Tumors of the parathyroid gland. Atlas of tumor pathology. 3rd series. Fascicle 6. Washington: AFIP; 1993.

Erikson LA, Lloyd RV. Familial disorders of the parathyroid gland. Diagn Histopathol. 2009;15:79–88.

Johnson SJ. Changing clinicopathological practice in parathyroid disease. Histopathology. 2010;56:835–51.

Johnson SJ, Sheffield EA, McNichol AM. Examination of parathyroid gland specimens. ACP best practice no 183. J Clin Pathol. 2005;58:338–42.

Stephenson TJ. Prognostic and predictive factors in endocrine tumours. Histopathology. 2006;48:629–43.

Part III

Respiratory and Mediastinal Cancer

- Lung Carcinoma
- Malignant Mesothelioma
- Mediastinal Cancer

Lung Carcinoma

17

The commonest worldwide cancer over 35,000 people die from lung cancer each year with 85–90 % attributed to tobacco smoking. The incidence has decreased in males but increased in females reflecting changes in smoking habits.

Lung cancer may present with persistent *cough*, *haemoptysis* secondary to ulceration of the tumour, *obstructive effects* (pneumonia), *local infiltration* (pleural effusion, chest wall pain/mass, hoarseness, Horner's syndrome due to apical Pancoast's tumour, superior vena cava syndrome), *systemic effects* (finger clubbing, paraneoplastic syndromes, weight loss), or as an *incidental finding* on radiology for other reasons. Urgent referral to a member of the lung cancer multidisciplinary team, initially a chest physician is required.

Investigation is by chest x-ray and staging by CT scan and endobronchial ultrasound to assess spread to locoregional lymph nodes, liver, adrenal glands and brain. MRI scan can detect invasion into the axilla, chest, vertebral column and spinal cord, and CT/PET scan has a role in defining small (<1–2 cm) intrapulmonary or distant metastases. High resolution CT (HRCT) can demonstrate lymphangitis carcinomatosa.

Tissue diagnosis is obtained in a high percentage (>90 %) of cases by a variety and combination of techniques depending on the tumour site, local infiltration and type. These include sputum cytology, bronchial brushings/washings/biopsy, transbronchial or percutaneous image guided (endobronchial ultrasound or CT) FNAC(fine needle aspirate cytology)/needle core biopsy, open lung wedge or mediastinoscopic/thoracoscopic biopsy. Thoracoscopic sampling of mediastinal lymph nodes is also used for staging purposes due to lack of sensitivity in CT scan assessment. In bronchogenic carcinoma diagnostic yield increases with the number of biopsy fragments. Transthoracic FNAC/needle biopsy is of particular use for peripheral lesions, and, transbronchial biopsy for lymphangitis carcinomatosa and cancers causing bronchostenotic extrinsic compression. Where a firm preoperative diagnosis of a peripheral lesion has not been obtained intraoperative frozen section is indicated as a prequel to opting for either a more radical cancer resection operation or a lung sparing wedge resection. Tracheal lesions may require assessment by rigid bronchoscopy. In the presence of extensive disease pleural fluid cytology or peripheral lymph node FNAC may provide a more accessible site for a positive diagnosis.

The histological tumour type of lung cancer (small cell or non-small cell carcinoma) is crucial in selection of appropriate non-surgical versus surgical primary treatment. Clinical staging determines suitability for surgical resection, neoadjuvant or palliative chemoradiotherapy. Pathological staging of the surgical specimen points to those patients that might benefit from postoperative adjuvant treatment. Subtyping of non-small cell carcinoma by a combination of routine morphology, immunohistochemistry and genetic analysis can indicate a potential role for targeted drug therapy in patients with advanced, recurrent or metastatic lung adenocarcinoma.

D.C. Allen, *Histopathology Reporting*,
DOI 10.1007/978-1-4471-5263-7_17, © Springer-Verlag London 2013

Peripheral wedge or segmental resection can be by either open surgery, or a closed video assisted technique, but recurrence rates for the latter tend to be higher than for more radical operations. Sleeve resections (bronchial or lobectomy) are lung sparing aimed at removal of a proximal endobronchial lesion, at or adjacent to the carina, with reanastomosis of the proximal major airway to the distal bronchial tree. Lobectomy resects one or more lobes with the draining hilar lymph nodes. Pneumonectomy comprises 20 % of lung resections and is indicated when there is tumour involvement of hilar structures or the oblique fissure is traversed. Segmentectomy, sleeve resections, lobar resections and pneumonectomy can all be extended to include en bloc excision of involved contiguous chest wall or thoracic structures. Extrapleural pneumonectomy encompasses removal of visceral and parietal pleurae, lung, ipsilateral hemidiaphragm and pericardium. Definition of an intrapericardial or extrapericardial plane of vascular resection is important in distinguishing T3 and T4 tumours.

The usual surgical approach is posterolateral thoracotomy with lobectomy and regional (hilar, mediastinal) lymphadenectomy. Patients require full clinical assessment of their fitness using a global risk score e.g. Thoracoscore prior to proceeding to radical treatment.

Patients with endobronchial obstruction may be managed by a variety of interventional techniques: brachytherapy, electrocautery, cryotherapy, thermal laser ablation, photodynamic therapy and airway stents. This can also be a prequel to further elective planned treatment.

17.1 Gross Description

Specimen

- Exfoliative cytology/aspiration cytology or needle biopsy (percutaneous/transbronchial/US or CT guided)/bronchial biopsy/thoracoscopic or mediastinoscopic biopsy/wedge resection/ sleeve resection/segmentectomy/(bi-)lobectomy/pneumonectomy (standard/

extrapleural/extra-/intrapericardial)±en bloc resection (may include mediastinal pleura, pericardium, great vessels, atrial wall).
- Resection can be either open or thoracoscopic (VATS: video assisted thoracoscopic surgery).
- Size (cm) and weight (g)/number of fragments.

Tumour

Site

- Central (main/segmental bronchus): <2 cm or ≥2 cm from the carina; RUL/RML/RLL/LUL/LLL.
- Hilar: at the hilum but not within a specific lobe.
- Peripheral (parenchymal/pleural).

Size

- Length × width × depth (cm) or maximum dimension (cm).
- Size is a TNM staging criterion.

Squamous cell carcinomas can attain a large size and remain localized, whereas small cell carcinomas can be small primary lesions but with extensive local mediastinal lymphadenopathy and distant spread and clinical symptoms reflecting disseminated disease.

Appearance

- Necrosis/haemorrhage/mucoid/cavitation.
- Polypoid/nodular/ulcerated/stenotic.
- Endobronchial/bronchial/extrabronchial.

Squamous cell carcinoma frequently cavitates, central carcinoid tumour is polypoid or nodular, small cell carcinoma is submucosal and bronchostenotic or shows extrinsic compression.

Edge

- Circumscribed/irregular.

Pulmonary Changes

- Scar: peripheral adenocarcinoma.
- Fibrosis/asbestosis.
- Partial and hilar, or total atelectasis/obstructive pneumonitis the extent of which helps

determine the pT stage. It is probably more accurately described radiologically but can be mapped in extent by sampling blocks of lung away from the tumour mass.

17.2 Histological Type

Crucial therapeutic distinction is made between *small cell carcinoma* and *non-small cell carcinoma* (*squamous cell/adenocarcinoma/large cell*). Typing is primarily *morphological* on routine H&E sections. An increasing proportion of cases require supplementary *immunohistochemistry* for designation of non-small cell carcinoma subtype (adenocarcinoma versus squamous cell carcinoma), neuroendocrine tumours/carcinomas (well differentiated/low-grade (carcinoid) tumour, or poorly differentiated/high-grade small cell/large cell carcinoma), and primary versus secondary carcinoma.

Squamous Cell Carcinoma

- *30–45% of cases*. It requires nuclear stratification, intercellular bridges, ± keratinisation.
- Large cell/small cell.
- Keratinising/non-keratinising.
- Variants:
- *Spindle cell* (*see carcinosarcoma*): cytokeratin positive ± vimentin positive.
- *Basaloid*: poor prognosis, nests of palisaded basaloid cells with central comedonecrosis, hyalinised stroma. More radiosensitive than other squamous cell carcinoma subtypes.
- *Papillary*: >70 % exophytic or papillary malignant epithelial fronds with focal invasion at the base and better prognosis (70 % 5 year survival).
- *Adenoidsquamous*: usual prognosis, acantholytic (pseudoglandular) pattern.
- *Adenosquamous*: mixed differentiation with the minor component at least 10 % of the tumour. It is of worse prognosis. The adenocarcinoma element may have obvious glands or is solid with mucin positive cells.
- *Clear cell*.

Small Cell Carcinoma

- *25% of cases*. A poorly differentiated/high-grade neuroendocrine carcinoma. Small round/fusiform nuclei (×2–3 lymphocyte size) with granular chromatin, moulding and an inconspicuous nucleolus. There is also DNA crush and vessel artifact (Azzopardi phenomenon), fir tree hyaline stroma, prominent apoptosis, necrosis and mitoses. The nuclear features are the diagnostic characteristic of small cell carcinoma. Note that there can be a scattered population of large bizarre (polyploid) cells.
- *Oat cell*: usual type.
- *Intermediate cell*: larger nucleus/more cytoplasm and most likely represents better preserved/fixed oat cell i.e. the same tumour.
- *Combined*: + non-small cell component (at least 10 %) e.g. squamous or adenocarcinoma.

Adenocarcinoma

- *15–25% of cases* (50 % of lung cancer in females and also in non-smokers) and showing a *progressive increase in incidence* with more accurate histological subtyping. Forty percent are endobronchial, 60 % peripheral, and 75 % involve the pleura at presentation and unusually can give an encasing pseudo-mesotheliomatous picture. There is commonly a central scar in peripheral lesions. Adenocarcinoma is more often suitable for resection than squamous cell carcinoma.
- Pulmonary adenocarcinoma is classified as either *non-mucinous* (acinar, papillary, micropapillary, solid, lepidic) or *mucinous* in type, although up to 85 % show *heterogeneity* with more than one, often multiple cell patterns.

Non-mucinous
- *Acinar*: gland forming.
- *Papillary*: frond forming with stromal cores.
- *Micropapillary*: papillary nodules without stromal cores. A papillary or micropapillary pattern indicates *more aggressive disease*, with a high incidence of lymph node and pleural metastases and venous invasion.

- *Solid*: with mucus formation (>5 PAS/AB-diastase positive cells in at least two high power fields).
- *Lepidic*: formerly bronchioloalveolar adenocarcinoma (BAC). Peripheral, single/multiple or a pneumonic infiltrate with lepidic spread along alveolar walls and no stromal, vascular or pleural invasion. Lepidic denotes use of the alveolar walls as a scaffold for growth giving a honeycomb appearance on microscopy.
- Prognosis of non-mucinous lung adenocarcinoma decreases in the following order: lepidic, acinar, solid, (micro)papillary.

Mucinous
- Colloid, goblet cell, columnar cell, signet ring cell, clear cell types.

For further discussion of lepidic/BAC and atypical adenomatous hyperplasia see Sect. 17.8.

Large Cell Carcinoma

- *5–10% of cases*.
- Shows no evidence of squamous cell or glandular differentiation although they probably represent undifferentiated forms of these.
- Variants: giant cell, rhabdoid, clear cell, lymphoepithelioma like, basaloid and neuroendocrine.

In primary clear cell carcinoma (rare) exclude: clear cell change in squamous cell or adenocarcinoma, secondary thyroid, salivary or renal cell carcinoma, malignant melanoma, and benign clear cell (sugar) tumour of lung (HMB-45 positive) – a perivascular epithelioid cell tumour (PEComa).

Miscellaneous

- *Pulmonary endodermal tumour or adenocarcinoma of fetal type*: young patients with a solitary mass, endometrioid type glands and better prognosis.
- *Pulmonary blastoma*: adults, peripheral, solitary and large. Well differentiated fetal type tubular glands in a cellular embryonal stroma and poor prognosis.

- *Carcinosarcoma*: forms a pulmonary or polypoid bronchial mass. Squamous cell or large cell/adenocarcinoma with fibrosarcoma like spindle cells (diffuse or focal cytokeratin (AE1/AE3)±TTF-1 positive) representing spindle cell carcinoma with or without heterologous mesenchymal differentiation, e.g. cartilage, bone, striated muscle. It has a *poor prognosis* and overlaps with pleomorphic (spindle/giant cell) carcinoma. Metastases can be epithelial, sarcomatoid or both.

Note that only about 40 % of primary lung carcinomas are of homogeneous histological type and *mixed differentiation and patterns* are reasonably common e.g. squamous cell and small cell components, acinar and papillary adenocarcinoma. The second component must comprise at least 10 % of the tumour volume to be regarded as a mixed tumour.

Neuroendocrine Tumours/ Carcinomas

- *5% of primary pulmonary neoplasms*. See also *small cell carcinoma* (above).
- Chromogranin, synaptophysin, CD56 (NCAM), TTF-1 positive. Well differentiated lesions stain more strongly with chromogranin than CD56, and poorly differentiated lesions the converse of this.
- A spectrum of tumours with *low-grade* well (carcinoid), moderately (atypical carcinoid) and *high-grade*/poorly differentiated (small cell/large cell) forms.
- *Carcinoid tumour*: in younger patients and polypoid/dumbbell shaped, either central or peripheral. Central cases present with haemoptysis and are dome shaped at bronchoscopy. Lymph node metastasis in 5–15 % and *70–90% 10 year survival*.
- *Atypical carcinoid tumour*: central/peripheral and spindle cells with cellular atypia, necrosis (usually punctate) and mitoses >2–10/10 high power fields. Lymph node metastasis in 40–60 % with *60% 5 year survival*.
- *Large cell neuroendocrine carcinoma*: *34% 5 year survival*. Significant numbers of endocrine

cells present rather than just a non-small cell carcinoma with focal endocrine differentiation. Shows solid sheets/nests/peripheral palisading/ moderate cytoplasm.

- High resolution CT scan has led to an increasing awareness of *diffuse idiopathic neuroendocrine cell hyperplasia* as both a reactive phenomenon in chronic inflammatory lung diseases e.g. bronchiectasis, and, as a possible indolent precursor to extraluminal carcinoid tumourlets/tumour. Carcinoid tumourlet is defined as <5 mm maximum dimension.

Salivary Gland Type Adenocarcinoma

- Bronchial mucosal gland origin.
- *Adenoid cystic carcinoma*: indolent growth but prognosis is poor with late metastases to nodes and lung parenchyma common. Along with squamous cell carcinoma it is the *commonest primary tracheal tumour*.
- *Mucoepidermoid carcinoma*: prognosis is determined by the histological grade.

Metastatic Carcinoma

Lung can be the *sole site of metastatic spread in 15–25 % of patients* with cancer. Tumours commonly metastasising to lung in order of frequency are: breast, colon, stomach, pancreas, kidney, malignant melanoma, prostate, thyroid and genital tract origin. Up to 40 % can be oligometastatic, in particular colorectum or kidney, *mimicking a primary lung lesion*.

Various *patterns of spread* are encountered

- Multiple/bilateral/well defined/rapid growth/ nodular or mass lesions: breast, gastrointestinal tract, kidney, sarcoma, malignant melanoma, ovary, germ cell tumour.
- Lymphangitis carcinomatosis: stomach, breast, pancreas, prostate, lung.
- Cavitation in a mass lesion: squamous cell carcinoma, gastrointestinal tract, leiomyosarcoma.
- Endobronchial polypoid mass: breast, kidney, gastrointestinal tract, sarcoma.

- Vasculoembolic: breast, stomach, liver, choriocarcinoma.
- Lepidic/bronchioloalveolar pattern of spread: gastrointestinal tract, pancreas (metastases are more pleomorphic and necrotic than bronchioloalveolar carcinoma), prostate.

Tissue Diagnosis

In limited biopsy material a positive diagnostic yield is increased by *multiple biopsies (5 or 6 minimum)* examined histologically through at least three levels, the aim being to *designate basic neoplastic categories* e.g. primary versus secondary cancer, small cell versus non-small cell carcinoma, other neuroendocrine (carcinoid) lesions and malignant lymphoma. This is due to *limited material, tumour heterogeneity and poor observer agreement* (50 % at best) at subclassifying moderately to poorly differentiated cancers of non-small cell type. Non-small cell carcinoma is a category of exclusion in that the tumour lacks distinctive morphological features of small cell, squamous cell or glandular differentiation. It comprises over *30 % of lung cancers* but there is evidence that this can be reduced to 5–10 % using a limited immunohistochemical panel for squamous cell carcinoma (CK5/6, p63) and pulmonary adenocarcinoma (CK7, TTF-1). This gives good biopsy to resection correlation despite some overlap in expression of these markers. Designation of small cell carcinoma is reasonably robust and it must be distinguished from carcinoid tumour (Ki-67 <2 %), malignant lymphoma (CAM5.2, CD56, CD45) and the small cell variant of squamous cell carcinoma. In this context the relatively *robust preservation of immunophenotypical expression* despite extensive biopsy crush artifact is a diagnostically useful tool.

Bronchial squamous cell carcinoma and basaloid carcinoma are preceded by a *squamous cell metaplasia – dysplasia – carcinoma in situ sequence*, often as a multifocal mucosal field change in the lower respiratory tract. The presence of carcinoma in situ and a lack of demonstrable invasion is not unusual in biopsies and must be *correlated with the clinical findings*. It may be representative of the lesion if derived from a segment of thickened, irregular mucosa. However, in the presence of an obvious *bronchoscopic abnormality* and *radiological mass lesion* it usually represents the edge of an invasive carcinoma. Squamous metaplasia may be entirely nonspecific, associated with a carcinoma or overlying a lesion such as carcinoid tumour or small cell carcinoma when it can be atypical and suggest an erroneous cytological diagnosis of non-small cell carcinoma in brushings material. Sometimes the main biopsy fragments are negative but dyscohesive clusters of cytologically malignant cells lie in mucus separate from the epithelial surface.

Close correlation with cytology preparations e.g. bronchial brushings and washings and transbronchial fine needle aspirates increases diagnostic yield and accuracy with *agreement rates of 70–90 %* for small cell carcinoma, well differentiated squamous cell carcinoma and adenocarcinomas. Cytology is particularly helpful where there is biopsy sampling error, extensive biopsy crush artifact e.g. small cell carcinoma, and extrabronchial or peripheral cancers. Cell yield and preservation can be high when biopsy fragments are negative or uninterpretable. Conversely the tissue pattern and capability for immunohistochemistry in a positive biopsy can be helpful in specific situations e.g. primary versus secondary adenocarcinoma, small cell carcinoma versus malignant lymphoma. Immunochemistry can now also be reliably applied to liquid based cytology preparations. Thoracoscopic biopsy is used for patients suspected of having malignancy but in whom bronchial biopsy and cytology are negative and in suspected bilateral disseminated disease. Other sources of a positive diagnosis are radiologically guided FNAC or core biopsy of peripheral lung tumours, pleural fluid cytology, and FNAC or biopsy of cervical or supraclavicular lymph nodes. These approaches should be considered when the tumour is difficult to diagnose by conventional means, the patient is unfit for bronchoscopy or there is suspected disseminated disease. Thus a *tissue diagnosis* is obtained providing *staging information, a basis for adjuvant therapy*, and *exclusion of unrelated non-respiratory malignancy*, e.g. malignant lymphoma.

The pulmonary nodule: a relatively common issue emerging at specialty multidisciplinary team meetings is the *significance of a solitary pulmonary nodule* detected at CT scan staging or follow up of a primary cancer originating at various organ sites. The nodule may be *benign* e.g. healed tuberculosis, abscess, rheumatoid nodule, aspergilloma, pulmonary chondroma, or, *malignant* e.g. a primary lung cancer, solitary metastasis or well differentiated endocrine (carcinoid) tumour. A range of *clinical and radiological features* help determine the *probability of malignancy* such as a history of haemoptysis, a previous high stage cancer with lymphovascular invasion, older age and smoking habit. *CT scan clues* include spiculated edges, size (2.1–3 cm: malignancy likelihood ratio of 3.67), and change in size over a period of time. *PET scan* metabolic activity has a high sensitivity and specificity for malignancy although lesions <1 cm are usually below its resolution. Indeterminate small lesions can be monitored by serial CT scans. Serum tumour markers may be of help. If suspected of being malignant, transbronchial or transthoracic biopsy may be required as the outcomes for the patient can differ significantly. The nodule could represent a new primary lung cancer amenable to resection, a potentially resectable solitary metastasis from a previously completely excised primary (e.g. colorectal cancer), or, result in exclusion from further radical treatment due to it being non-regional metastatic (pM) disease with an adverse outlook e.g. oesophagogastric carcinoma.

17.3 Differentiation

Well/moderate/poor/undifferentiated or Grade 1/2/3/4.

- For squamous carcinoma based on cellular atypia, keratinisation and intercellular bridges.
- For adenocarcinoma based on percentage tumour gland formation (well/G1: >95 %: moderate/G2 50–95 %: poor/G3 <50 %).

Small cell carcinoma and large cell carcinoma are by definition undifferentiated (grade 4) and have poor prognosis.

Fig. 17.1 Lung carcinoma (Reproduced, with permission, from Wittekind et al. (2005), © 2005)

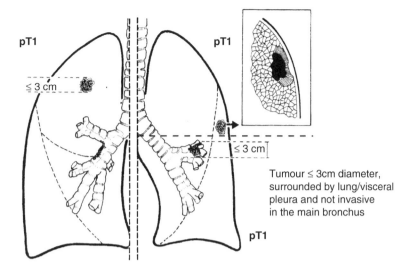

pT1

pT1

≤ 3 cm

≤ 3 cm

Tumour ≤ 3cm diameter, surrounded by lung/visceral pleura and not invasive in the main bronchus

pT1

17.4 Extent of Local Tumour Spread

Border: pushing/infiltrative.

Lymphocytic reaction: prominent/sparse.

Distance to the proximal bronchial limit (mm).

Distance to the mediastinal limit (mm).

Distance to the pleura (mm).

- Visceral pleural invasion is recognised by direct perforation of the mesothelium and also infiltration of the inner elastin layer in the submesothelial plane. Note that the pleura can be distorted without actual true invasion and use of an elastin stain is helpful. Under TNM7 pleural invasion can be substaged as none (PL0), visceral pleura (PL1), surface of visceral pleura (PL2) or parietal pleura (PL3).

Distance to the pericardium (mm).

Mucosa, cartilage plates, parenchyma.

Tumour necrosis.

The TNM7 classification applies to non-small cell carcinomas, small cell carcinomas (of limited disease extent only), and bronchopulmonary carcinoid tumours.

pTx	Positive cytology
pTis	Carcinoma in situ
pT1	Tumour ≤3 cm diameter, surrounded by lung/visceral pleura and not invasive proximal to a lobar bronchus
pT1a	Tumour ≤2 cm diameter
pT1b	2 cm < tumour ≤3 cm diameter

pT2	Tumour >3 cm diameter but ≤7 cm, or involves main bronchus 2 cm or more distal to the carina, or visceral pleura. Partial atelectasis, extending to hilum but not the entire lung
pT2a	3 cm< tumour ≤5 cm diameter
pT2b	5 cm< tumour ≤7 cm diameter
pT3	Tumour >7 cm or invading any of: chest wall, diaphragm, mediastinal pleura, parietal pericardium, or, tumour of main bronchus <2 cm distal to the carina, or, total lung atelectasis/obstructive pneumonitis, or separate tumour nodule(s) in the same lobe as the lung primary
pT4	Tumour of any size invading the mediastinum, heart, great vessels, trachea, recurrent laryngeal nerve, oesophagus, vertebral body, carina, or, tumour with separate tumour nodule(s) in different ipsilateral lobe to that of the primary.

See Figs. 17.1, 17.2, 17.3, and 17.4

Note that for accurate postsurgical staging *clinical details are required* e.g. anatomical proximity of the tumour to the carina (pT2 vs pT3) in central lesions. Relevant clinical information may be supplied on the bronchoscopy specimen request form, or it may only be finalised after discussion at the multidisciplinary team meeting.

Involvement of parietal pericardium, rib and phrenic nerve are pT3.

Vocal cord paralysis, superior vena cava syndrome, compression of trachea or oesophagus, or involvement of visceral pericardium are classified as pT4.

Fig. 17.2 Lung carcinoma (Reproduced, with permission, from Wittekind et al. (2005), © 2005)

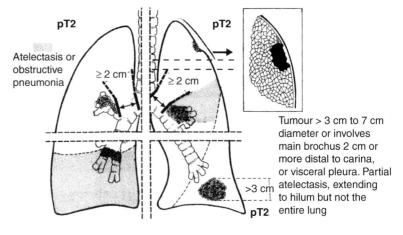

Tumour > 3 cm to 7 cm diameter or involves main brochus 2 cm or more distal to carina, or visceral pleura. Partial atelectasis, extending to hilum but not the entire lung

Fig. 17.3 Lung carcinoma (Reproduced, with permission, from Wittekind et al. (2005), © 2005)

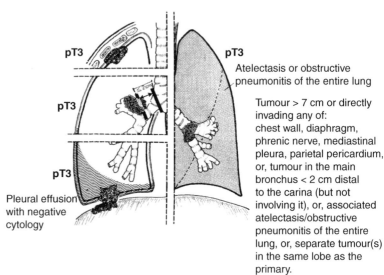

Atelectasis or obstructive pneumonitis of the entire lung

Tumour > 7 cm or directly invading any of: chest wall, diaphragm, phrenic nerve, mediastinal pleura, parietal pericardium, or, tumour in the main bronchus < 2 cm distal to the carina (but not involving it), or, associated atelectasis/obstructive pneumonitis of the entire lung, or, separate tumour(s) in the same lobe as the primary.

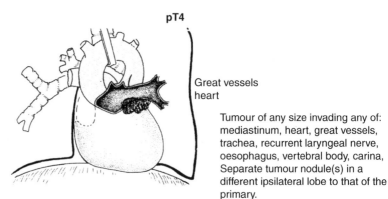

Fig. 17.4 Lung carcinoma (Reproduced, with permission, from Wittekind et al. (2005), © 2005)

Great vessels heart

Tumour of any size invading any of: mediastinum, heart, great vessels, trachea, recurrent laryngeal nerve, oesophagus, vertebral body, carina, Separate tumour nodule(s) in a different ipsilateral lobe to that of the primary.

Some *60–75% of lung cancers are incurable at presentation* due to extensive local or distant spread with symptoms developing late in the disease course. Spread is by endobronchial polypoid growth, direct extension along the bronchus (proximally and distally) either with in situ

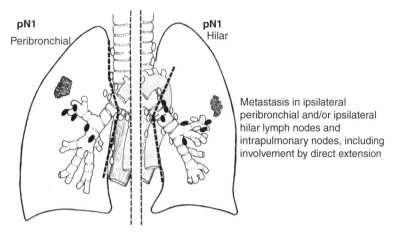

Fig. 17.5 Lung carcinoma: regional lymph nodes (Reproduced, with permission, from Wittekind et al. (2005), © 2005)

pN1
Peribronchial

pN1
Hilar

Metastasis in ipsilateral peribronchial and/or ipsilateral hilar lymph nodes and intrapulmonary nodes, including involvement by direct extension

or penetrating submucosal invasion, or direct into the lung parenchyma, and to the mediastinum and pleura when diaphragm and chest wall may be involved. Distant metastases are commonly seen in the liver, lung elsewhere (by lymphovascular or aerogenous spread), adrenals, bone, skin, kidney and central nervous system (particularly adenocarcinoma). A *majority of small cell carcinomas have extensive metastatic spread at the time of diagnosis* and they are regarded clinically as being either limited (confined to one hemithorax: use TNM7) or extensive disease.

17.5 Lymphovascular Invasion

Present/absent.
Intra-/extratumoural.
Common (80 %) in lung cancer and along with lymph node metastases is an *adverse prognostic indicator*.

17.6 Lymph Nodes

Site/number/size/number involved/limit node/extracapsular spread.

Regional nodes: intrathoracic, scalene, supraclavicular.

A regional lymphadenectomy will ordinarily include a minimum of 6 lymph nodes. The surgeon will often submit separately dissected and labelled lymph node stations. Three of these

lymph nodes/stations should be mediastinal, including the subcarinal nodes and three from N1 nodes/stations. Lymph node metastases are unusual for primary tumours <2 cm in diameter.

pN0	No regional lymph node metastasis
pN1	Metastasis in ipsilateral peribronchial/hilar/intrapulmonary nodes including involvement by direct extension (node stations 10–14)
pN2	Metastasis in ipsilateral mediastinal/subcarinal nodes (node stations 1–9)
pN3	Metastasis in contralateral mediastinal, contralateral hilar, ipsi-/contralateral scalene or supraclavicular nodes.

See Figs. 17.5, 17.6, and 17.7

pM1 is distant metastasis and includes (pM1a) separate tumour nodule(s) in a contralateral lobe, or tumour with pleural nodules or malignant pleural or pericardial effusion. M1b disease is distant metastases.

Cervical, scalene or mediastinal lymph node FNAC or biopsy is sometimes used to establish a diagnosis of carcinoma in patients suspected of having a malignancy but in whom bronchial biopsy and cytology are negative, when it represents recurrent disease, or who are medically unfit for invasive procedures.

17.7 Excision Margins

Distances (mm) to the proximal bronchial, vascular, mediastinal soft tissue and chest wall limits and pleura. *Completeness of surgical resection*

Fig. 17.6 Lung carcinoma: regional lymph nodes (Reproduced, with permission, from Wittekind et al. (2005), © 2005)

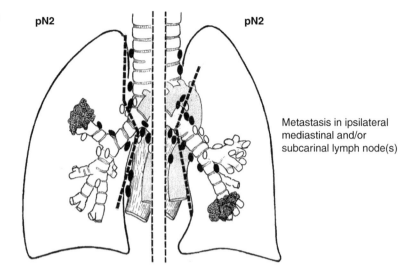

Metastasis in ipsilateral mediastinal and/or subcarinal lymph node(s)

Fig. 17.7 Lung carcinoma: regional lymph nodes (Reproduced, with permission, from Wittekind et al. (2005), © 2005)

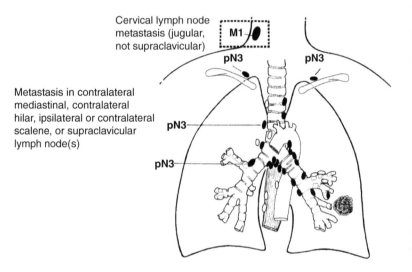

Cervical lymph node metastasis (jugular, not supraclavicular)

Metastasis in contralateral mediastinal, contralateral hilar, ipsilateral or contralateral scalene, or supraclavicular lymph node(s)

and lymph node status are the most important determinants of prognosis.

The presence of significant dysplasia at the bronchial mucosal limit can be a marker of potential local recurrence. Carcinoma in situ at the proximal bronchial margin is considered to represent residual disease.

17.8 Other Pathology

Lymphangitis carcinomatosa: can be diagnosed on transbronchial biopsy and is characterised by involvement of peribronchial and perivascular lymphatics.

Asbestos bodies/asbestosis/malignant mesothelioma: 5 % of lung cancer deaths. Asbestos exposure can also be a co-factor for development of bronchogenic carcinoma.

Scar/fibrosis: in lung periphery can occur within, predispose to, harbor or arise secondary to pulmonary adenocarcinoma.

Synchronous or metachronous lung cancers: in up to 5 % of cases and associated with independent cancers of the head and neck region in 10–20 % of cases. Upper aerodigestive tract panendoscopy may be required, often guided by relevant findings on CT scan.

Metastatic carcinoma: distribution varies greatly and may be single or multifocal, diffuse or nodular, endobronchial, parenchymal, lymphovascular, vasculoembolic or pleural. *Knowledge of the clinical history and direct comparison of morphology with the previous primary tumour are important.* This can be supplemented by cytokeratin profile expression (CK7/20) and specific immune markers e.g. thyroglobulin (thyroid), PSA/PSAP (prostate), CA 125/WT1 (ovary), ER/GCDFP-15 (breast), CK20/CDX-2 (colorectal), TTF-1/napsin A (lung adenocarcinoma) and CA19-9 (pancreatic and upper gastrointestinal cancers). Surgical resection of germ cell tumour and carcinomatous (e.g. colorectum) pulmonary metastases is not infrequent, the appearances of which can be greatly altered by adjuvant therapy i.e. tumour necrosis, inflammation, fibrosis and tissue maturation. Similarly chemotherapy of metastatic osteosarcoma can result in pulmonary nodules of mature bone with no residual malignant tissue.

Atypical adenomatous hyperplasia: usually <5 mm dia and well demarcated from adjacent lung parenchyma, it is regarded as *a precursor of malignancy* with a *proposed AAH-lepidic/BAC-invasive adenocarcinoma sequence.* It is seen in 10–40 % (often multifocal) of resected lung carcinomas especially peripheral or *lepidic/bronchioloalveolar carcinoma (BAC).* BAC (usually >1 cm) is either of type II pneumocyte or peripheral Clara cell origin and is generally *non-mucinous* in character (solitary, hob nail cells, good prognosis, 60–75 % of cases). *Mucinous adenocarcinoma* (multifocal, bilateral, worse prognosis) is characterised as either *in situ (mucinous BAC), minimally invasive,* or *invasive.* The latter is characterized by size >3 cm, extent of invasion >0.5 cm, multiple nodules, an irregular border and miliary spread into adjacent lung parenchyma. BAC has a better prognosis than other lung cancers, particularly when <3 cm diameter when it is regarded as an in situ adenocarcinoma. It is being increasingly detected by CT/PET/FNAC investigations. Thorough sampling is necessary to detect any central prognostically adverse fibrous scar that may harbour more usual type invasive adenocarcinoma, or a micropapillary pattern. Their presence decreases 5 year survival rates from 78–100 % down to 53–67 %. CK7/TTF–1 and napsin A positivity are useful in distinguishing pulmonary adenocarcinoma from secondary carcinoma, e.g. large bowel and pancreas.

Extrapulmonary effects: inappropriate or ectopic hormone secretion e.g. small cell carcinoma and Cushings syndrome (ACTH), carcinoid syndrome, diabetes insipidus (ADH), gynaecomastia, hypercalcaemia.

Immunophenotype

- *Small cell carcinoma:*
  Chromogranin ±, positive for synaptophysin, CD56 (NCAM), CAM 5.2 (paranuclear dot reactivity), TTF-1, Ki67 >90 %.
- *Squamous cell carcinoma:*
  Cytokeratins (AE1/AE3, CK5/6, CK14, 34βE12) and p63 positive, ± EMA, vimentin, CEA, CK7, CAM 5.2.
- *Spindle cell carcinoma:*
  Cytokeratin (focal AE1/AE3, CK5/6, 34βE12) positive, vimentin positive, ± CEA, TTF-1.
- *Adenocarcinoma:*
  CAM 5.2, CK7, TTF-1, napsin A, EMA, CEA, vimentin, CD15, MOC-31, Ber EP4 positive.
- *Lepidic/bronchioloalveolar carcinoma:*
  TTF-1, napsin A, cytokeratin (CAM 5.2) positive. Non-mucinous is CK7 +/CK20–, mucinous CK7 +/CK20 +/TTF-1 ±.
- *Specificity:* note that no one immunomarker is distinctive and that there can be considerable overlap between various non-small cell carcinoma subtypes and expression for cytokeratins, TTF-1 and p63. Some squamous cell carcinomas can be CK7/TTF-1 positive and 20 % of lung adenocarcinomas can be TTF-1negative. Similarly 50 % of large cell carcinomas can be TTF-1 positive.
- *Well differentiated neuroendocrine (carcinoid) tumour:*
  Chromogranin, TTF-1, synaptophysin, CAM5.2, Ki67 ≤2 %.

Prognosis

Prognosis in lung cancer (overall 13% 5 year survival) relates to weight loss, performance status, cell type (small cell carcinoma has 2 % long-term survival and 90 % present with locally advanced or systemic disease), cell differentiation (well differentiated is better than poorly differentiated), completeness of surgical resection and tumour stage, in particular nodal status. *Only 10–25 % of non-small cell carcinomas are potentially curable by resection with a majority treated non-surgically.* An important therapeutic distinction must be made between *small cell carcinoma (chemoradiotherapy)* and *non-small cell carcinoma (surgery ± radiotherapy).* This can be achieved with a relatively high level of consistency (kappa = 0.86) whereas subtyping of non-small cell carcinoma shows poor inter-observer agreement (kappa = 0.25). A general *guide to suitability for surgical resection* is non-small cell cancer >2 cm from the carina and without mediastinal lymph node involvement i.e. ≤*pT2 N1.* International trials are currently examining the role of neoadjuvant therapy in non-small cell carcinoma more advanced than stage pT2 N1.

Adjuvant or front line radical radiotherapy ± chemotherapy may be offered to patients with a poor performance status. *Palliative chemo-/radiotherapy* can be given to patients with high stage disease, or *local ablation* treatment if there is impending endoluminal airway obstruction. An important development in *pulmonary adenocarcinoma* is the determination of *epidermal growth factor receptor (EGFR) mutation status.* Some 15 % of cases, in particular females and never smokers, are positive by *genetic mutation analysis* and a proportion of these patients with locally advanced, recurrent or metastatic disease respond to *targeted oral erlotinib or gefitinib therapy* – an EGFR tyrosine kinase inhibitor. The role of the pathologist is to ascertain a firm diagnosis of pulmonary adenocarcinoma and to select an appropriate block rich in tumour for genetic mutation analysis. Conversely anti-endothelial growth factor therapy (bevacizumab) is contraindicated in squamous cell carcinoma due to the potential risk of haemorrhage. Other potential drug targets, mutation status (EGFR, ALK, KRAS) in non-small cell lung carcinoma and the effects on the differential tumour response to

various chemotherapeutic agents are being explored e.g. EML4/ALK translocation in lung adencocarcinoma and a positive response to crizotinib therapy. Surgery is only considered for small cell carcinoma if it is *limited in extent* i.e. ≤3 cm diameter without lymph node metastases – otherwise *chemoradiation* is indicated. The significance of occult bone marrow micrometastases detected by immunohistochemistry is uncertain. Prognosis improves if the carcinoma is "early" or "occult" with positive cytology but negative chest radiology: preoperative chemotherapy may also be beneficial.

Operable (localised)	5 year survival (%)
Squamous/large cell adenocarcinoma	35
Well differentiated	75
Poorly differentiated	35
Overall	50
Small cell	10

Non-operable (extensive)	5 year survival (%)
Squamous cell	6
Small cell	2

17.9 Other Malignancy

Leukaemia

- 50–60 % of acute leukaemias.
- 15–40 % of chronic leukaemias.
- Pleural, peribronchial and perivascular lymphangitic spread.
- Rarely, there is a granulocytic sarcoma mass lesion; CD34/CD43/CD 68/CD117/chloroacetate esterase/myeloperoxidase positive.

Malignant Lymphoma

- Primary *MALToma* or *diffuse large B cell lymphoma (5–20 % of cases)* or secondary to nodal/systemic disease. Pulmonary involvement is present in up to 38 % of patients with lymph node based malignant lymphoma. Designation depends on the constituent cell type and clinicopathological staging of the extent of disease. There may also be a previous history of nodal lymphoma.

MALT Lymphoma

- *The commonest primary lung lymphoma.*
- Sixth/seventh decade.
- ± Sjögren's syndrome or rheumatoid arthritis.
- Central mass with peripheral tracking along septa, bronchovascular bundles and pleura.
- Solitary or multifocal ± spread to other MALT sites.
- Limited resection ± chemo-/radiotherapy.
- 5 year survival is 80–90 %, most are low-grade but can transform to high-grade (40–60 % 5 year survival).
- Some large B cell (high-grade) pulmonary lymphomas probably originate in low-grade MALToma.

High-grade lesions are easily assessed as malignant but must be distinguished from other tumours e.g. non-small cell carcinoma, using immunohistochemistry. *Low-grade lesions* are characterised by a dense monomorphic interstitial population of centrocyte like cells, absence or colonisation of reactive follicles, lymphoepithelial lesions and local invasion. B cell predominance, light chain restriction and *immunoglobulin heavy/light chain monoclonal gene rearrangements* are confirmatory in distinction from a lymphoid interstitial pneumonitis or follicular bronchiolitis. Mass lesions previously designated pseudolymphoma are now considered to be low-grade MALTomas.

Primary or Secondary Hodgkin's Lymphoma

- Usually secondary to spread from mediastinal disease.
- Parenchymal nodules, endobronchial plaque/nodules or miliary interstitial spread.

T Cell Rich Large B Cell Lymphoproliferative Disorder/ Malignant Lymphoma (EBV Related)

- On a spectrum with B cell lymphomatoid granulomatosis/angiocentric immunoproliferative lesion and associated with EBV.
- Polymorphous (lymphocytes, plasma cells, histiocytes) angiocentric/destructive infiltrate containing atypical lymphoid cells.
- Clonal immunoglobulin heavy chain gene rearrangements are present in 50 % of cases.
- *Prognosis (poor)* is dictated by the *histological grade* (number of atypical cells) and extrapulmonary lesions are common (kidneys, liver, brain, spleen).

Intravascular Malignant Lymphoma

- Malignant angioendotheliomatosis or *angiocentric large B cell lymphoma*: skin, central nervous system and adrenal gland involvement with poor prognosis.

Post Transplant Lymphoproliferative Disorder (PTLD)

- An EBV associated spectrum of lymphoproliferation (immortalised B cells) following (first 2 years) immunosuppression for solid organ or bone marrow transplantation. It occurs in the native or transplant lung affecting 2 % of patients.
- Can respond to *reduction of immunosuppression* and antiviral therapy.
- *Early* (plasma cell hyperplasia), *polymorphous* (infectious mononucleosis-like) or *monomorphic* (as in large B cell lymphoma) stages. Also shows angioinvasion and necrosis.
- *Monomorphic/monoclonal lesions* are worse prognosis than *polymorphic/polyclonal lesions*.
- Diagnosis by chest X-ray, CT scan, transthoracic needle biopsy, morphology, immunophenotype, clonality (PCR: 50 % of monomorphic cases

are monoclonal) and EBV status (in situ hybridisation).

Other Haematopoietic Malignancy

- *Anaplastic large cell lymphoma*: CD30/ALK positive. Null phenotype but T cell receptor gene rearrangements in 90 % of cases.
- *Extramedullary plasmacytoma*: peri-/intrabronchial mass, amyloid, light chain restriction, 40 % 5 year survival.

Epithelioid Haemangioendothelioma (Intravascular Sclerosing Bronchioloalveolar Tumour (IVSBAT))

- A vascular tumour of intermediate-grade malignancy (CD 31/CD34 positive) in young adult females. Slow progression and association with liver and skin lesions.

Kaposi's Sarcoma

- HIV.

Angiosarcoma

- Primary or secondary.

Malignant Melanoma

- Usually secondary, intraparenchymal or endobronchial.

Sarcomas Including Synovial Sarcoma, Leiomyosarcoma, Rhabdomyosarcoma (Embryonal Children, Pleomorphic Adults)

In any lung sarcoma it is important to exclude the more common possibilities of either metastatic disease from a primary elsewhere, a lung carcinoma with sarcoma like morphology, or a spindle cell malignant mesothelioma. Endobronchial sarcoma presents earlier with better prognosis than intrapulmonary sarcoma. Sarcoma may also arise as an intraluminal mass within the pulmonary artery. Synovial sarcoma can be lung or pleura based, leiomyosarcoma, angiosarcoma and intimal sarcoma centred on major vessels, while chondrosarcoma, osteosarcoma and malignant small blue cell tumours can arise from rib or chest wall and invade underlying lung.

Bibliography

Association of Directors of Anatomic and Surgical Pathology. Recommendations for the reporting of resected primary lung carcinoma. Hum Pathol. 1995; 26:937–9.

Baldwin DR, White B, Schmidt-Hansen M, Champion AR, Melder AM on behalf of the Guideline Development Group. Diagnosis and treatment of lung cancer: summary of updated NICE guidance. BMJ. 2011;343:1019–22.

Beasley MB. Pulmonary neuroendocrine tumours and proliferations: a review and update. Diagn Histopathol. 2008;14:465–73.

Burnett RA, Swanson Beck J, Howatson SR, Lee FD, Lessells AM, McLaren KM, Ogston S, Robertson AJ, Simpson JG, Smith GD, Tavadia HB, Walker F. Observer variability in histopathological reporting of malignant bronchial biopsy specimens. J Clin Pathol. 1994;47:711–3.

Colby TV, Koss MN. Tumors of the lower respiratory tract. Atlas of tumor pathology. 3rd series. Fascicle 13. Washington: AFIP; 1995.

Corrin B, Nicholson AG. Pathology of the lungs. 3rd ed. London: Churchill Livingstone; 2011.

Flieder DB. Recent advances in the diagnosis of adenocarcinoma: the impact of lung cancer screening on histopathologists. Curr Diagn Pathol. 2004;10:269–78.

Guinee Jr DG. Update on pulmonary and pleural lymphoproliferative disorders. Diagn Histopathol. 2008;14: 474–98.

Kerr KM. Morphology and genetics of pre-invasive pulmonary disease. Curr Diagn Pathol. 2004;10:259–68.

Kerr KM. Pulmonary adenocarcinomas: classification and reporting. Histopathology. 2009;54:12–27.

Kerr KM. Personalized medicine for lung cancer: new challenges for pathology. Histopathology. 2012;60:531–46.

Lantuejoul S, Brambilla E. Prognostic biomarkers in non-small-cell lung carcinoma. Curr Diagn Pathol. 2006;12:418–28.

Lantuejoul S, Salameire D, Salon C, Brambilla E. Pulmonary preneoplasia – sequential molecular carcinogenetic events. Histopathology. 2009;54:43–54.

Marson JV, Mazieres J, Groussard O, Garcia O, Berjaud J, Dahan M, Carles P, Daste G. Expression of TTF-1 and cytokeratins in primary and secondary epithelial lung tumours: correlation with histological type and grade. Histopathology. 2004;45:125–34.

McLean EC, Monaghan H, Salter DM, Wallace WA. Evaluation of adjunct immunohistochemistry on reporting patterns of non-small cell lung carcinoma diagnosed histologically in a regional pathology centre. J Clin Pathol. 2011;64:1136–8.

McNulty M, Cox G, Au-Yong I. Investigating the solitary pulmonary nodule. BMJ. 2012;344:44–6.

Salter DM. Pulmonary and thoracic sarcomas. Curr Diagn Pathol. 2006;12:409–17.

The Royal College of Pathologists. Lung Cancer Dataset and Tissue Pathways for Pulmonary Pathology and Cardiovascular Pathology. Accessed at http://www.rcpath.org/index.asp?PageID=254.

Travis WD. Reporting lung cancer pathology specimens. Impact of the anticipated 7th edition TNM classification based on recommendations of the IASLC Staging Committee. Histopathology. 2009;54:3–11.

Travis WD, Colby TV, Koss MN, Rosado-de-Christenson ML, Muller NL, King TE. Non-neoplastic disorders of the respiratory tract. Atlas of nontumor pathology. Fascicle 2. Washington: AFIP; 2002.

Travis WD, Brambilla E, Muller-Hermelink HK, Harris CC. WHO classification of tumours, Pathology and genetics. Tumours of the lung, pleura, thymus and heart. Lyon: IARC Press; 2004.

Wallace WAH. The challenge of classifying poorly differentiated tumours in the lung. Histopathology. 2009;54:28–42.

Wittekind CF, Greene FL, Hutter RVP, Klimpfinger M, Sobib LH. TNM atlas: illustrated guide to the TNM/pTNM classification of malignant tumours. 5th ed. Berlin: Springer; 2005.

Yeh Y-C, Wu Y-C, Chen C-Y, Wang L-S, Hsu W-H, Chou T-Y. Stromal invasion and micropapillary pattern in 212 consecutive surgically resected stage 1 lung adenocarcinomas: histopathological categories for prognosis prediction. J Clin Pathol. 2012;65:910–8.

Zhang J, Liang Z, Gao J, Luo Y, Liu T. Pulmonary adenocarcinoma with a micropapillary pattern: a clinicopathological, immunophenotypic and molecular analysis. Histopathology. 2011;59:1204–14.

Malignant Mesothelioma

Malignant mesothelioma is a major asbestos related worldwide health problem with a peak of some 250,000 deaths predicted in Europe over the next 10 years.

Pleural disease can be asymptomatic or present with pain, breathlessness or general systemic effects e.g. weight loss. Pleural plaques, fibrotic thickening, calfcification and pleural effusion are demonstrated by chest x-ray and CT scan. Pleural thickening >1 cm, nodularity and extension on to the mediastinal surfaces make malignancy more likely.

Ultrasound localised thoracentesis or pleural fluid aspiration can be diagnostic or therapeutic for symptomatic relief. Percutaneous closed needle biopsy is insufficient in up to 30 % of cases and only diagnostic in a minority (16–40 %) of patients. It may need to be supplemented by CT guided or video assisted thoracoscopic (VATS) biopsy or open pleural biopsy. The latter may be allied to decortication or stripping of the constricting visceral peel carried out for the dual purpose of making a diagnosis and to expand the underlying lung. Diagnostic rates increase to over 90 %. Specimen size is important with a positive diagnosis in a majority of specimens >10 mm. Histological subtype also affects diagnostic yield with paucicellular desmoplastic and sarcomatoid mesotheliomas giving the lowest accuracy. Chest wall biopsy site seeding is a potential problem for which preventative radiotherapy is used.

Pleurectomy attempts to debulk the malignant mesothelioma providing multiple strips of pleural membrane. Extrapleural pneumonectomy is en bloc resection of the pleurae, lung, ipsilateral hemidiaphragm and pericardium. Peritoneal disease may present with ascites and a tissue diagnosis is obtained by peritoneal fluid cytology, laparoscopic or open biopsy.

18.1 Gross Description

Specimen

- Pleural, peritoneal or laparoscopic aspiration cytology or biopsy/ thoracoscopic or open biopsy/pleurectomy/extrapleural pneumonectomy/omentectomy.
- Size (cm) and weight (g).

Tumour

Site
- Pleural (visceral/parietal)/pericardial/peritoneal.
- Pleura (>80 %) is the commonest site then peritoneum (10–15 %).

Size
- Length × width × depth (cm) or maximum dimension (cm).

Appearance
- Localised (solitary)/diffuse/nodular/plaque/ infiltrative/cystic change.

Edge
- Circumscribed/irregular.

18.2   Histological Type

Adenomatoid Tumour

- Benign: a circumscribed pale nodule in the epididymis, fallopian tube or uterine myometrium with or without a serosal connection. It usually comprises a microcystic pattern of mesothelial cell proliferation with prominent intervening smooth muscle.

Localised Solitary Fibrous Tumour

- Rare/solitary/visceral pleura, circumscribed/ smooth or bossellated.
- "Patternless" fibroblasts and vessels with bland cytology, 90 % are benign, and CD 34/ bcl2/CD99 positive.
- Now regarded as arising from subserosal fibroblasts/mesenchymal cells rather than from mesothelial cells, and is encountered in other organs.

Multilocular Peritoneal Inclusion Cysts (Multicystic Peritoneal Mesothelioma)

- On the surfaces of the uterus, ovary, bladder, rectum and pouch of Douglas it is *potentially locally recurrent*, and rarely, invasive into retroperitoneum, bowel mesentery and wall. Differential diagnosis is lymphagitic (lining cells are cytokeratin negative) and unilocular peritoneal inclusion cysts, and cystic adenomatoid tumour and malignant mesothelioma. About 50 % recur over many years and some

have a previous history of surgery, endometriosis or pelvic inflammatory disease.

Well Differentiated Papillary Peritoneal Mesothelioma

- In middle aged women, it is rare, with most being an incidental finding at hysterectomy. Localised and benign but can be extensive and diffuse nodular serosal/omental disease with ultimately progression and ascites.

Diffuse Malignant Mesothelioma

- The main variants are *epithelial* (*epithelioid*), *sarcomatoid* and *biphasic*. Rarer types are desmoplastic, small cell, lymphohistiocytoid, deciduoid and undifferentiated or anaplastic.
- *Epithelial* (*60 %*):
  Tubulopapillary
  Microglandular
  Solid (epithelioid)
  Small cell 6 %
  Pleomorphic (large cell)
  Lymphohistiocytoid 1 %: aggressive
  Deciduoid
  Rhabdoid
  Clear cell
  Signet ring cell.
- *Sarcomatoid* (*15 %*):
  Fibrosarcomatous like/cellular storiform patterns
  Fibrous (desmoplastic) 5–10 %
  Angiomatoid
  Chondroid/osteoblastic/rhabdomyoblastic/ leiomyoid.
- *Mixed* (*biphasic*) (*25 %*).

Metastatic Carcinoma

- *The commonest malignant tumour of the pleura.*

- Lung/breast/stomach/ovary/prostate/kidney carcinomas, malignant melanoma, soft tissue sarcoma and germ cell tumours can all *mimic malignant mesothelioma* on histology, and even gross distribution of disease resulting in an encasing pseudomesotheliomatous picture. Knowledge of a *relevant previous history* and close clinicopathological correlation with *comparison of tumour morphology* and *immunohistochemistry* are needed.

- Metastatic malignant melanoma occasionally involves the pleura. It can be spindle cell in type mimicking lung cancer and malignant mesothelioma. Standard malignant melanoma markers (S100, melan-A, HMB-45) may be only variably positive. A *previous clinical history* is important to think of the diagnosis and *comparison of the initial malignant melanoma histology* is helpful in confirmation.

18.3 Differentiation

Well/moderate/poor.

- *No formal grading system* is used, and probably best regarded as a minority of well differentiated lesions (e.g. papillary and multicystic peritoneal variants), and others which are not graded. *Sarcomatoid lesions* are considered *poorly differentiated, epithelial lesions* as *well to moderately differentiated*. A high mitotic rate is an adverse indicator.

18.4 Extent of Local Tumour Spread

Border: pushing/infiltrative.

Lymphocytic reaction: prominent/sparse.

The TNM7 classification applies to pleural malignant mesothelioma only.

pT1	Tumour involves ipsilateral parietal (mediastinal, diaphragmatic) pleura
	(a) No involvement of visceral pleura
	(b) Focal involvement of visceral pleura
pT2	Tumour involves ipsilateral pleural surfaces with also any of: confluent visceral pleural tumour, invasion of the diaphragmatic muscle or lung parenchyma
pT3[a]	Tumour involves ipsilateral pleural surfaces with also any of: invasion of endothoracic fascia, mediastinal fat, solitary chest wall soft tissue focus, non-transmural pericardial involvement
pT4[b]	Tumour involves ipsilateral pleural surfaces with also any of: contralateral pleura, peritoneum, rib, extensive chest wall or mediastinal invasion, myocardium, brachial plexus, spine, transmural pericardium, malignant pericardial effusion

[a]Locally advanced but potentially resectable tumour
[b]Locally advanced but technically non-resectable tumour
See Figs. 18.1, 18.2 and 18.3

Spread is typically pleural, encasing the lung with extension along fissures and septa and into subpleural lung parenchyma. *Lymph node spread* and *distant metastases* (up to 30 % of cases) occur *late in the disease course*.

Contiguous spread through the diaphragm with involvement of abdominal organs is not infrequent.

Peritoneal disease is usually secondary to pleural tumour but can also be primary and asbestos related. *Pericardial disease* usually represents spread from pleural tumour.

Flat or granular pleura adjacent to tumour nodules may show cytological atypia constituting "*mesothelioma in situ*" and although unusual in pleural biopsies this can be a useful indicator of potential for progression to invasion or the presence of concurrent malignant mesothelioma not sampled by the biopsy needle.

18.5 Lymphovascular Invasion

Present/absent.
Intra-/extratumoural.

Fig. 18.1 Pleural malignant
mesothelioma (Reproduced,
with permission, from
Wittekind et al.
(2005), © 2005)

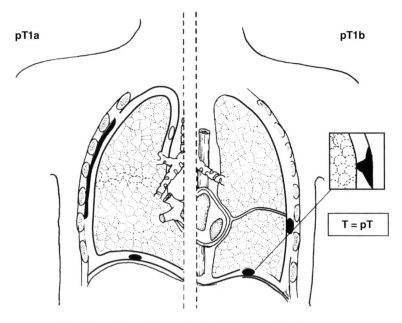

Tumour involves ipsilateral parietal pleura with or without focal
involvement of visceral pleura

a. Tumour involves ipsilateral parietal (mediastinal, diaphragmatic)
   pleura. No involvement of visceral pleura

b. Tumour involves ipsilateral parietal (mediastinal, diaphragmatic)
   pleura, with focal involvement of visceral pleura

Tumour involves any of the ipsilateral pleural surfaces, with at least one of the
following:

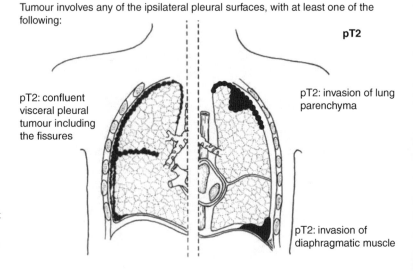

Fig. 18.2 Pleural malignant
mesothelioma (Adapted
from Wittekind et al. (2005),
© 2005)

Fig. 18.3 Pleural malignant mesothelioma (Adapted from Wittekind et al. (2005), © 2005)

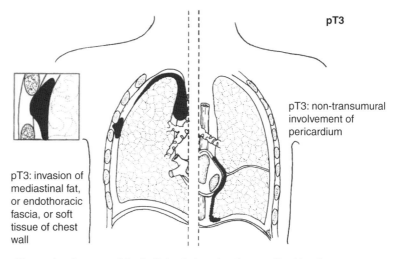

pT3

pT3: non-transumural involvement of pericardium

pT3: invasion of mediastinal fat, or endothoracic fascia, or soft tissue of chest wall

Tumour involves any of the ipsilateral pleural surfaces, with at least one of the above:

18.6   Lymph Nodes

Site/number/size/number involved/limit node/extracapsular spread.

Regional nodes: intrathoracic, internal mammary, scalene, supraclavicular.

pN0	No regional lymph node metastasis
pN1	Metastasis in ipsilateral bronchopulmonary and/or hilar lymph node(s), including involvement by direct extension
pN2	Metastasis in subcarinal lymph node(s) and/or ipsilateral internal mammary or mediastinal lymph node(s)
pN3	Metastasis in contralateral mediastinal, internal mammary, hilar node(s), and/or ipsilateral or contralateral scalene or supraclavicular lymph node(s).

18.7   Excision Margins

Distance (mm) to the nearest painted excision margin of local resection for limited disease.

18.8   Other Pathology

Pleural plaques, subpleural fibrosis, asbestosis, bronchogenic carcinoma: requiring increasing levels of *asbestos exposure*, respectively.

About 2–3 % of people with exposure to significant amounts of asbestos develop malignant mesothelioma. The consequences of asbestos exposure depend on the *fibre type* (amphiboles e.g. crocidolite are particularly pathogenic), and can be both *dose related* and *idiosyncratic*. Some individuals require less exposure to develop asbestos-related disease while others with extensive fibre burden do not. Classically there is a *long lag period* of 20–50 years until illness develops. *Exposure can also be second-hand* e.g. washing a spouse's contaminated clothing. Fibre burden can be assessed by incineration of lung tissue and quantitation by scanning electron microscopy. Identification of ferruginous asbestos bodies by light microscopy correlates with a significant fibre load. Exposure is usually *occupation related*. A typical clinical history of malignant mesothelioma is a unilateral opaque chest radiograph with necessity for multiple, repeated pleural taps. Note that the tumour may infiltrate chest wall through the biopsy needle track.

Metastatic malignancy: a number of *malignant tumours metastatic to the pleura can mimic malignant mesothelioma*. These include, amongst others, breast carcinoma, adenocarcinoma of lung, spindle cell carcinoma/carcinosarcoma of lung, renal cell carcinoma, malignant melanoma, malignant lymphoma and leukaemia, ovarian carcinoma, thymoma and sarcoma. There is no one specific marker for malignant mesothelioma and diagnosis often relies on exclusion of metastatic carcinoma and sarcoma by *clinical history, examination, radiology, comparative morphology and immunohistochemistry* of cytology or biopsy material. *Radiology* is very useful in demonstrating the distribution of disease e.g. diffuse pleural thickening of malignant mesothelioma versus an intrapulmonary/hilar mass with pleural thickening (lung carcinoma), or multiple discrete lung nodules with pleural thickening (metastatic carcinoma).

Diagnostic immunohistochemistry: positivity with one or more of CEA, BerEP4, MOC-31, TTF-1, E-cadherin and Leu M1 (CD 15) (Table 18.1), indicating *pulmonary adenocarcinoma* and excluding malignant mesothelioma (although some cases can be BerEP4 positive). Putatively positive *mesothelioma markers* that are negative in lung adenocarcinoma are CK 5/6, calretinin, thrombomodulin, HBME-1, N-cadherin and WT-1. EMA usually shows strong membranous positivity in epithelial malignant mesothelioma. *A practical panel for diagnostic use is CEA, BerEP4, TTF-1, EMA, CK5/6, calretinin* and *WT-1*. Note that immunoreactivity for various of these markers can be reduced in poorly differentiated epithelioid and spindle cell malignant mesotheliomas. Adenocarcinoma may also be mucicarmine positive/PAS-diastase resistant for mucin (60 % of cases). Distinction of malignant mesothelioma from other non-small cell lung cancers is usually by morphology as there can be overlap in cytokeratin profiles e.g. squamous cell carcinoma is CK5/6 positive although it should be calretinin/ WT-1 negative.

Sarcomatoid mesothelioma: may co-express cytokeratins, vimentin and muscle-specific actin. Differential diagnosis is spindle cell lung carcinoma and primary or secondary sarcoma with similar immunophenotypic co-expression e.g. epithelioid vascular tumours, leiomyosarcoma or synovial sarcoma. *Desmoplastic mesothelioma* (>50 % of the tumour is poorly cellular fibrous tissue) must be distinguished from *fibrous pleurisy* (inflammatory and reactive looking) and pleural plaque (acellular basket weave pattern of collagen) neither of which show parenchymal or chest wall infiltration, or strongly cytokeratin positive spindle cells distributed diffusely throughout the full depth of the fibrous tissue. *Solitary fibrous tumour* (CD34 positive, cytokeratin negative) should also be considered.

Mesothelial malignancy versus reactive mesothelial hyperplasia: morphological markers are *cytological atypia* and *cellularity, necrosis* and *invasion* of subpleural connective tissue i.e. *the extent, degree of atypia*, and *invasiveness of the mesothelial cell population* in an adequate specimen. Malignant mesothelial cells also express p53 and EMA but unlike reactive mesothelial cells are negative for desmin. However *immunohistochemistry is of limited diagnostic use in making this distinction* and the emphasis should be on morphology. In a significant minority of cases diagnosis may not be able to be made at first presentation, but the possibility raised from a constellation of atypical features in the pleural fluid cytology and biopsies over a series of medical admissions with attendant investigations.

Reactive mesothelial hyperplasia and dense inflammatory fibrosis do not clinically progress as does malignant mesothelioma with *repeated clinical presentations* and *the need for symptomatic relief by paracentesis*. Some well differentiated lesions pursue such a biological course over a span of several years but normally the *clinical progression is relatively rapid* indicating a malignant diagnosis. Reactive mesothelial hyperplasia may be seen in pulmonary infarction, tuberculous pleuritis, rheumatoid arthritis, systemic lupus erythematosus, and overlying primary or secondary neoplasms.

Table 18.1 Immunoexpression in mesothelial cell proliferations

Antibody	Epithelial mesothelioma	Reactive mesothelial cells	Pulmonary adenocarcinoma
CAM5.2	+	+	+
Vimentin	+	±	±
EMA	+	−	+
CK 5/6	+	+	−
HBME-1	±	+	−
Thrombomodulin	±	−	−
WT-1	+	+	−
CEA	−	−	+
Leu M1 (CD15)	−	−	+
Ber EP4	−	−	+
TTF-1	−	−	+
E-cadherin	−	−	+
N-cadherin	+	−	

Other markers include:

 S100, HMB-45, melan-A (malignant melanoma).

 CD 45, CD 20, CD 3 (B/T cell malignant lymphoma).

 Thyroglobulin, CK 19, TTF-1, RET (thyroid papillary carcinoma).

 CA125, CK 7, WT-1 (ovarian serous carcinoma).

 EMA, vimentin, CD10, abdominal ultrasound/CT scan (renal cell carcinoma).

 PSA, PSAP (prostate carcinoma).

 βHCG, AFP, CD30, PLAP, CD117, OCT3/4, SALL4 (germ cell tumour).

 ER/PR, GCDFP-15, CK 7 (breast carcinoma).

 CEA, CK 20, CDX-2 (gut carcinomas).

 CA 19-9, CK 7, CK 20, CA125 (pancreatic carcinoma).

Prognosis

Prognosis of diffuse malignant mesothelioma relates to stage but is generally poor with the majority of patients dead from their disease within 1–3 years: 4–12 months for pleural mesothelioma, less than 18 months for peritoneal mesothelioma. Spindle cell tumours are more aggressive than epithelioid variants. Malignant mesothelioma is variably sensitive to *chemoradiation. Adjuvant chemotherapy* combined with *resection of limited disease* (pleural decortication or pleuropneumonectomy) can occasionally result in prolonged remission with 15–30 % 3 year survival rates, but only a small minority of patients are suitable. *Symptomatic relief* may be gained by multiple paracenteses of malignant pleural or peritoneal fluid supplemented by *intracavitary chemotherapy*. This may act either directly on the tumour cells reducing secretions or produce a loculated, sclerosant effect. *Pallative*

radiotherapy and *chemical* (*talc*) *pleurodesis* also have roles to play. The former can induce bizarre multinucleated tumour cell forms and the latter a pseudosarcomatous biphasic pattern. Iatrogenic *wound site implantation* metastases can also occur in 15–20 % of cases. Well-differentiated multicystic and papillary peritoneal mesotheliomas are regarded as being of borderline or low malignant potential.

18.9   Other Malignancy

- Epithelioid haemangioendothelioma, angiosarcoma, synovial sarcoma.
- Thymoma.
- Malignant small cell tumour of thoracopulmonary region (Askin tumour).
- Desmoplastic small cell tumour.
- Malignant lymphoma: secondary to a lymphoproliferative disorder (e.g. CLL), nodal

or systemic disease, or, primary e.g. the rare pyothorax, or, effusion associated malignant lymphomas (large B cell lymphomas: EBV and HHV 8/immunodeficiency associated, respectively).

Bibliography

Abutaily AS, Addis BJ, Roche WR. Immuno-histochemistry in the distinction between malignant mesothelioma and pulmonary adenocarcinoma: a central evaluation of new antibodies. J Clin Pathol. 2002;55:662–8.

Addis B, Roche H. Problems in mesothelioma diagnosis. Histopathology. 2009;54:55–68.

Attanoos RL, Gibbs AR. Asbestos-related deaths. Curr Diagn Pathol. 2002;8:373–83.

Attanoos RL, Gibbs AR. Asbestos-related neoplasia. In: Lowe DG, Underwood JCE, editors. Recent advances in histopathology, vol. 20. London: RSM Press; 2003. p. 73–8.

Attanoos RL, Gibbs AR. The pathology associated with therapeutic procedures in malignant mesothelioma. Histopathology. 2004;45:393–7.

Attanoos RL, Gibbs AR. The comparative accuracy of different pleural biopsy techniques in the diagnosis of malignant mesothelioma. Histopathology. 2008;53: 340–4.

Battifora H, McCaughey WT. Tumors of the serosal membranes. Atlas of tumor pathology. 3rd series. Fascicle 15. Washington: AFIP; 1995.

Corrin B, Nicholson AG. Pathology of the lungs. 3rd ed. London: Churchill Livingstone; 2011.

Downer NJ, Ali NJ, Au-Yong ITH. Investigating pleural thickening. BMJ. 2013;346:35–7.

Guinee Jr DG. Update on pulmonary and pleural lympho-proliferative disorders. Diagn Histopathol. 2008;14: 474–98.

Nash G, Otis CN. Protocol for the examination of specimens from patients with malignant pleural mesothelioma. Arch Pathol Lab Med. 1999;123:39–44.

Ordonez NG. The immunohistochemical diagnosis of mesothelioma. A comparative study of epithelioid mesothelioma and lung adenocarcinoma. Am J Surg Pathol. 2003;27:1031–51.

Rena O. Extrapleural pneumonectomy in malignant mesothelioma. BMJ. 2011;343:1186.

Travis WD, Brambilla E, Muller-Hermelink HK, Harris CC, WHO Classification of Tumours. Pathology and genetics. Tumours of the lung, pleura, thymus and heart. Lyon: IARC Press; 2004.

Wittekind CF, Greene FL, Hutter RVP, Klimpfinger M, Sobib LH. TNM atlas: illustrated guide to the TNM/ pTNM classification of malignant tumours. 5th ed. Berlin: Springer; 2005.

Mediastinal Cancer

Mediastinal neoplasms are often asymptomatic (50 % of cases) particularly if benign. Malignant tumours are more often associated with both local and systemic symptoms.

Mediastinal neoplasms can present in a number of ways:

1. During staging or follow up (chest x-ray, CT or MRI scans) of a patient with a known cancer elsewhere e.g. lung carcinoma, colorectal carcinoma, non-Hodgkin's/Hodgkin's malignant lymphoma, or testicular/ovarian germ cell tumour.

2. As an incidental finding on chest x-ray in a patient who may or may not have ill-defined symptoms e.g. dyspnoea, cough, dysphagia.

3. As a finding in the investigation of a patient with other presenting features e.g. pneumonia or pleural effusion.

4. As superior vena cava (SVC) syndrome due to malignant infiltration or compression of local structures e.g. lung carcinoma (primary or secondary), malignant lymphoma.

5. As a paraneoplastic syndrome, e.g. myasthenia gravis, Cushings disease (ACTH: adrenocorticotrophic hormone) or secretion of inappropriate antidiuretic hormone (SIADH).

Therefore, knowledge of a relevant past medical history is fundamental in determining the nature of the underlying abnormality. Further clinical investigations are viewed in light of this and can include: CT/MRI scans to determine local invasion and solid/cystic features, angiography, blood tests[1] (AFP, HCG, LDH, parathormone, alkaline phosphatase, acetylcholine receptor antibodies), electromyography and tensilon test, oesophagoscopy and bronchoscopy. Age is also indicative in that thymomas are the commonest thymic tumours in adults followed by malignant lymphoma, whereas the converse applies to thymic based tumours in children. Tissue diagnosis is often obtained by thoracoscopic, CT guided percutaneous/transbronchial FNAC (fine needle aspiration cytology) or needle core biopsy. Material is provided not only for routine morphology, but, importantly, ancillary techniques such as immunohistochemistry to aid in the distinction between diagnoses such as metastatic carcinoma, lymphoblastic or large cell malignant lymphoma and thymoma. However, in some cases, due to the limitations of these sampling techniques, invasive mediastinal incisional biopsy may be required via cervical mediastinoscopy or anterior mediastinotomy. This can improve diagnostic yields from 60 % to over 80 %. Prior to this it should be determined whether a more convenient source of tissue diagnosis is available e.g. palpable supraclavicular or cervical lymphadenopathy, or pleural fluid cytology. Needle core biopsy of a thymoma is also contentious due to disruption of the tumour capsule and the possibility of seeding into the operative site.

---

[1]AFP: α-fetoprotein, HCG: β subunit human chorionic gonadotrophin, LDH: lactate dehydrogenase.

Tumour site within the mediastinum is an important clue to tumour type e.g. middle mediastinal disease is most likely to be metastatic carcinoma or malignant lymphoma, whereas anterosuperior mediastinal lesions are more likely to be thymus based cancers e.g. thymoma, germ cell tumours and malignant lymphoma. Thus *a diagnostic short list is created based on clinical presentation, patient age, gender and tumour location.*

19.1   Gross Description

Specimen

- Percutaneous or mediastinoscopic/thoracoscopic FNAC/(needle core) biopsy/resection (cervical thymectomy or thoracotomy).
- Number of fragments and their length (mm).
- Size (cm) and weight (g).

Tumour

Site
- Mediastinal boundaries:

Lateral	Pleural cavities
Anterior	Sternum
Posterior	Spine
Superior	Thoracic inlet
Inferior	Diaphragm.

- Superior:
  Thymoma and thymic cysts.
  Malignant lymphoma.
  Nodular goitre thyroid.
  Ectopic parathyroid lesions.
- Anterior:
  Thymoma (75 % of cases) and thymic cysts.
  Well differentiated neuroendocrine (carcinoid) tumours.
  Malignant lymphoma.
  Germ cell tumours.
  Metastatic carcinoma.
  Thyroid/parathyroid lesions.
  Mesenchymal lesions – lipoma, lymphangioma, haemangioma.

- Middle:
  Metastatic carcinoma.
  Malignant lymphoma.
  Pericardial/bronchogenic cysts.
  Primary cardiac tumours.
- Posterior: neural tumours – neurilemmoma, neurofibroma, ganglioneuroma, ganglioneuroblastoma, malignant schwannoma, neuroblastoma, paraganglioma, and, gastroenteric cysts.

Size
- Length × width × depth (cm) or maximum tumour dimension (cm).
- Size of thymoma can be a prognostic indicator.

Appearance
- Circumscribed/encapsulated/infiltrative/ fleshy/pale/pigmented/cystic/ necrotic/haemorrhagic e.g. thymoma can be encapsulated or infiltrative, solid/cystic or multiloculated, whereas malignant lymphoma is fleshy and pale ± necrosis and sclerosis. Teratoma can be cystic, solid, necrotic or haemorrhagic. Neurilemmoma is encapsulated ± cystic degeneration.

Edge
- Circumscribed/irregular.

19.2   Histological Type

Metastatic Carcinoma

- The *commonest malignant mediastinal tumour* (particularly in the middle mediastinum). It can mimic a primary thymic tumour both clinically and radiologically e.g. small cell carcinoma lung can have a small primary lesion with extensive direct or lymph node spread to the mediastinum.
- *Direct spread*: lung, oesophagus, pleura, chest wall, vertebra, trachea.
- *Distant spread*: breast, thyroid, nasopharynx, larynx, kidney, prostate, testicular (or ovarian) germ cell tumour, malignant melanoma.

Identify a residual rim of lymphoid tissue at the tumour edge to indicate a lymph node metastasis.

Malignant Lymphoma

- *10–15 % of mediastinal masses* in the adult and occurs in decreasing order of frequency in the anterior, superior and middle mediastinum. Thymic or lymph node based. It is the *commonest primary neoplasm of the middle mediastinum*.

Specific thymic/mediastinal features are:

Hodgkin's lymphoma: young females. Nodular sclerosis in type and fibrotic/lobulated ± thymic epithelial cysts and granulomas with lacunar cells (CD15/30 positive). Treatment is radiotherapy with or without chemotherapy and prognosis depends on the stage of disease.

Lymphoblastic lymphoma: acute dyspnoea in adolescent males due to compression of large airways by bulky disease, and sometimes SVC syndrome. Mediastinal plus cervical/supraclavicular and axillary disease; ± Hassall's corpuscles and can therefore mimic a thymoma. Small to medium sized lymphoid cells, apoptosis, tdt positive – usually T cell (CD3: 80 % of cases) and a high Ki-67 index (>95 %). Bone marrow, peripheral blood and central nervous system involvement are common. It is treated with aggressive intent.

Mediastinal large B cell lymphoma: young females presenting with SVC syndrome, airway obstruction, pleural/pericardial effusion or systemic symptoms. There is sclerosis/fibrosis – banded and pericellular. Immunophenotype is CD 45, CD 20 positive, Ki-67 positive in >70 % of cells; also CD30, bcl-6 and CD10 the latter suggesting a follicle centre cell origin. Spread to pericardium, pleura, lung, sternum and chest wall are common. An initial response to chemotherapy is a good prognostic indicator.

MALToma/anaplastic large cell lymphoma: occasionally.

Germ Cell Tumours

- *Up to 20 % of mediastinal tumours/cysts* and commoner than in other extragenital sites

e.g. retroperitoneum or the sacrococcygeal region.

- Thymus based with a primary origin in extragonadal germ cells. *Type I neoplasms* ((immature) teratoma/yolk sac tumours) occur in neonates and young children, and *type II neoplasms* (non-seminomatous germ cell tumours) in young adults.
- Exclude metastases from a clinical or occult testicular/ovarian germ cell tumour, particularly if there is associated retroperitoneal disease.
- *Mature cystic teratoma*: the *commonest mediastinal germ cell tumour* and similar to that in the ovary.
- *Immature teratoma*: rare; immature epithelium, mesenchyme (cartilage) or neural elements.
- Mature and immature teratoma generally have a *benign course if completely resected* although adult immature teratoma is more aggressive and mature teratoma in the postpubertal patient is potentially malignant.
- *Mature teratoma ± yolk sac tumour*: encountered in infany and early childhood the former is generally resectable and benign, the latter achieves 80 % 5 year survival with appropriate treatment.
- *Embryonal carcinoma, yolk sac tumour, choriocarcinoma* (third decade, gynaecomastia): all require *chemotherapy* and are less responsive with a higher relapse rate and lower survival than equivalent testicular lesions. There is also a higher rate of *somatic malignant transformation* e.g. adenocarcinoma, angiosarcoma, rhabdomyosarcoma and *myeloid malignancies* than in gonadal germ cell tumours. Serum HCG and AFP levels are raised in >90 % of non-seminomatous germ cell tumours and high levels are an adverse prognostic indicator.
- *Seminoma*: PLAP, CD117, OCT3/4, SALL4 positive, cytokeratin negative and 69 % 10 year survival. The seminoma cells can be obscured by granulomatous inflammation, reactive lymphoid follicular hyperplasia or thymic epithelial cysts, and immunohistochemical markers are helpful.
- *Chemotherapy*: of germ cell tumour results in necrosis. Residual tumour can regrow and

follow up radiology, serum tumours markers and surgical excision or additional chemotherapy are carried out. As with retroperitoneal disease from gonadal germ cell tumours, this can be further malignant germ cell tumour, or, tissue maturation and growing teratoma syndrome with pressure effects on adjacent organs.

- *Metastases*: are seen overall in 20 % of mediastinal germ cell tumours; seminoma 41 % and non-seminomatous germ cell tumours 85–95 %. Blood borne spread is to lung, bone, liver, brain and retroperitoneum.

Neurogenic Tumours

- Posterior mediastinum.
- *Children*: tumours derived from the sympathetic nervous system; neuroblastoma, ganglioneuroblastoma, ganglioneuroma.
- *Adults*: tumours derived from the peripheral nervous system; neurilemmoma, neurofibroma ± cystic degeneration. Malignant peripheral nerve sheath tumour: de novo or in von Recklinghausen's disease, ± enteric glands, ± rhabdomyoblasts (malignant Triton tumour). Poor prognosis with pleural and pulmonary spread.

Sarcoma

- Rarely primary: *liposarcoma, synovial sarcoma.*
- *Rhabdomyosarcoma* especially the alveolar subtype (desmin/myo D1/myogenin positive).

Thymoma

- *Anterosuperior mediastinum (80% of cases)* but can occur in other anatomical compartments e.g. neck, thyroid, lung and pleura.
- Solid, yellow/grey, lobulated ± cystic change: *80% are encapsulated and easily excised, 20% are infiltrative*. It comprises a dual population of cytokeratin positive epithelial cells and T marker (CDs 1, 3, 4, 8, 99, 1a)

positive lymphocytes of variable maturity. Classification which can reflect invasiveness and prognosis relies on:

1. The character of the epithelial cells and lymphocytes
2. The relative proportion of these cells
3. Their cellular atypia, and,
4. The organoid architecture: lobulated corticomedullary differentiation; epithelial lined glands and cysts; Hassall's-like corpuscles; perivascular spaces.

Individual tumours can show some heterogeneity in these features. The classification according to Müller-Hermelink is:

Medullary (6%):
  Spindle shaped epithelial cells.
  Scanty to moderate numbers of mature lymphocytes.
  Thick capsule.
  Excellent prognosis.

Mixed (composite) (20%):
  Elderly patients, thick capsule, excellent prognosis.
  Biphasic, lobulated.
  Medullary plus a component of round to stellate epithelial cells (vesicular nucleus, inconspicuous nucleolus) with numerous lymphocytes.

Predominantly cortical (organoid) (7%):
  Lymphocyte rich, organoid corticomedullary areas (thymus like).
  Less prominent epithelial component and an expansile edge with local invasion common.

Cortical (42%):
  Young patients.
  Large round/polygonal epithelial cells with vesicular nucleus.
  Lesser component of intervening immature lymphocytes.
  Lobulated, fibrous septa, locally invasive.

Well differentiated thymic carcinoma (17%):
  Predominantly epithelial (small cells with mild nuclear atypia).
  Few lymphocytes.
  Lobulated, sclerotic, invasive.

Thymic carcinoma (8%):
  Clear cut cytological features of malignancy.
  Exclude metastasis from lung or elsewhere.

90 % are squamous cell carcinoma (±keratini-sation): also lymphoepithelioma like carcinoma (similar to that of nasopharyngeal carcinoma).

Others:

Spindle cell carcinoma (sarcomatoid carcinoma/carcinosarcoma).

Clear cell carcinoma.

Basaloid carcinoma.

Mucoepidermoid carcinoma.

Papillary carcinoma.

Adenocarcinoma.

Small cell carcinoma (grade 3 neuroendocrine thymic tumour).

Undifferentiated and neuroendocrine large cell carcinoma.

Carcinoid tumour (classic/spindle cell/pigmented/with amyloid, or, atypical: grade 1, or, grade 2 neuroendocrine thymic tumours).

Comparison of the above with the *WHO classification (types A, B, C)* is as follows:

Type A	Medullary
Type B	Predominantly cortical (B1), cortical (B2) and well differentiated thymic carcinoma (B3)
Type AB	Mixed
Type C	Thymic carcinoma and its variants.

19.3 Differentiation/Grade

Metastatic Carcinoma

- Well/moderate/poor/undifferentiated.

Malignant Lymphoma

- Low-grade: MALToma.
- High-grade: diffuse large B cell lymphoma; lymphoblastic lymphoma.

Germ Cell Tumours

- Seminoma.

- Non-seminomatous: mature/immature teratoma with or without somatic malignancy, embryonal carcinoma, yolk sac tumour, choriocarcinoma.
- Mixed germ cell tumour (35 % of cases).

Neurogenic Tumours

- Small round blue cell: neuroblastoma component.
- Low-grade/high-grade: sarcoma.

Thymoma

- See above.

19.4 Extent of Local Tumour Spread

Border: pushing/infiltrative.

Lymphocytic reaction: prominent/sparse.

For all tumours:

- Confined to the mediastinal nodes.
- Confined to the thymus.
- Into the mediastinal connective tissues.
- Into other organs e.g. pleura, lung, pericardium, main vessels.

I	Completely encapsulated macroscopically and microscopically. Can include invasion into but not through the capsule, and no invasion into surrounding tissues.
II	Minimally invasive: with either a. microscopic transcapsular invasion <3 mm in extent into surrounding tissues, or, b. macroscopic adhesion, or, invasion into surrounding fatty tissues but not breaking through mediastinal pleura or pericardium.
III	Widely invasive and/or implants: into neighbouring organs e.g. pleura, pericardium, great vessels and lung
IV	Metastatic: with either a. widespread discontinuous pleural or pericardial dissemination, or , b. lymphogenous or haematogenous disease.

I–IV equate to pT1–pT4 under a proposed TNM staging system with III encompassing pT3, IVa equating to pT4, and IVb including pN1-3 and pM1.

Lymphohaematogenous metastases e.g. cervical lymph nodes, lung, liver, bone and ovary can occur after a lag period of months to years post diagnosis.

19.5 Lymphovascular Invasion

Present/absent.
    Intra-/extratumoural.

19.6 Lymph Nodes

Site/number/size/number involved/limit node/extracapsular spread.
    Regional nodes: intrathoracic, scalene, supraclavicular nodes

Thymoma

pN0	No regional lymph nodes involved
pN1	Metastasis to anterior mediastinal lymph nodes
pN2	Metastasis to intrathoracic lymph nodes other than the anterior mediastinal lymph nodes
pN3	Metastasis to extrathoracic lymph nodes.

19.7 Excision Margins

Distances (mm) to the nearest painted margins of excision.

19.8 Other Pathology

Associations

About 30–45 % of thymoma patients have *myasthenia gravis* – muscular fatigability of the proximal limbs and head and neck including extraocular, masticatory, speech and facial expression muscles. Acetylcholine receptor antibody is positive. These patients can also have a range of other *haematological, dermatological* and *systemic autoimmune diseases* which can either precede or follow surgical resection. Other *paraneoplastic syndromes* relate to the mediastinal cancer type e.g. small cell lung carcinoma with secretion of ACTH or IADH.

Thymic carcinoid tumour is associated with *carcinoid tumour* at other sites e.g. bronchus, ileum and type I multiple endocrine neoplasia (MEN I) syndrome. Typically ribbons, rosettes, and balls of cells with central necrosis and calcification.

Immunophenotype

- *Metastatic carcinoma*: cytokeratins, CEA, EMA, BerEP4, TTF-1, CA125, CA19-9, ER.
- *Hodgkin's lymphoma*: CD 15, CD 30.
- *Non-Hodgkin's lymphoma*: CD 45, CD 20, CD 3, CD 30, ALK1, κ/λ light chain restriction, molecular gene rearrangements.
- *Lymphoblastic lymphoma*: tdt, CD 10, CD 99, CD 3, Ki-67 >95 %.
- *Seminoma*: PLAP, CD117, OCT3/4, SALL4 (cytokeratin negative).
- *Embryonal carcinoma/yolk sac tumour*: cytokeratins, HCG, AFP, CD 30, CD117 and OCT3/4 (negative in yolk sac tumour), SALL4 (±PLAP – in embryonal carcinoma).
- *Thymoma*: cytokeratins, EMA, CEA, S100 positive interdigitating reticulum cells; variably mature T lymphocytes CDs 1, 3, 4, 8, 99, 1a. Thymic carcinoma retains CD 5 positivity – also CD117 positive.
- *Carcinoid*: chromogranin, synaptophysin, CD56±CAM 5.2. Ki-67 index 440 ≤2 %.

Cystic Change

- *Unilocular thymic cysts*: developmental and thin non-inflamed wall with cubocolumnar epithelial lining.

- *Multilocular thymic cysts*: multilocular and adherent to mediastinal structures due to inflammation and fibrosis mimicking an invasive thymic tumour. There is a cubocolumnar or squamous epithelial lining.
- 50 % of thymic *nodular sclerosing Hodgkin's lymphomas*.
- *Thymic seminoma* or *non-seminomatous germ cell tumour*.
- Cystic change can lead to a non-representative sample on needle core biopsy.

Prognosis

Prognosis relates to the nature of the underlying pathological abnormality and as to whether it represents primary or secondary disease. Cancer subtype also determines the choice of therapy e.g. surgery, chemotherapy or radiotherapy. Note that prebiopsy or presurgical radiotherapy and chemotherapy can induce tumour apoptosis, necrosis and hyalinisation which can lead to difficulties in accurate classification of disease.

In *thymoma several rules apply*:
1. Tumours with predominantly bland *spindle/oval cells* are usually encapsulated and of excellent prognosis,
2. Tumours with predominantly *round/polygonal epithelial cells* have a course related to the relative predominance of epithelial cells over lymphocytes and any cellular atypia that is present, and
3. The *encapsulation of the tumour*, or its lack of encapsulation and any *signs of invasion at surgery* along with *completeness of excision* are, irrespective of the histological subtype, the best markers of future clinical behaviour. Macroscopic adherence in the mediastinum may be the only sign of capsular penetration – the surgeon should mark it and refrain from incising the capsule to allow full histological assessment.

Medullary (type A) and mixed thymoma tend to present at stages I or II, predominantly cortical (type B1) or cortical (type B2) more often stages III or IV. However, *prognosis is usually 90–100 % 5 year survival*, patients with myasthenia gravis doing worse than those without. *Treatment is surgical* with small localised lesions removed via a *transcervical route*. The usual surgical approach is *median sternotomy*. This is supplemented by *radiotherapy* if there is any possibility of residual tumour or local recurrence (2–10 % of cases, more usually the predominantly cortical and cortical types). *Distant metastases* may need *chemotherapy*. Well differentiated thymic carcinoma (type B3) has an 80 % 5 year survival. Thymic carcinoma (type C) may require a combination of *surgery, radiotherapy and chemotherapy* for bulky local disease or distant spread. Disease course relates to tumour type being either aggressive (death in 6 months to 2 years in non-keratinising carcinoma, sarcomatoid/clear cell/undifferentiated carcinomas), intermediate (squamous cell carcinoma, carcinoid tumour) or indolent (muco-epidermoid/basaloid carcinomas).

Bibliography

Anastasiadis K, Ratatunga C. The thymus gland: diagnosis and surgical management. 1st ed. Berlin/New York: Springer; 2007.

Burke A, Jeudy Jr J, Virmani R. Cardiac tumours; an update. Heart. 2008;94:117–23.

Den Bakker MA, Oosterhuis JW. Tumours and tumour-like conditions of the thymus other than thymoma: a practical approach. Histopathology. 2009;54:69–89.

Detterbeck F. International thymic malignancies interest group: a way forward. J Thorac Oncol. 2010;5: S365–70.

Detterbeck FC, Nicholson AG, Kondo K, Van Schil P, Moran C. The Masaoka-Koga stage classification of thymic malignancies: clarification and definition of terms. J Thorac Oncol. 2011a;6:S1710–6.

Detterbeck FC, Moran C, Huang J, Suster S, Walsh G, Kaiser L, et al. Which way is up? Policies and procedures for surgeons and pathologists regarding resection specimens of thymic malignancy. J Thorac Oncol. 2011b;6:S1730–8.

Masaoka A, Monden Y, Nakahara K, Tanioka T. Follow-up study of thymomas with special reference to their clinical stages. Cancer. 1981;48:2485–92.

Muller-Hermelink HK, Marx A, Kircher T. Advances in the diagnosis and classification of thymic epithelial tumours. In: Anthony PP, MacSween RNM, editors. Recent advances in histopathology, vol. 16. Edinburgh: Churchill Livingstone; 1994. p. 49–72.

Salter DM. Pulmonary and thoracic sarcomas. Curr Diagn Pathol. 2006;12:409–17.

The Royal College of Pathologists. Dataset for the histological reporting of thymic epithelial tumours. Accessed at http://www.rcpath.org/index. asp?PageID=254.

Travis WD, Brambilla E, Muller-Hermelink HK, Harris CC. WHO classification of tumours. Pathology and genetics. Tumours of the lung, pleura, thymus and heart. Lyon: IARC Press; 2004.

Part IV

Skin Cancer

- Non-melanocytic Skin Carcinoma
- Malignant Melanoma

Non-melanocytic Skin Carcinoma

Actinic keratosis, Bowen's disease (in situ or intraepidermal carcinoma), squamous cell carcinoma and basal cell carcinoma are the commonest solar induced non-melanocytic tumours, other skin malignancy being relatively unusual. They arise either as red, scaly patches or non-healing sore nodular lesions on the sun exposed head and neck areas and hands of fair skinned people, who have a 10–20 fold increased risk over people with dark skin. Some 75 % are basal cell carcinomas and 75 % of these arise on the head and neck areas with exposure to ultraviolet irradiation a key aetiological factor. With an increasingly elderly population lifetime risk of developing cutaneous carcinoma is estimated at 30–50 %. A minority are associated with genetic disorders, or areas of chronic scarring and ulceration e.g. Marjolin's ulcer of the leg. Delay in presentation of cutaneous carcinoma is associated with increased tumour growth, local tissue destruction (e.g. spread to the orbit requiring exenteration), and, with squamous cell carcinoma potential for lymphovascular metastases.

Curettage, shave and punch biopsies are often small, processed intact and embedded in toto. Curettage removes the lesion in fragments and is followed by electrothermal cautery to its base. Diathermy excision distorts the tissue making accurate histological assessment problematic. Shave biopsy excises benign surface lesions. Punches can be either diagnostic or therapeutic in intent, and the submitting clinician should indicate this clearly on the request form. They can also be deep if it is necessary to visualise the subcutaneous fat. Slightly larger shaves and punches may be bisected and similarly all processed. In general, margins are not marked and this is also so for incision biopsies which are for diagnostic purposes from the edge of a larger lesion. Histological levels are usually examined. Excisional biopsies attempt to remove the lesion with clear margins of normal skin. Assessment is aided by painting the deep and lateral limits and use of serial transverse slices or quadrant blocks tailored to local protocols. Attached orientation sutures can aid assessment of specific anatomical margins. This is particularly useful when it is only feasible to achieve minimal clearance e.g. on the face, ear, lip, nasal or periorbital areas. Thus, cases are handled individually according to the specimen size, type of lesion and its size and position within the specimen. If initial histological sections fail to reveal a tumour when an experienced dermatologist has given a strong clinical suspicion that there is one present the pathologist must always be prepared to take extra blocks or carry out further levels for examination. Additional histological clues can be evident e.g. epidermal dysplasia, dermal inflammation/hyalinisation or retraction artifact that would suggest the possibility of an adjacent carcinoma. This is particularly so for recurrences which can be small and difficult to demonstrate.

Tumours arising in the face around the eyes, ears, nose and mouth (the so called "H-zone") are more difficult to treat with a tendency for wider subclinical spread and a higher incidence of local recurrence and metastasis. A more complex

D.C. Allen, *Histopathology Reporting*,
DOI 10.1007/978-1-4471-5263-7_20, © Springer-Verlag London 2013

oncoplastic dermatological surgical technique may be required with intraoperative frozen section checking of circumferential surgical margins and wound reconstruction (Moh's micrographic surgery). Sometimes primary or secondary excision specimens are submitted with a central circular deficiency due to prior sampling for diagnosis or research by the clinician. Care must be taken in orientation of the specimen and accurate assessment of tumour diameter and margin distances can be somewhat problematic. In secondary excision for scar recurrence the tumour may be small or macroscopically difficult to define and eccentrically located within the specimen. Serial slices and total processing of the tissue may be required.

In general treatment of cutaneous carcinoma is by wide local excision, or if indicated Moh's micrographic surgery. Other modalities are: radiotherapy, photodynamic therapy, topical imiquimod (Aldara: an immune response modifier mediating cell death), curettage and cautery, cryotherapy and laser. Choice of therapy is determined by patient age and preference, comorbidities, and, tumour type, site, size, and whether it is a primary or recurrent lesion.

20.1   Gross Description

Specimen

- Smear cytology/curettage/shave biopsy/punch biopsy/incision biopsy/excision biopsy/Mohs' surgery.
- Size: length × width × depth (mm).

Tumour

Site
- Anatomical site: limbs/trunk/head/neck/perineum/epidermal/dermal/subcutaneous.
- Sun exposed areas of the head and neck, scalp and back of hands are the preferred sites for the common cancers. The central face, periorbital areas, lips and ears are clinical high risk anatomical sites prone to local recurrence due

to difficulties in obtaining adequate primary margins.

Size
- Length × width × depth (mm) or maximum dimension (mm).
- Tumour size ≤2 or >2 cm is a pT1/pT2 stage determinant for the common skin cancers. Clinical low risk basal cell carcinomas are usually <1 cm diameter. Size >1 cm and tumour thicknesses >2 and >4 mm are clinical high risk factors in cutaneous squamous cell carcinoma. Prognosis of Merkel cell carcinoma >5 mm in thickness is poor. Cutaneous adnexal carcinoma >2 mm in thickness is a high risk feature.

Appearance
- Verrucous/warty/nodular/exophytic/sessile/ulcerated/invaginated/cystic/plaque/haemorrhagic/necrotic/pigmented.

Edge
- Circumscribed/irregular.

20.2   Histological Type

Squamous Cell Carcinoma

- Forehead, face, ears, scalp, lip, neck, back of hands.
- Keratinising/non-keratinising.
- *80 % are well to moderately differentiated and keratinising.*
- Variants with adverse prognosis and higher rates of local recurrence and/or metastasis:

  Acantholytic (pseudoglandular or adenoid): metastasis in 5–19 % of cases >2 cm diameter. Overlaps with *pseudoangiosarcomatous (pseudovascular) squamous cell carcinoma* which has a mortality of up to 50 %.

  Spindle cell (sarcomatoid): accounts for over 30 % of metastatic squamous cell carcinomas.

  Desmoplastic: >30 % of the tumour area is desmoplastic.

  Small cell or *basaloid.*

  Post traumatic (e.g. Marjolin's ulcer).

Adenosquamous (mixed differentiation) arising from pluripotential acrosyringium cells.

Squamous cell carcinoma associated with adjacent in situ change (Bowens disease).

- Others:

  Verrucous: high rate of local recurrence on the sole of foot and at the anal margin. It is locally invasive, exophytic with "church spire" hyperkeratosis and a pushing deep margin of cytologically bland bullous processes.

  Clear cell (elderly, scalp).

  Papillary.

  Lymphoepithelial.

  Keratoacanthoma: rapid clinical growth over 1–3 months with potential for involution over 3–9 months and even complete regression. It is crateriform with a central keratin plug and lipped rim of hyperplastic squamous epithelium. It is sometimes regarded as and difficult to distinguish from a well differentiated variant of squamous cell carcinoma. A designation of keratoacanthoma is excluded by adjacent in situ change, dermal invasion or desmoplasia, significant cellular pleomorphism, and plentiful or atypical mitoses.

Basal Cell Carcinoma

- *The commonest non-melanocytic cutaneous carcinoma* comprising a proliferation of basaloid/germinative cells and characterised by *local tissue infiltration, destruction* and *recurrence* and, very rarely, metastasis. Circumscribed, local or expansile tumours have a low risk of local recurrence but there is a high risk for those with a diffuse, multifocal or infiltrative *growth pattern*. Note that there is often more than one growth pattern in any given lesion and the level of clinical risk is determined by the highest risk growth pattern present. Basosquamous *cellular differentiation* is also a notable clinical risk factor.
- *Nodular*: the commonest subtype (60–80 % of cases, often head and neck area) with nodules of varying size, ± tumour necrosis and cystic spaces (nodulocystic), peripheral palisading,

mitoses and dermal retraction artifact. Includes adenoid, (trabecular/ribbons of cells), keratotic (horn cysts, squamous metaplasia), pigmented, fibroepithelial (Pinkus tumour) variants, and, those with adnexal (follicular, sebaceous or eccrine) differentiation.

- *Superficial multifocal*: 10–20 % of cases comprising multifocal nests of tumour budding off the epidermal or hair follicle basal layer. Recurrence is due to inadequate primary excision of peripheral margins. Often occur on the trunk.
- *Infiltrative/morphoeic*: small, irregular infiltrating groups in a fibrous, scirrhous or amyloid like hyaline stroma in a poorly circumscribed lesion. The pattern resembles a tree trunk with spreading roots which can be deeply infiltrative jeopardising the deep margin. Usually occurs on the upper trunk or face.
- *Micronodular*: multiple small round nests less than 25 cells in diameter, with an asymmetrical, infiltrative growth pattern.
- *Metatypical/basosquamous carcinoma*: metatypical is a poorly defined term describing a tumour with the configuration of a basal cell carcinoma but with more cytonuclear atypia and a fibroblastic response. If there are foci of moderately to severely atypical or malignant squamous cell differentiation the tumour is designated basosquamous cell carcinoma. This is an intermediate tumour between basal cell and squamous cell carcinomas of usual type with potential for local recurrence and metastatic spread. A general rule is that most lesions are simply keratotic basal cell carcinomas with abrupt keratinisation. If the carcinoma has squam*oid* foci it is metatypical basal cell carcinoma whereas if it has distinct squam*ous* foci it is basosquamous carcinoma.
- Metastasis in basal cell carcinoma is extremely rare. *Low risk tumours* can be adequately treated in *primary care* by suitably trained personnel, whereas *high risk tumours* are dealt with in *secondary care*. High risk lesions prone to local recurrence are characterised by: *anatomical site* (face, eyes, nose, lips, ears), *growth pattern* (infiltrative/morphoeic/

micronodular), *cellular differentiation* (baso-squamous), the presence of *perineural or lymphovascular invasion, Clark level V invasion,* and *stage ≥pT2.*

Adnexal Carcinoma

- These are *rare tumours* best dealt with by a pathologist with dermatopathological expertise in the context of a multidisciplinary meeting. Diagnostic clues are cellular atypia, necrosis, mitoses, perineural/lymphovascular invasion and an unusually deep and infiltrative margin. Benign adnexal tumours are either in continuity with the epidermis (e.g. eccrine poroma), or classically form nodular, smooth bordered, vertically orientated "blue (haematoxyphilic) balls" in the dermis. Often there is a dual cell population or epithelial bilayer. Their malignant counterparts form horizontally orientated, irregularly shaped plaques that are sometimes ulcerated. Low power patterns are solid-cystic, papillary-tubular or sclerosing. Low-grade carcinomas show considerable cellular differentiation, uniform cell size with infrequent mitoses and little pleomorphism: they do well if small and completely excised. Examples are microcystic adnexal carcinoma, syringoid eccrine carcinoma, adenoid cystic carcinoma and mucinous eccrine carcinoma. High-grade cancers show poor differentiation, necrosis and mitoses, and they can metastasise widely. Examples are malignant hidradenoma, malignant spiradenoma/cylindroma, aggressive digital papillary adenocarcinoma and porocarcinoma.
- Adnexal tumours can be of *hair follicle, sebaceous or ductal (eccrine/apocrine) differentiation.*
- Hair follicle differentiation: tricholemmocarcinoma, malignant pilomatrixoma.
- Sebaceous differentiation: epithelioma/carcinoma.
- Ductal differentiation: apocrine or eccrine – including syringomatous carcinoma, microcystic adnexal carcinoma, malignant chondroid syringoma/nodular hidradenoma/spiradenoma subtypes, porocarcinoma, mucinous carcinoma, aggressive digital papillary adenoma/adenocarcinoma and adenoid cystic carcinoma.

Paget's Disease

- Extramammary sites are vulva, perineum, scrotum, axillae: see Chaps. 7 and 27.

Neuroendocrine Carcinoma: Merkel Cell or Small Cell Neuroendocrine Carcinoma of Skin

- On the head/neck, extremities, in the elderly, it is a poorly differentiated/high-grade neuroendocrine carcinoma comprising small blue cells with increased apoptosis and a high mitotic rate.
- Chromogranin/synaptophysin/CD56 and paranuclear dot CAM 5.2, AE1/AE3, CK20 positive. Ki-67, CD117, CD99 and Fli-1 positive, but TTF-1 negative.
- There can be overlying basal or squamous cell carcinoma (in situ or invasive) in 30 % of cases. Rarely the tumour can also show components of squamous cell or eccrine differentiation.
- *Clinically exclude secondary small cell carcinoma of lung* (CK 20 negative/TTF-1 positive). *Histologically exclude malignant lymphoma* (CD45 positive) and a *small cell variant of malignant melanoma* (S100, melan-A positive). There is a reported association of Merkel cell carcinoma with polyoma virus infection (SV40 antibody positive).
- Of *poor prognosis*, local recurrence and lymph node metastases are common. Treatment is *primary excision with wide margins. Adverse indicators* are: size >2 cm, thickness >5 mm, mitoses >10/10 high power fields or Ki-67 >50 %, an infiltrative border, extensive lymphovascular or subcutaneous fat (level V) invasion, lymph node involvement or positive primary excision margins. Some Merkel cell carcinomas can regress and present as metastatic disease of unknown primary origin.

Dermal Tumours

- Adnexal, fibrohistiocytic, neural, muscular, vascular, adipose.

Metastatic Carcinoma

Skin metastases occur in up to *10% of malignancies* and can *predate*, *occur synchronously, or after the primary lesion*. Clinical presentation with a skin metastasis (2 % of cases) is seen particularly with lung, kidney and ovarian cancer. *Late metastases* (at 10 years or more) come from breast carcinoma, malignant melanoma, and kidney, bladder, colon and ovarian cancers. Some metastases are by *direct local extension* to overlying skin e.g. breast carcinoma, others by *distant vascular spread* e.g. kidney carcinoma and malignant melanoma. In males the commonest skin metastases are: lung, colon, malignant melanoma and head and neck squamous cell carcinomas. In females: breast (70 %), colon, malignant melanoma and ovarian cancers. Stomach cancer should also be considered in both sexes.

- Single/multiple nodule(s) commonly on the trunk and head and neck regions (especially umbilicus and scalp), sometimes *in the vicinity of the primary lesion*.
- Some metastases can be epidermotropic and *simulate a primary lesion* e.g. malignant melanoma. Most are dermal and show nodular, interstitial and intravascular patterns necessitating distinction from primary adnexal carcinoma. *Previous clinical history, comparative morphology* and relevant *immunohistochemical profiles* are important in this respect. Clear cell hidradenoma and ductal eccrine adenocarcinoma are the commonest primary lesion mimicking skin metastases.
- Secondary small cell carcinoma of lung or gastrointestinal carcinoid can mimic Merkel cell carcinoma although both are CK20 negative.

20.3 Differentiation

Well/moderate/poor/undifferentiated, or, Grade 1/2/3/4.

- Basal cell carcinomas are usually not graded but subtyped according to low or high risk growth patterns with comment made on any unusual cellular differentiation features e.g. basosquamous carcinoma.
- For squamous cell carcinoma based on cellular atypia (pleomorphism/mitoses), keratinisation and intercellular bridges. Broders grade I (>75 % differentiated), II (25–75 %), III (<25 %) and IV (no differentiation). High grade tumours show poor differentiation, frequent spindle cell change, necrosis and high mitotic activity.
- For adnexal carcinoma grade is based on the tumour cell lineage, the degree of appendage differentiation, cellular atypia, mitoses and necrosis.
- Undifferentiated carcinomas are grade 4. Dedifferentiation correlates with an increasing risk of recurrence and metastasis.

20.4 Extent of Local Tumour Spread

Border: pushing/infiltrative.
Lymphocytic reaction: prominent/sparse.
The TNM7/AJCC7 classification applies to any skin carcinoma except Merkel cell carcinoma, but not carcinomas of the eyelid, vulva and penis.

pTis	Carcinoma in situ
pT1	Tumour ≤2 cm in greatest dimension
pT2	Tumour >2 cm in greatest dimension
pT3	Tumour invades deep extradermal structures (cartilage, skeletal muscle, bone, jaws and orbit)
pT4	Tumour with direct or perineural invasion of skull base or axial skeleton

Depth of dermal invasion for squamous cell carcinoma can also be expressed in anatomical Clark levels I-V (see chap. 21). *High risk types* correspond to: Clark levels IV and V (reticular dermis, subcutaneous fat), depth of invasion >2 and >4 mm, perineural or lymphovascular invasion, poor tumour differentiation, high risk anatomical sites (i.e. ear, lip, periorbital, central face) and stage ≥pT2. AJCC7 also incorporates <2 or ≥2 of these high risk factors into stages pT1 and pT2, respectively.

Merkel cell carcinoma: pT1≤2 cm, pT2>2–5 cm, pT3>5 cm, pT4 into deep extra-dermal structures such as bone, muscle, fascia or cartilage. This staging classification applies to Merkel cell carcinoma of the skin, penis, vulva and vermillion lip, but not the eyelid. A *tumour thickness >5 mm is particularly adverse*.

20.5 Lymphovascular Invasion

Present/absent.

Intra-/extratumoural.

- Perineural and lymphovascular invasion are not commonly seen (sometimes in squamous cell carcinoma, rarely in high risk basal cell carcinoma) but when present correlate with higher rates of local recurrence and metastases. Also an adverse indicator in Merkel cell carcinoma.

20.6 Lymph Nodes

Site/number/size/number involved/limit node/extracapsular spread.

Regional nodes: those appropriate to the site of the primary tumour i.e. head and neck (preauricular, submandibular, cervical and supraclavicular), thorax and upper limb (axillae), and abdomen, loins, buttocks, lower limbs, perianal/anal margin (all inguinal nodes). Although not usually submitted a regional lymphadenectomy will ordinarily include a minimum of six lymph nodes. Involvement of iliac, pelvic, abdominal or intrathoracic nodes is classified as pM1.

pN0	No regional lymph node metastasis
pN1	Metastasis in a single regional lymph node ≤3 cm diameter
pN2	Metastasis in a single regional lymph node >3–6 cm, or, multiple nodes ≤6 cm
pN3	Metastasis in a regional lymph node >6 cm

Merkel cell carcinoma: pN1a microscopic and pN1b macroscopic regional lymph node metastasis. Distant metastasis is: pM1a skin, subcutaneous tissue or non-regional nodes, pM1b lung and pM1c other visceral sites.

20.7 Excision Margins

Distances (mm) to the nearest painted deep and peripheral excision margins, either of serial transverse slices (toast racked) or quadrant blocks according to local protocols. Comment should also be made on the presence of dysplasia or in situ change at the margins.

Adequate treatment is based on successful *complete primary excision* or, if there is initial margin involvement, on *secondary re-excision*. Involved is tumour at (=0 mm) a margin; close to is ≤1 mm; clear of is >1 mm. A further quality indicator of adequacy of excision is *stratification of margin clearance* as either ≤1, 1–5 or >5 mm. It is estimated that 4 and 3 mm margins will adequately clear 95 and 85 % of basal cell carcinomas respectively – particular caution must be exercised for those subtypes that can show extensive subclinical spread. Risk of local recurrence for basal cell carcinomas can be as high as 30–40 % if optimal margins are not achieved. Cutaneous adnexal carcinomas can have ill-defined infiltrative lateral and deep margins compromising complete primary excision e.g. microcystic adnexal carcinoma.

20.8 Other Pathology

Squamous cell carcinoma: more prone to lymph node metastases particularly if >2 cm diameter or >2 mm in thickness, poorly differentiated or with perineural spread. Morphologically it shows nuclear stratification, intercellular bridges ± keratinisation. General *prognostic indicators* for squamous cell carcinoma are stage, level of dermal invasion and tumour thickness. *Recurrent tumours* tend to be ≥4 mm thick with involvement of the deep dermis, and *fatal tumours* at least 1 cm thick with extension into subcutaneous fat. Tumours arising in non-sun exposed sites e.g. trunk, perineum, penis and areas of trauma e.g. burns, Marjolin's ulcer have a higher risk of metastasis.

Predisposing lesions to cutaneous carcinoma are:

- Actinic keratosis/solar elastosis: sun exposure.
- Psoralen plus ultraviolet A (PUVA) treatment for psoriasis.
- Varicose ulcers (Marjolin's), lichen planus, hidradenitis suppurativa.
- Immunosuppression post transplant or chemotherapy, HIV.
- Bowen's disease: indolent progression to carcinoma.
- Condyloma accuminatum, Bowenoid papulosis, HPV infection: perineum/perianal margin squamous carcinoma.
- Epidermodysplasia verruciformis, xeroderma pigmentosum.
- Naevus sebaceous of Jadassohn.
- Naevoid basal cell carcinoma (Gorlins) syndrome.

Double pathology: may be encountered e.g. basal or squamous cell carcinoma overlying Merkel cell carcinoma, basal cell carcinoma and syringocystadenoma papilliferum in naevus sebaceous of Jadassohn, basal cell carcinoma and dermatofibroma.

Pseudoepitheliomatous (pseudocarcinomatous) hyperplasia: may be seen in association with: chronic venous stasis, ulceration, chronic inflammation e.g. pyoderma gangrenosum, and overlying neoplasms e.g. granular cell tumour.

Actinic keratosis, carcinoma in situ and invasive squamous carcinoma: distinction can be difficult and some of these lesions may have to be designated "best regarded as squamous cell carcinoma". Treatment (primary surgical excision ± radiotherapy) is the same for both.

Sebaceous carcinoma: may be periocular and aggressive or extraocular and non-aggressive. It forms a spectrum of behaviour with sebaceous epithelioma (local recurrence). It is usually solitary, but if multiple in a younger patient consider Muir Torre syndrome (FAP associated).

Immunophenotype

Skin carcinoma varies greatly in its immunophenotypic expression –

Squamous cell carcinoma: high molecular weight cytokeratins, AE1/AE3, CK5/6, EMA, p63, CEA positive; BerEP 4 negative.

Basal cell carcinoma: low molecular weight cytokeratins, BerEP 4 positive; EMA, CEA negative.

A combination of CEA and BerEP 4 can help to distinguish between squamous cell carcinoma and basal cell carcinoma.

Adnexal carcinomas: usually EMA and CEA positive, and differential molecular weight cytokeratin expression according to their differentiation. In general they are CK7, CAM 5.2 (low molecular weight), AE1 (intermediate molecular weight), HMFG1 and GCDFP-15 positive.

Some centres use smear cytology with immediate reporting to distinguish basal cell from non-basal cell cutaneous carcinoma to facilitate a one-stop assessment and institution of treatment.

20.9 Other Malignancy

Leukaemia

- *5–10 % of leukaemia cases*: sometimes as a first manifestation of disease but more often secondary to widespread systemic or recurrent disease.
- Children: acute lymphoblastic leukaemia (ALL). CD79a, CD10 (CALLA) positive ± tdt, Ki-67 >90 %.
- Adults: chronic lymphocytic leukaemia (CLL) – CD5/CD23 positive, or, chronic myeloid leukaemia (CML: syn myeloid sarcoma/chloroma) – CD34/CD43/CD68/CD117/chloroactetate esterase/myeloperoxidase positive. Also multiple myeloma (CD79a, CD138, κ, λ light chain restriction, Bence Jones proteinuria, monoclonal gammopathy, lytic skull lesions).

Malignant Lymphoma: Primary

- Defined as disease confined to skin for at least 6 months after complete clinicopathological staging.
- T cell 68 %: B cell 30 %.

Immunohistochemistry (for cell lineage and light chain restriction) and *molecular studies (T cell receptor gene and immunoglobulin heavy chain gene rearrangements)* are also of use in cutaneous malignant lymphoma. *T cell malignant lymphomas* show *epidermotropism* while *B cell malignant lymphomas* often have a *dermal grenz zone* and a *"bottom-heavy" infiltrate extending into the subcutaneous fat*. Note that the latter can also show reactive germinal centres and a polymorphous reactive cellular infiltrate. Low-grade T cell malignant lymphomas have a horizontal band like dermal growth pattern while high-grade lesions and B cell malignant lymphomas are sharply demarcated with a nodular, vertical and three-dimensional growth. Molecular studies are particularly helpful in inflammatory conditions simulating cutaneous malignant lymphoma e.g. lymphocytoma cutis, lupus erythematosus profundus, and lymphomatoid reactions to drugs and insect bites. Designation of malignant lymphoma can sometimes be difficult and should always be clinicopathological in the context of a multidisciplinary meeting. In some cases the subsequent clinical progression or lack of it is the final arbiter.

Some malignant lymphomas present in the skin and never as a primary lesion in lymph node or extracutaneous site e.g. mycosis fungoides. Others can resemble their lymph node counterparts but show a different clinical behaviour. Cutaneous lymphoproliferative disorders can be grouped as: *reactive* ("pseudolymphomas"), *prelymphomatous* (e.g. parapsoriasis), or established *malignant lymphoma* of either low- or high-grade malignancy.

T cell, indolent behaviour:

Mycosis fungoides ± follicular mucinosis: comprising 60–70 % of cutaneous lymphomas MF has overlapping patch, plaque, tumour, erythrodermic and poikilodermic stages with late lymph node, blood and extracutaneous involvement. It forms 50 % of cutaneous T cell malignant lymphomas and comprises medium sized cerebriform, epidermotropic CD3/CD4 positive CD8 negative lymphoid cells.

Pagetoid reticulosis: intraepidermal T cell infiltrate.

Granulomatous slack skin disease: T cell infiltrate with giant cell elastophagocytosis in the major skin folds. Malignant lymphoma may occur years later.

Anaplastic large cell, CD 30 positive: >30 % of the cells are blasts and >75 % of these are CD30 positive. Usually T cell, sometimes null, 40 % spontaneously regress and a 5 year survival of 90 %. There is a small/medium cell variant: <30 % CD30 positive blasts in the infiltrate.

Lymphomatoid papulosis: recurring self-healing papulonodular eruption of uncertain malignant potential with variable polymorphous/monomorphous pictures including CD30 positive large cells. A wedge shaped infiltrate at low power.

T cell, aggressive behaviour:

Sézary syndrome: the leukaemic phase of erythrodermic cutaneous T cell lymphoma.

Anaplastic large cell, CD 30 negative.

Pleomorphic medium/large cell.

Cutaneous γδ T cell lymphoma.

Subcutaneous panniculitis like lymphoma: multiple subcutaneous lumps in the extremities of young adults. Honeycomb panniculitic infiltrate of the subcutaneous fat. CD8 positive, αβ T cell gene rearrangements.

NK, NK/T cell: CD56 positive, occasionally T cell positive and angiocentric/destructive.

B cell, indolent behaviour (95 % 5 year survival):

Follicle centre lymphoma: trunk, head and neck (scalp). CD20/CD10/bcl-6 positive but bcl-2 negative. Widely spaced follicles in the deep dermis and subcutaneous fat. Includes a good prognosis large cell variant.

Marginal zone lymphoma: good prognosis – a minority have *Borrelia burgdorferi* organism as a chronic antigenic stimulus. Nodular perivascular/periadenexal, or diffuse infiltrate of centrocytoid/monocytoid cells including reactive germinal centres. Lymphoplasmacytoid forms, plasma cells and eosinophils, rare lymphoepithelial lesions. Immunoglobulin light chain restriction and monoclonality aid distinction from reactive lymphoid tissue. On the trunk, head and neck, upper limbs.

B cell, intermediate behaviour:

Mantle cell lymphoma: rare and exclude spread from systemic disease.

Large cell lymphoma of the lower legs in elderly women: grenz zone, with a dermal/subcutaneous, perivascular/periadnexal infiltrate. It is CD20/CD10/bcl- 6 positive. Variable 58–95 % 5 year survival. Multiplicity of lesions is adverse.

B cell, aggressive behaviour:

Large cell lymphoma in other clinical settings: e.g. diffuse cutaneous or intravascular large B cell lymphoma (angiotrophic lymphoma).

Lymphoblastic lymphoma in children and adults: tdt positive.

The behaviour of *lymphomatoid granulomatosis* (EBV positive large B cells, with reactive small T cells) depends on the content of blasts, grade 3 equating to diffuse large B cell lymphoma.

Maligant Lymphoma: Secondary

• Secondary to nodal/systemic disease.

For details on the classification, immunophenotyping and staging of malignant lymphoma refer to Chap. 35.

Sarcoma

Soft tissue sarcomas are outnumbered 100–1 by benign soft tissue tumours. There are over 50 different histological types often with more than one subtype. They vary in their behaviour from indolent to aggressive but *cutaneous sarcomas are more favourable* than their deep sited fascial counterparts. In general *5 year survival is 65–75 %* with *complete local excision being the most important determinant*. A majority are locally infiltrative and a minority potentially metastatic.

The latter depends on tumour type, grade, size and depth from the skin surface. They usually arise in older patients in the extremities (particularly thigh), trunk, head and neck and retroperitoneum. Cutaneous sarcomas form an elevated plaque or nodule that can ulcerate. Investigation is by ultrasound, CT and MRI scans. Superficial lesions smaller than 2–5 cm can be *excised in their entirety*. Larger, deeper tumour may require initial diagnostic sampling by *needle core* or *deep punch biopsy* prior to *radical extirpative surgery*. *Molecular genetic analysis* has a *diagnostic* and *prognostic role* to play in select cases and to determine any indication for *neoadjuvant therapy*.

Dermal and subcutaneous soft tissue tumours may have classical clinical features, e.g. angiosarcoma of the scalp in the elderly and Kaposi's sarcoma in HIV. However, they are classified according to their cell of origin and malignancy is assessed by cellularity, cellular atypia, mitotic activity, necrosis and infiltrative margins. *Immunohistochemistry* is often very useful in determining histogenesis e.g. desmin, h-caldesmon, actin, myogenin (muscular), S100 (neural, melanocytic (also HMB-45, melan-A), chondroid, adipose), CD 31, CD34, factor VIII (vascular), CD 68 ((fibro-)histiocytic) and CD 34 (dermatofibrosarcoma). Examples are: cutaneous leiomyosarcoma, dermatofibrosarcoma protuberans, angiosarcoma, epithelioid haemangioendothelioma, malignant nerve sheath tumour, liposarcoma and extraskeletal myxoid chondrosarcoma (usually extending from deep soft tissues). See Chap. 36 for further details.

Kaposi's sarcoma is found in the elderly (solitary) or young (HIV, multiple). The early patch/plaque phase is subtle, characterised by linear "vascular" slit-like spaces in the dermal collagen orientated parallel to the epidermis. Later there is a sieve-like pattern with extravasation of red blood cells and nodular spindle cell proliferation. Associated with human herpes virus 8 (HHV-8).

Immunohistochemistry: is also important in the differential diagnosis of *cutaneous spindle cell lesions*, viz. spindle cell squamous carcinoma versus malignant melanoma, leiomyosarcoma, sarcoma and atypical fibroxanthoma (AFX).

A working panel is CAM5.2, AE1/AE3, CK5/6, p63, S100, melan-A, desmin, h-caldesmon, smooth muscle actin and CD68. Other morphological clues are dysplasia of the surface squamous epithelium (carcinoma), junctional activity and melanin pigmentation (melanoma), Touton-like giant cells (AFX) and eosinophilic fusiform spindle cells (leiomyosarcoma). *Clinical history* is important to exclude a metastatic spindle cell carcinoma or malignant melanoma. Hence AFX is a diagnosis of clinical, morphological and immunohistochemical exclusion. It arises on the sun exposed head and neck area of elderly patients, is a *low-grade malignant tumour* regarded by some as a spindle cell squamous carcinoma, but behaves in a benign fashion if completely excised. It can show false positive melan-A staining in the pleomorphic cells. There is also a monomorphic spindle cell variant. AFX is excluded by the following: perineural, lymphovascular or subcutaneous invasion, or, necrosis. If any of these are present it is designated *pleomorphic dermal sarcoma* with 30 % recurrence and 10 % metastasis rates.

A further indication for immunohistochemistry is in the distinction between Merkel cell tumour (CK20/synaptophysin/CD56/EMA/CD99/ Fli-1), malignant lymphoma (CD 45 (lymphoblastic – tdt/CD 99)), PNETs (CD99±NSE/ neurofilament) and small cell malignant melanoma (S100/melan-A/HMB-45).

Miscellaneous

Langerhans cell histiocytosis: a S100/CD1a positive clonal, epidermotropic dendritic cell proliferation. Can be solitary but also potentially in bone, lung and lymph nodes. Multifocal unisystem disease has good prognosis, but multisystem disease a poor prognosis – 10 % with multifocal disease die, 30 % remit completely and 60 % pursue a chronic course.

Mastocytosis: either solitary mastocytoma, indolent cutaneous mastocytosis (formerly urticaria pigmentosa), or, in a small minority progressive systemic mastocytosis. A clonal mast cell infiltrate with a "fried egg" appearance, toluidine blue/CD117 positive.

Bibliograghy

Alsaad KO, Obaidat NA, Ghazarian D. Skin adnexal neoplasms – part 1: an approach to tumours of the pilosebaceous unit. J Clin Pathol. 2007;60:145–59.

Baxter JM, Patel AM, Varma S. Facial basal cell carcinoma. BMJ. 2012;345:37–42.

Calonje JE, Brenn T, Lazar AJ, McKee PH. McKee's pathology of the skin with clinical correlations. 4th ed. Philadelphia: Elsevier/Saunders; 2012.

Cerroni L. Lymphoproliferative lesions of the skin. J Clin Pathol. 2006;59:813–26.

Goh SGN, Calonje E. Cutaneous vascular tumours: an update. Histopathology. 2008;52:661–73.

Leonard M. Cutaneous metastases: where do they come from and what can they mimic? Curr Diagn Pathol. 2007;13:320–30.

Llombart B, Monteagudo C, Lopez-Guerrero JA, Carda C, Jorda E, Sanmartin O, Almenar S, Molina I, Martin JM, Llombart-Bosch A. Clinicopathological and immunohistochemical analysis of 20 cases of Merkel cell carcinoma in search of prognostic markers. Histopathology. 2005;46:622–34.

Motley R, Kersey P, Lawrence C. Multiprofessional guidelines for the management of the patient with primary cutaneous squamous cell carcinoma. Br J Dermatol. 2002;146(1):18–25.

Murphy GF, Elder DE. Non-melanocytic tumors of the skin. Atlas of tumor pathology. 3rd series. Fascicle 1. Washington: AFIP; 1991.

Obaidat NA, Alsaad KO, Ghazarian D. Skin adnexal neoplasms – part 2: an approach to tumours of cutaneous sweat glands. J Clin Pathol. 2007;60:129–44.

Shriner DL, McCoy DK, Goldberg DJ, Wagner Jr RF. Mohs' micrographic surgery. J Am Acad Dermatol. 1998;39(1):79–97.

Slater DN. Classification and diagnosis of cutaneous lymphoproliferative disorders. In: Lowe DG, Underwood SCE, editors. Recent advances in histopathology 20. London: RSM Press; 2003. p. 53–72.

Telfer NR, Colver GB, Morton CA. Guidelines for the management of basal cell carcinoma. Br J Dermatol. 2008;159:35–48.

The Royal College of Pathologists. Cancer Datasets (Basal cell carcinoma, Malignant Melanoma, Squamous Cell Carcinoma, Primary Cutaneous Adnexal Carinomas) and Tissue Pathways (Inflammatory and Non-neoplastic Dermatoses and Non-neoplastic Lesions). Accessed at http://www.rcpath.org/index.asp?PageID=254.

Van Roggen JFG, Lim TK, Hogendoorn PCW. The histopathological differential diagnosis of mesenchymal tumours of the skin. Curr Diagn Pathol. 2005;11: 371–89.

Weedon D. Skin pathology. 3rd ed. London: Churchill Livingstone; 2009.

Weedon D, LeBoit P, Burg G, Sarasin A, editors. World Health Organisation classification of tumours. Pathology and genetics. Tumours of the skin. Lyon: IARC Press; 2005.

Malignant Melanoma

21

Malignant melanoma remains less common than the usual cutaneous basal cell and squamous cell carcinomas but is more frequently encountered in young people aged 15–45 years. If left untreated it can be fatal due to a propensity for lymphatic and haematogenous metastases, and it causes the majority of deaths related to skin cancer. Primary prevention and screening should see a reduction in overall incidence and mortality. The former is characterised by the Australian "slip/slop/slap/seek/slide" campaign viz slip on a long sleeved top, slop on sunscreen, slap on a hat, seek shade and slide on sunnies (sunglasses)! Any recent change in a melanocytic lesion such as irregularity of profile, border or pigmentation, and spontaneous ulceration should be assessed by a dermatologist and regarded with suspicion. The clinical appearances at dermoscopy, which magnifies the lesion by 5–100 fold, are a help in this regard: irregularity of margins, variation in pigmentation network with streaks and punctation. The ABCDE rule (Asymmetry, irregular Border, uneven Colour, Diameter >6 mm, Enlarging or Evolving) is clinically useful but has its limitations for early lesions.

Diathermy and curettage are avoided as this distorts interpretive histological detail and endangers margin clearance. Rather, primary cold knife excision with clear (at least 2 mm) margins should be attained for initial histological designation which will usually require examination through multiple levels. The deep and lateral margins are painted prior to blocking into serial transverse slices or quadrant blocks, taking into account any attached orientation sutures. Some pathologists will either photograph the lesion surface or take a face-down photocopier image for a record of its outline or proximity to a margin. Re-excision specimens for wider margins usually have a central longitudinal scar, and quadrant blocks with a double central transverse slice will generally suffice. Some malignant melanomas require a significantly complex plastics procedure for full excision depending on the anatomical site and lesion type e.g. lentigo maligna of the face. Full clinical staging of malignant melanoma can involve ultrasound of superficial and deep abdominal lymph nodes, CT, MRI and PET scans, and serum lactate dehydrogenase (LDH). CT/PET scan is indicated according to local protocols but in general for pT3b/pT4 lesions. With increasing sun exposure in fair skinned people and heightened public awareness the range of melanocytic lesions incorporating malignant melanoma,"early" and borderline lesions e.g. melanoma in situ and dysplastic naevi has increased in incidence presenting challenges for the diagnostic surgical pathologist.

For patients with metastatic disease the presence of tumour cell BRAF mutation (60 % of cases) is predictive of response to vemurafinib targeted therapy. If there is no obvious primary

D.C. Allen, *Histopathology Reporting*,
DOI 10.1007/978-1-4471-5263-7_21, © Springer-Verlag London 2013

lesion on the skin, or clinical history of excision of a melanocytic lesion, ocular or mucosal malignant melanoma e.g. anorectal, oesophageal, vulval or penile must be considered as a potential source for the locoregional or disseminated disease.

21.1   Gross Description

Specimen

- Curettage/shave biopsy/punch biopsy/incision biopsy/excision biopsy.
- Size: length × width × depth (mm).

Tumour

Site
- Anatomical location – trunk, limbs, head/neck, perineum, mucosal, ocular, multifocal (1–5 %).
- Epidermal/dermal/subcutaneous.
- Commonly face, ear, head and neck with back and shoulders in males and legs in females.

Size
- Length × width × depth (mm) or maximum dimension (mm).

Appearance
- Verrucous/nodular/sessile/ulcerated/pigmented or non-pigmented/halo/satellite lesions/scarring.

Edge
- Circumscribed/irregular.

21.2   Histological Type

Malignant Melanoma in Situ

- Intraepidermal: spread can be lentiginous (continuous basal layer) or upward (single cells, nests, "buck-shot" or Pagetoid) in this non-invasive radial growth phase.

Lentigo Maligna Melanoma

- Elderly patients/face/Hutchinson's melanotic freckle: a lentiginous single cell and nested proliferation of melanocytes along the surface epidermal and appendageal basal layer. They show cytological atypia (enlarged, hyperchromatic angular nuclei and cytoplasmic vacuolation) ± architectural atypia (expanded junctional nests) on a background of dermal solar elastosis. Expansion and spindling of junctional nests and any clinically nodular areas should raise a suspicion of invasion. The clinical term lentigo maligna encompasses any degree of proliferation that is confined to the epidermis (i.e. it includes Clark level I or melanoma in situ) while lentigo maligna melanoma implies the presence of dermal invasion (at least Clark level II). In general it has a favourable prognosis if completely excised.

Superficial Spreading Malignant Melanoma

- Radial phase of spread.[1]
  Usually an asymmetrical lateral border of atypical junctional cell nests with a central segment of epidermis showing upward melanocytic spread (single cells/nests/"buck-shot" patterns). Moderate dusty pigmentation ± a dermal component related to the growth phase i.e. lateral growth before vertical invasion. Often intermittently on sun exposed sites of young patients.

---

[1]Radial growth phase includes melanoma in situ (i.e. intraepidermal) ± microinvasion of the papillary dermis. The radial phase may be indolent with no metastatic potential and 95–100 % survival rate. The dermal component is usually <1 mm thick i.e. the lesion is wider than it is deep and can have morphologically bland cell nests (usually <10 cells across) of uniform size and cytological appearance. Mitotic figures are absent. This may be accompanied by signs of regression with a brisk lymphocytic response. The radial phase potentially progresses by clonal expansion to the vertical phase.

Nodular Malignant Melanoma

- Vertical phase of spread.[2]

Often exophytic/nodular/ulcerated and thick ± pigmentation, with ≤2 or 3 rete pegs showing atypical junctional nests at the lateral border of the lesion. This is the most aggressive form of malignant melanoma, seen in older patients and exclusively in vertical growth phase.

Acral/Mucosal/Lentiginous Malignant Melanoma

- Sole of foot, palm of hand, nail bed, mucosal membranes. The most frequent malignant melanoma in heavily pigmented people. Features are often a combination of lentigo maligna and superficial spreading patterns ± a nodular, vertical growth phase component. Prognosis is poor due to delay in diagnosis with increased thickness at presentation.

In general, these main subtypes show prognostic differences and there is correlation with recurrence and metastases e.g. nodular malignant melanoma is often thick (with a significant Breslow depth) and ulcerated. Knowledge of the various clinicopathological subtypes is an important aid in their diagnostic recognition.

Others

- e.g. Desmoplastic, neurotropic, verrucous, balloon cell, signet ring cell, small cell, myxoid, minimal deviation, metastatic malignant melanoma, malignant blue naevi.

---

[2] Vertical growth phase tumour comprises expansive nests, nodules or plaques of cytologically atypical melanoma cells in the dermis; it implies a biological potential for metastatic spread and is the main determinant of prognosis. The cell nests are usually larger than the biggest intraepidermal nest, ≥10–25 cells in dimension, show variation throughout the lesion, mitoses and a variable host dermal lymphocytic response. Vertical growth phase melanomas are often at least Clark level III and thicker than 1 mm with an inconstant relationship between the width and depth of the lesion.

21.3   Differentiation/Cell Type

- Epithelioid.
- Spindle cell.
- Mixed.
- Knowledge of the constituent cell type in the primary lesion is useful for the subsequent diagnostic confirmation of recurrent or metastatic lesions.

21.4   Extent of Local Tumour Spread

Border: pushing/infiltrative.

Lymphocytic reaction: prominent/sparse/absent – an increased number of tumour infiltrating lymphocytes (TILs) has a positive association with survival.

Regression: paradoxically, in thin melanomas >75 % lesion regression (partial or full thickness destruction of melanoma cells, lymphohistiocytic infiltrate, fibrosis, melanophages, vascular ectasia) is an *adverse prognostic factor*. It is a hallmark of where malignant melanoma cells were once sited and its extent should be recorded. It is also regarded by some as an explanation for an *occult cutaneous primary in the presence of widespread metastatic disease*. It is also partly responsible for the unevenness of pigmentation that is such a useful clinical sign.

TMN7 classification: applies to malignant melanoma of skin at all sites including eyelid, vulva, penis, anal margin and scrotum but not those arising in mucous membranes (oral cavity, nasopharynx, vagina, urethra, anal canal), conjunctiva or uvea. Visceral melanomas do not have a separate classification although malignant melanoma of the upper aerodigestive tract is aggressive and is regarded as either moderately advanced (pT3 mucosal) or very advanced (pT4 beyond the mucosa) disease.

Prognosis: the TNM7 classification of malignant melanoma incorporates three main prognostic features: *tumour thickness, anatomical Clark levels* (in pT1 category only) and the *absence or presence of ulceration* (defined as the histological absence of an intact epidermis overlying a major portion of the primary melanoma without recent trauma or a surgical procedure). The American Joint Committee on Cancer has modified stage pT1 to include *mitotic counts* as a *mitotic rate ≥1/mm² is an adverse prognostic indicator*.

Breslow Depth or Thickness (mm)

- Ocular micrometer, Vernier scale or eyepiece graticule measurement of *tumour maximum vertical diameter* to the first decimal point, from the top of the granular layer or ulcerated tumour surface to the deepest point of invasion (Fig. 21.1). Malignant melanoma cells in adjacent pilosebaceous unit epithelium do not count. S100 or melan-A immunostains can help highlight malignant melanoma cells in the dermis that might otherwise be obscured by a heavy lymphocytic infiltrate at the base of the lesion.

Anatomical Clark level

- Increasing levels of invasion are associated with decreased survival although it may simply reflect thickness of the lesion.

I	Intraepithelial/intraepidermal
II	Papillary dermis or periadnexal connective tissue sheath
III	Papillary-reticular interface: papillary dermis filled and expanded down to an interface marked by the position of the superficial vascular plexus and horizontal orientation of the collagen fibres.
IV	Reticular dermis
V	Subcutaneous fat. Where fat is absent e.g. lip, this includes extension into other structures e.g. striated muscle

pTis	Melanoma in situ (Clark level I)/severe melanocytic dysplasia
pT1	Tumour ≤1 mm in thickness
	(a) Clark level II or III, without ulceration
	(b) Clark level IV or V, or, with ulceration
pT2	1 mm < tumour ≤2 mm in thickness
	(a) Without ulceration
	(b) With ulceration

pT3	2 mm < tumour ≤4 mm in thickness
	(a) Without ulceration
	(b) With ulceration
pT4	Tumour >4 mm in thickness
	(a) Without ulceration
	(b) With ulceration

See Fig. 21.2

AJCC modification: pT1a – without ulceration and mitoses <1/mm², pT1b – with ulceration and/or mitoses ≥1/mm². For practical purposes 1 mm² equates to four high power fields (×40 objective) but this does vary according to the field diameter of the microscope. A *mitotic "hot spot"* in the invasive tumour is selected and counts made over contiguous fields.

Tumour related ulceration: (particularly if >3–5 mm or 70 % of the lesion) is an *independent adverse prognostic factor*, with 50 % 10 year survival versus 78 % if non-ulcerated. It can also result in understaging of Breslow thickness although there is a strong correlation between them. It is an index of rapid tumour growth.

Definition: MIN (melanocytic intraepithelial neoplasia)=severe melanocytic atypia (dysplasia) and melanoma in situ (level I) pTis. This nomenclature is not widely used in practice. Levels are examined to exclude any associated microinvasion (single cells, small groups of cells in the papillary dermis).

21.5   Lymphovascular Invasion

Present/absent.

Intra-/extratumoural.

Rarely seen, but perineural or intraneural invasion is commonly present in neurotropic desmoplastic malignant melanomas with a subsequent high recurrence rate necessitating wide primary or secondary excision. Lymphovascular invasion and angiotropism (malignant melanoma cells cuffing small vessels) are adverse prognostic indicators.

21.6   Lymph Nodes

Site/number/size/number involved/limit node/extracapsular spread.

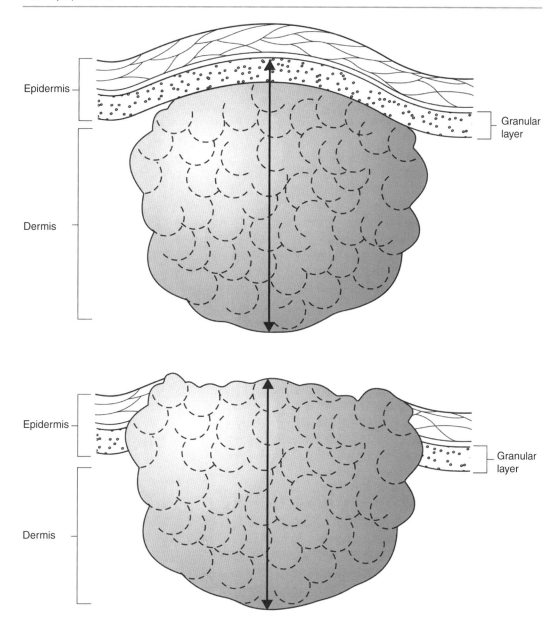

Breslow depth or thickness (mm) = the maximum vertical depth from the top
of the granular layer or ulcerated surface to
the deepest point of invasion

Fig. 21.1   Malignant melanoma (Reproduced, with permission, from Allen (2006), © 2006)

Regional nodes: those appropriate to the site of the primary tumour. A regional lymphadenectomy will ordinarily include a minimum of six lymph nodes. Classification based on sentinel node biopsy alone is designated (sn) e.g. pN0 (sn).

pN0	No regional lymph node metastasis
pN1	Metastasis in one regional lymph node
	(a) Micrometastasis (clinically occult)
	(b) Macrometastasis: detected clinically with confirmation after lymphadenectomy, or, gross extracapsular invasion

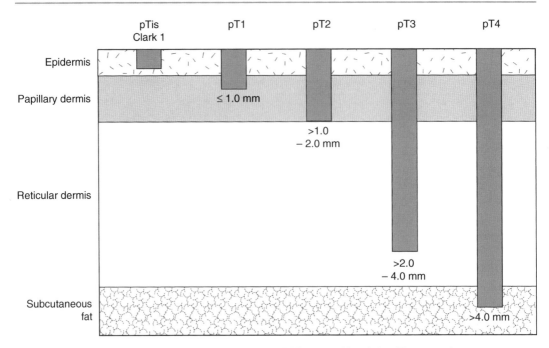

In case of discrepancy between tumour thickness and level, the pT category is based on the less favourable finding

Fig. 21.2 Malignant melanoma (Reproduced, with permission, from Allen (2006), © 2006)

pN2	Metastasis in two to three regional lymph nodes
	(a) Micrometastasis
	(b) Macrometastasis
	(c) In-transit metastases/satellite(s) without metastatic lymph nodes
pN3	Four or more metastatic lymph nodes, or matted lymph nodes, or in-transit metastases/satellite(s) plus metastatic lymph node(s)

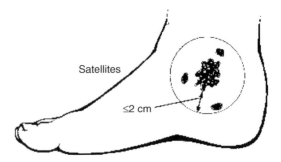

Fig. 21.3 Malignant melanoma (Reproduced, with permission, from Wittekind et al. (2005), © 2005)

Satellites: are tumour nests or nodules (macroscopic or microscopic (>0.05 mm)) within 2 cm of the primary tumour but not contiguous with it (at least 0.3 mm away) and are *prognostically adverse*. Levels are recommended to demonstrate lack of continuity (Fig. 21.3).

In-transit metastases: involve skin or subcutaneous tissue more than 2 cm from the primary tumour but not beyond the regional lymph nodes (Fig. 21.4).

Spread of malignant melanoma: is to regional lymph nodes, skin (satellite nodules and in-transit metastases), liver, lungs, gastrointestinal tract, bone and central nervous system. Distant metastases can be *late (>10–25 years)* representing regrowth of "dormant" seedlings.

pM1a	Skin, subcutaneous tissue or lymph node(s) beyond the regional nodes
pM1b	Lung
pM1c	Other sites, or any site with elevated serum lactic dehydrogenase (LDH)

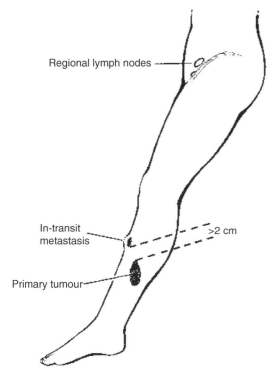

Regional lymph nodes

In-transit metastasis

>2 cm

Primary tumour

Fig. 21.4 Malignant melanoma (Reproduced, with permission, from Wittekind et al. (2005), © 2005)

21.7 Excision Margins

Distances (mm) to the nearest painted deep and peripheral excision margins either of serial transverse slices (toast racked) or quadrant blocks according to local protocols – of the vertical and radial disease phases and any in situ change.

Minimum recommended margins of clearance: these vary according to the tumour depth of invasion

Depth	Minimum margin
0 mm (in situ)	5 mm
<1 mm	10 mm
1–2 mm	10–20 mm
>2 mm	20–30 mm.

Adequate treatment is based on successful *complete primary excision* or, if there is initial margin involvement, *secondary re-excision* to avoid any possibility of locally persistent malignant melanoma or scar related local metastasis. This is supplemented by *regional lymph node dissection* and *systemic therapy* for metastatic disease. *Sentinel lymph node biopsy* may be used in patients with clinically negative regional lymph nodes and a vertical growth phase malignant melanoma ≥1 mm thick. It involves 2 mm serial transverse slices of the lymph node with preparation of multiple haematoxylin and eosin (H&E) and matching immunohistochemical stains for S-100 and HMB-45. Differential diagnoses include sinus histiocytes, capsular naevus cell nests and benign ductal epithelial inclusions. If positive a regional lymphadenectomy is carried out.

21.8 Other Pathology

- *Pigmentation*: none/light/moderate/heavy. Often patchy in distribution due to regression or clonal growth of pigmented melanocytic cells. Amelanotic malignant melanoma is more frequent in the face and head and neck areas.
- *Mitoses*: number/10 high-power fields (×40 objective), or <1 or ≥1/mm^2.
- *Ulceration*: present/absent and extent (mm/% of the lesion).
- *Elastosis*: present/absent.
- *Regression*: present/absent – inflammation/ fibrosis/telangiectasia/melanophages.
- *Pre-existing lesion*: present/absent and less common than de-novo malignant melanoma (60–70 % of cases) although this proportion may shift as screening yields more early lesions.
- *Satellite lesions*: present/absent; distance (mm) from the primary.

Primary versus secondary/recurrence: secondary tumour tends to be nodular and dermal/ subcutaneous ± vascular invasion with no epidermal component. Occasionally secondary melanoma may show epidermal changes but usually the dermal disease is more extensive in width. Some malignant melanomas can develop multiple locoregional cutaneous recurrences over many years and do not develop lymph node or distant metastatic disease, although such satellite nodule and in-transit metastases are an indicator of potential systemic dissemination. They are regarded as tumour emboli arrested in lymphatics which then grow to form a tumour mass. They are seen in about 5 % of malignant melanomas >1 mm thick. They are surgically excised.

Dysplastic naevus: variable reports of sporadic and familial predisposition to malignant melanoma. Strict criteria (clinical and pathological) must be adhered to (see below) as there is a range of *benign naevi with active junctional components that can mimic dysplastic naevus or malignant melanoma* (*pseudomelanoma*). These include: junctional/Pagetoid Spitz naevus, pigmented spindle cell naevus of Reed, halo naevus, traumatised and partially excised or recurrent naevi, irradiated naevus, mitotically active, desmoplastic, clonal and deep penetrating naevi, cellular blue naevus, acral and genital naevi. Age, anatomical site, lesion type and clinical history e.g. a previous malignant melanoma or change (pigment/profile/margin) in a naevus must all be considered along with the morphology.

- Single or multiple (dysplastic naevus syndrome).
- ≥4 mm with variable pigmentation and irregular borders.
- Nested and lentiginous melanocytic proliferation.
- Architectural and cytological atypia.
- Elongation/lateral fusion of rete pegs.
- Dermal lamellar fibroplasia with vascularisation and chronic inflammation in the dermis.

Morphological clues to a diagnosis of malignant melanoma: lesion *asymmetry*, *extension of atypical melanocytes* up into the epidermis and lateral to the lesion, *melanocytic atypia* and *lack of dermal maturation* (diminution in cell size with dermal depth), *deeply placed mitoses* (deeper than the superficial dermis), and a *dermal lymphocytic infiltrate*. Melanocytic cell nests also vary in size, shape and cytological atypia within a lesion.

Mimics: there are also a number of *pigmented non-melanocytic tumours* that can mimic melanocytic neoplasms clinically and histologically and that need to be considered in the differential diagnosis. These can be

Epithelial: seborrhoeic keratosis, melanoacanthoma, basal cell carcinoma, skin appendage tumours, Bowen's and Paget's disease, melanotic non-cutaneous carcinomas (e.g. renal, anorectum).

Mesenchymal: dermatofibroma, atypical fibroxanthoma, dermatofibrosarcoma protuberans, angiosarcoma.

Neural: neurilemmoma, neurofibroma, neurothekoma, and,

Neuroendocrine: Merkel cell carcinoma, medullary carcinoma thyroid.

Immunophenotype

- Useful in the distinction between *maligant melanoma* and *non-melanocytic tumours* but not reliable for separating benign and malignant melanocytic lesions. In general there are no immunohistochemical or molecular biomarkers with sufficient sensitivity or specificity to clearly separate diagnostically ambiguous melanocytic lesions into benign and malignant categories. Note also that some malignant melanomas are cytokeratin (CAM5.2), CEA and EMA positive.
- S100 protein, HMB-45 and melan-A. Used in combination as other tumours can show positivity for these individual markers.
- Masson Fontana for pigment.
- Ki-67 proliferation index and p53: increased (>5 %) in malignant melanocytic lesions. Ki-67 index is regarded as a more accurate prognostic indicator in established malignant melanoma than mitotic count.

Prognosis

Prognosis: of malignant melanoma is unpredictable but relates strongly to the *vertical component or thickness/depth of invasion* and *adequacy of excision* with the width of margins tailored accordingly. Estimated overall 5 year survival rates are about 60 % but *tumour stage/thickness* is the most powerful prognostic determinant:

Stage I	Up to 1 mm thick with ulceration, or 2 mm without	85–99 % survival
Stage II	>1–2 mm thick with ulceration, or >2 mm thick	40–85 % survival
Stage III	Any thickness with involvement or regional lymph node(s) or adjacent skin	25–60 % survival
Stage IV	Distant metastasis	9–15 % survival

Recurrence rates: vary from 15–70 % for stage II malignant melanomas, and more than 50 % for stage III disease.

Other adverse indicators: patient age (>50 years), sex (male), histological regression, histological type (nodular), vascular invasion, tumour phase (vertical), satellitosis, necrosis, ulceration, mitotic activity and anatomical site (hands, sole of foot, head, neck, trunk and back are worse). One study found that a prognostic index of tumour thickness multiplied by the number of mitoses/mm^2 was the most accurate method of predicting patients who would remain disease free. Occasionally malignant melanoma may *present as metastatic disease* e.g. axillary nodes due to complete regression of a cutaneous lesion leaving no obvious primary tumour on examination. Other possible occult sources are the eye and mucosal surfaces of the upper aerodigestive tract (including oesophagus), vagina and anal canal. These mucosal, acral lentiginous and subungal malignant melanomas have poor prognosis due to late presentation. This is recognized in the upper aerodigestive tract by TNM7 regarding them as either moderately (pT3: mucosal) or very advanced (pT4: beyond the mucosa) disease. In general, factors such as age, pregnancy, lesion diameter, histological type and inflammatory infiltrate are outweighed by *tumour thickness* and *stage*. However, even in thick (>5 mm) melanomas there is a subset of patients who may survive 10 years or more. Their tumours tend to be of spindle cell or Spitz like cell type with a lack of mitoses and vascular invasion. Conversely occasional thin melanomas can metastasise. Select patients with metastatic disease are treated with *chemotherapy* and *immunotherapy*. The presence of *tumour cell BRAF mutation* (60 % of cases) is predictive of response to vemurafinib targeted therapy.

Balloon cell malignant melanoma tends to develop multiple cutaneous and subcutaneous metastases. The inter-related desmoplastic (myofibroblastic differentiation) and neurotropic (Schwann cell differentiation) variants arise mostly on the head and neck of elderly patients (particularly the lip) and show a high incidence of local recurrence, and potentially metastases. Diagnosis requires an index of suspicion to distinguish from a dermal scar, recognition of tumour infiltrate in the deep dermis and accompanying clues in the form of an epidermal component. Immunohistochemistry (S100) is important in confirmation although it may be negative (HMB-45/melan A). Perineural invasion (30 % of cases) is a feature.

Bibliography

Allen DC. Histopathology reporting: guidelines for surgical cancer. 2nd ed. Springer: London; 2006.

Balch CM, Gershenwald JE, Soong SJ, Thompson JF, Atkins MB, Byrd DR, Buzaid AC, Cochran AJ, Coit DG, Ding S, Eggermont AM, Flaherty KT, Gimotty PS, Kirkwood JM, McMasters KM, Mihn MF, Morton DL, Ross MI, Sober AJ, Sandak VK. Final version of 2009 AJCC melanoma staging and classification. J Clin Oncol. 2009;27:6199–202.

Banerjee SS, Harris M. Morphological and immunophenotypic variations in malignant melanoma. Histopathology. 2000;36:387–402.

Bhawan J. Non-melanocytic mimics of melanocytic neoplasms. Histopathology. 2012;60:715–30.

Brenn T. Pitfalls in the evaluation of melanocytic lesions. Histopathology. 2012;60:690–705.

Calonje JE, Brenn T, Lazar AJ, McKee PH. McKee's pathology of the skin with clinical correlations. 4th ed. Philadelphia: Elsevier/Saunders; 2012.

Cook MG, Di Palma S. Pathology of sentinel lymph nodes for melanoma. J Clin Pathol. 2008;61:897–902.

Culpepper KS, Granter SR, McKee PH. My approach to atypical melanocytic lesions. J Clin Pathol. 2004;57:1121–31.

DeWit NJW, Van Muijen GNP, Ruiter DJ. Immunohistochemistry in melanocytic proliferative lesions. Histopathology. 2004;44:517–41.

Elder DE, Murphy GF. Melanocytic tumors of the skin. Atlas of tumor pathology. 3rd series. Fascicle 2. Washington: AFIP; 1991.

Kirkham N. The differential diagnosis of thin malignant melanoma. Curr Diagn Pathol. 2003;9:281–6.

Marsden JR, Newton-Bishop JA, Burrows L, Cook M, Corrie PG, Cox NH, Gore ME, Lorigan P, MacKie R, Nathan P, Peach H, Powell B, Walker C. Revised UK guidelines for the management of malignant melanoma. Br J Dermatol. 2010;163:238–56.

Moore DA, Pringle JH, Saldanha GS. Prognostic tissue markers in melanoma. Histopathology. 2012;60:679–89.

Shriner DL, McCoy DK, Goldberg DJ, Wagner Jr RF. Mohs' micrographic surgery. J Am Acad Dermatol. 1998;39(1):79–97.

The Royal College of Pathologists. Cancer Datasets (Basal cell carcinoma, Malignant Melanoma, Squamous Cell Carcinoma, Primary Cutaneous Adnexal Carcinomas) and Tissue Pathways (Inflammatory and Non-neoplastic Dermatoses and Non-neoplastic Lesions). Accessed at http://www.rcpath.org/index.asp?PageID=254.

Weedon D. Skin pathology. 3rd ed. London: Churchill Livingstone; 2009.

Weedon D, LeBoit P, Burg G, Sarasin A, editors. World Health Organisation classification of tumours. Pathology and genetics. Tumours of the skin. Lyon: IARC Press; 2005.

Wittekind C, International Union against Cancer, et al. TNM atlas: illustrated guide to the TNM/pTNM classification of malignant tumours. 4th ed. Berlin: Springer; 2005.

Part V

Breast Cancer

- Breast Carcinoma

Breast Carcinoma

22

Breast cancer accounts for 25 % of all cancers in females. It is associated with Western lifestyle and other risk factors include early menarche, late first childbirth, and a marked genetic susceptibility particularly a strong family history or positivity for BRCA1/BRCA2 genes. Involvement of regional lymph nodes is the strongest prognostic indicator of locoregional and systemic disease relapse, and, overall survival. Lymph node status along with determination of predictive markers such as oestrogen receptor (ER) and Her-2 status are instrumental in selection of hormonal or systemic chemotherapy for patients with localised, recurrent or advanced disease. High risk breast cancers include ER negative, Her-2 positive, basal and apocrine type lesions. Recent research has proposed that breast cancer may be subclassified into as many as ten different genetic types that can more accurately predict response to treatment and survival. The genetic profiles stratified ER positive cancers according to survival, and identified Her-2 positive and triple marker negative (ER/PR (progesterone)/Her-2 receptor) cases.

Bilateral cancer occurs in younger women and is more often lobular in type. There is also a definite familial risk for development of breast cancer, some 20 % of which can be attributed to BRCA1 and BRCA2 gene abnormalities with associated ovarian, uterine, pancreatic and colon cancers.

Male breast carcinoma (1 % of cases) occurs in older men, presents late and has a poor prognosis. It shows the same range of morphological characteristics as female breast cancer.

Symptomatic breast cancer usually presents with a palpable lump, skin tethering, or nipple rash (Paget's disease), retraction or discharge (due to an intraductal epithelial proliferation). Asymptomatic in situ or invasive lesions are detected at two- view mammography (80–90 % sensitivity) as either linear branching microcalcifications, a discrete mass or an area of stromal distortion and spiculate density. Mammographic screening is at 3 yearly intervals for patients aged 50–70 years in the United Kingdom. It detects a higher yield of smaller invasive cancers and "earlier" lesions with a greater proportion of in situ carcinoma than in the symptomatic population.

Diagnosis of breast disease is based on the triple approach viz clinical examination, mammography (± ultrasound), and radiologically guided or free hand fine needle aspiration cytology (FNAC) and/or needle core biopsy. This has superseded frozen section examination of suspected breast cancers allowing a one stop diagnosis, counselling of the patient and progression to a one stage therapeutic procedure. It involves complete local excision of the primary tumour and an axillary lymph node procedure. This is either sentinel lymph node excision biopsy or sampling for a clinically node negative axilla, or clearance lymphadenectomy for a clinically or FNAC proven node positive axilla. In a small minority of cases the non-operative diagnosis is inconclusive and open biopsy is required e.g. radial scar or papillary lesions. Screening detected impalpable lesions and areas of microcalcification require radiological guide wire localisation to ensure adequate excision. MRI scan is only indicated where there is discrepancy between clinical and imaging disease extent, or breast density, particularly in the younger patient, precludes accurate mammographic assessment. It may have a role to play in mapping the extent of ductal carcinoma in situ (DCIS) that is present or to detect satellite lesions in infiltrating lobular carcinoma. Full clinical staging (CT/PET scans, radioisotope bone scan) can be undertaken when there is significant lymph node disease (N2:$\geq$4 nodes involved), or for other indicators such as bone pain or altered liver function tests.

Localisation biopsies should be accompanied by a post-operative specimen x-ray, and, have attached orientation sutures/clips in place according to a pre-agreed protocol. There may also be an in situ guide wire(s). Breast conserving surgery by wide local excision removes the tumour with a 1 cm rim of normal tissue or a more extensive cylindrical (superficial to deep) excision (segmentectomy/quadrantectomy). Partial mastectomy involves removal of the tumour and surrounding breast with an overlying ellipse of non-nipple bearing skin. Again, orientation sutures are attached allowing differential painting of surgical margins. Mastectomy removes the breast tissue and overlying skin including the nipple with the chest wall left intact. A subcutaneous mastectomy leaves the skin intact for reconstructive procedures but removes the breast tissue and nipple-areolar-complex (NAC). The axillary fat and contents may be submitted in continuity, or, separately as either a sentinel node(s), axillary sampling, or a multipart clearance procedure. Sentinel lymph nodes (1–2 in number) are demonstrated in-vivo by injection of a vital blue dye and/or radiocolloid around the area of the tumour prior to surgery. A small axillary incision with both direct visual inspection and use of a gamma probe allows identification of stained lymphatics leading to a "hot blue" sentinel lymph node(s). The excised lymph node is serially sliced transverse to its long axis at 2 mm intervals and all processed for histology, supplemented by

levels of the paraffin block and cytokeratin immunohistochemistry where indicated. Some centres also use intraoperative imprint cytology or frozen section to allow definitive treatment at the one procedure. Needle core biopsies are usually 19 gauge providing three or four thin cores of tissue measuring up to 1.5–2 cm long. Gentle painting with alcian blue allows visualization at the paraffin block cutting stage. One representative section is usually sufficient for lesions other than radiological calcifications. The latter often require examination of multiple histological levels until any represented mammographic abnormality is detected. Specimen x-ray is used to check for the presence of calcifications to ensure that there has been sampling of the mammographically abnormal area. They are usually seen histologically in about 80 % of cases and about 50 % are due to in situ or invasive disease, the rest being associated with benign changes in the breast parenchyma.

22.1 Gross Description

Specimen

- FNAC/needle core biopsy/localisation biopsy/ open biopsy/segmental excision/quadrantectomy/partial mastectomy/mastectomy. Optimal fixation is important in assessing tumour type, grade, lymphovascular invasion and hormone receptor expression. This can be facilitated by receiving the specimen fresh and making an initial cut for fixation purposes.
- Axillary lymph nodes: sentinel biopsy/sampling/clearance.
- Size (cm) and weight (g).

Tumour

Site
- Right/left/bilateral.
- Quadrant: 50 % upper outer (UOQ), 15 % upper inner (UIQ), 10 % lower outer (LOQ), 17 % central, 3 % diffuse (massive or multifocal). Breast cancer occurs either as a localised

lesion, or multiple invasive foci not connected by DCIS and clearly separated by normal breast tissue. The latter may arise from multifocal field change within a number of abnormal ductulolobular units or as a result of seeding from involved lymphovascular channels. *Multifocality* is a quadrant based discontinous tumour growth usually arising simultaneously within different lobular units. *Multicentricity* is the presence of carcinoma in a breast quadrant other than the one containing the dominant mass. Some estimates of multicentricity are up to 13 % of cases and more frequently seen in lobular carcinoma than ductal. A general rule of thumb for *multicentricity and bilaterality is 10–15%*. Some 5–10 % of cases have synchronous or subsequent (metachronous) tumours.

- Distances (cm) from the nipple and resection limits.

Size

- Maximum dimension of invasive lesion (cm).
- Maximum dimension of whole tumour (invasive + DCIS) (cm).
- Microscopic measurement updates and takes precedence over gross measurement. This is particularly so for small and poorly defined cancers e.g. infiltrating lobular, the latter sometimes requiring specimen mapping and blocking to determine its extent.
- In multifocal or multicentric carcinoma the largest tumour is used to designate the pT category (Fig. 22.1).
- Tumour size in a biopsy with positive margins is added to any residue in the mastectomy specimen to determine the pT category.
- Tumour regression due to neoadjuvant therapy may necessitate size determination by prior findings on clinical examination and imaging.

Appearance

- Scirrhous/fleshy/mucoid/cystic/diffuse thickening.

Ductal carcinoma tends to form a discrete mass lesion whereas lobular carcinoma can be difficult to define clinically, radiologically, cytologically and at the laboratory dissection bench.

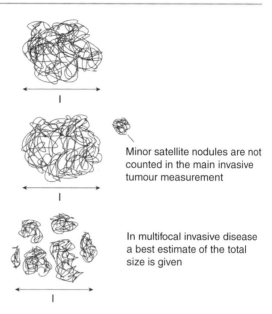

Minor satellite nodules are not counted in the main invasive tumour measurement

In multifocal invasive disease a best estimate of the total size is given

Fig. 22.1 Breast carcinoma: invasive tumors measurements (Reproduced, with permission, from Allen (2006), © 2006)

This has obvious implications for completeness of excision in patients treated with breast conserving surgery and the pathological assessment of the surgical margins. If the core biopsy types the breast cancer as infiltrating lobular, breast MRI scan may be performed to detect any satellite lesions that could preclude opting for conservative surgery.

Edge

- Circumscribed/irregular. Mucinous and medullary carcinomas often have circumscribed pushing margins.

22.2 Histological Type

In Situ Carcinoma

Ductal Carcinoma in Situ (DCIS)

- Bound by basement membrane involving ≥ 2 ducts or $\geq 2–3$ mm diameter. Epithelial proliferation of lesser extent is designated *atypical ductal hyperplasia* (*ADH*) unless of high cytological grade or with comedonecrosis (Fig. 22.2).

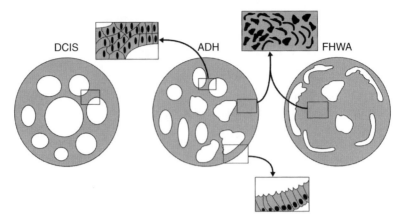

Fig. 22.2 Ductal carcinoma in-situ (*DCIS*) versus atypical ductal hyperplasia (*ADH*) versus florid hyperplasia without atypia (*FHWA*): cytology and histology. DCIS features smooth, punched-out luminal borders within involved basementmembrane-bound space. The cytological features are regular and present throughout the entire population of at least two basement-membrane-bound spaces. FHWA is the most densely cellular and extensive of the proliferative disease without atypia lesions, also called "papillomatosis". There are ragged, often slit-like luminal borders. The nuclei throughout the involved area show variablity and tendency to a swirling pattern, as illustrated. ADH has features predominantly of non-comedo, cribriform DCIS, but also some features of proliferative disease without atypia or normally polarized cells within the same basement-membrane-bound space (Page and Rogers (1992), ©1992. Reproduced, with permission, from Elsevier)

- *Nuclear grade*: low, intermediate, high.
  - Low is monomorphic evenly spaced cells with small central nuclei, few mitoses and necrosis is rare.
  - High is pleomorphic irregularly spaced cells with large irregular nuclei, coarse chromatin, ≥ 1 nucleolus, mitoses and often necrosis. There is loss of cell polarisation.
- Necrosis: comedo or punctate. Comedo = central eosinophilic necrosis containing five or more pyknotic nuclei.
- Cell polarisation: present or absent.
- *Architectural patterns*:
Comedo
Solid
Cribriform
Papillary
Micropapillary.

Rarer forms include encysted papillary, clinging, signet ring cell, apocrine (rare: needs atypia/necrosis/mitoses), clear cell, cystic hypersecretory and neuroendocrine variants.

Lobular Carcinoma in Situ (LCIS)

- Uniform cells populating the lobule.
- No lumen in the acini.

- $\geq 50~\%$ of the acini in the lobule are expanded and filled (Fig. 22.3).
- ± Pagetoid spread into ducts.
- Potentially multifocal (70 %) and bilateral (30–40 %).
- Epithelial proliferation of lesser extent (e.g. with preservation of lumina) is designated *atypical lobular hyperplasia (ALH)*.

The morphological spectrum of *LN* (*Lobular Neoplasia*) comprising ALH and LCIS can be encountered in a needle core biopsy, but is often not diagnosed preoperatively and is seen as an incidental finding in excision specimens. It is a *marker for an increased risk of malignancy* (greater for LCIS) and has a peak incidence between the ages of 40–50 years, some 10 years younger than that of DCIS. If a concurrent carcinoma is not present current recommendations are long term follow up with or without tamoxifen treatment.

Distinction between DCIS and LCIS is not always easy e.g. lobular cancerisation by low-grade DCIS and, rarely, mixed lesions occur. Loss of E-cadherin expression favours a lobular proliferation which comprises a uniform population of dyscohesive cells associated with intracytoplasmic lumina.

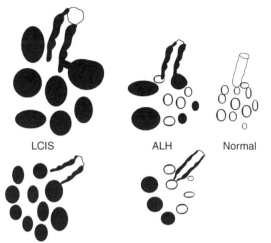

Fig. 22.3 Schematic demonstration of diagnostic criteria for lobular carcinoma in-situ (*LCIS*). There is distention and distortion of more than half the acini, and an absence of central lumina. When these changes are less well developed (i.e. <50 % of acini involved) atypical lobular hyperplasia (*ALH*) is diagnosed. Note that the pagetoid spread into adjacent ducts is more common in LCIS, but may be seen in ALH (Page et al. (1991), © 1991, reproduced, with permission, from Elsevier)

Microinvasion

- ≤1 mm from the adjacent basement membrane with infiltration of non-specialised interlobular/interductal stroma.
- The presence of multiple foci of microinvasion should be noted, but, it is classified according to the largest focus and not the sum total of them.

Minimal Invasive Cancer

- Variably defined as <0.5 or <1 cm maximum dimension and not a term in common clinical use.

Invasive Carcinoma

Regarded as either *low-grade* or *high-grade* invasive breast cancers based on their morphological, genetic, immunophenotype and ER profiles. *Low-grade disease* includes tubular, tubulolobular, cribriform, mucinous, papillary, classical infiltrating lobular and grade 1/2 invasive ductal carcinomas. *High-grade disease* includes grade 3 invasive ductal, basal type, apocrine type, metaplastic, and pleomorphic infiltrating lobular cancers.

Ductal

- No special type (NST): *70–75 % of breast cancer.*

Lobular

- *15 % of breast cancer.*
- *Classical*: 40 %; single files of small cells in a targetoid periductal pattern, and with AB-PAS positive intracytoplasmic lumina.
- *Alveolar*: a nested pattern of 20 or more cells.
- *Solid*: sheets of tumour cells.
- *Trabecular*: bands of cells two to four across.
- *Signet ring cell.*
- *Pleomorphic*: classical pattern but with cytological atypia and *aggressive* clinical behaviour. Regarded by some as having mixed lobular and ductal characteristics.
- *Mixed*: 40 %; more than one component of these types but each is <80 % of the tumour area.
- *Tubulolobular*: classical pattern with focal microtubules which are less distinct than in tubular carcinoma.

Special Types

- *Tubular*: round, ovoid, angular tubules with a single cell layer, cytoplasmic apical snouts and a fibrous/desmoplastic stroma.
- *Cribriform*: invasive cords and islands with the morphology of cribriform DCIS comprising punched out lumina and cytoplasmic apical snouts.
- *Colloid (mucinous)*: pushing margins, extracellular mucin with small clusters (10–100 cells) of uniform epithelial cells.
- *Papillary*: solid or encysted (intracystic). There is absence of a peripheral myoepithelial layer and increased expression of invasion

associated biomarkers (e.g. matrix metallo-proteinases). Because of this, papillary carcinoma is generally regarded as a *low-grade invasive encapsulated carcinoma* with an expansile growth pattern and indolent behaviour, rather than an in situ carcinoma. Invasion is either (a) a solid, dominantly invasive carcinoma with a pushing margin and papillary pattern, or (b) an encysted papillary carcinoma with focal invasion (the invasive component can be papillary or ductal, NST). Note also and distinguish from *invasive micropapillary carcinoma* (micropapillae without cores set in clear spaces – the "inside-out" tumour with an external rim of apical cytoplasm), which correlates with *lymphovascular* and *axillary node metastases*. This pattern can also can be seen as a component of 5 % of ductal, NST tumours.

- *Medullary, classical*: with a sharply circumscribed margin, >75 % is a patternless tumour cell syncytium with grade 3 cytology. There is a prominent peri-/intratumoural stromal lymphoplasmacytic infiltrate and an absence of glands and scant fibrous stroma.
- *Medullary, atypical*: contains up to 25 % ductal, NST, or an irregular margin with focal infiltration, or adjacent DCIS. Probably better regarded as invasive ductal, NST, with medullary features. The term medullary like carcinoma has been suggested to encompass both classical and atypical medullary cancers, particularly as the observer reproducibility rates are so low.

Mixed Types

- *10% of breast cancers.*
- *Mixed differentiation ductal and lobular.*
- *Tubular mixed*: stellate mass, central tubules with peripheral less differentiated adenocarcinoma.

Others

- *Metaplastic*: biphasic epithelial (ductal in situ/invasive NST grade 2/3, or, squamous cell) and sarcomatous elements (carcinosarcoma), or pure monophasic spindle cell carcinoma (cytokeratin/EMA/p63 positive). The sarcomatous element is either fibrosarcomatous/malignant fibrous histiocytoma like or chondro-, osteo-, leiomyo-, rhabdomyo- or liposarcomatous. Represents carcinoma with a spectrum of malignant spindle cell stroma which can be homologous or heterologous in character. *It behaves as a high-grade carcinoma*. The epithelial component may be minor and require multiple blocks to demonstrate. Metaplastic carcinoma often presents at a *more advanced stage* than high risk ("triple marker negative") infiltrating duct cancer, with a tendency for *recurrence* and *decreased survival*. This relates particularly to lymph node status and the presence of a squamous cell component. Metastases can comprise either the squamous cell or spindle cell elements.

- *Pleomorphic carcinoma*: high-grade ductal cancer with background spindle cells and >50 % bizarre giant cells (cytokeratin positive). Presents with advanced disease.
- *Carcinoma with osteoclast giant cells (CD68 positive).*
- *Signet ring cell carcinoma*: gastric carcinoma analogue.
- *Small cell*: rare, a poorly differentiated/high-grade neuroendocrine carcinoma, aggressive, chromogranin ±/synaptophysin/CD56/Ki-67 positive.
- *Other neuroendocrine*: invasive ductal carcinoma with neuroendocrine differentiation (variable nests, spindle cells or large cells), or, low-grade/well differentiated neuroendocrine (carcinoid) tumour. Note that metastatic neuroendocrine carcinoma from lung (TTF-1 positive) or gastrointestinal tract (CDX-2 positive) can mimic both in situ and invasive primary mammary carcinoma.
- *Secretory*: one-third are in children, indolent, and of good prognosis. Two-thirds are in adults and more aggressive. Shows tubular/solid/honeycomb patterns and PAS/AB-diastase positive luminal secretions.
- *Squamous cell*: primary, or secondary from breast skin, or metastatic e.g. lung. Also

distinguish from metaplastic breast carcinoma which often has an identifiable component of usual in situ or invasive breast cancer.

- *Clear cell*: glycogen rich and worse prognosis.
- *Mucoepidermoid*: grade determines the prognosis with cystic/mucin secreting better than solid/epidermoid variants.
- *Adenoid cystic*: indolent with late recurrence. As for mucoepidermoid carcinoma it is a salivary gland tumour analogue.
- *Apocrine*: rare, cytoplasmic apical snouts, GCDFP-15 positive. Aggressive.
- *Adenomyoepithelioma*: in the elderly, of low malignant potential and characterised by sheaths of proliferating clear myoepithelial cells around epithelial lined spaces. Occasionally malignant myoepithelioma (spindle cells with mitoses).

Pure Carcinoma

- ≥90 % of the tumour volume.

Mixed Carcinoma

- 50–90 % of the tumour comprises a special type component.

Metastatic Carcinoma

- Often solitary and in the UOQ at a late stage in known carcinomatosis. The majority of childhood breast malignancy is metastatic e.g. alveolar rhabdomyosarcoma. In adults, it is usually lung (small cell carcinoma), malignant melanoma, malignant lymphoma/leukaemia, but also ovary, contralateral breast (usually this represents a metachronous primary), gastrointestinal tract, kidney, thyroid carcinomas and small intestinal carcinoid tumour. *A relevant clinical history, absence of in situ change and multiple intravascular deposits are pointers to metastases.* Specific combinations of antibodies e.g. CK7/

TTF-1/napsin-A (lung adenocarcinoma), paranuclear dot CAM 5.2/synaptophysin/CD56 (small cell carcinoma), S100/HMB-45/melan-A (malignant melanoma), CD45/CD20/CD3/CD68/myeloperoxidase (malignant lymphoma/myeloid leukaemia), CA125/CK7/WT-1 (ovary), CK20/CDX-2 (colorectal), RCC ab/EMA/CD10/vimentin (kidney), thyroglobulin/TTF-1 (thyroid) and markers of breast profile (e.g. ER/PR, cytokeratin 7, CEA, GCDFP-15) may be helpful in distinguishing between primary breast from non-mammary disease. *Metastatic tumour should be considered in any breast lesion with unusual clinical, radiological, gross or histological features.*

22.3   Differentiation/Grade

Well/moderate/poor, or, Grade 1/2/3.

See protocol: Grading of Invasive Breast Carcinoma.

22.4   Extent of Local Tumour Spread

Border: pushing/infiltrative.

Lymphocytic reaction: prominent/sparse.

Quadrant(s):

- Paget's disease.
- Skin involvement (direct extension or lymphatics).

pT is based on the maximum dimension of invasive cancer and not whole size measurements that include adjacent DCIS.

The TNM7 classification applies to carcinoma of the female and male breast

pTis	Carcinoma in situ: DCIS, LCIS or Paget's with no tumour
pT1	Tumour ≤2 cm
T1 mic	≤0.1 cm
T1 a	0.1 cm < tumour ≤0.5 cm
T1 b	0.5 cm < tumour ≤1 cm
T1 c	1 cm < tumour ≤2 cm
pT2	2 cm < tumour ≤5 cm
pT3	Tumour >5 cm

pT4   Tumour any size with direct extension to
       chest wall (ribs, intercostal muscles,
       serratus anterior but not pectoral muscle)
       or skin[a]
         (a) Chest wall
         (b) Oedema including peau d'orange,
             skin ulceration or satellite nodules[b]
             in the same breast
         (c) (a) and (b)
         (d) Inflammatory carcinoma: clinically
             sore and red due to tumour
             involvement of dermal lymphatics
             and often without an underlying
             palpable mass. It can be difficult to
             obtain tissue proof on FNAC or
             needle core biopsy. The malignant
             cells are usually ductal, NST,
             grade 3

[a]Clinical or grossly apparent skin satellite nodules, not
just histological foci
[b]Clinically apparent=detected by clinical examination or
by imaging studies (excluding lymphoscintigraphy) or
grossly visible pathologically.
(See Figs 22.4, 22.5, 22.6, 22.7, 22.8, 22.9, 22.10 and
22.11)

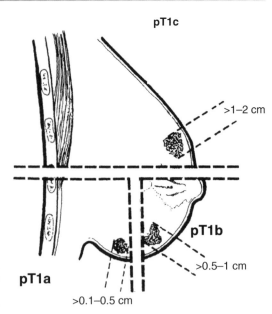

Fig. 22.5 Breast carcinoma (Reproduced, with permission, from Wittekind et al. (2005), © 2005)

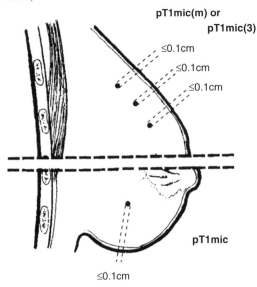

Fig. 22.4 Breast carcinoma (Reproduced, with permission, from Wittekind et al. (2005), © 2005)

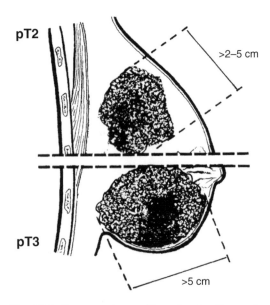

Fig. 22.6 Breast carcinoma (Reproduced, with permission, from Wittekind et al. (2005), © 2005)

In Situ Change

- Present/absent.
- Intra-/extratumoural: >1 mm outside the main tumour mass and its extent.
- Pure DCIS of limited size (<4 cm) tends to be

unicentric, albeit ramifying through the involved duct system. It is treated by breast conserving surgery, either *microdochectomy* or *wide local excision* depending on its site and extent, and *adjuvant radiotherapy*. If >4 cm axillary sentinel lymph node biopsy may be carried out to exclude the small incidence of occult invasive disease that occurs. If it is mammographically extensive *mastectomy* is done. If it forms more than 25 % of an invasive cancer and is present away from it in a local excision specimen it constitutes an extensive intraductal component (EIC). This is an indication for considering proceeding to mastectomy and/or *radiotherapy*. DCIS is also assessed for ER status (>80 % are positive) as a guide to potential *hormonal treatment* response e.g. tamoxifen, aromatase inhibitors. Note that ER negative high-grade DCIS is not hormone responsive and has a higher recurrence rate.

- *Architectural pattern*: solid/cribriform/(micro-) papillary/comedo.
- *Cytonuclear grade*: shows less heterogeneity and higher inter-observer agreement than architectural pattern. It is now the favoured method for grading DCIS using either nuclear features alone (NHS Breast Screening Programme) or combined with the presence of comedonecrosis (Van Nuys classification). *High-grade correlates with a greater frequency of recurrence, concurrent or subsequent invasive carcinoma.* Other significant risk factors include: an involved or close (<1 mm) margin after local excision, younger age (< 40 years), symptomatic presentation, and ER negativity.

Not infrequently there is correlation between DCIS architectural pattern and cytonuclear grade e.g. comedonecrosis is high-grade and cribriform low-grade. However, this is not always the case e.g. solid or micropapillary although usually low- to intermediate-grade can be high-grade.

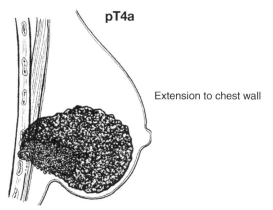

pT4a

Extension to chest wall

Fig. 22.7 Breast carcinoma (Reproduced, with permission, from Wittekind et al. (2005), © 2005)

22.5 Lymphovascular Invasion

Present/absent.

Intra-/extratumoural: >1 mm outside the main tumour mass.

The commonest site for vascular invasion is at the tumour edge and it is present in about

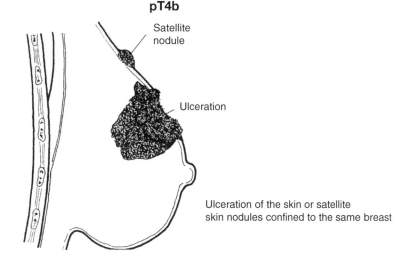

pT4b

Satellite nodule

Ulceration

Ulceration of the skin or satellite skin nodules confined to the same breast

Fig. 22.8 Breast carcinoma (Reproduced, with permission, from Wittekind et al. (2005), © 2005)

pT4b

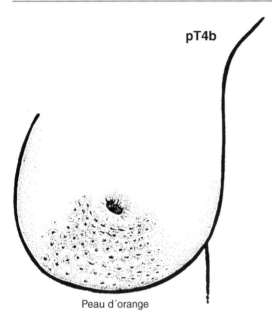

Peau d´orange

Fig. 22.9 Breast carcinoma (Reproduced, with permission, from Wittekind et al. (2005), © 2005)

pT4c

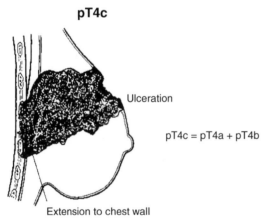

Ulceration

pT4c = pT4a + pT4b

Extension to chest wall

Fig. 22.10 Breast carcinoma (Reproduced, with permission, from Wittekind et al. (2005), © 2005)

25–35 % of cases. Its presence can *double the risk of local recurrence.*

22.6 Lymph Nodes

Site/number/size/number involved/apical node/extracapsular spread.

Regional nodes: axillary (levels I, II, III and intramammary), ipsilateral infraclavicular[2], internal mammary[3] and supraclavicular[4]. Any other

pT4d

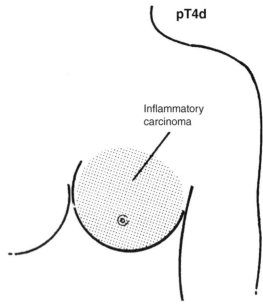

Inflammatory carcinoma

Fig. 22.11 Breast carcinoma (Reproduced, with permission, from Wittekind et al. (2005), © 2005)

lymph node metastasis is regarded as a distant metastasis pM1, including cervical or contralateral internal mammary. A regional lymphadenectomy will ordinarily include a minimum of six lymph nodes (level I) and in practice more often between 15 and 30 (levels I, II and III).

Axillary Lymph Nodes

They receive ≥75 % of the lymphatic flow.

Level I	Low axilla. Lymph nodes lateral to the border of pectoralis minor muscle
Level II	Mid-axilla. Lymph nodes between the medial and lateral borders of the pectoralis minor muscle
Level III	Apical axilla. Lymph nodes medial to the medial margin of the pectoralis minor muscle

See Fig. 22.12

pN0	No regional lymph nodes metastasis
pN1	(a) Metastasis in 1–3 ipsilateral axillary lymph node(s)
	(b) Internal mammary lymph node(s) with microscopic metastasis by sentinel lymph node biopsy but not clinically apparent[a]
	(c) = a + b

pN2   (a) Metastasis in 4–9 ipsilateral axillary lymph nodes

(b) In clinically apparent internal mammary lymph node(s) but without axillary lymph nodes

pN3   (a) Metastasis in ≥10 axillary or infraclavicular lymph node(s)

(b) Metastasis in clinically apparent ipsilateral internal mammary lymph node(s) with axillary lymph nodes, or, metastasis in >3 axillary lymph nodes and in internal mammary lymph nodes with microscopic metastasis by sentinel lymph node biopsy but not clinically apparent.

(c) Metastasis in ipsilateral supraclavicular lymph node(s)

ᵃClinically apparent = detected by clinical examination or by imaging studies (excluding lymphoscintigraphy) or grossly visible pathologically

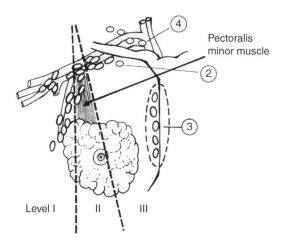

Fig. 22.12 Breast carcinoma: axillary lymph nodes (Reproduced, with permission, from Wittekind et al. (2005), © 2005)

Sentinel lymph node staging is designated as a suffix in brackets e.g. pN1(sn).

Cytokeratin markers are useful where the morphological appearances are suspicious, but not diagnostic of metastatic carcinoma e.g. sinusoidal lobular carcinoma cells versus sinus histiocytosis. The significance of lymph node *micrometastases* (≤2 mm: pN1 (mi)) remains uncertain with some regarding it as an adverse prognostic indicator but others less convinced. From a practical viewpoint it does influence choice of systemic adjuvant chemotherapy and hormonal therapy and should be reported. The biological status of *isolated tumour cells* (≤0.2 mm: pN0 (i+)) is not established.

Histological levels of serial slices and cytokeratin immunostains may be necessary particularly if *sentinel lymph node biopsy* (95 % positive predictive value for axillary lymph node metastasis) alone is used for staging purposes in clinically node negative patients. Other recommended approaches to axillary disease are *axillary lymph node sampling* (3 or 4 level I lymph nodes for staging only), particularly if operative identification of a sentinel lymph node is uncertain, or *axillary lymph node clearance* (for staging and treatment). Axillary lymph node involvement is seen in *30–40% of cases*. The Nottingham group has shown that a *threshold of three involved lymph nodes* is associated with *decreased breast cancer specific survival* and *distant metastasis free survival*. Of patients with axillary lymph node disease there can also be involvement of the internal mammary chain (22 %), and supraclavicular lymph nodes (20 %). *Distant metastases* are to the skeleton, lung and pleura, liver, ovary, adrenal gland and central nervous system. *Presentation with metastatic tumour in axillary lymph nodes* is usually due to either breast carcinoma or malignant melanoma and this can be resolved with immunohistochemistry. The source of the breast carcinoma is usually the ipsilateral breast or axillary tail of breast and the lesion can be clinically occult and difficult to locate as its size is often less than 2 cm in diameter. Invasive lobular carcinoma has a greater tendency than ductal tumours to metastasise to retro-/peritoneum, meninges, gastrointestinal and female genital tracts.

22.7 Excision Margins

Measure the distances (mm) to the nearest and other painted margins (superficial, deep, lateral, medial, inferior, superior). Differential block labelling and use of multi-coloured inks are important. Separate orientated cavity margin samples may also be submitted by the surgeon.

Adequate clearance of margins:
- Invasive carcinoma 5 mm.
- In situ carcinoma 10 mm (ductal only as lobular can be multifocal).
- In practice a minimal margin of 1–2 mm is targeted, with follow up radiotherapy for wide local excision specimens.

Involved margins (defined as carcinoma cells *at* the ink) can *triple the risk of local recurrence* and can be an indication for either *radiotherapy* (deep, superficial margins), or *further surgery* as a local re-excision (site orientated cavity shavings) or conversion to a mastectomy. Note that margins can be particularly difficult to define and assess in lobular carcinoma when distinction from fibrous breast tissue can be problematic. *Margin involvement in DCIS* is a *strong predictor of local recurrence* about *50 % of which will be as invasive disease*, particularly so for high cytonuclear grade DCIS and often correlating with high-grade cancer. The presence of lobular neoplasia (LN) at a surgical margin should be recorded but does not require re-excision.

22.8 Other Pathology

Assess breast tissue away from the tumour for:

Atypical hyperplasia, carcinoma in situ, satellite invasive foci, lymphovascular invasion (LVI).

Carcinoma in situ and LVI: when present away from (>1 mm) the tumour they are *strong prognostic indicators of local and lymph node recurrence* and are important in selecting appropriate postoperative adjuvant therapy or further surgical excision. Relationship of *satellite invasive foci* to resection margins must also be assessed and they occur more frequently in infiltrating lobular carcinoma.

Atypical hyperplasia (ductal and lobular: ADH/ALH): regarded as having ×4–5 increased risk of subsequent carcinoma, and in situ change ×10–11 increased risk over control populations. The precancerous nature of atypical hyperplasia is illustrated by its shared molecular abnormalities with carcinoma in situ. There is also evidence for a *FEA (flat epithelial atypia/columnar cell hyperplasia with atypia) – ADH – DCIS – low-grade cancer sequence*. These risk lesions and *lobular neoplasia (LN)* have a strong association with *low-grade breast cancer*. Conversely *high-grade DCIS* tends to progress to *high-grade invasive disease*. LCIS is usually an incidental microscopic finding e.g. adjacent to a simple cyst, or present (60 %) in the vicinity of invasive lobular cancer, and it is potentially

multifocal and bilateral. DCIS may present as Paget's disease ± nipple discharge, a tumour forming mass (especially comedo type with a greater propensity for invasive carcinoma), or adjacent to a symptomatic invasive breast cancer. In many cases it is an incidental finding on open biopsy or an impalpable lesion detected on radiological screening (15–20 % of screening cancers). This can be either as linear, branching calcifications, or within the context of a radiologically suspicious but histologically benign lesion e.g. radial scar/complex sclerosing lesions (RS/CSLs). Immunohistochemical markers calponin, p63, CK5/6 and CK14 are useful in demonstrating a myoepithelial cell layer as an aid to distinction from invasive carcinoma. These *RS/CSLs are often associated with foci of ADH/DCIS* and are regarded as *an independent marker of increased risk* for subsequent development of carcinoma.

Clinicopathological correlation: it is essential to *correlate the clinical mammographic abnormality with the excised specimen*. This requires *dissection guided by the postoperative specimen radiograph* demonstrating the lesion in question, with or without an in situ guide wire localisation needle. The histological slides must contain the abnormality e.g. carcinoma or microcalcification, and if not, all of the residual tissue processed or further blocks selected according to radiographic study of the specimen serial slices. Usual calcification (calcium phosphate) is easily recognisable as basophilic in routine sections. A minority (10 %) is oxalate in character, can be partially removed by tissue processing and is recognised by being doubly refractile on polarisation. It is usually seen in benign disease, e.g. fibrocystic disease. Similarly *needle core biopsy for microcalcification requires x-ray of the cores* to ensure that the relevant area has been sampled.

Paget's disease: affects 2 % of breast cancer patients and is distinguished immunohistochemically from malignant melanoma and Bowen's disease by being mucin, CEA, EMA, ER, Her-2 (50 %) and cytokeratin 7 positive, and S100, HMB-45 and melan-A negative. *DCIS of large cell type* is nearly always identified in the subareolar duct system and there is associated *invasive breast carcinoma in 35–50 % of cases*.

Depending on the mammographic extent of the underlying lesion (size, in situ versus invasive disease) breast conserving surgery with removal of the nipple-areolar-complex (NAC), partial or total mastectomy is carried out.

Microinvasion: defined as <1 mm from the nearest basement membrane and requiring infiltration of non-specialised interlobular/interductal stroma. It must be distinguished from the more frequent *cancerisation of lobules* (lobular architecture/intact basement membrane), and clinically is managed similarly to DCIS as the incidence of axillary lymph node metastases is very low. The likelihood of invasion increases with the grade of DCIS and presence of comedonecrosis, and extra blocks and levels should be assessed. Usually the type of invasive carcinoma correlates with the type of DCIS but LCIS can be associated with invasive carcinoma of ductal or lobular type.

Neoadjuvant chemo-/radiotherapy: effects include tumour cell necrosis, degeneration, apoptosis, vacuolation, inflammation and fibrosis. It tends to be reserved for large *clinically advanced cT3/cT4 tumours*, or where surgery is contraindicated due to *poor general health*. It may then be followed by *surgical resection* as it improves resectability and may have a role to play in *downstaging* of the tumour, although this is not yet clarified. It also makes tumour typing and grading difficult, features that are perhaps better assessed on the pre-treatment needle core biopsy. Tumour size may also need to be based on the radiographic or ultrasound measurements. Tumour response to neoadjuvant therapy can be gauged by assessing residual cancer burden as a proportion of the estimated original tumour bed. *Postoperative radiotherapy* is used for the control of local recurrence of breast cancer in the presence of positive deep or superficial margins of excision. It can result in diagnostically confusing cytological atypia in native ductulolobular unit epithelium. The presence of widespread metastatic disease should be clinically determined prior to surgical resection so that *palliative systemic therapy* can be considered instead.

Treatment of localised disease: is by *wide local excision* ensuring 10–20 mm palpable margins of clearance around the tumour. Conversion to *mastectomy* (10–15 % of cases) is undertaken

in the following combination of circumstances: if the patient is <50 years of age, has a tumour diameter >2 cm, has lymphovascular invasion or involvement of the surgical margins. Otherwise the residual breast receives *radiotherapy*. *Mastectomy* (*about 30 % of cases*) is indicated as initial treatment if the tumour is centrally situated (behind the nipple), >3 cm in diameter and/or associated with radiological evidence of extensive DCIS, or if it is the patient's preference. *Adjuvant hormonal therapy* is determined by the tumour ER/PR status. *Radiotherapy* after mastectomy is indicated for a large tumour, when there are more than four lymph nodes positive or there is vascular invasion. *Chemotherapy* is usually indicated in high-grade and lymph node positive patients particularly in the younger age group. Her-2 tumour status also determines choice of chemotherapy and any indication for *trastuzumab therapy* in locally recurrent disease or distant metastases.

Triple assessment: concordance of its three modalities (*clinical examination, radiology, FNAC/needle core biopsy*) has replaced frozen section and the majority of open biopsies in the diagnosis of breast carcinoma. This allows a one stop assessment and progression to definitive breast conserving or more radical surgery. Open biopsy may still be required where there is discordance between the parameters. *FNAC* cannot accurately distinguish between in situ and invasive malignant cells and *core biopsy* is advantageous e.g. high-grade DCIS. Note that diagnostic core biopsy can underestimate cancer grade and may not accurately reflect tumour subtype compared with the resection specimen e.g. for reasons of tumour heterogeneity in both cellularity and differentiation. Core biopsy is also advantageous, when FNAC is either insufficient (e.g. scirrhous or lobular carcinoma) or inconclusive (e.g. some well differentiated grade I cancers), for some benign lesions, non-palpable lesions and mammographic calcifications. In addition, it is of use in the neoadjuvant setting for determination of tumour grade and ER/PR/Her-2 receptor status. The *trend towards core biopsy over FNAC* is predicated upon these factors and the limited availability of cytopathological expertise for the interpretation of the latter. FNAC advantages are convenience to the patient and clinician, speed of results, low cost and ease of access to determining the axillary lymph node status. Potential *diagnostic pitfalls in core biopsies* are overcall of: RS/CSL as tubular carcinoma, apocrine atypia as DCIS, chronic inflammation (cytokeratin negative) as lobular carcinoma and radiotherapy changes as carcinoma. *False negative diagnoses* include the reverse of the above, metaplastic carcinoma mistaken for a fibrous scar, undercalling of DCIS as ADH, and, invasive cancer due to sampling limitations. The latter is the outcome in up to 20 % of subsequent resection specimens for ADH/DCIS.

Prognosis

Prognosis relates to patient age, tumour type, size, grade, lymphovascular invasion, lymph node and hormonal status. ER negative, lymph node positive and Her-2 positive cancers equate to high risk. Overall 5 year survival is 60% for clinically localised disease and 34% for regional disease.

Nottingham Prognostic Index (NPI) = 0.2 × invasive tumour size (cm) + stage + tumour grade.

		Score
StageA	No nodes involved	1
StageB	≤3 low axillary nodes involved	2
StageC	≥4 nodes and/or the apical node involved	3

NPI score	Prognosis	5 year survival
<3.4	Good	88 %
3.4–5.4	Intermediate	68 %
>5.4	Poor	21 %

Dutch workers advocate a morphometric index based on tumour size, mitotic activity index and lymph node status as giving practical clinical prognostic data. Average age <35 years is also adverse.

Prognosis according to *histological type* (10 year survivals):

Excellent (>80 %)	Tubular, cribriform, mucinous, tubulolobular, encysted papillary
Good (60–80 %)	Tubular mixed, alveolar lobular, mixed ductal NST/special type

Intermediate (50–60 %)	Classical lobular, medullary, invasive papillary
Poor (<50 %)	Ductal (NST), mixed ductal and lobular, solid and pleomorphic lobular, metaplastic

Higher stage of disease at presentation, decreased response to conventional chemotherapy and lower patient survival are associated with tumours that are ER/PR negative, DNA aneuploid, over express p53 and Her-2, and have a high Ki-67 proliferation index. These are usually high-grade ductal cancers, no special type.

Breast cancer subtypes with reference to genetic and immunophenotypical expression of luminal and basal epithelial antigens are:

Luminal A	ER/PR positive Her-2 negative
Luminal B	ER/PR positive Her-2 positive
Non-luminal	ER/PR negative Her-2 positive, or, basal type (ER/PR/Her-2 triple marker negative and CK5/6, 34βE12 positive)

These morphological and immunophenotypical categories of breast cancer are also reflected in *differing molecular developmental pathways related to ER expression*. ER positive cancers include low-grade luminal A and high-grade luminal B tumours. ER negative cancers encompass high risk Her-2 positive, basal type and apocrine lesions. Recent research proposes up to ten genetic subtypes of breast cancer with differing response to treatment and survival rates. Thus low-grade/risk breast cancers are characterized by showing glandular differentiation, low nuclear pleomorphism and mitotic activity, strongly express ER, and include good prognosis subtypes such as tubular, invasive cribriform, mucinous and classical lobular carcinomas.

Hormonal and Her-2 Receptor Status

Oestrogen/Progesterone Receptor (ER/PR) Expression

Positive in 70–80 % of ductal (usually grade 1/2) cancers and 80–90 % of infiltrating lobular carcinomas.

Most postmenopausal patients receive the anti-oestrogen tamoxifen but positive ER status in premenopausal patients is important so that consideration can be given to hormonal treatment. PR expression is a prognostic marker and may also indicate hormone responsiveness.

Scoring System: "Category Score"

Staining characteristics	Microscopic assessment	ER status
Negative	No staining	ER−
Weak	×25, ×40 objective	ER+
Moderate	×10 objective	ER+
Strong	×10 objective	ER+

Scoring System: "Histo Score"

In the Histo score, each cell is assessed as:

0	No staining
1	Weak staining
2	Moderate staining
3	Strong staining

The percentage of cells showing each intensity of staining is estimated over as much of the section as possible and the Histo Score is calculated by multiplying the intensity score by the percentage of tumour cells showing that intensity: e.g. a tumour with 50 % of cells strongly stained, 25 % moderately stained and 25 % weakly stained would score $(50×3)+(25×2)+(25×1)=225$. Histo Scores less than 75 are considered to be ER negative and those above 75 are considered to be ER positive.

Scoring System: Allred or "Quick Score"

In the Quick score, the proportion of cells staining and their intensity are assessed as:

Proportion	
	0=no nuclear staining
	1=<1 % nuclei staining
	2=1–10 % nuclei staining
	3=11–33 % nuclei staining
	4=34–66 % nuclei staining
	5=67–100 % nuclei staining

Intensity	
	0=no staining
	1=weak staining
	2=moderate staining
	3=strong staining

Adding the 2 scores together gives a maximum score of 8 with the likelihood of anti- oestrogen responsiveness being

0	Hormonal therapy will not work
2–3	A small (20 %) chance of treatment response
4–6	An even (50 %) chance of treatment response
7–8	A good (75 %) chance of treatment response

Currently the Quick score is the recommended method of assessment.

Individual cancers can show heterogeneity of ER expression and in some respects the Histo and Quick Scores can take this into account. Carcinoma in situ (low- to intermediate-grade), infiltrating lobular carcinoma, low-grade invasive ductal carcinoma and postmenopausal cancers tend to be ER positive, while high-grade in situ and invasive ductal lesions and a significant number of premenopausal carcinomas (grade related) are ER negative. In practice with improved immunohistochemistry the vast majority of breast cancers are either strongly positive or completely negative for ER and assessable visually at a glance. PR expression can be less clear cut. Expression is also amenable to quantitation by automated image analysis. Hormonal therapy is also considered in patients with low ER but high PR scores.

Her-2 neu (c-erbB2) Expression

Her-2 over expression (*15–30% of breast cancers*) is associated with high-grade in situ and grade 3 invasive ductal cancers, pleomorphic infiltrating lobular cancers, and, ER negative, recurrent or metastatic tumours. It can indicate *potential resistance to tamoxifen and CMF (Cyclophosphamide, Methotrexate, Fluorouracil) chemotherapy* but *benefit from high dose adriamycin or Herceptin/trastuzumab monoclonal antibody therapy*. When combined with neoadjuvant chemotherapy trastuzumab treatment can potentially double the rate of complete pathological response, and in the adjuvant setting reduces recurrence and improves survival. Her-2 status is assessed immunohistochemically (IHC) as negative (0–1+), equivocal (2+) or positive (3+). Equivocal cases (2+) are then subjected to fluorescent, chromogenic or dual colour dual hapten in situ hybridisation (FISH/CISH/DDISH) analysis for Her-2 gene amplification (25–30 % of cases positive), therapy being indicated in IHC 2+/ISH positive cases.

0	No membrane staining
1+	Weak incomplete membrane staining in >10 % of cells
2+	Weak or moderate complete membrane staining in >10 % of cells
3+	Strong complete membrane staining in >30 % of cells

ER, PR and Her-2 status tends to be performed on the *diagnostic core biopsy* due to better fixation and antigen preservation compared to resection specimens, and also the timeliness of availability of results for discussion at the next scheduled multidisciplinary meeting. An equivocal or negative core biopsy result can be repeated on the resection to exclude any possibility of heterogeneous expression. ER, PR and Her-2 status are also determined on recurrent carcinoma deposits e.g. skin, chest wall muscle, liver.

Immunophenotype: Miscellaneous Markers for Breast Cancer

- Ki-67 proliferation index (percentage positive cells), Her-2, p53, DNA ploidy.
- Cytokeratin (CAM 5.2, AE1/AE3, CK7), GCDFP-15, EMA, CEA positive. Variably positive for HMB-45, S100 and vimentin.
- CK7 positive/CK20 negative: the reverse of this is seen in intestinal tract tumours and this can be useful in metastatic carcinoma of uncertain origin, e.g. signet ring cell carcinoma.
- Myoepithelial markers to distinguish RS/CSLs from tubular carcinoma and in situ from

invasive ductal cancer: CK5/6, CK14, calponin, p63.
- E-caldherin: loss of expression in ALH/LCIS and infiltrating lobular carcinoma but retention in ductal lesions. Conversely 34βE12 is expressed in LCIS but lost in DCIS.
- Usual ductal epithelial hyperplasia is 34βE12, CK5/6 and CK 14 positive. ADH/DCIS is negative for these basal epithelial markers but positive for luminal epithelial antigens CK 8 and CK 18, indicating an absence of the mixed luminal/basal epithelial differentiation that is present in usual hyperplasia. ADH and DCIS are also uniformly ER positive whereas usual epithelial hyperplasia shows heterogeneous expression.

22.9   Other Malignancy

Leukaemia

- Single/multiple, uni-/bilateral.
- During the course of known disease or as a primary clinical presentation.
- Acute lymphoblastic leukaemia (ALL)/chronic lymphocytic leukaemia (CLL)/myeloma (κ, λ light chain restriction and clinical evidence of systemic disease).
- Myeloid/granulocytic sarcoma (CD34/CD43/CD68/CD117/chloroacetate esterase/myeloperoxidase positive) can mimic infiltrating lobular carcinoma (cytokeratins, cellular mucin) and malignant lymphoma (CD 45, CD 20, CD 3).

Malignant Lymphoma

- Usually secondary to known lymph node/systemic disease and not biopsied.
- *0.5% of primary malignant breast tumours.*
- May *clinically* and *radiologically mimic a carcinoma* and *immunohistochemistry* of aspirate and/or biopsy material will be necessary.

Primary malignant lymphoma (by exclusion of systemic lymphoma after staging):

1. *Commonest*: *aggressive large B cell non-Hodgkins lymphoma* usually unilateral in elderly women.
2. Secondly: aggressive Burkitt's/Burkitt's like lymphoma in young pregnant or lactating women. Bilateral with central nervous system and ovarian involvement.
3. Rarely: indolent low-grade MALToma (?prior lymphocytic lobulitis).
4. Differential diagnosis: infiltrating lobular carcinoma, medullary carcinoma; immunohistochemistry – cytokeratins, CD 45, CD 20, CD 3. ER can be positive in carcinoma and malignant lymphoma.
5. *Prognosis*: *overall 48% 5 year survival*; Burkitt's, poor.

Phyllodes Tumour

- Benign, borderline or malignant comprising a *biphasic proliferation* of double layered hyperplastic *epithelium* and abundant, cellular *stromal* mesenchymal elements with a *leaf like architecture*.

Designation is based on:

1. Circumscribed or infiltrative margins
2. Stromal cellularity
   Overgrowth (absence of epithelium in one low power field)
   Atypia
   Mitoses >5–10/10 high-power fields = probably malignant when combined with overgrowth and atypia
   Mitoses >10/10 high-power fields = malignant
   Overexpression of p53.

Most are benign, but *local recurrence is not uncommon* (*21% of cases*) and a small number develop haematogenous metastases to lung and bone. Axillary lymph node metastases are rare. At the benign end of the spectrum the differential diagnosis is cellular fibroadenoma, and at the malignant end metaplastic breast carcinoma (cytokeratin positive) and sarcoma. Mammography and FNAC are not particularly accurate at diagnosing phyllodes tumour. Patients are usually at least 40–50 years of age and diagnostic core biopsies show characteristic high percentage (>85 %) stromal content with variable cellularity, pleomorphism and mitotic activity. *Wide local excision* (*1 cm margins*) is needed for histological designation and prevention of local recurrence, which can occur even with benign and borderline lesions. Those classified as malignant have metastatic potential.

Sarcoma

Sarcoma forms <1 % of breast malignancies e.g. angiosarcoma (± post radiotherapy), and other primary soft tissue sarcomas (in decreasing order of frequency): malignant fibrous histiocytoma, fibrosarcoma, rhabdomyosarcoma, liposarcoma, leiomyosarcoma. Prognosis relates to high histological grade, mitotic counts and infiltrating margins. Important and more common differential diagnoses are *metaplastic breast carcinoma* (identify an epithelial component, cytokeratin positive), and *malignant phyllodes tumour* (biphasic and typical architecture).

Angiosarcoma is the commonest primary breast sarcoma, occurs in middle aged to elderly women, and usually in the field of *prior irradiation* after a period of three or more years. It is on average 5 cm in diameter with poorly defined margins. It must be distinguished from haemangioma, pseudoangiomatous stromal hyperplasia (PASH), and atypical vascular proliferation occurring in the dermis after recent breast conserving surgery. Grade 1 lesions (40 %) have an 81 % 10 year survival. Grade 3 lesions (40 %) mimic poorly differentiated carcinoma and have 10 % 10 year survival with metastases to lungs, liver, skin, bone and brain. Diagnosis can be difficult on FNAC and biopsy is required. Angiosarcoma is variably factor VIII, CD 34 and CD 31 positive.

Other spindle cell lesions of the breast to be considered in a differential diagnosis are: metastatic malignant melanoma and sarcomatoid renal cell carcinoma, fibromatosis and myofibroblast-related lesions (inflammatory myofibroblastic tumour, myofibroblastoma).

Reporting Categories for Breast Fine Needle Aspirates and Wide Bore Needle Core Biopsies

FNAC is highly efficient and accurate at diagnosing a wide range of breast disease when interpreted in conjunction with the patient's age, clinical history, clinical features of the lesion and its radiological appearances. Two basic patterns are encountered:

1. Benign
   A biphasic pattern of cohesive breast epithelium and background bare nuclei
   Low to moderate cellularity (except fibroadenoma which is of high cellularity)
2. Malignant
   Dyscohesive clusters and singles of variably atypical epithelial cells
   Cytoplasmic preservation in dispersed cells
   Absence of bare nuclei
   Stripped (bare) malignant nuclei
   Moderate to high cellularity for the patient's age.

FNAC reporting categories are:

C1	An inadequate specimen: insufficient epithelial cells, epithelial cell content obscured by inflammation or a technically poorly prepared smear
C2	An adequate benign specimen: of sufficient cellularity and showing a benign biphasic pattern
C3	Atypia, benign: showing some mild nuclear change or cellular dissociation but within an essentially benign pattern
C4	Atypia, suspicious: a pattern and cell constitution suspicious but not diagnostic of malignancy for quantitative (inadequate cellularity) or qualitative (insufficient atypia) reasons
C5	Malignant: a cellular specimen showing an unequivocally malignant pattern and individual malignant cells

FNAC is supplemented by wide bore needle core biopsy which is particularly helpful in certain circumstances: in the diagnosis of various benign breast lesions (e.g. RS/CSLs), phyllodes tumour, infiltrating lobular carcinoma (which may be scanty on FNAC), the distinction between in situ and invasive malignancy (the latter being an indication for an axillary lymph node procedure), and for determination of tumour grade and receptor status in the neoadjuvant setting.

Wide bore needle core biopsy reporting categories are:

B1	Unsatisfactory/normal tissue only
B2	Benign: e.g. fibroadenoma, sclerosing adenosis, columnar cell change, apocrine metaplasia, epithelial hyperplasia of usual type
B3	Benign but of uncertain malignant potential: benign lesions associated with the presence of cancer and/or the risk of developing it e.g. flat epithelial atypia (FEA), radial scar/complex sclerosing lesion (RS/CSL), ADH, ALH/LCIS, phyllodes tumour, papillary lesions
B4	Suspicious of malignancy: epithelial proliferation suspicious but not diagnostic of malignancy for quantitative or qualitative reasons
B5	Malignant: (a) In situ (b) Invasive

Reporting categories are a useful tool in the day-to-day management of individual cases and crucial for clinicopathological audit purposes. It is imperative that FNAC and wide bore needle core biopsy material are closely correlated with their respective surgical specimens. There is an increasing trend towards the use of needle core biopsy alone. This is partly because of a lack of widespread cytopathological expertise in interpretation of FNACs, but also because of its higher sensitivity and specificity for designating benign, indeterminate, non-palpable and calcified lesions. Assay of hormonal and Her-2 receptor status is also facilitated.

Grading of Invasive Breast Carcinoma

Grading is most relevant to infiltrating duct carcinoma, no special type and although more difficult to apply to special cancer types can give additional prognostic information. Infiltrating lobular carcinoma tends to be given grade 2 although the classical and pleomorphic variants score as grades 1 and 3 respectively. The Elston-Ellis modification of the Scarff-Bloom-Richardson system is used. There can be tumour grade heterogeneity and tubule formation takes this into account as it is based on the whole tumour area. However nuclear features and mitoses are assessed on the least differentiated area.

Three parameters are assessed and scored:

	Score
1. Tubule formation	
Majority of tumour (>75 %)	1
Moderate (10–75 %)	2
Little or none (<10 %)	3
2. Nuclear pleomorphism	
Small regular, uniform	1
Larger with variation	2
Marked variation in size and shape (± multiple nucleoli)	3

3. Mitoses (tumour periphery and most active areas rather than the paucicellular centre). The mitotic count (number of mitoses per ten high-power fields) is related to the objective field diameter:

Leitz Diaplan	Leitz Ortholux	Nikon Labophot	
×40 obj.	×25 obj.	×40 obj.	
0–11	0–9	0–5	1
12–22	10–19	6–10	2
>22	>19	>10	3

Total score	Grade	
3–5	1	Well differentiated
6–7	2	Moderately differentiated
8–9	3	Poorly differentiated

Bibliography

Abdel-Fatah TMA, Powe DG, Hodi Z, Lee AHS, Reis-Filho JS, Ellis IO. High frequency of coexistence of columnar cell lesions, lobular neoplasia, and low grade ductal carcinoma in situ with invasive tubular carcinoma and invasive lobular carcinoma. Am J Surg Pathol. 2007;31:417–26.

Abdel-Fatah TMA, Powe DG, Hodi Z, Reis-Filho JS, Lee AHS, Ellis IO. Morphologic and molecular evolutionary pathways of low nuclear grade invasive breast cancers and their putative precursor lesions: further evidence to support the concept of low nuclear grade breast neoplasia family. Am J Surg Pathol. 2008;32:513–23.

Allen DC. Histopathology reporting: guidelines for surgical cancer. 2nd ed. Springer: London; 2006.

Alvarenga CA, Paravidino PI, Alvarenga M, Gomes M, Dufloth R, Zeferino LC, Vassallo J, Schmitt FC. Reappraisal of immunohistochemical profiling of special histological types of breast carcinomas: a study of 121 cases of eight different subtypes. J Clin Pathol. 2012;65:1066–71.

Barnes NLP, Ooi JL, Yarnold JR, Bundred NJ. Ductal carcinoma in situ of the breast. BMJ. 2012;344:38–43.

Bloom HJG, Richardson WW. Histological grading and prognosis in breast carcinoma: a study of 1049 cases of which 359 have been followed for 15 years. Br J Cancer. 1957;11:359–77.

Brodie C, Provenzano E. Vascular proliferations of the breast. Histopathology. 2008;52:30–44.

Collins LC, Schnitt SJ. Papillary lesions of the breast: selected diagnostic and management issues. Histopathology. 2008;52:20–9.

Dixon M. ABC of breast diseases. 2nd ed. London: BMJ books; 2000.

Dixon JM, Wilson V, Verrill M, Symmans WF. Her2 testing in patients with breast cancer. Must be performed in a timely manner to facilitate treatment decisions. BMJ. 2012;344:9.

Douglas-Jones AG, Gupta SK, Attanoos RL, Morgan JM, Mansel RE. A critical appraisal of six modern classifications of ductal carcinoma in situ of the breast (DCIS): correlation with grade of associated invasive carcinoma. Histopathology. 1996;29:397–409.

Doyle EM, Banville M, Quinn CM, Flanagan F, O'Doherty A, Hill ADK, Kerin MJ, Fitzpatrick P, Kennedy M. Radial scars/complex sclerosing lesions and malignancy in a screening programme: incidence and histological features revisited. Histopathology. 2007;50:607–14.

Ellis IO, Humphreys S, Michell M, Pinder SE, Wells CA, Zakhour HD. Guidelines for breast needle core biopsy handling and reporting in breast screening assessment. Best practice no 179. J Clin Pathol. 2004;57:897–902.

Elston CW, Ellis IO, editors. The breast. Systemic pathology, vol. 13. 3rd ed. Edinburgh: Churchill Livingstone; 1998.

Feely L, Quinn CM. Columnar cell lesions of the breast. Histopathology. 2008;52:11–9.

Fulford LG, Reis-Filho JS, Lakhani SR. Lobular in-situ neoplasia. Curr Diagn Pathol. 2004;10:183–92.

Fulford LG, Easton DF, Reis-Filho JS, Sofronis A, Gillett CE, Lakhani SR, Hanby A. Specific morphological features predictive for the basal phenotype in grade 3 invasive ductal carcinoma of breast. Histopathology. 2006;49:22–34.

Guidelines for non-operative diagnostic procedures and reporting in breast cancer screening. Non-operative diagnosis subgroup of the National Coordinating Group for breast screening pathology. NHSBSP publication no 50. 2001.

Habashy HO, Powe DG, Abdel-Fatah TM, Gee JMW, Nicholson RI, Green AR, Rakha EA, Ellis IO. A review of the biological and clinical characteristics of luminal-like oestrogen receptor-positive breast cancer. Histopathology. 2012;60:845–63.

Hanby AM, Hughes TA. In situ and invasive lobular neoplasia of the breast. Histopathology. 2008;52:58–66.

Harris G, Pinders S, Ellis I. Ductal carcinoma in-situ: diagnosis and classification. Curr Diagn Pathol. 2004;10:204–10.

Kennedy M, Masterson AV, Kerin M, Flanagan F. Pathology and clinical relevance of radial scars: a review. J Clin Pathol. 2003;56:721–4.

Lagios MD, Westdahl PR, Margolin FR, Roses MR. Duct carcinoma in-situ; relationship of extent of non-invasive disease to the frequency of occult invasion, multicentricity, lymph node metastases, and short-term treatment failures. Cancer. 1982;50:1309–14.

Lee AHS. The histological diagnosis of metastases to the breast from extramammary malignancies. J Clin Pathol. 2007;60:1333–41.

Lee AHS. Recent developments in the diagnosis of spindle cell carcinoma, fibromatosis and phyllodes tumour of the breast. Histopathology. 2008;52:45–57.

Lee AHS, Denley HE, Pinder SE, Ellis IO, Elston CW, Vujovic P, Macmillan RD, Evans AJ, Nottingham Breast Team. Excision biopsy findings of patients with breast needle core biopsies reported as suspicious of malignancy (B4) or lesion of uncertain malignant potential (B3). Histopathology. 2003;42:331–6.

Lee AHS, Salinas NMV, Hodi Z, Rakha EA, Ellis IO. The value of examination of multiple levels of mammary needle core biopsy specimens taken for investigation of lesions other than calcification. J Clin Pathol. 2012a;65:1097–9.

Lee H, Yung S-Y, Ro JY, Kwon Y, Sohn JH, Park IH, Lee KS, Lee S, Kim SW, Kang HS, Ko KL, Ro J. Metaplastic breast cancer: clinicopathological features and its prognosis. J Clin Pathol. 2012b;65:441–6.

Lerwill MF. Current practical applications of diagnostic immunohistochemistry in breast pathology. Am J Surg Pathol. 2004;28:1076–91.

Lloyd J, Flanagan AM. Mammary and extramammary Paget's disease. J Clin Pathol. 2000;53:742–9.

Lopez-Garcia MA, Geyer FC, Lacroix-Triki M, Marchio C, Reis-Filho JS. Breast cancer precursors revisited: molecular features and progression pathways. Histopathology. 2010;57:171–92.

Mohammed ZMA, Going JJ, McMillan DC, Orange C, Mallon E, Doughty JC, Edwards J. Comparison of visual and automated assessment of Her2 status and their impact on outcome in primary operable invasive ductal breast cancer. Histopathology. 2012;61:675–84.

Nadji M, Gomez-Fernandez C, Ganjei-Azar P, Morales AR. Immunohistochemistry of estrogen and progesterone receptors reconsidered. Experience with 5993 cases. Am J Clin Pathol. 2005;123:21–7.

O'Malley FP, Bane A. An update on apocrine lesions of the breast. Histopathology. 2008;52:3–10.

Page DL, Rogers LW. Combined histologic and cytologic criteria for the diagnosis of mammary atypical ductal hyperplasia. Hum Pathol. 1992;23:1095–7.

Page DL, Kidd TE, Dupont WD, Simpson JF, Rogers LW. Lobular neoplasia of the breast: higher risk for subsequent invasive cancer predicted by more extensive disease. Hum Pathol. 1991;22:1232–9.

Pathology Reporting of Breast Disease. A joint document incorporating the third edition of the NHS Breast Screening Programme Guidelines for Pathology Reporting in Breast Cancer Screening and the second edition of the Royal College of Pathologists Minimum Dataset for Breast Cancer Histopathology. NHSBSP Publication No 58. January 2005. Accessed at http://www.rcpath.org/index.asp?PageID=695.

Pinder SE, Ellis IO, Elston CW. Prognostic factors in primary breast carcinoma. J Clin Pathol. 1995;48:981–3.

Pinder SE, Elston CW, Ellis IO. The role of the preoperative diagnosis in breast cancer. Histopathology. 1996;28:563–6.

Pinder SE, Provanzano E, Earl H, Ellis IO. Laboratory handling and histology reporting of breast specimens from patients who have received neoadjuvant chemotherapy. Histopathology. 2007;50:409–17.

Provenzano E, Johnson N. Overview of recommendations of Her2 testing in breast cancer. Diagn Histopathol. 2009;15:478–82.

Provenzano E, Pinder SE. Guidelines for the handling of benign and malignant surgical breast specimens. Curr Diagn Pathol. 2007;13:96–105.

Purdie CA. Sentinel lymph node biopsy. Review of the literature and guidelines for pathological handling and reporting. Curr Diagn Pathol. 2007;13:106–15.

Rakha EA, Ellis IO. An overview of assessment of prognostic and predictive factors in breast cancer needle core biopsy specimens. J Clin Pathol. 2007;60:1300–6.

Rakha EA, El-Sayed ME, Reis-Filho JS, Ellis IO. Expression profiling technology: its contribution to our understanding of breast cancer. Histopathology. 2008;52:76–81.

Rakha EA, Morgan D, Macmillan D. The prognostic significance of early stage lymph node positivity in operable invasive breast carcinoma: number or stage. J Clin Pathol. 2012a;65:624–30.

Rakha EA, Tun M, Junainah E, Ellis IO, Green A. Encapsulated papillary carcinoma of the breast: a study of invasion associated markers. J Clin Pathol. 2012b;65:710–4.

Reis-Filho JS, Tutt ANJ. Triple negative tumours: a critical review. Histopathology. 2008;52:108–18.

Rosen PP. Rosen's breast pathology. 3rd ed. Philadelphia: Lippincott, Williams and Wilkins; 2009.

Rosen PP, Obermann HA. Atlas of tumor pathology. 3rd series. Fascicle 7. Washington: AFIP; 1993.

Sainsbury JRC, Anderson TJ, Morgan DAL. ABC of breast diseases. Breast cancer. BMJ. 2000;321:745–50.

Schnitt SJ. Columnar cell lesions of the breast: pathological features and clinical significance. Curr Diagn Pathol. 2004;10:193–203.

Tan PH, Tse GMK, Bay BH. Mucinous breast lesions: diagnostic challenges. J Clin Pathol. 2008;61:11–9.

Tavassoli F, Devilee P. WHO classification of tumours. Tumours of the breast and female genital organs. Lyon: IARC Press; 2003.

The Royal College of Pathologists. Breast Cancer Dataset and Tissue Pathways. Accessed at http://www.rcpath.org/index.asp?PageID=254.

Torjesen I. Landmark study classifies breast cancer into 10 genetic types. BMJ. 2012;344:1.

Tse GM, Tan P-H, Pang ALM, Tang APY, Cheung HS. Calcification in breast lesions: pathologists' perspective. J Clin Pathol. 2008;61:145–51.

Tse GM, Tan P-H, Lacambra MD, et al. Papillary lesions of the breast – accuracy of core biopsy. Histopathology. 2010;56:481–8.

Walker RA. Immunohistochemical markers as predictive tools for breast cancer. J Clin Pathol. 2008;61: 689–96.

Walker RA, Bartlett JMS, Dowsett M, Ellis IO, Hanby AM, Jasani B, Miller K, Pinder SE. Her2 testing in the UK: further update to recommendations. J Clin Pathol. 2008;61:318–24.

Walker RA, Hanby A, Pinder SE, Thomas J, Ellis IO, National Coordinating Committee for Breast Pathology Research. Current issues in diagnostic breast pathology. J Clin Pathol. 2012;65:771–85.

Westenend PJ, Meurs CJC, Damhuis RAM. Tumour size and vascular invasion predict distant metastases in stage I breast cancer. Grade distinguishes early and late metastases. J Clin Pathol. 2005; 58:196–201.

Willems SM, van Deurzen CHM, van Diest PJ. Diagnosis of breast lesions: fine-needle aspiration cytology or core needle biopsy? A review. J Clin Pathol. 2012;65:287–92.

Wittekind C, International Union against Cancer, et al. TNM atlas: illustrated guide to the TNM/pTNM classification of malignant tumours. 5th ed. Berlin: Springer; 2005.

Part VI

Gynaecological Cancer

- Ovarian Carcinoma (with Comments on Fallopian Tube Carcinoma)
- Endometrial Carcinoma
- Cervical Carcinoma
- Vaginal Carcinoma
- Vulval Carcinoma
- Gestational Trophoblastic Tumours

Ovarian Carcinoma (with Comments on Fallopian Tube Carcinoma)

23

Ovarian cancer accounts for 30 % of female genital tract malignancies and some 50 % of its cancer related deaths. High parity and use of oral contraceptives are protective, while long term oestrogen replacement therapy in postmenopausal women is a risk factor. About 10 % of cases are on the basis of hereditary susceptibility, germline mutations in BRCA1 and BRCA2 genes conferring 20–50 % and 10–25 % lifetime risks of developing ovarian cancer, respectively. Serous carcinoma is the commonest ovarian epithelial malignancy overall (70–80 % of cases) and responsible for 90 % of deaths from ovarian cancer.

Ovarian cancer has a poor prognosis with an average 5 year survival of 35–40 %, although this is improving due to screening, more effective chemotherapy and changes in surgical practice. This adverse outlook is due to late presentation in 70 % of cases at an advanced stage of disease (FIGO II-IV), and with non-specific symptoms such as abdominal fullness or swelling. A high risk malignancy index equates to postmenopausal status, a solid or cystic lesion with septation, papillae or nodules on ultrasound scan, and elevated serum CA125 > 35kU/L. The UKCTOCS (United Kingdom Collaborative Trial of Ovarian Cancer Screening) is currently assessing the feasibility of using these criteria in detecting earlier stage disease. Low elevated levels of serum CA125 can also be seen in pregnancy, menstruation and endometriosis, and, other cancers e.g. breast, uterus, lung and pancreas. Further investigations include MRI scan, CT scan chest/abdomen/pelvis, and peritoneal fluid aspiration for cytology.

Radiological imaging is an effective tool for detection of ovarian neoplasia but cannot distinguish between primary and metastatic disease. If a benign cyst is suspected FNAC (fine needle aspiration cytology) may be used, and cystectomy or unilateral salpingo-oophorectomy considered, particularly in a young woman of child bearing age. Percutaneous biopsy is only used where there is an adnexal mass associated with extensive peritoneal disease that is considered inoperable, and a definite tissue diagnosis would provide a basis for neoadjuvant or palliative chemotherapy. Otherwise suspected malignant ovarian lesions are treated by total abdominal hysterectomy and bilateral salpingo-oophorectomy with omentectomy and peritoneal cytology. If diagnostic ascitic fluid has not been previously submitted or is not present at operation, peritoneal staging washings are carried out. The pathologist should integrate the histological and cytological findings to determine an appropriate tumour stage. Distinction between hyperplastic mesothelial cells and borderline/malignant serous epithelial cells can be particularly problematic emphasising the need for close correlation. Pelvic and retroperitoneal lymph nodes are clinically and radiologically assessed but not usually resected in stage I disease. Intraoperative frozen section may be necessary to determine lymph node status prior to undertaking radical surgery inclusive of lymphadenectomy, as it may be precluded by the presence of metastatic

D.C. Allen, *Histopathology Reporting*,
DOI 10.1007/978-1-4471-5263-7_23, © Springer-Verlag London 2013

disease. More limited surgery and staging are options in young women who wish to preserve their fertility. Appendicectomy can be indicated particularly with bilateral cystic ovarian tumours and any clinical suggestion of pseudomyxoma peritonei or an appendiceal mucocoele.

As commented on above, radiologically guided needle core biopsy of omental disease may be required for a definitive diagnosis, and also in patients not suitable for primary surgical debulking. Neoadjuvant chemotherapy can then be given, and if there is a good tumour response in a medically fit patient, subsequent cytoreductive salvage surgery or clearance of macroscopic abdominopelvic disease undertaken. Optimal debulking is defined as ≤10 mm of residual disease after completion of surgery. Due to changes of tumour regression after neoadjuvant chemotherapy it is difficult to subtype, grade and stage the ovarian cancer, although immunophenotypical expression similar to that of the chemonaieve tumour is often retained. Designation and staging is therefore based on the pre-treatment needle core sample and clinical disease distribution. Tumour type may also be an indicator as to potential chemoresponsiveness e.g. mucinous and clear cell adenocarcinomas and low-grade serous carcinomas respond less. Postoperative chemotherapy is used for tumours that have spread beyond the ovary, or, if ovary confined but with any of: high-grade, capsule rupture, ascites or positive peritoneal washings.

In general ovarian cancer is split into two types based on morphological subtype and tumour grade. Type 1 or low-grade cancers show more indolent behaviour and early stage disease with good to intermediate prognosis (endometrioid/mucinous: 90 % 5 year survival: clear cell: 70 % 5 year survival), and can be treated by optimal surgical debulking. The much commoner Type 2 or high-grade cancers are more aggressive with advanced stage (III/IV) disease, poor prognosis (high-grade serous: 20–40 % 5 year survival, <1 % ovary confined), and require a combination of radical surgery and chemotherapy.

23.1   Gross Description

Specimen

- FNAC/wedge biopsy/oophorectomy and/or cystectomy/uni-/bilateral salpingo-oophorectomy ± hysterectomy/omentectomy/lymphadenectomy.
- Weight (g) and size (cm).

Tumour

Site

- Ovarian (cystic, cortical, medullary, hilar or serosal)/paraovarian/broad ligament.
- Serosal tumour is associated with a worse prognosis than an equivalent cortical or intracystic lesion. Medullary, hilar or paraovarian tumour nodules may indicate a metastatic deposit rather than a primary lesion.
- Unilateral/bilateral (30–40 % of serous epithelial lesions).

Size

- Length × width × depth (cm) or maximum dimension (cm).

Appearance
Capsule: intact/deficient, smooth/rough.
Cut surface:
- Cystic:
  Uni-/multilocular
  Warty growths/nodules
  Fluid contents: serous/mucoid
  Sebaceous content: hair/teeth/colloid (struma ovarii)
- Solid:
  Partially/totally (cm)
  Necrosis/haemorrhage.
- Ovarian cancer tends to have a mixed cystic and solid appearance. The former comprises uni-/multilocular thin walled cysts with warty, nodular, papillary or solid areas of tumour growth which can be internal (endophytic) or serosal (exophytic). In lesions with a smooth external surface, areas of capsular deficiency

should be actively sought and the relationship to any tumour noted, either caused by it (due to capsular infiltration), or, overlying or away from it. The latter may be due to surgical dissection through a plane of adhesions or intra-operative rupture because of the size/cystic nature of the lesion, respectively. It is therefore important to determine the mechanism and part of the tumour that is deficient or ruptured in assessing potential spillage of benign, borderline or malignant cells into the peritoneal cavity so that the multidisciplinary meeting can assign an appropriate FIGO stage. The solid component of ovarian cancer tends to be somewhat friable and pale in appearance. Other visual diagnostic clues include: granulosa cell tumour (pale/fleshy/cystic), steroid cell and carcinoid tumours (yellow), thecoma/fibroma (white, whorled cut surface with yellow areas, lobulated), metastatic malignant melanoma (pigmented), immature teratoma (dermoid cyst with solid areas other than calcification/teeth), malignant lymphoma (pale/fleshy) and metastases (multiple, necrosis, nodular corticomedullary/serosal/hilar/para-ovarian/paratubal deposits).

Edge
- Circumscribed/irregular.

Fallopian tube: length (cm); infiltration of paratubal connective tissue. Tumour nodules in tubal mucosal fimbriae.

Omentum: weight (g) and size (cm); tumour nodules: number/maximum dimension (cm).

23.2 Histological Type

Epithelial and sex cord stromal lesions form 60–70 % of ovarian tumours (75 % of which are benign) and *90–95 % of primary ovarian malignancy*. These have traditionally been considered to arise from the surface (coelomic) epithelium or cortical epithelial inclusion cysts. More recent evidence points towards an origin from the *fallopian tube fimbrial epithelium* for a high proportion of ovarian serous adenocarcinomas. Epithelial

tumours are classified according to their *cell type*, *growth pattern* (solid, cystic, surface), *amount of fibrous stroma* and *neoplastic potential of the constituent epithelium* (benign, borderline or malignant/invasive). *Germ cell tumours comprise 25 % of ovarian tumours* and the vast majority of these are benign. They form 60–70 % of childhood ovarian tumours and while the majority of these are benign (cystic teratoma) there is a greater proportion of malignant germ cell tumours (immature teratoma, yolk sac tumour) than in adults.

Epithelial

Serous	55 %	
Mucinous	5–10 %	
Endometrioid	15 %	benign, borderline or
Clear cell	10 %	malignant lesions
Brenner	2 %	

- The *commonest primary ovarian carcinomas* are high-grade serous carcinoma (70 %), clear cell carcinoma (10 %), endometrioid carcinoma (10 %), mucinous carcinoma (2–4 %) and low-grade serous carcinoma (2 %).
- *Mixed*: either of different epithelial subtypes or differentiation within one subtype
  - Mucinous cystadenoma/Brenner tumour: a relatively common finding.
  - Clear cell/endometrioid (both can arise ex-endometriosis), serous/endometrioid or serous/clear cell adenocarcinomas. Classification is subject to considerable observer variation and true mixed differentiation is relatively rare with the common epithelial subtypes. Each component must comprise at least 10 % of the tumour area. The prognosis is often determined by the nature of the major component. However, the presence of a minor component of serous or undifferentiated carcinoma in an otherwise endometrioid adenocarcinoma adversely affects prognosis with the latter probably representing dedifferentiation from the low-grade endometrioid

adenocarcinoma. High-grade serous adenocarcinomas may also show endometrioid and clear cell like areas mimicking these two subtypes.

– Endometrioid adenocarcinoma with squamous cell differentiation (benign or malignant cytology).

- *Undifferentiated*:
  – Small cell carcinoma of either a. hypercalcaemic type (young, bilateral, small cells with follicle like structures), or, b. pulmonary type (lung small cell carcinoma analogue), both of which are of poor prognosis and show variable EMA/cytokeratin positivity ± chromogranin/synaptophysin/CD56. There is also a large cell neuroendocrine carcinoma variant.
  – Non-small cell: immunohistochemistry may be necessary to distinguish it from malignant lymphoma, malignant melanoma, epithelioid variants of sarcoma, granulosa cell tumour and rare ovarian cancers e.g. transitional cell carcinoma or squamous cell carcinoma.
  – Osteoclast like.
  – Trophoblastic differentiation.

Malignant Mixed Mesodermal Tumour (Carcinosarcoma)

- Old age, *poor prognosis, <1 % of ovarian tumours*.
- Homologous: ovarian type adenocarcinoma (serous, endometrioid, clear cell, undifferentiated) with cytokeratin positive spindle cells indicating that this lesion is a carcinoma with variable malignant mesenchymal differentiation.
- Heterologous: ovarian type adenocarcinoma with foci of immature/malignant cartilage, striated muscle, osteoid.

Sex Cord/Stromal

- *8 % of ovarian neoplasms*.
- *Fibroma/thecoma* (85 %): fibroma (storiform spindle cells/collagenous stroma) is one of the commonest ovarian tumours. Thecomatous elements are fat stain positive. Fibroma/thecoma can be associated with Meig's syndrome and endometrial hyperplasia. Sclerosing stromal tumour is a related variant. Fibrosarcoma shows cytological atypia and increased mitoses and is very rare.

- *Granulosa cell tumour* (12 %):
  Adult: micro-(macro)follicular (Call-Exner bodies), trabecular, insular, watered-silk, solid, sarcomatoid patterns, and longitudinal nuclear grooves.
  Juvenile: solid or cystic, follicular patterns of small cells ± mitoses. It is less aggressive than the adult counterpart with tumour recurrence and metastases rare.

- *Sertoli-Leydig tumour*: well/moderate/poor differentiation with varying proportions of tubules lined by Sertoli cells, Leydig cells and spindle cells ± heterologous elements e.g. mucin secreting glands. Sertoli cells are cytokeratin positive, and the stroma is inhibin positive.

- *Mixed and unclassified variants* (10 % of cases).

- *Gynandroblastoma*: an equal mix of android and gynaecoid elements i.e. granulosa-theca/Sertoli-Leydig.

- *Gonadoblastoma*: mixed germ cell/sex cord cell elements usually dysgerminoma/ Sertoli/granulosa like cells.

- *Sex cord tumour with annular tubules* (*SCTAT*): associated with Peutz-Jeghers syndrome and adenoma malignum of the cervix.

- *Immunohistochemistry*: the sex cord stromal tumours are variably inhibin/melan-A/calretinin/WT-1/SF-1/FOXL2 and CAM5.2/CD99(both focal) positive, but CA125/CK7/EMA/BerEP4 negative.

Steroid Cell Tumours

- Rare (0.1 %), hormonally active with virilisation (75 %).
- Polygonal eosinophilic cells, inhibin/calretinin/melan-A/SF-1 positive.
- 30 % are malignant based on size (>7 cm), mitoses, atypia, and necrosis.

Germ Cell Tumours

- *Teratoma*: mature/cystic.
  Immature/solid.
  Monodermal e.g. carcinoid tumour, struma ovarii (thyroid tissue).
  Malignant transformation, e.g. squamous cell carcinoma (80 % of malignant cases), carcinoid tumour, adenocarcinoma (no specific type or mucinous), thyroid papillary carcinoma.
- *Dysgerminoma* (seminoma analogue: PLAP/CD117/OCT3/4/SALL4 positive), *yolk sac tumour* (children/young adults, reticular/microcystic/endodermal sinus/tubulopapillary patterns, AFP/glypican 3/SALL 4 positive, chemosensitive), *embryonal carcinoma* (CD30/CAM5.2/OCT3/4/SALL 4/SOX 2 positive). SALL4 is a robust pluripotential pan-germ cell marker. It is positive in normal germ cells, immature teratoma, embryonal carcinoma, dysgerminoma and yolk sac tumour. OCT3/4 shows similar immunoexpression but is negative in yolk sac tumour.
- *Mixed germ cell tumour* (8 % of cases) e.g. dysgerminoma and yolk sac tumour.
- *Choriocarcinoma*
  Primary: rarely, primary prepubertal or as part of a mixed germ cell tumour.
  Secondary: to gestational uterine, tubal or ovarian lesions (better prognosis).

Metastatic Carcinoma

- *10–15 % of malignant ovarian tumours* often *mimicking a primary lesion* clinically and pathologically: especially from colorectum, appendix, stomach, pancreas, endocervix, endometrium and breast (infiltrating lobular). With any *ovarian mucinous tumour metastases from elsewhere is a more common finding* and must be excluded by past medical history, clinical and radiological investigation.
- *Krükenberg tumours*: classically bilateral signet ring cell metastases from stomach and mucin positive with a reactive fibrous ovarian stroma±luteinisation. Spread is transperitoneal and rare differential diagnoses include primary ovarian signet ring cell carcinoma, ovarian goblet cell carcinoid tumour (syn: crypt cell adenocarcinoma), and sclerosing stromal tumour. Other sources for Krükenberg tumours are large bowel, appendix, gall bladder, pancreas and breast.
- *Direct spread*: colorectal carcinoma, carcinoma of fallopian tube, endometrium and cervix.
- *Distant spread*: lung, malignant melanoma, breast, kidney, thyroid. Small cell ovarian tumours (juvenile granulosa, small cell carcinoma±hypercalcaemia) must be distinguished from metastatic small cell carcinoma of lung.

Features favouring an ovarian primary are: unilaterality, large size (>12 cm) with a smooth external surface and an expansile microscopic growth pattern. Other indicators to a primary lesion are associated ovarian pathology e.g. benign cystic teratoma (dermoid cyst), Brenner tumour, Sertoli-Leydig tumour, or a mural nodule (see Sect. 23.8). *Approximately 70 % of secondary carcinomas* are bilateral most of which are <10 cm in diameter. Additional clues are solid, discrete, corticomedullary nodular deposits, surface or hilar deposits, prominent infiltrative stromal desmoplasia, lymphovascular invasion, extensive necrosis, colloid and signet ring carcinomas, pseudomyxoma peritonei, and lack of CK7 positivity. *Prognosis of metastatic carcinoma to the ovary is poor as this represents advanced disease.* Conversely primary ovarian mucinous carcinomas are usually low-grade and have limited extent early stage disease. A number of metastases mimic primary ovarian carcinoma histologically e.g. gastrointestinal tract (endometrioid/mucinous), renal cell (mesonephroid/clear cell), thyroid (struma ovarii) and hepatocellular (yolk sac tumour) carcinomas. A relevant clinical history is crucial in designation and further clinical investigation e.g. CT scan abdomen, serum AFP or CEA may be necessary to discover an occult primary lesion. See Sect 23.8 for further discussion.

23.3   Differentiation

Adenocarcinoma

- Well/moderate/poor/undifferentiated, or, Grade 1/2/3/4.
- Grading for epithelial ovarian tumours is based on the degree of architectural differentiation (glandular/papillary/solid), cytological pleomorphism, and mitotic activity ± overt invasion of the stroma or capsule. The *presence and extent of stromal invasion is a strong prognostic indicator*.
- In serous adenocarcinoma there is usually correlation between cytoarchitectural differentiation features. Poorly differentiated tumours form the majority of cases, and are solid with tubulopapillary slit like spaces and high nuclear grade. Less common patterns are pseudoendometrioid, transitional cell like and microcystic. Well to moderately differentiated tumours are much less common (2 % of cases), and are partially cystic with glands, papillae and lower nuclear grade. An exception to this with cytoarchitectural disparity is the grade 1 solid/nested psammomatous serous adenocarcinoma. In general, on morphological, molecular and behavioural grounds, ovarian serous adenocarcinomas are regarded as being either *low-grade* or *high-grade*, with the distinguishing features of *marked cytological atypia*, and, a threshold of *≤12 or >12 mitoses per 10 high power fields*. This model has been extended to postulate *two pathogenetic types of ovarian carcinoma*.
  - *Type 1* (*low-grade*): including borderline epithelial lesions, low-grade serous adenocarcinoma, mucinous, low-grade endometrioid and clear cell adenocarcinomas, malignant Brenner tumour
  - *Type 2* (*high-grade*): including high-grade serous adenocarcinoma, undifferentiated carcinomas and carcinosarcomas.
  - *Type 1 cancers* have an indolent transition to malignancy from benign Mullerian neoplasia (e.g. cystadenoma/adenofibroma), metaplasia (e.g. endometriosis) or potentially fallopian tube fimbrial epithelial implants on the ovarian surface. They present with early stage disease, are treated by total surgical debulking, and are in general non-chemoresponsive. They show a variety of gene mutations such as BRAF, KRAS, PTEN and microsatellite instability.
  - *Type 2 cancers* undergo abrupt malignant change usually from a fallopian tube fimbrial epithelial precursor (*STIC – serous tubal intraepithelial carcinoma*), and occasionally ovarian cortical inclusion cysts or surface coelomic epithelium. They show p53 mutations and spread throughout the surfaces of the peritoneal cavity. They form >90 % of advanced stage ovarian cancers requiring a combination of radical surgery and chemotherapy.
- A suggested scheme for endometrioid carcinoma is similar to its uterine counterpart based on the percentage of non-squamous/non-morular solid growth pattern: grade 1 (≤5 %), 2 (6–50 %), 3 (>50 %).
- In endometrioid and mucinous tumours disproportionate nuclear atypia raises the grade by one level e.g. 1 → 2. In serous and clear cell carcinomas (both grade 3) *high nuclear grade* and *tumour subtype* take precedence over architecture.
- In mucinous tumours the *presence of invasion* outweighs cytoarchitectural grading features.

Borderline (Low Malignant Potential)

- *Serous borderline epithelial lesions* are of excellent prognosis regardless of stage and are bilateral in 20–25 % occurring in a younger age group (40–50 years) than established carcinoma. They form 10–15 % of epithelial tumours comprising epithelial complexity with budding, atypia, mitoses and nuclear layering but no destructive stromal invasion. There is peritoneal recurrence in 10–15 % of cases. The outlook for *mucinous epithelial borderline tumours* (≤3 nuclei deep) depends on the subtype i.e. the rare Mullerian endocervical (good outlook), or the much commoner intestinal variant (worse outlook). This is due to the latter being associated with appendiceal mucinous lesions (see pseudomyxoma peritonei).

Micropapillary serous carcinoma: requires no demonstrable invasion but is designated on the degree of micropapillary/cribriform epithelial complexity. It is an exophytic lesion often associated with invasive peritoneal implants, bilaterality and advanced stage. It is of worse prognosis than usual serous borderline tumours, *behaving in effect as a low-grade adenocarcinoma.*

Sex Cord/Stromal

- Well/moderate/poor differentiation but weak correlation with prognosis, and grading is more dependent on the specific tumour type.

Functional: e.g. oestrogenic drive to endometrium in thecoma (25 % of cases) and granulosa cell tumour. Virilisation in Sertoli-Leydig tumour.

Prognosis: of sex cord/stromal tumours relates to size (< or >5 cm), an intact or deficient capsule, bulk of extraovarian disease, atypia, mitoses (per 10 high power fields), necrosis and bilaterality.

Recurrence: in 30 % of patients and tends to be local. It may be extra-pelvic and after a considerable *lag period of 10–20 years* although recurrent juvenile granulosa and Sertoli-Leydig tumours recur within 3 years. Raised serum inhibin levels may be useful in detecting recurrent granulosa cell tumour. Note that artifactual displacement of granulosa cells due to surgical trauma or cut up can mimic vascular invasion.

Germ Cell

- *Mature*: cystic (95 % of cases). Common tissues represented are skin and appendage structures, muscle, fat, ganglia, neuroglia, respiratory, gastrointestinal and pancreatic glandular tissue, retinal elements, cartilage, teeth and bone.
- *Immature*: solid with histologically identifiable immature tissues especially cartilage, neuroepithelium, striated muscle and immature cellular mesenchyme.
- Grade 1: mostly mature tissue, loose mesenchyme, immature cartilage, focal (<1 low power field/slide) immature neuroepithelium.
- Grade 3: scant mature tissue, extensive (>3 low power fields/slide) immature neuroepithelium ± peritoneal implants which can be mature (e.g. gliomatosis peritonei) or immature, and are graded separately.
- ± carcinoma (e.g. squamous cell, adenocarcinoma) or sarcoma (e.g. rhabdomyosarcoma, sarcoma of no specific type) in mature or immature lesions. *Development of a somatic type malignancy is an adverse indicator.*
- GFAP, synaptophysin and SALL 4 can help in identification of immature neuroepithelial elements.
- Combination chemotherapy for grade 2/3 tumours and those with peritoneal implants gives 90–100 % survival.

23.4 Extent of Local Tumour Spread

Border: pushing/infiltrative.

Lymphocytic reaction: prominent/sparse.

Capsule/serosa/paratubal connective tissue/ contiguous fallopian tube/uterus. Involvement of fallopian tube was traditionally considered to be secondary to primary ovarian disease wherein the bulk of tumour resided. Extension of tumour along the tubal mucosa was regarded as a mimic of carcinoma in situ and a tubal origin. Current evidence indicates *an origin for a significant majority of ovarian and primary peritoneal serous cancers from fallopian tube fimbrial serous tubal intraepithelial carcinoma (STIC)*. Spread to uterus is usually as a serosal plaque of friable tumour with invasion of outer myometrium and/or its underlying vessels.

Extensive sampling of ovarian epithelial cystic lesions is necessary (1 block/cm diameter) as there can be marked *heterogeneity* and *coexistence of benign, borderline and malignant features* e.g. mucinous lesions. In this respect more blocks are required than in an obviously malignant homogeneous tumour, and nodular/solid areas should be preferentially sampled in an otherwise cystic lesion. *Microinvasion ≤10 mm² (or approximately 3 mm diameter)* can be difficult to distinguish from crypt epithelial complexity and invagination into stroma (desmoplasia is a useful feature in adenocarcinoma). It is occasionally seen in otherwise borderline serous tumours but does not alter the prognosis. *Invasion >5 mm* may help to discriminate between mucinous and endometrioid borderline and adenocarcinoma lesions with a worse clinical outcome.

Invasion of stroma and/or capsule remains the hallmark of adenocarcinoma but not infrequently its presence is difficult to assess or it is not evident. This is particularly problematic in mucinous lesions, where a designation of non-invasive carcinoma or intraepithelial carcinoma may be made on the basis of *epithelial complexity* and *cellular atypia* alone e.g. nuclear stratification ≥4 deep, a confluent glandular or cribriform epithelial pattern, or stroma-free papillae of epithelial cells. Further sampling is necessary to exclude frankly invasive areas warranting the more usual designation of adenocarcinoma. A 'destructive' infiltrative pattern of invasion also has a poorer outlook than an 'expansive' confluent invasive edge.

Minimal staging requires removal of the ovarian primary lesion, biopsy of the contralateral ovary, biopsy of omentum and peritoneal surfaces, and peritoneal washings for cytology if ascitic fluid is not present.

FIGO

FIGO staging is recommended and is broadly comparable to TNM7. The classification applies to malignant surface epithelial-stromal tumours including those of borderline malignancy. Non-epithelial ovarian cancers may also be classified using this scheme.

I	Growth limited to the ovaries
	(a) One ovary, capsule intact, no serosal disease or malignant cells in ascites or peritoneal washings
	(b) Two ovaries, capsule intact, no serosal disease or malignant cells in ascites or peritoneal washings
	(c) One or both ovaries with any of: capsule rupture[a], serosal disease or malignant cells in ascites or peritoneal washings
II	Growth involving one or both ovaries with pelvic tumour extension and/or implants
	(a) Uterus, and/or tube(s)
	(b) Other pelvic tissues
	(c) II(a) or II(b) with malignant cells in ascites or peritoneal washings
III	Growth involving one or both ovaries with metastases to abdominal peritoneum[b], and/or regional nodes
	(a) Microscopic peritoneal metastasis beyond pelvis
	(b) Macroscopic peritoneal metastasis ≤2 cm in greatest dimension beyond pelvis
	(c) Peritoneal metastasis >2 cm in greatest dimension and/or regional lymph node metastasis (N1)
IV	Growth involving one or both ovaries with distant metastases e.g. liver parenchyma or positive pleural fluid cytology.

[a]Rupture of the capsule can be spontaneous or surgical
[b]Peritoneal metastasis outside the pelvis includes involvement of the omentum (Figs. 23.1, 23.2 and 23.3)

The commonest pattern of spread is the *contralateral ovary, peritoneum, para-aortic and pelvic lymph nodes and liver. Lung is the preferred extra-abdominal* site and occasionally presentation can be at other abdominopelvic e.g. sigmoid colon, or unusual sites e.g. breast, clinically mimicking primary intestinal and mammary disease, respectively.

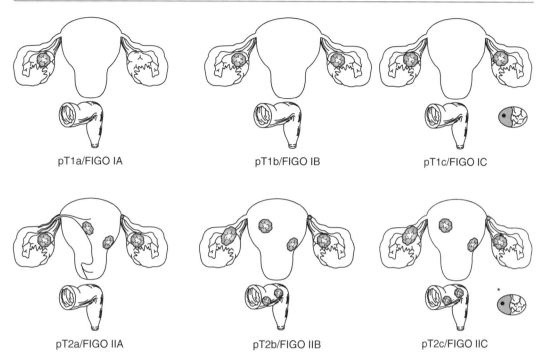

Fig. 23.1 Ovarian carcinoma (Reproduced, with permission, from Allen (2006), © 2006)

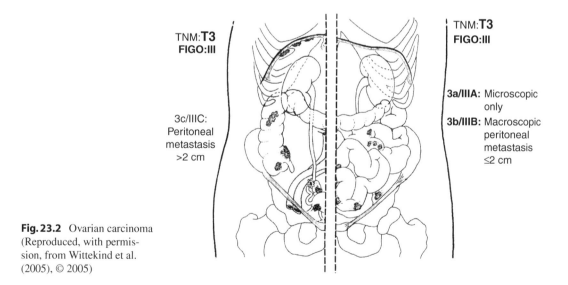

Fig. 23.2 Ovarian carcinoma
(Reproduced, with permis-
sion, from Wittekind et al.
(2005), © 2005)

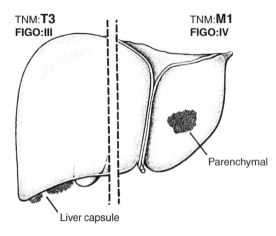

TNM:**T3**
FIGO:**III**

TNM:**M1**
FIGO:**IV**

Parenchymal

Liver capsule

Fig. 23.3 Ovarian carcinoma (Reproduced, with permission, from Wittekind et al. (2005), © 2005)

23.5　Lymphovascular Invasion

Present/absent.

Intra-/extratumoural.

Look for particularly in the paraovarian/paratubal connective tissues.

23.6　Lymph Nodes

Site/number/size/number involved/extracapsular spread.

Regional nodes: obturator (hypogastric), common iliac, external iliac, lateral sacral, paraaortic, inguinal. A regional lymphadenectomy will ordinarily include a minimum of ten lymph nodes.

- Beware of overcalling intranodal endosalpingiosis or Müllerian inclusions which can be associated with borderline changes and difficult to distinguish from microscopic metastases. Comparison with the index ovarian lesion and disease elsewhere e.g. peritoneum is important in designation. They are not thought to be associated with an adverse outcome.

23.7　Omentum/Peritoneum

Some 40 % of serous borderline tumours, especially exophytic lesions, are associated with foci of peritoneal serous epithelial proliferation particularly in the omental and pelvic peritoneum.

Endosalpingiosis

- *No epithelial atypia*: ± a benign or borderline ovarian lesion.
- A metaplastic process in serosal epithelial inclusions.

Implants

- *Epithelial atypia*: usually associated with a *borderline ovarian serous lesion* (rarely, mucinous). The implants are assessed independently of the ovarian tumour as: *non-invasive* or *invasive* (destructive infiltration of underlying tissue disrupting the omental lobular architecture), and, *epithelial* (proliferative) or *desmoplastic/stromal* (>50–75 % loose stroma/granulation tissue with small nests or papillae of epithelial cells).
- Probably represents *multifocal neoplasia* arising in peritoneal inclusions. Endosalpingiosis, desmoplastic and non-invasive proliferating implants should be noted and follow up recommended. *Invasive proliferating implants are regarded as low-grade carcinoma* as they progress in 80 % of cases with a 10 year survival of about 35 %. Non-invasive proliferating implants are distinguished from surface serous adenocarcinoma by greater epithelial architectural and nuclear atypia in >25 % of the lesion area in adenocarcinoma.

Primary Peritoneal Carcinoma

- young to middle aged females.
- *Serous adenocarcinoma in type*: CK7/WT1/p53/p16/ER positive.
- There is *extensive peritoneal disease±an ovarian serosal component* with otherwise normal ovaries (any ovarian invasion <5 mm²). It may arise from fallopian tube STIC or surface coelomic epithelium. It can also be

associated with EIC (endometrial intraepithelial carcinoma), or low volume high-grade endometrial serous carcinoma.

- Treated by surgical cytoreduction and chemotherapy. The psammomatous-rich adenocarcinoma variant has a better prognosis and indolent course.

Pseudomyxoma Peritonei

Pseudomyxoma peritonei is strongly associated with *appendiceal mucinous neoplasia* and there can be *concomitant cystic ovarian mucinous borderline tumours of intestinal type*. The peritoneal cavity fills with abundant mucin with or without a component of either cytologically bland, proliferating or malignant epithelium. *Prognosis of generalized pseudomyxoma peritonei is poor* as it is refractory to treatment, *slowly progressive* and leads to *bowel obstruction*. It usually arises due to rupture or spread from an appendiceal mucinous lesion – either a *low-grade appendiceal mucinous neoplasm* (*LAMN*), or less often, a *high-grade mucinous adenocarcinoma* (*MACA*). Appendiceal and ovarian lesions coexist in 90 % of pseuodmyxoma peritonei cases and the latter are now considered to represent direct implantation from the former due to spillage of neoplastic appendiceal epithelium into the peritoneal cavity. Immunohistochemistry may be of help in that ovarian lesions of appendiceal origin may be CK20 positive/CK7 negative but primary ovarian tumours CK7 positive/CK20 negative. A CK20 positive/CK7 positive phenotype can indicate either origin as 50 % of LAMNs are of this immunophenotype and ovarian mucinous tumours can show patchy CK20 positivity. In this case consideration also has to be given to a cystic metastasis from the pancreaticobiliary tree which can also co-express CA125 and show 'maturation phenomenon' with coexistence of benign, borderline and malignant morphology. In addition comment should be made as to whether pseudomyxoma peritonei is free mucinous ascites, organising mucin fluid or mucin dissection with fibrosis. The latter, *abundant mucin in the peritoneal cavity*, and the presence of *epithelial cells in the mucin* and *atypical cytological appearances* are also adverse prognostic parameters. Mucinous tumour confined to the right lower quadrant of the abdomen is regarded as being localized (pT4a) disease, whereas if beyond it is metastatic (pM1a) in distribution. Because of the strength of association *appendicectomy should be considered particularly when mucinous ovarian tumours are bilateral and there is extraovarian peritoneal disease*.

Metastatic Adenocarcinoma

- From primary ovarian adenocarcinoma usually forms either macroscopically obvious confluent tumour nodules, or a diffusely thickened omental cake.

23.8   Other Pathology

Hereditary factors: responsible for 5–10 % of ovarian carcinomas. Mutations in the *BRCA1* and *BRCA2* genes carry a *20–50% risk* of ovarian cancer up to the age of 70 years. The tumours occur 5 years earlier than sporadic ovarian carcinoma, are mainly of serous histological type, and have a strong association with breast cancer (BRCA1: 87 % risk). Affected patients have a higher proportion of solid undifferentiated serous cancers with increased mitoses and prominent tumour infiltrating lymphocytes (TILs). There is also an increased 9 % lifetime risk of ovarian cancer in *hereditary non-polyposis colorectal cancer* (*HNPCC*) due to abnormality in DNA mismatch repair genes (usually MSH2/MSH6), and typical ovarian cancer types are endometrioid and clear cell. Prognosis of hereditary ovarian cancer is grade and stage dependent similar to that of sporadic ovarian carcinoma. There is some evidence of a slightly better prognosis due to a better response to chemotherapy. Lesions in hereditary tubo-ovarian neoplasia may be early or microscopic and require serially slicing and processing in-toto of both ovaries and fallopian tubes (STIC).

Meig's syndrome: ascites, ovarian fibroma and right sided pleural effusion.

Contralateral ovary and tube: *synchronous/metastatic disease* of parenchyma or serosa (e.g. 40 % of serous papillary lesions). Clues to metastatic disease in the non-dominant ovary are multiple nodules, surface implants and lymphovascular invasion. Synchronous primary lesions will tend to show similar tumour distribution and appearance e.g. size and cystic with solid components.

Uterus: *synchronous/metastatic disease* of endometrium, endocervix or serosa i.e. multifocal Müllerian neoplasia. When tumour is present in the ovary and endometrium (usually endometrioid adenocarcinoma, sometimes serous adenocarcinoma) it can be difficult to tell which is the primary/metastatic site or if they are independent primary tumours i.e. stage II/III versus synchronous stage I disease. The *tumour site* and *distribution* (dominant bulk/depth of invasion/multiple serosal nodules/hilar involvement/lymphovascular invasion), and evidence of any *precancerous lesions* (endometrial hyperplasia/fallopian tube fimbrial STIC/ovarian endometriosis) are useful clues. The good prognosis of endometrioid adenocarcinomas confined to the endometrium and one or both ovaries suggests that they usually represent independent synchronous tumours, but in other cases with extensive disease distinction can be somewhat arbitrary and best attributed in light of full clinicopathological details. Ovarian carcinoma metastasizing to endometrium is rare but involvement of the outer myometrium is not uncommon.

Endometriosis: concurrent *ovarian endometriosis* (± atypical hyperplasia) and endometrial carcinoma are seen in up to 25 % of ovarian endometrioid adenocarcinomas. The frequency of associated disease is lower in ovarian clear cell (mesonephroid) adenocarcinoma which may also be related to foci of ovarian endometriosis (10–20 %), with the latter now considered in some cases to be a potentially premalignant lesion. Clear cell adenocarcinoma should be distinguished from yolk sac tumour, dysgerminoma and metastatic renal cell carcinoma (see below).

Ploidy: DNA aneuploidy in borderline ovarian epithelial lesions and ovarian adenocarcinoma is generally regarded as an adverse prognostic indicator, although it is not routinely assessed in daily practice.

Mucinous borderline tumours: these are either *intestinal* (85 % of cases: associated with appendiceal mucinous neoplasia ± pseudomyxoma peritonei), or *Müllerian* (endocervical; 30 % are associated with endometriosis) in type. They have differing pathological and clinical features representing *high-grade* and *low-grade proliferating mucinous tumours*, respectively. A wide spectrum of benign/borderline/malignant intestinal differentiation can be seen and *metastases* from appendix, colon, stomach, and pancreas need to be excluded clinically. *Primary ovarian lesions are now recognised to comprise only a minority (2–10%) of ovarian mucinous tumours* of borderline or malignant character. Primary mucinous tumours can also rarely show a spectrum of *mural nodules* of varying size and appearances ranging from anaplastic carcinoma (cytokeratin positive large/spindle cells: aggressive) and sarcoma (fibrosarcoma, rhabdomyosarcoma) to benign behaving sarcoma like (pseudosarcomatous) lesions with cytokeratin negative giant cells and spindle cells. Pseudomyxoma ovarii is commoner in borderline and malignant lesions, particularly those with pseudomyxoma peritonei of appendiceal origin. Mucinous (intestinal type) and endometrioid ovarian carcinomas and Sertoli-Leydig tumours can closely mimic or be imitated by colorectal and other gastrointestinal adenocarcinomas. These secondary tumours can occur after, concurrently or even predate the detection of the primary tumour.

Immunophenotype in the Differential Diagnosis of Ovarian Tumours

Colorectal metastases to the ovary tend to be bilateral, solid with areas of necrosis, and on microscopy show crescentic garland type strips of tumour with segmental and dirty necrosis. There is diffuse cellular staining with CEA,

CA19-9 and βcatenin and CA125 is usually negative. *Ovarian serous and endometrioid carcinomas* tend to be cystic with solid areas, uni- or bilateral, show cell apex CEA staining, ± CA125/WT1 and variable CA19-9. βcatenin is negative but CDX-2 can be positive in intestinal phenotype ovarian lesions making it unsuitable in this context for distinction from colorectal cancer. *Ovarian mucinous lesions* are also often ER, PR, WT1 and CA125 negative negating the use of these markers in the distinction from secondary carcinoma. Mucin is scanty in endometrioid variants and negative in Sertoli-Leydig tumours.

The *clinical and radiological anatomical distribution of disease* is important and commonly a rectosigmoid primary cancer will also show locoregional mesenteric lymph node disease and peritoneal involvement. At *intraoperative frozen section* the site of origin of a mucinous adenocarcinoma cannot be given with confidence, whereas this distinction can be made on morphological grounds for ovarian serous or clear cell adenocarcinoma invading large bowel. Despite this the differential diagnosis between ovarian and colorectal cancer can still be difficult and *in any ovarian mucinous or endometrioid tumour the possibility of a gastrointestinal origin must be excluded clinically*. *Differential cytokeratin expression* may be of use with intestinal tumours showing a different profile (CK20 positive/7 negative) to ovarian tumours (CK7 positive/CK20±, patchy). Gastrointestinal cancers are usually p53 positive. Note that *gastric and pancreaticobiliary cancers* are also variably CK7/20 positive and may even express CA125 as do some endometrial cancers. There is loss of DPC4 (SMAD4) in 50 % of pancreaticobiliary cancers but not in ovarian lesions. *Endocervical adenocarcinoma* is often p16 (HPV surrogate marker) positive. Metastatic *breast carcinoma* shows a similar cytokeratin profile (CK7+/CK20-, ER/PR positive) but is also GCDFP-15 positive. Infiltrating lobular breast cancer is particularly prone to gynaecological tract metastasis and a relevant clinical history is important. Other metastatic tumours mimicking primary ovarian cancer are *renal cell carcinoma* (CT abdomen, sinusoidal vascular pattern, less hob-nail cells, RCC ab/CD10/EMA/

vimentin positive) and *transitional cell carcinoma of the urinary tract* (uroplakin III/ CK7/ CK20 positive). In peritoneal fluid cytology specimens BerEP4 is helpful in distinguishing between mesothelial and epithelial cells.

Serum levels and tissue expression of various antigens are detectable in a range of ovarian neoplasms but characteristically strong associations are:

CK7/CA125/WT-1/p53/p16	Tubal/ovarian/ peritoneal adenocarcinoma (serous type)
HNF-1β	Ovarian clear cell carcinoma
AFP/glypican 3/SALL 4	Ovarian yolk sac tumour
βHCG/cytokeratins	Ovarian choriocarcinoma
PLAP/CD117/OCT3/4/SALL 4	Dysgerminoma
Inhibin/CD99/calretinin/SF-1	Granulosa cell tumour

SALL4 is a robust pluripotential pan-germ cell marker. It is positive in normal germ cells, immature teratoma, embryonal carcinoma, dysgerminoma, yolk sac tumour. OCT3/4 is similar but is negative in yolk sac tumour.

Prognosis

Prognosis of ovarian carcinoma relates to morphological features such as histological type and grade, volume percentage epithelium and mitotic activity index as well as large volume of disease after cytoreduction, high volume ascites, high postoperative CA125 levels, the age and BRCA gene status of the patient. Over expression of markers such as p53 and Her-2 may also be adverse. However, *the predominant factor is stage of disease* and the *degree of extra-ovarian spread and omental involvement*. *Early stage disease* confined to the ovary or pelvis has an *80 % 5 year survival rate* whereas the *majority (70 %) of patients present late* with widespread metastatic disease (FIGO III/IV) and *20–30 % 5 year survival*. Undoubtedly there are different types of ovarian adenocarcinoma according to their origins and behaviour i.e. *type 1/low-grade cystadenocarcinoma* arising from a cystic ovarian neoplasm/Mullerian metaplasia with indolent behaviour and early stage disease, or, *type 2/high-grade adenocarcinoma* arising from fallopian tube fimbrial epithelium or a thin rim of outer cortex and showing aggressive behaviour with disproportionately extensive local spread and involvement of adjacent structures. *Overall survival probability at 5 years is about 35–40 %.* Serum CA 125 levels are useful for monitoring disease progression and response to treatment but will be elevated in only 50 % of early, curable disease. A suggested screening strategy is a combination of clinical examination, serum CA125 levels and abdominopelvic ultrasound examination. FNAC has a role to play in the distinction between functional cysts (e.g. granulosa/luteal – inhibin positive) and benign or malignant epithelial lesions (cytokeratin/BerEp4 positive). Accurate surgical assessment is needed to avoid understaging of ovarian cancer, with *surgical excision* the mainstay of treatment. Cytoreductive surgery is also used for extensive disease with *adjuvant therapy*. The majority of patients with high volume and high-grade serous carcinoma initially respond to treatment but *70–80 % eventually relapse with local recurrence*. In some cases a subsequent "second-look" operation is carried out to assess the response to therapy and as a prequel to further chemotherapy. Borderline serous and endocervical mucinous ovarian epithelial neoplasms are uniformly of excellent prognosis (95–100 % 5 year survival), even if microinvasion (<1–3 mm diameter) is present, with uni- or bilateral adnexectomy as effective as radical surgery. Prognosis is worse with invasive peritoneal implants, and poor for intestinal type borderline mucinous lesions associated with appendiceal mucinous neoplasia and pseudomyxoma peritonei. Stage I mucinous adenocarcinoma has a good prognosis but may metastasise if extensive stromal invasion is present. The possibility of an ovarian mucinous tumour representing spread from appendix, colorectum, endocervix or pancreaticobiliary tree should always be considered. Clear cell adenocarcinoma is intermediate-grade with a worse outlook than mucinous or endometrioid ovarian cancer e.g. 70 % 5 year survival for stage I disease. Undifferentiated carcinoma and malignant mixed mesodermal tumour (carcinosarcoma) have a poor prognosis. The vast majority of *sex cord/stromal tumours are stage I with 85–95 % 5 year survival*. Higher stage and tumour rupture are adverse indicators but only about *10–30 % of cases subsequently recur*, often at a late stage with 10 and 20 year survivals of 60–90 % and 40–60 % respectively. Malignant ovarian germ cell tumours are unusual and occur mainly in children, adolescents and young adults. Sixty percent present with stage I disease (5 year survival 90 %) with a 70–80 % 5 year survival rate for all stages of disease. Serum βHCG and AFP levels are useful in postoperative monitoring and postoperative chemotherapy is used for tumours other than stage I, grade I immature teratoma.

23.9 Other Malignancy

Malignant Lymphoma

- *Primary* or more commonly *secondary* to systemic disease, particularly if low-grade B cell malignant lymphoma.
  Burkitt's/Burkitt's-like: childhood, young adults, and associated with bilateral breast lymphoma in young women.
  Non-Hodgkin's diffuse large B cell: average survival 3 years, often shows sclerosis.
- *Differential diagnoses*: includes the full range of malignant small blue cell tumours as well as granulosa cell tumour and dysgerminoma. Confirm by immunohistochemistry for lymphoid markers and negativity for inhibin, calretinin, PLAP, OCT3/4, SALL4, desmin, CD99, and neuroendocrine markers (neurofilament/synaptophysin/chromogranin).

Leukaemia

- Granulocytic sarcoma (CD34/CD43/CD68/CD117 and chloroacetate esterase/myeloperoxidase positive).

- 10–20 % of acute and chronic leukaemias; a site of relapse for ALL during bone marrow remission.

Sarcoma

- *Leiomyo-rhabdomyo-/angio-/chondro-/osteo-/neurofibrosarcoma*: these are all rare and more often part of a malignant mixed mesodermal tumour or (immature) teratoma.
- *Endometrioid stromal sarcoma*: granulosa like cells with distinctive vascular pattern of spiral arteriole type vessels. CD10 positive and smooth muscle actin/desmin focally positive, and, inhibin/h-caldesmon negative. Exclude spread from a uterine lesion.
- *Undifferentiated* (*high-grade*) *sarcoma*: fibro-/rhabdomyosarcoma like with atypia and mitoses.

Malignant Melanoma

- *Secondary*: present in 20 % of fatal cases.
- *Primary*: within the wall of a dermoid cyst.

Others

Secondary involvement or clinical mimicry of an ovarian tumour by peritoneal *malignant mesothelioma* (well-differentiated papillary/multicystic, or of no special type), *intra-abdominal desmoplastic small round blue cell tumour* (with divergent differentiation: cytokeratin, EMA, vimentin, synaptophysin, desmin positive; in the pelvis and abdomen of young people), *Ewing's sarcoma/PNET, neuroblastoma* (neurofilament/synaptophysin), *rhabdomyosarcoma* (desmin/myoD1/myogenin) and retroperitoneal liposarcoma.

23.10   Comments on Fallopian Tube Carcinoma

Primary carcinoma of the fallopian tube has traditionally been considered to be rare (<1 % of primary genital tract malignancy: increased risk in BRCA1/BRCA2 gene mutations), and greatly outnumbered by direct tubal extension from ovarian carcinoma (where the bulk of tumour is in the ovary) and uterine carcinoma (where the bulk of tumour is in the uterus). However previous comments (above) on the *fallopian tube fimbrial epithelial origin (STIC) for a significant proportion of ovarian/peritoneal serous carcinomas* should be noted. The tumour should be located macroscopically within the tube or its fimbriated end, and the uterus and ovaries should be grossly normal with any malignancy conforming to features of metastases or, alternatively, in keeping with the size and distribution of an independent primary. In primary fallopian tube carcinoma the tumour may be microscopic or the tube is distended by a solid or papillary tumour. Histologically the cancer is *invasive papillary adenocarcinoma usually similar to ovarian serous adenocarcinoma*. However, the full spectrum of Müllerian subtypes has been reported e.g. endometrioid, mucinous, clear cell, transitional and unusual tumours e.g. squamous cell carcinoma. Prognosis depends mostly on the stage of disease, with 5 year survival rates of 77 % for stage I and 20 % for stage III. Tumour recurrence is intra-abdominal and spread is similar to that of ovarian carcinoma. Other rare malignant tumours recorded are malignant mixed mesodermal tumour, leiomyosarcoma and gestational choriocarcinoma. Benign adenomatoid tumour is the commonest neoplasm occurring within the wall usually near the uterine cornu.

Broad ligament lesions include female Wolffian adnexal tumour (solid, sieve like trabecular/tubular pattern and CK7/inhibin/calretinin/androgen receptor positive, benign), and cystic lesions lined by Müllerian epithelium of variable type (e.g. serous, mucinous etc.) and character (usually benign/occasionally borderline or malignant).

FIGO

For details see ovarian carcinoma.

I	Tumour limited to the fallopian tube(s)
II	Tumour involving tube(s) with pelvic extension
III	Tumour involving tube(s) with metastases to abdominal peritoneum, and/or regional nodes
IV	Tumour involving tube(s) with distant metastases, e.g. liver parenchyma or positive pleural fluid cytology.

Bibliography

Allen DC. Histopathology reporting: guidelines for surgical cancer. 2nd ed. Springer: London; 2006.

Al-Nafussi A. Ovarian epithelial tumours: common problems in diagnosis. Curr Diagn Pathol. 2004;10:473–99.

Carlson J, Roh MH, Chang MC, Crum CP. Recent advances in the understanding of the pathogenesis of serous carcinoma: the concept of low- and high-grade disease and the role of the fallopian tube. Diagn Histopathol. 2008;14:352–65.

Deen S, Thomson AM, Al-Nafussi A. Histopathological challenges in assessing borderline ovarian tumours. Curr Diagn Pathol. 2006;12:325–46.

DeLair D, Soslow RA. Key features of extrauterine pelvic serous tumours (fallopian tube, ovary, and peritoneum). Histopathology. 2012;61:329–39.

Folkins AK, Longacre TA. Hereditary gynaecological malignancies: advances in screening and treatment. Histopathology. 2013;62:2–30.

Fox H, Wells M, editors. Haines and Taylor obstetrical and gynaecological pathology. 5th ed. Edinburgh: Churchill Livingstone; 2003.

Gurung A, Hung T, Morin J, Gilks CB. Molecular abnormalities in ovarian carcinoma: clinical, morphological and therapeutic correlates. Histopathology. 2013;62:59–70.

Heatley MK. Dissection and reporting of the organs of the female genital tract. J Clin Pathol. 2008;61:241–57.

Herrington CS. Recent advances in molecular gynaecological pathology. Histopathology. 2009;55:243–9.

Kasprzak L, Foulkes WD, Shelling AN. Hereditary ovarian carcinoma. BMJ. 1999;318:786–9.

Khoo U-S, Shen D-H, Wong RW-C, Cheung AN-Y. Gynaecological cancers in genetically susceptible women: new thoughts on tubal pathology. Diagn Histopathol. 2009;15:545–9.

Kurman RJ, Seidman JD, Shih IM. Expert opinion. Serous borderline tumours of the ovary. Histopathology. 2005;47:310–8.

Leen LMS, Singh N. Pathology of primary and metastatic mucinous ovarian neoplasms. J Clin Pathol. 2012;65:591–5.

Lerwill MF, Young RH. Mucinous tumours of the ovary. Diagn Histopathol. 2008;14:366–87.

McCluggage WG. My approach to and thoughts on the typing of ovarian carcinomas. J Clin Pathol. 2008a;61:152–63.

McCluggage WG. Immunohistochemical markers as a diagnostic aid in ovarian pathology. Diagn Histopathol. 2008b;14:335–51.

McCluggage WG. Ten problematic issues identified by pathology review for multidisciplinary gynaecological oncology meetings. J Clin Pathol. 2012a;65:293–301.

McCluggage WG. Immunohistochemistry in the distinction between primary and metastatic ovarian mucinous neoplasms. J Clin Pathol. 2012b;65:596–600.

McCluggage WG, Wilkinson N. Metastatic neoplasms involving the ovary: a review with an emphasis on morphological and immunohistochemical features. Histopathology. 2005;47:231–47.

McCluggage WG, Hirschowitz L, Ganesan R, Kehoe S, Nordin A. Which staging system to use for gynaecological cancers: a survey with recommendations for practice in the UK. J Clin Pathol. 2010;63:768–70.

Miller K, McCluggage WG. Prognostic factors in ovarian adult granulosa cell tumour. J Clin Pathol. 2008;61:881–4.

Rabban JT, Zaloudek CJ. A practical approach to immunohistochemical diagnosis of ovarian germ cell tumours and sex cord-stromal tumours. Histopathology. 2013;62:71–88.

Redman C, Duffy S, Bromham M, Francis K on behalf of the Guideline Development Group. Recognition and initial management of ovarian cancer: summary of NICE guidance. BMJ. 2011;342:973–5.

Robboy SJ, Bentley RC, Russell R, Anderson MC, Mutter GL, Prat J. Pathology of the female reproductive tract. 2nd ed. London: Churchill Livingstone Elsevier; 2009.

Roth LM. Two-tier grading system for ovarian epithelial cancer. Has its time arrived? Am J Surg Pathol. 2007;31:1285–7.

Russell P, Farnsworth A. Surgical pathology of the ovaries. 2nd ed. New York: Churchill Livingstone; 1997.

Scully RE, Young RH, Clement PB. Tumors of the ovary, maldeveloped gonads, fallopian tube and broad ligament. Atlas of tumor pathology. 3rd series. Fascicle 23. Washington: AFIP;1998.

Singh N. Synchronous tumours of the female genital tract. Histopathology. 2010;56:277–85.

Stewart CJR, McCluggage WG. Epithelial-mesenchymal transition in carcinomas of the female genital tract. Histopathology. 2013;62:31–43.

Tavassoli F, Devilee P. WHO classification of tumours. Pathology and genetics. Tumours of the breast and female genital organs. Lyon: IARC Press; 2003.

The Royal College of Pathologists. Cancer Datasets (Vulval Neoplasms, Cervical Neoplasia, Endometrial Cancer, Uterine Sarcomas, Neoplasms of the Ovaries and Fallopian Tubes and Primary Carcinoma of the Peritoneum), and Tissue Pathways for Gynaecological Pathology. Accessed at http://www.rcpath.org/index.asp?Page ID=254.

Vang R, Shih IM, Kurman RJ. Fallopian tube precursors of ovarian low- and high-grade serous neoplasms. Histopathology. 2013;62:44–58.

Wilkinson N, Osborn S, Young RH. Sex cord-stromal tumours of the ovary: a review highlighting recent advances. Diagn Histopathol. 2008;14:388–400.

Willmott F, Allouni KA, Rockall A. Radiological manifestations of metastasis to the ovary. J Clin Pathol. 2012;65:585–90.

Wittekind C, International Union against Cancer, et al. TNM atlas: illustrated guide to the TNM/pTNM classification of malignant tumours. 5th ed. Berlin: Springer; 2005.

Young RH, Gilks CB, Scully RE. Mucinous tumors of the appendix associated with mucinous tumors of the ovary and pseudomyxoma peritonei: a clinicopathologic analysis of 22 cases supporting an origin in the appendix. Am J Surg Pathol. 1991;15:415–29.

Endometrial Carcinoma

The uterus and the ovary are the commonest sites for female genital tract cancer with risk factors for endometrial cancer including obesity, diabetes, nulliparous status, hypertension and late menopause. The majority (>80 % of cases) are type I endometrial adenocarcinoma arising as a result of unopposed exogenous or endogenous oestrogens from a background of endometrial hyperplasia, and presenting confined to the endometrium with a good prognosis. Type II cancers occur in older women, are oestrogen independent and >50 % present with extrauterine spread due to early lymphatic dissemination. Prognosis is poor worsening in the order: clear cell adenocarcinoma, serous adenocarcinoma and carcinosarcoma.

Most endometrial cancers present with abnormal vaginal bleeding and this is particularly significant in a postmenopausal patient with 88 % of patients over 50 years and a peak incidence of 60–64 years of age. Other symptoms include an abdominopelvic mass, feeling of fullness in the abdomen and uterine prolapse. There may also be constipation or urinary frequency. Investigation is by dilatation and curettage under general anaesthetic, but now more commonly outpatient pipelle endometrial sampling. The retrieved fragments are usually very scanty and may require filtering from the formalin fixative. The role of the pathologist is not to phase the endometrium but to comment on whether any functional endometrium is actually represented, and if so, if it is benign, atypical or malignant. Atypical endometrium may represent a false negative sample of a concurrent adenocarcinoma. Investigation also includes transvaginal ultrasound scan which can relate the endometrial stripe thickness to the menopausal status (postmenopausal is usually <5 mm), and detect any focal lesions e.g. polyps. Hysteroscopy allows direct visualisation of the uterine cavity and more extensive sampling. Transcervical resection of the endometrium (TCRE) is reserved for benign dysfunctional endometria in premenopausal patients. If there are histological features suspicious of or diagnostic of malignancy in biopsy material, MRI scan is used to assess tumour stage, in particular the depth of myometrial invasion, and the presence of cervical or extrauterine involvement. CT scan assesses more distant spread.

A significant proportion of patients with atypical hyperplasia and early stage well differentiated endometrioid adenocarcinoma may respond to progesterone therapy, although this is excluded by radiological evidence of myoinvasive disease. In general treatment of uterine cancers (adenocarcinoma, carcinosarcoma, sarcoma) is by hysterectomy and bilateral salpingo-oophorectomy, with peritoneal washings as part of the staging procedure. The surgical approach is often laparoscopic and vaginal. Modified radical hysterectomy (inclusive of vaginal cuff, parametria, omentectomy and limited regional lymphadenectomy) is considered for deeply myoinvasive cancers, those with cervical involvement, or high-grade cancers (serous, clear cell, undifferentiated, squamous cell). They, and cancers with lymphovascular invasion, may also require

D.C. Allen, *Histopathology Reporting*,
DOI 10.1007/978-1-4471-5263-7_24, © Springer-Verlag London 2013

preoperative chemotherapy and/or post-operative chemoradiotherapy. Occasional locally advanced tumours are not amenable to resection and chemo-/radiotherapy is used as the first line of management. This can result in marked cytological changes e.g. radiation atypia mimicking serous intraepithelial carcinoma, or taxane induced ring mitoses. Furthermore, significant tumour regression can lead to only microscopic residual foci of tumour masked by a necroinflammatory response, making assessment of pathological stage difficult. Vaginal vault recurrence of uterine cancer is relatively common and treated with further local surgery and/or radiotherapy. A rare, late complication is post irradiation sarcoma or carcinoma, within the field of treatment after a latent period of several years.

24.1 Gross Description

Specimen

- Curettage/pipelle sample (on an outpatient basis: some cases are also detected by routine cervical smear)/TCRE (transcervical resection of endometrium) chippings.
- Subtotal/total/radical hysterectomy/bilateral salpingo-oophorectomy/limited pelvic lymph node dissection, omentectomy .
- Size (cm) and weight (g).
- Suboptimal fixation of the endometrium in a hysterectomy specimen can make accurate histological assessment problematic. This can be countered by post-surgical injection of formalin with a narrow caliber plastic stylet through the cervical os.

Tumour

Site

- Fundus, body, isthmus. Involvement of the lower uterine segment is unfavourable.

Size

- Length × width × depth (cm) or maximum dimension (cm).

Appearance

- Polypoid/papillary/solid/ulcerated/infiltrative/necrotic/haemorrhagic.
- Malignant mixed mesodermal tumours are typically fundal and polypoid in an elderly patient and may protrude inferiorly through the internal cervical os.

Edge

- Circumscribed/irregular.

Extent

- Infiltration   endometrium,   myometrium, serosa, cervix, parametrium.

Adjacent Endometrium

- Atrophic, hyperplastic, polypoid.

24.2 Histological Type

The vast majority of uterine cancers are *adenocarcinoma of two main types*, although there is overlap between the categories

- *Type I* (*prototype: endometrioid adenocarcinoma*): peri-/postmenopausal, low parity, high socio-economic status, obesity, diabetes, hypertension, hyperoestrogenism (hormonal therapy, endogenous or secreting tumour e.g. ovarian sex cord-stromal), ER positive, background endometrial hyperplasia. Microsatellite instability/PTEN (phosphatase and tensin homologue) mutations.
- *Type II* (*prototypes: serous and clear cell adenocarcinomas, carcinosarcoma*): older patients, more aggressive, atrophic endometrium with precursor serous EIC (endometrial intraepithelial carcinoma), ER±. p53 mutations.

A minority of endometrial cancers are *familial*, or associated with *hereditary non-polyposis colorectal cancer* (*HNPCC*) where incidence (2 %) approximates that of bowel cancer. Adenocarcinoma is usually of endometrioid type, but distinctive clues to these microsatellite unstable cancers are tumour in the lower uterine segment and of undifferentiated morphology with a prominent   infiltrate   of   peri-/intratumoural lymphocytes (TILs). This can be further explored with mismatch repair immunohistochemistry. Significance as to prognosis is uncertain. Cumulative dose of *tamoxifen in patients with breast cancer* is also a risk factor for endometrial carcinoma.

Endometrioid Adenocarcinoma

- *70–80 % of cases.*
- Typical: low-grade well differentiated endometrial type glandular pattern, in perimenopausal patients, and due to unopposed oestrogenic drive ± adjacent endometrial hyperplasia.
- Variants:
  - *With squamous differentiation* – up to 30 % of cases. The tumour is graded on the glandular component as it can be difficult to tell if the squamous cell element is benign or malignant. Where both elements are well differentiated the previous designation of adenocanthoma is now rarely used.
  - *Secretory carcinoma* – the cells resemble secretory endometrium.
  - *Ciliated carcinoma* – rare, the cells resemble tubal epithelium.
  - *Villoglandular carcinoma* – low-grade, well differentiated and papillary. Exclude high-grade serous carcinoma (high-grade nuclear characteristics with a tufted papillary pattern).
  - *Sertoliform carcinoma.*

Serous (Papillary) Adenocarcinoma

- *5–10 % of cases.*
- *High-grade* in the elderly and de-novo with no adjacent hyperplasia but associated with *serous EIC.*
- Typically shows *disproportionate lympho-vascular/myometrial invasion* and *omental spread* relative to the amount of endometrial disease. This means that EIC or stage I serous carcinoma can be associated with *extensive extrauterine spread* and present as a *primary peritoneal serous adenocarcinoma* but no

clinically or radiologically obvious uterine or ovarian mass lesion.
- Potentially *multifocal* with extrauterine lesions e.g. ovary, fallopian tube.
- High-grade nuclear characteristics, usually a papillary pattern but occasionally tubuloglandular.
- Necrosis and psammoma bodies are often seen. Over expresses p53, Her-2, p16, PTEN, HMGA2 and Ki-67. ER ±/PR-. It is also WT-1 negative in distinction from ovarian papillary serous adenocarcinoma which is positive and this is a useful feature in differential diagnosis and staging.
- *Poor prognosis* with *30 % 5 year survival.*

Clear Cell Adenocarcinoma

- *1–5 % of cases*; postmenopausal. Not related to diethylstilboestrol and *aggressive* with myometrial invasion.
- >50 % of the cells are clear cell, mixed solid/glandular/tubulocystic/papillary architecture.

Mucinous Adenocarcinoma

- >50 % cells have stainable mucin.
- *Usually low-grade, minimally invasive and good prognosis.*
- Distinguish from cervical adenocarcinoma by differential biopsy/curettage, and exclude a gastrointestinal primary (clinical history, CK20/CDX-2 positive/CK7 negative).

Squamous Cell Carcinoma

- In old age often with cervical stenosis and pyometra; exclude spread from a cervical carcinoma.

Mixed

- Second component is >10 % of the tumour area e.g. composite endometrioid/serous/clear cell adenocarcinoma. Any carcinoma with *5–10% serous characteristics* tends to behave more aggressively and should be designated as such. Adenocarcinoma with squamous cell differentiation is excluded. Adenosquamous carcinoma (where both components are obviously malignant) is a mixed lesion with a poor prognosis.

Undifferentiated Carcinoma

- Small cell/not otherwise specified: *aggressive*.
- Spread from a cervical primary or lung primary must be excluded in small cell carcinoma.
- It can be difficult to distinguish between *high-grade endometrioid, serous and undifferentiated uterine carcinomas* and more recognisable foci should be sought using extra blocks. *Undifferentiated carcinoma* shows a sheeted dyscohesive pattern of large, monomorphic, mitotically active cells sometimes with rhabdoid cells, giant cells, necrosis and myxoid stroma. It lacks a minor component of more usual serous or endometrioid cancer and is only focally cytokeratin positive. More than *50% present with advanced stage* and *ultimately fatal disease*. Occasional cases are in younger patients, in the lower uterine segment and associated with DNA mismatch repair abnormalities.

Malignant Mixed Müllerian Tumours (MMMT)

- *Low-grade malignancy*: adenosarcoma; carcinofibroma. Both are rare.
- *High-grade malignancy*: carcinosarcoma/sarcomatoid carcinoma is a carcinoma comprising either serous or endometrioid endometrial adenocarcinoma with a *biphasic pattern* and component of vimentin/cytokeratin positive malignant spindle cells. Lesions can be either *homologous* or *heterologous* (containing tissues alien to the uterus, commonly immature/

malignant cartilage, striated muscle, bone). Carcinosarcoma is the commonest malignant mixed tumour and 50 % contain heterologous elements (see Sect. 24.8 for further discussion).

Metastatic Carcinoma

- *Direct spread*: cervix, bladder, rectum.
- *Distant spread*: infiltrating lobular breast carcinoma, kidney, malignant melanoma, stomach, pancreas. The commonest are breast, stomach, colon, pancreas carcinomas. Often myometrial with an endometrial component, metastases can mimic primary endometrial disease e.g. infiltrating lobular breast carcinoma (endometrial stromal sarcoma), renal carcinoma (clear cell adenocarcinoma), and colorectal carcinoma (mucinous adenocarcinoma). A relevant *clinical history* and *comparison with previous histology* are crucial in making the distinction. Metastases should be considered in any endometrial cancer of unusual appearance, multinodular growth pattern, with prominent lymphovascular involvement or lack of precancerous endometrial changes.

24.3 Differentiation

Well/moderate/poor/undifferentiated.

- 80–85 % are well to moderately differentiated. Grade I/II/III for endometrioid adenocarcinoma.

The glandular component of endometrioid adenocarcinomas is graded I <5 %, II 6–50 %, and III >50 % non-squamous, non-morular solid growth pattern. Nuclear grading can also raise the architectural grade e.g. II→III: grade 1 (oval nuclei, even chromatin, inconspicuous nucleolus, few mitoses) and grade 3 (irregular, rounded nuclei, prominent nucleoli, frequent mitoses). Grade 2 nuclear grade is intermediate between grades 1 and 3. Some cancers show grade heterogeneity indicative of tumour progression. In tumours with squamous cell differentiation grading is based on the glandular component. Serous, clear cell, carcinosarcoma and undifferentiated carcinomas are considered high-grade with nuclear grade taking precedence over architecture. Mucinous carcinomas are generally grade 1.

24.4   Extent of Local Tumour Spread

Border: pushing/infiltrative.

Lymphocytic reaction: prominent/sparse.

Endometrium

- *EIN (endometrial intraepithelial neoplasia)* is an umbrella term encompassing and highlighting the diagnostic difficulties there are in distinguishing between entities on the overlap spectrum of complex endometrial hyperplasia with atypia, and, intra-endometrial adenocarcinoma. Progression along this spectrum is characterised by increased *glandular crowding and complexity*, *intraglandular necrosis* and *cytological atypia* with *reduction in intervening stroma*. An important differential diagnosis is a benign mimic with focal glandular crowding e.g. endometrial polyp (look for covering epithelium and prominent vascular stroma with thick walled vessels). Another possible consideration is atypical polypoid adenomyoma arising from the isthmus in younger patients (look for a glandular proliferation in abundant smooth muscle).
- *EIC (endometrial intraepithelial carcinoma)* is effectively serous adenocarcinoma in situ of the endometrial surface epithelium and is present *adjacent to or overlying 90 % of serous adenocarcinomas*. It over expresses p53 and Ki-67. It is also occasionally seen with clear cell carcinoma and even extrauterine peritoneal disease in the absence of invasive endometrial cancer.
- *EIN* and *EIC* are to be distinguished from the range of relatively commonly occurring *endometrial metaplasias* and *reactive epithelial changes*. These include ciliated tubal, mucinous, squamous morular and intestinal metaplasias,

and surface syncytial, papillary, eosinophilic and clear cell changes.

Myometrium

- Proportion of wall involved <50 %, ≥ 50 %.
- If ≥50 % on MRI scan a radical hysterectomy is considered. Outer myometrial involvement is seen in about 25 % of cases.

Extent of myometrial invasion relates to the histological type and grade of carcinoma. True myometrial invasion must be distinguished from both a normal irregular outline or expansion of the endo-/myometrial junction (look for a continuous line of myometrial vascular structures in a compressed atrophic myometrium), and, abnormal epithelium in pre-existing adenomyosis (look for periglandular endometrial stroma – CD10 positive). Invasive stromal desmoplasia and inflammation are useful diagnostic clues although often not present in carcinoma. Alternative patterns of invasion should also be considered e.g. diffuse along a broad pushing front, or, MELF (microcystic, elongated, fragmented). Endometrial/myometrial junction and endometriosis containing carcinoma usually have a broad or lobulated front and smooth outline associated with native endometrial stroma. To some extent this dilemma is superseded by FIGO staging with stage I disease encompassing any carcinoma confined to the endometrium or up to <50 % of the myometrium. An approximate landmark for the latter is invasion less than or beyond the myometrial vascular arcuate plexus. Occasionally a patient is a non-operable surgical candidate due to co-morbidity and a TCRE specimen is provided – assessment of myoinvasion can be problematic due to the random orientation of the chippings.

Serosa

- Distance (mm) of the deepest point of invasion from the nearest serosal surface. Direct serosal spread is relatively unusual but is associated with a 40 % 5 year survival rate and a tendency for recurrences in extra-abdominal sites.

Vagina

- Vaginal recurrences are not uncommon and treated by further local surgery or radiation therapy. The rare situation of clinical presentation of endometrial carcinoma with a vaginal metastasis is adverse with a median survival of 1–2 years.

Parametrium

- Parametrial involvement either by direct extension or lymphatic invasion is an *indicator of poor prognosis*. It can only be assessed when there has been a modified radical hysterectomy i.e. for a preoperative diagnosis of a high-grade cancer or where imaging has suggested cervical or deep myometrial involvement.

Endocervix/Exocervix

- *10 % of cases* usually by direct invasion, lymphatic spread or occasionally by implantation following curettage. *Stromal invasion* increases the *risk of pelvic lymph node metastases*. It must not be confused with post biopsy or cut-up artifactual 'carry-in', florid reactive changes following biopsy sampling or curettage, or other benign mimics of neoplasia e.g. mesonephric remnants or tuboendometrial metaplasia. There is considerable interobserver variation in assessing whether there is tumour involvement of endocervical glands versus cervical stroma. Distinction between an *endometrial* and *cervical origin for a tumour* can be difficult clinically, radiologically and histologically in curettage samples. Some reliance is placed on the *nature of the tissue from which the carcinoma appears to be arising* e.g. dysplastic cervix or hyperplastic endometrium. *Immunohistochemistry* may also be of help in *low-grade adenocarcinomas* in that uterine endometrioid adenocarcinoma is usually vimentin/ER positive and CEA negative while cervical adenocarcinoma is the opposite of this. In addition, p16 antibody also stains more strongly in cervical

adenocarcinoma. Alternatively with high-grade or undifferentiated carcinoma endometrial lesions may be p53+/p16- and cervical cancers the converse of this. Cervical squamous carcinoma may also be strongly p63 positive.

Fallopian Tubes/Ovaries

- Either by direct extension or metastatic spread. Lymphovascular invasion favours the latter. If extrauterine disease is confined to the ovaries or fallopian tubes 5 year survival is still relatively favourable at 75 %.

Omentum

FIGO
FIGO staging is recommended and applicable to uterine carcinoma and carcinosarcoma.

I	Tumour confined to the corpus:
	(a) Invades endometrium or less than half of the myometrium
	(b) Invades half or more of the myometrium
II	Tumour invades cervical stroma but does not extend beyond the uterus
III	Local and/or regional lymph node tumour spread:
	(a) Invades uterine serosa and/or adnexa(e)
	(b) Vaginal and/or parametrial involvement
	(c) Metastasis to pelvic (C1) and/or paraaortic (C2) lymph nodes
IV	Tumour invades
	(a) Bladder and/or bowel mucosa[a] and/or
	(b) Distant metastases including intraabdominal and/or inguinal lymph nodes.

[a]Requires histological confirmation by biopsy. Invasion of the rectal wall or bladder wall is pT3. Positive peritoneal cytology is reported separately without changing the stage. "Frozen pelvis" is a clinical term meaning tumour extension through the parametrium to the pelvic wall(s) i.e. IIIB (See Figs. 24.1, 24.2 and 24.3)

24.5 Lymphovascular Invasion

Present/absent.

Intra-/extratumoural. Usually at the invasive front of the carcinoma.

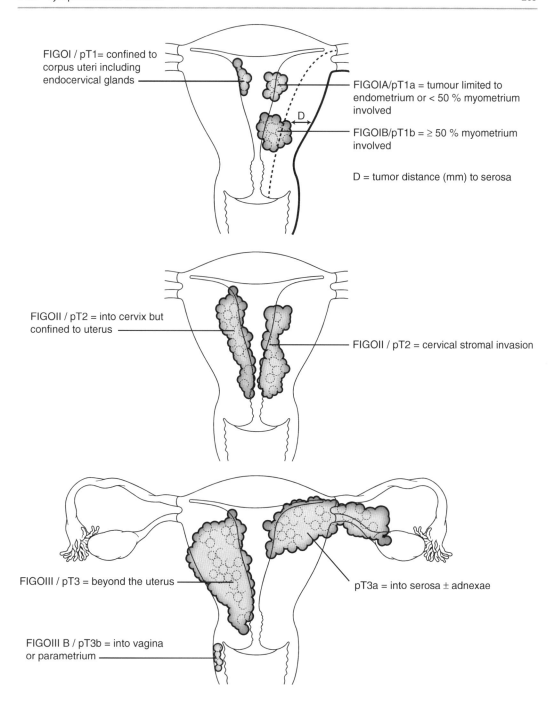

Fig. 24.1 Uterine carcinoma (Reproduced, with permission, from Allen (2006), © 2006)

- Seen particularly in *serous* and deeply *myo-invasive endometrioid adenocarcinomas*. Lymphovascular invasion in the outer myometrium is an adverse prognostic indicator but it does not upstage an otherwise superficially invasive (FIGO IA) carcinoma.

- Beware vascular *pseudoinvasion* in laparoscopic hysterectomy (LAH) specimens and autolysis related cut-up *smear artifact*. It can also be difficult to separate true lymphovascular invasion from intramyometrial peritumoural *retraction artifact*. These distinctions

Fig. 24.2 Uterine carcinoma (Reproduced, with permission, from Wittekind et al. (2005), © 2005)

TNM: **T4**
FIGO:IVA

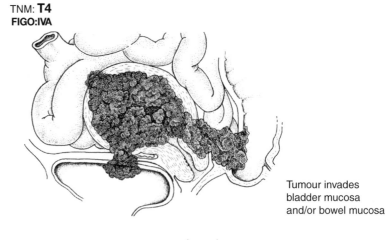

Tumour invades
bladder mucosa
and/or bowel mucosa

Fig. 24.3 Uterine carcinoma: regional lymph nodes (Reproduced, with permission, from Wittekind et al. (2005), © 2005)

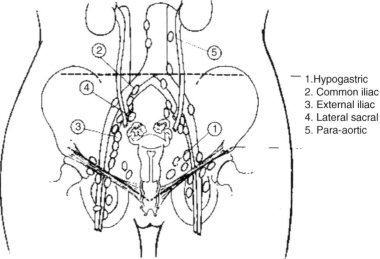

1.Hypogastric
2. Common iliac
3. External iliac
4. Lateral sacral
5. Para-aortic

are important as *lymphovascular invasion* is an *indicator for postoperative adjuvant therapy*. The presence of red blood cells, a perivascular lymphocytic infiltrate and a demonstrable endothelial lining (CD34, D2-40) are useful pointers. True vascular invasion is also unusual in early stage low-grade cancers. Note that it can also be mimicked by the cystic spaces (lined by epithelium rather than endothelium) of the MELF pattern of myometrial invasion.

24.6 Lymph Nodes

Site/number/size/number involved/extracapsular spread.

Regional nodes: pelvic (obturator and internal iliac), common and external iliac, parametrial, sacral and para-aortic. A regional lymphadenectomy will ordinarily include a minimum of ten lymph nodes.

The commonest sites of *extrauterine spread* are the *regional lymph nodes* and *ovaries*. Lymph node disease relates to the tumour grade, type, depth of invasion and lymphovascular involvement. *Invasion of the outer third of the myometrium* is associated with *lymph node metastasis in up to 33 % of cases*. Pelvic and paraaortic lymph node metastases are associated with 65–85 % and 35–45 % 5 year survivals respectively. Initial spread is to pelvic lymph nodes but there can be skip metastasis to involve paraaortic lymph nodes alone. *Recurrences* are in the pelvis and vaginal vault. High-grade serous carcinoma tends to show extensive omental and pelvic disease. *Distant metastases* of uterine carcinoma are to lung, liver, bone, central nervous system and skin of the scalp.

24.7   Excision Margins

Distances (mm) to the serosa, tubal and inferior vaginal limits.

24.8   Other Pathology

Uterus

*   *Polyp(s)*, *hyperplasia* (*simple*, *or*, *complex with architectural±cytological atypia*), *adenomyosis*. Carcinoma occasionally develops within a preexisting *endometrial polyp* although this is increased in *tamoxifen therapy* (see below). It can be of either usual low-grade endometrioid or high-grade serous type.
    About *25% of untreated atypical hyperplasias progress to adenocarcinoma* and up to *40% are associated with concurrent disease*. Features favouring *adenocarcinoma* over complex hyperplasia with cytological atypia are: *intraglandular epithelial bridges*, *stroma free papillary and cribriform epithelial patterns*, *intraglandular polymorphs and necrosis*, *cytological atypia*, *mitoses and stromal elimination and invasion*. Criteria for stromal invasion include a. irregularly infiltrating glands associated with a fibroblastic or desmoplastic response, and/or, b. extensive papillary or confluent glandular (cribriform) growth patterns. Stromal and superficial myometrial invasion are useful in distinguishing between intra-endometrial and invasive adenocarcinoma in curettage specimens. Inhabitation of *adenomyosis* by complex hyperplasia or adenocarcinoma usually shows circumscribed foci with surrounding native endometrial stroma.

Ovary

*   *Thecoma* and *granulosa cell tumour*: can result in oestrogenic drive to the endometrium

resulting in simple or complex hyperplasia, or adenocarcinoma.

*   *Accompanying ovarian carcinoma*: this is seen in 5–10 % of endometrial carcinomas. Distinction between *synchronous primary lesions* and *ovarian secondaries* rests on the latter being bilateral, multinodular, often serosal and with ovarian stromal lymphovascular invasion. The uterine primary will usually be high-grade with deep myometrial and lymphovascular invasion. There is a higher frequency of *concurrent early stage primaries in endometrioid adenocarcinoma of the uterus and ovary* (*25%*) than in the other cancer subtypes.

Other Comments

Tamoxifen effects: tamoxifen related polyps, hyperplasia, adenocarcinoma, adenosarcoma, carcinosarcoma (MMMT). Tamoxifen is an antioestrogen but has paradoxical oestrogenic effects on the endometrium leading to an increased frequency of a range of endometrial neoplasms some of which are prognostically adverse. Polyps can be large, multiple, necrotic, have areas of glandular, papillary or clear cell metaplasia, and may even harbour adenocarcinoma, often serous in type.

Carcinosarcoma: is often polypoid at the fundus of an elderly patient with deep myometrial and lymphovascular invasion. About *30% present with stage III/IV disease*. The carcinomatous component is usually *high-grade glandular* (endometrioid, clear cell, serous or undifferentiated), and the *sarcomatous element homologous* (cf. endometrial stroma, leiomyosarcoma, fibrosarcoma) or *heterologous* (striated muscle, cartilage, bone, fat). Immunohistochemistry for epithelial and mesenchymal markers e.g. desmin may be necessary to confirm the diagnosis. This *aggressive neoplasm has a 20–40% 5 year survival*.

Adenosarcoma: the majority (80 %) of adenosarcomas arise in the postmenopausal endometrium. They are polypoid with proliferative type glands and usually homologous stromal type sarcoma distributed in a condensed periglandular cambium layer. *Recurrence* (*30%*) relates to mitoses, stromal overgrowth and myoinvasion in this *low- to intermediate-grade malignancy.*

Immunophenotype

Endometrioid adenocarcinoma usually co-expresses cytokeratins (7, 8, 18, 19) and vimentin. Oestrogen and progesterone marking is common relating to histological type and grade, and is of some use in assessing potential response to hormonal therapy in disseminated disease. CEA stains weaker than in cervical carcinoma. In contrast to grade 3 endometrioid adenocarcinomas, high-grade *serous adenocarcinomas* over express p53, p16, PTEN, HMGA2 and may be negative for ER/PR. These immunoprofiles may be of use in distinguishing high-grade endometrioid adenocarcinoma from serous adenocarcinoma with a tubuloglandular pattern. Uterine serous adenocarcinoma is also WT1 negative in contrast to ovarian serous adenocarcinoma. DNA aneuploidy is an index of high-grade, advanced stage tumours and over expression of Ki-67, p53 and Her-2 (20–40 % of cases) is adverse.

Prognosis

Radical hysterectomy is considered for endometrial carcinoma if there is ≥50 % myometrial invasion with grade II or III histology, invasion of the cervix, undifferentiated, clear cell or serous adenocarcinoma, lymphovascular invasion or suspicious lymph nodes on CT scan. *Preoperative adjuvant chemo-/radiotherapy* may also be used in these circumstances. *Intraoperative frozen section* of suspicious lymph nodes is an important prequel to radical resection, and if positive a more conservative approach adopted.

Overall 5 year survival for endometrial carcinoma is *80–85%* with *type I* oestrogen-related cases arising from a background of hyperplasia typically presenting with stage I disease, and doing better than *type II* non-oestrogen-dependent lesions (*30–70% 5 year survival*). Serous, undifferentiated, squamous cell and clear cell carcinomas are more aggressive than equivalent stage endometrioid tumours. *Lymphovascular invasion,*

which correlates with progressing tumour grade, myometrial invasion and stage (cervical and extra-uterine spread), is an *adverse prognostic factor* (70–75 % 5 year survival). Prognosis also relates strongly to *tumour stage*: I, 82–95 % 5 year survival; II, 60–80 %; III, 30–50 %. *Tumour grade* has an influence in that grade I tumours (87 % 5 year survival) fare better than grade III cancers (58 % 5 year survival).

24.9   Other Malignancy

Endometrial stromal lesions can be benign (stromal nodule) or malignant, the latter having infiltrating margins. Biopsy or curettage samples impose limitations in making this assessment, which is more appropriately done on a hysterectomy specimen.

Endometrial Stromal Sarcoma

- A *low-grade malignancy resembling endometrial stroma* (stromal cells/spiral arteriole vascular pattern) with infiltrative margins and variable mitoses (usually <5–10/10 high-power fields). Shows characteristic *lymphovascular invasion* (previously called endolymphatic stromal myosis). It comprises 20 % of uterine sarcomas and 2 % of uterine malignancies. An *80–90% 5 year survival rate* if confined to the uterus, but prone to *local pelvic or abdominal recurrence (30%) after a lag period of many years*, and may cause pressure effects e.g. hydronephrosis. *High stage tumours* have a *40% 10 year survival rate*. Sometimes hormone responsive to adjuvant progesterone therapy.

Undifferentiated Uterine Sarcoma

- Previous and current alternate designation as high-grade endometrial stromal sarcoma. Characterised by cellular pleomorphism, mitoses (>10/10 high-power fields) and destructive myometrial invasion with infiltrating margins and aggressive behaviour. *Size of tumour (>4 cm)* and *extrauterine extension* are adverse indicators in low- and high-grade lesions. Treatment is surgical although there is some evidence for partial response to chemotherapy and hormonal manipulation in metastatic disease.

FIGO staging for uterine sarcomas

I	Tumour confined to the uterine corpus
	(a) ≤5 cm
	(b) >5 cm
II	Tumour extends beyond the uterus
	(a) To adnexa(e)
	(b) To extrauterine pelvic tissues
III	Tumour invades abdominal tissues
	(a) One site
	(b) Two sites
	(c) Pelvic and/or paraaortic lymph nodes
IV	Tumour invades
	(a) Bladder and/or rectum, or
	(b) Distant metastases.

Immunophenotype of mesenchymal tumours: endometrial stromal sarcomas are CD10, WT1, ER, PR and vimentin positive. Up to 50 % are desmin positive but they are h-caldesmon negative. Low-grade lesions also preserve a pericellular reticulin pattern. Differential diagnosis of endometrial stromal sarcoma is leiomyomatous tumour (strongly desmin/h-caldesmon positive ± CD10), and that of undifferentiated uterine sarcoma is undifferentiated carcinoma (cytokeratin, EMA positive).

Leiomyomatous Tumours

- *Malignancy relates to a combination of*:
  infiltrative margins.
  cellular atypia.
  coagulative tumour cell necrosis.
  mitoses >10/10 high-power fields.
  Leiomyosarcoma (1–3 % of uterine malignancies/40–50 % of uterine sarcomas) is usually a *high-grade* lesion with a bulky mass, satellite nodules, areas of necrosis and *variably poor outlook (20–70 % 5 year survival)*. *Surgical excision* with or without adjuvant chemotherapy is the mainstay of treatment.

Variants are typical (spindle cells), epithelioid and myxoid. Tumour cells are smooth muscle actin, desmin, h-caldesmon, calponin and vimentin positive with cross reactivity for cytokeratin (CAM 5.2) and variable ER expression.

- *Uncertain malignant potential*:
  Cellular atypia and mitoses 5–10/10 high-power fields indicate probable malignancy if the atypia is moderate or severe.
- *Cellular leiomyoma*:
  Benign; identify thick walled vessels and strong desmin positivity to distinguish from an endometrial stromal tumour.
- *Mitotically active leiomyoma*:
  Benign if no significant cytological atypia, abnormal mitoses or coagulative tumour cell necrosis.
- *Cell type*:
  Myxoid and epithelioid leiomyosarcomas have less tumour cell necrosis, cytological atypia and mitotic activity. Relatively bland myxoid lesions can locally recur and metastasise. An infiltrative growth pattern is a useful diagnostic feature.
- *Beware pseudomalignancy*:
  1. Bizarre *symplastic leiomyoma*. Benign if the symplastic nuclear change is focal, the mitotic count is low (<3/10 high-power fields) and coagulative tumour cell necrosis is absent.
  2. Changes after *gonadotrophin analogue treatment*, viz. haemorrhage and necrosis, symplastic type nuclear atypia and apparent hypercellularity. Extensive coagulative necrosis after uterine artery embolisation can also confuse, but other features of malignancy such as atypia and mitoses are usually absent.
  3. *Intravenous leiomyomatosis* with vascular invasion and "metastases" but not malignant.

Choriocarcinoma/Placental Site Trophoblastic Tumour (PSTT)

- After abortion, normal or molar pregnancy.
- See Chap. 28.

Malignant Lymphoma/Leukaemia

- See Chap. 25.

Others

- Haemangiopericytoma, angiosarcoma, soft tissue sarcomas and germ cell tumours are all rare.

Bibliography

Al – Nafussi A. Uterine smooth muscle tumours: practical approach to diagnosis. Curr Diagn Pathol. 2004;10:140–56.

Allen DC. Histopathology reporting: guidelines for surgical cancer. 2nd ed. Springer: London; 2006.

Ambros RA, Sherman ME, Zahn CM, Bitterman P, Kurman RJ. Endometrial intraepithelial carcinoma: a distinctive lesion specifically associated with tumors displaying serous differentiation. Hum Pathol. 1995;26:1260–7.

Baak JPA, Mutter GL. EIN and WHO 94. J Clin Pathol. 2005;58:1–6.

Baker P, Oliva E. Endometrial stromal tumours of the uterus: a practical approach using conventional morphology and ancillary techniques. J Clin Pathol. 2007;60:235–43.

Burch DM, Tavassoli FA. Myxoid leiomyosarcoma of the uterus. Histopathology. 2011;59:1144–55.

Catasus L, Gallardo A, Prat J. Molecular genetics of endometrial carcinoma. Diagn Histopathol. 2009;15:554–9.

Chiang S, Oliva E. Recent developments in uterine mesenchymal neoplasms. Histopathology. 2013;62:124–37.

Clarke BA, Gilks CB. Endometrial carcinoma: controversies in histopathological assessment of grade and tumour cell type. J Clin Pathol. 2010;63:410–5.

Clarke B, McCluggage WG. Iatrogenic lesions and artefacts in gynaecological pathology. J Clin Pathol. 2009;62:104–12.

Darvishian F, Hummer AJ, Thaler HT, Bhargava R, Linkov I, Soslow RA. Serous endometrial cancers that mimic endometrial adenocarcinoma. Am J Surg Pathol. 2004;28:1568–78.

Ferguson SE, Tornos C, Hummer A, Barakat RR, Soslow RA. Prognostic features of surgical stage 1 uterine carcinosarcoma. Am J Surg Pathol. 2007;31:1653–61.

Folkins AK, Longacre TA. Hereditary gynaecological malignancies: advances in screening and treatment. Histopathology. 2013;62:2–30.

Fox H, Wells M, editors. Haines and Taylor. Obstetrical and gynaecological pathology. 5th ed. Edinburgh: Churchill Livingstone; 2003.

Garg K, Soslow RA. Lynch syndrome (hereditary nonpolyposis colorectal cancer) and endometrial carcinoma. J Clin Pathol. 2009;62:679–84.

Grayson W, Cooper K. Application of immunohistochemistry in the evaluation of neoplastic epithelial lesions of the uterine cervix and endometrium. Curr Diagn Pathol. 2003;9:19–25.

Heatley MK. Dissection and reporting of the organs of the female genital tract. J Clin Pathol. 2008;61:241–57.

Herrington CS. Recent advances in molecular gynaecological pathology. Histopathology. 2009;55:243–9.

Hirschowitz L, Nucci M, Zaino RJ. Problematic issues in the staging of endometrial, cervical and vulval carcinomas. Histopathology. 2013;62:176–202.

Ismail SM. Gynaecological effects of Tamoxifen. J Clin Pathol. 1999;52:83–8.

Ismail SM. Histopathological challenges in the diagnosis of endometrial hyperplasia and carcinoma. Curr Diagn Pathol. 2006;12:312–24.

Loddenkemper C, Foss HD, Dallenbach FE, Stein H. Recent advances in the histopathology of stromal tumours of the endometrium. Curr Diagn Pathol. 2005;11:125–32.

Matias-Guiu X, Prat J. Molecular pathology of endometrial carcinoma. Histopathology. 2013;62:111–23.

McCluggage WG. My approach to the interpretation of endometrial biopsies and curettings. J Clin Pathol. 2006;59:801–12.

McCluggage WG. Problematic areas in the reporting of endometrial carcinomas in hysterectomy specimens. Diagn Histopathol. 2009;15:571–81.

McCluggage WG. Ten problematic issues identified by pathology review for multidisciplinary gynaecological oncology meetings. J Clin Pathol. 2012;65:293–301.

McCluggage WG, Hirschowitz L, Ganesan R, Kehoe S, Nordin A. Which staging system to use for gynaecological cancers: a survey with recommendations for practice in the UK. J Clin Pathol. 2010;63:768–70.

McCluggage WG, Connolly LE, McBride HA, Kalloger S, Gilks CB. HMGA2 is commonly expressed in uterine serous carcinomas and is a useful adjunct to diagnosis. Histopathology. 2012;60:547–53.

Nicolae A, Preda O, Nogales FF. Endometrial metaplasias and reactive changes: a spectrum of altered differentiation. J Clin Pathol. 2011;64:97–106.

Pecorelli S, FIGO Committee on Gynecologic Oncology. Revised FIGO staging for carcinoma of the vulva, cervix and endometrium. Int J Gynecol Obstet. 2009;105:103–4.

Prat J. FIGO Committee on Gynecologic Oncology. FIGO staging for uterine sarcomas. Int J Gynecol Obstet. 2009;104:177–8.

Robboy SJ, Bentley RC, Russell R, Anderson MC, Mutter GL, Prat J. Pathology of the female reproductive tract. 2nd ed. London: Churchill Livingstone Elsevier; 2009.

Saso S, Chatterjee J, Georgiou E, Ditri AM, Smith RJ, Ghaem-Maghami S. Endometrial cancer. BMJ. 2011;342:84–9.

Scurry J, Patel K, Wells M. Gross examination of uterine specimens. J Clin Pathol. 1993;46:388–93.

Silverberg SG. Protocol for the examination of specimens from patients with carcinomas of the endometrium. Arch Pathol Lab Med. 1999;123:28–32.

Silverberg SG, Kurman RJ. Tumors of the uterine corpus and gestational trophoblastic disease. Atlas of tumor pathology. 3rd series. Fascicle 3. Washington: AFIP; 1992.

Singh N. Synchronous tumours of the female genital tract. Histopathology. 2010;56:277–85.

Soslow RA. Uterine mesenchymal tumors: a review of selected topics. Diagn Histopathol. 2008;14:175–88.

Soslow RA. High-grade endometrial carcinomas – strategies for typing. Histopathology. 2013;62:89–110.

Stewart CJR, McCluggage WG. Epithelial-mesenchymal transition in carcinomas of the female genital tract. Histopathology. 2013;62:31–43.

Tavassoli F, Devilee P. WHO classification of tumours. Pathology and genetics. Tumours of the breast and female genital organs. Lyon: IARC Press; 2003.

The Royal College of Pathologists. Cancer Datasets (Vulval Neoplasms, Cervical Neoplasia, Endometrial Cancer, Uterine Sarcomas, Neoplasms of the Ovaries and Fallopian Tubes and Primary Carcinoma of the Peritoneum), and Tissue Pathways for Gynaecological Pathology. Accessed at http://www.rcpath.org/index.asp?PageID =254.

Wittekind C, International Union against Cancer, et al. TNM atlas: illustrated guide to the TNM/pTNM classification of malignant tumours. 5th ed. Berlin: Springer; 2005.

Cervical Carcinoma

Cervical cancer is the second commonest cancer in females worldwide. Its incidence in Western Society is decreasing due to screening programmes and this will be improved upon by HPV (Human Papilloma Virus) vaccination schemes. A majority of deaths related to cervical cancer are in developing countries. Cervical dysplasia and cancer are predisposed to by HPV infection, early age at onset of sexual intercourse, multiple sexual partners, and smoking.

Cervical epithelial lesions are often detected because of an abnormal smear as part of a cervical screening programme. A persistent or high-grade abnormality is referred for colposcopic visualisation of the squamocolumnar epithelial transformation zone to delineate abnormal areas of mucosa characterised by punctation, mosaicism and loss of uptake of iodine (AWE: acetowhite epithelium). Cervical punch biopsy determines the nature of the abnormality, which if localised, is thermally ablated or resected by large loop or cone biopsy depending on its extent. The aim is to completely excise any precancerous lesion. Specimens are orientated, serially sliced and all processed with standard step sections to establish the nature (squamous cell or glandular) and grade of the lesion, the presence of any invasive component, and relationship to the exocervical, endocervical and deep margins. Close histocytological correlation is required for accurate reporting and smear follow up of completely excised lesions is for 5–10 years with subsequent return to usual screening programme intervals. A proportion of established cervical cancers are asymptomatic, in the older age group and undiscovered due to non-attendance at cervical smear appointments. Some result from misinterpretation and undercalling, or non-representative sampling of previous smears in what is a screening programme with inevitable false negative cases. Symptomatic disease (e.g. postcoital bleeding) requires clinical examination, and if a cancer is suspected, a targeted wedge biopsy rather than a punch biopsy taken as this has a greater chance of establishing invasive disease. Tumour staging is by MRI scan (for local spread) and CT scan (for distant spread). Occasionally PET scan is done for distant metastases, and if imaging cannot exclude bladder or bowel involvement, cystoscopy and sigmoidoscopy may be required.

Cold cone knife biopsy may be considered for small cancers or if a cervical glandular lesion is suspected. However, in general, with tumours greater than FIGO stage IA, radical hysterectomy inclusive of pelvic lymphadenectomy is carried out. Laparoscopic vaginal hysterectomy is used for tumours ≤2 cm. Intraoperative frozen section of clinically suspicious lymph nodes or sentinel lymph node mapping is sometimes indicated before proceeding to radical surgery. In occasional cases in young women with a FIGO IB tumour ≤2 cm a fertility sparing radical trachelectomy (upper vagina, cervix, parametria) with laparoscopic lymphadenectomy is performed. It can be associated with up to a 50 % chance of successful subsequent pregnancy. Postoperative chemoradiation is indicated for patients with positive pelvic lymph nodes, and, radiotherapy for

D.C. Allen, *Histopathology Reporting*,
DOI 10.1007/978-1-4471-5263-7_25, © Springer-Verlag London 2013

lymph node negative patients but with more than one-third depth stromal invasion, lymphovascular invasion or tumour diameter >4 cm. Indications for pelvic exenteration are invasion of adjacent organs, recurrent disease and severe pelvic irradiation necrosis, in the absence of distant extrapelvic metastases on CT/PET scan. Advanced disease may present with ureteric obstruction and chronic renal failure, haematuria or rectal symptoms. It can be treated by primary chemoradiation with subsequent salvage hysterectomy, or exenteration if deemed appropriate by the clinical multidisciplinary team. Less than 5 % of patients with recurrent disease are alive at 5 years.

25.1   Gross Description

Specimen

- Cervical smear/punch or wedge biopsy/diathermy (hot) or knife (cold) cone biopsy/ LLETZ (large loop excision of transformation zone)/hysterectomy/trachelectomy with laparoscopic lymphadenectomy/radical (Wertheim's) hysterectomy with vaginal cuff, parametria and lymphadenectomy/ pelvic (anterior/posterior/total) exenteration (components: bladder, ureters, uterus, vagina, tubes and ovaries, rectum)
- Size (cm) and weight (g).

Tumour

Site
- Endocervix/exocervix.
- Anterior/posterior.
- Lateral (right/left).

Size
- Length × width × depth   (cm)   or   maximum dimension (cm).
- Early stromal invasion is breech of the basement membrane with scant stromal penetration <1 mm in depth.

- Microinvasion is a term that was inconsistently used and is no longer favoured. *Early cancer* is more appropriately designated by FIGO stage as defined by the depth and horizontal extent of invasive disease:
  Depth – ≤3 mm (FIGO IA1) or ≤5 mm (FIGO IA2) depth of invasion from the nearest (surface or glandular) basement membrane, usually involved by CIN/CGIN (cervical intraepithelial neoplasia/cervical glandular intraepithelial neoplasia).
  Horizontal extent - ≤7 mm.
  Vessels – venous or lymphatic permeation *does not alter the staging* but is taken into account for management decisions by the gynaecological oncologist.

Appearance
- Polypoid/papillary/nodular/solid/ulcerated/ burrowing. Ulcerated cancers generally infiltrate more deeply than polypoid ones.

Edge
- Circumscribed/irregular.

Extent
- Infiltration cervical wall, parametria/paracervix, corpus uteri, vagina.

25.2   Histological Type

Squamous Cell Carcinoma

- *80 % of cases.*
- Classical:
  Keratinising
  Non-keratinising – large cell/small cell. Non-keratinising large cell is recognisably squamous in character with cell stratification and intercellular bridges but no keratin pearls are present.
  variants:
- *Verrucous*: exophytic and locally invasive, it may recur after excision and radiotherapy. It shows bland cytology with bulbous processes and a pushing deep margin.

- *Warty*: surface koilocytosis and an invasive deep margin.
- *Spindle cell*: upper aerodigestive tract analogue with tumour cell fibroplasia (sarcomatoid carcinoma).
- *Papillary*: two types of papillary neoplasm with either CIN like dysplastic/in situ squamous cell epithelium, or, squamotransitional cell type epithelium. The latter occurs in post menopausal women and is associated with late recurrence and metastases (25 %). Invasion at the base may be superficial or associated with more usual squamous cell carcinoma.
- *Basaloid*: an aggressive neoplasm comprising nests of basaloid cells with peripheral palisading and central keratinisation or necrosis.
- *Lymphoepithelioma like*: circumscribed margin, lymphocytic infiltrate, large uniform cells with a prominent nucleolus. It may have a better prognosis and is radiosensitive. ±EBV (Epstein Barr Virus) positive.

Adenocarcinoma

- *10–15 % of cases.*
- *Endocervical*: 70 % of cervical adenocarcinomas and variably glandular/mucinous related to the degree of differentiation which is usually well to moderate.
- *Endometrioid*: 25 % of cervical adenocarcinomas, and exclude a uterine adenocarcinoma extending to cervix. Typically at the junctional zone arising from endometriosis/tuboendometrial metaplasia, and may coexist with usual endocervical type adenocarcinoma. A minimal deviation variant exists.
- *Minimal deviation* (*adenoma malignum*): late presentation and poor prognosis with bland epithelium showing mitoses and irregular gland extension deep (>50 %) into the cervical stroma. CEA and p53 over expression may be of diagnostic help. It is associated with Peutz-Jeghers syndrome.
- *Villoglandular*: good prognosis in young females. Papillary with CGIN type covering epithelium, connective tissue cores and indolent invasion at the base. More aggressive moderately differentiated variants occur and it can be associated with more usual cervical cancer subtypes. Also consider implantation from an endometrial primary.
- *Clear cell*: clear, hobnail cells, glycogen PAS positive, solid, tubules, papillae. Some are associated with in utero exposure to diethylstilboestrol.
- *Serous papillary*: poor prognosis and potentially multifocal in endometrium and ovary. High-grade cytological appearances ± psammoma bodies – exclude low-grade villoglandular adenocarcinoma.
- *Mesonephric*: from mesonephric duct remnants deep in the posterior or lateral cervical wall. Small glands with eosinophilic secretions.
- *Non-Müllerian mucinous*: intestinal including colloid and signet ring cell carcinomas. There is also a gastric type. Poor prognosis compared to usual endocervical-type adenocarcinoma (30 % vs 70 % 5 year survival), and exclude a gastrointestinal secondary adenocarcinoma.

Poorly Differentiated Carcinoma

- *Scirrhous, undifferentiated.*
- In undifferentiated carcinomas also consider differential diagnoses such as sarcoma (epithelioid leiomyosarcoma), malignant melanoma and malignant lymphoma.

Mixed Tumours

- *Mixed type* (e.g. squamous cell/adenocarcinoma) and *differentiation* (e.g. endocervical/endometrioid adenocarcinoma).
- *Adenosquamous, solid with mucus production*: varies from well differentiated glandular and squamous cell components, to solid poorly differentiated squamous cell carci-

noma with stainable PAS positive mucin production (up to 30 % of cases) and which is *more aggressive* than usual squamous cell carcinoma.

Miscellaneous Carcinoma

- *Glassy cell*: a poorly differentiated adenosquamous carcinoma in young women.
- *Adenoid basal*: indolent and often an incidental finding at hysterectomy or cone biopsy. Organoid lobules and nests of cells with punched out lumina ± eosinophilic secretions. Strong association (90 %) with overlying high-grade CIN or microinvasive squamous cell carcinoma.
- *Mucoepidermoid* and *adenoid cystic*: low-grade and indolent behaviour although recurrence/metastasis if incompletely removed.

Small Cell Carcinoma

- *Primary* or *secondary*. A poorly differentiated/high-grade neuroendocrine carcinoma. Chromogranin(focal)/synaptophysin/CD56 positive with poor prognosis. High Ki-67 index, TTF-1/CD99/p16/p63±. Treated by chemotherapy and not surgery.

Other Neuroendocrine Tumours

- *Atypical carcinoid* like tumour of intermediate-grade malignancy as well as classical well differentiated/low-grade *carcinoid tumour* (rare), and high-grade *large cell neuroendocrine carcinoma*.

Metastatic Carcinoma

- *Direct spread*: endometrium (commonest), colorectum, bladder.
- *Distant spread*: breast (especially infiltrating lobular), stomach, ovary.

25.3 Differentiation

Well/moderate/poor/undifferentiated, or, Grade 1/2/3/4.

Varies according to lesion type e.g. keratinising squamous cell carcinoma is well to moderately differentiated, non-keratinising large cell moderate, and non-keratinising small cell poorly differentiated. About 60 % are moderately differentiated. Tumour grade does not reliably predict prognosis and is only broadly indicative. However, grade 1 (small amount (≤10 %) of solid growth with mild nuclear atypia) has a better prognosis than grade 3 (solid pattern (>50 %) with severe nuclear atypia) adenocarcinoma. Undifferentiated carcinomas show no squamous cell or glandular differentiation (grade 4). Small and large cell neuroendocrine carcinomas are high-grade or poorly differentiated.

25.4 Extent of Local Tumour Spread

Border: pushing/infiltrative.
  Lymphocytic reaction: prominent/sparse.
  Infiltration
- Cervical wall, parametria, endometrium, myometrium, vagina.
- Depth through the cervical stroma and parametrium and distance to the nearest parametrial resection margin (mm).
- Infiltration of the superficial and deep thirds of the cervix have average disease free intervals of 94 and 73 % respectively.

FIGO/TNM

FIGO staging is recommended with additional TNM7 comments on the lymph node status. The classifications are applicable to cervical carcinomas.

I	Carcinoma confined to the uterus (extension to the corpus is disregarded)
IA	Lesions detected only microscopically; maximum size 5 mm deep and 7 mm across; venous or lymphatic permeation does not alter the staging

IA1	≤3 mm deep, ≤7 mm horizonal axis
IA2	3 mm < tumour depth ≤5 mm, ≤7 mm horizontal axis
IB	Clinically apparent lesions confined to the cervix or preclinical lesions larger than stage IA (occult carcinoma)
IB1	Clinical lesions ≤4 cm in size
IB2	Clinical lesions >4 cm in size
II	Invasive carcinoma extending beyond the uterus but has not reached either lateral pelvic wall. Involvement of upper two-thirds of vagina, but not lower third
IIA	Without parametrial invasion (IIA1 ≤4 cm in size: IIA2 >4 cm)
IIB	With parametrial invasion
III	
IIIA	Invasive carcinoma extending to either lower third of vagina and/or
IIIB	Lateral pelvic wall and/or causes hydronephrosis/non-functioning kidney
IV	Invasive carcinoma involving mucosa[a] of urinary bladder mucosa and/or rectum or extends beyond the true pelvis. Adjacent organ involvement (IVA) or distant metastases (IVB).

[a]Bladder/rectal mucosal involvement requires confirmation by biopsy and involvement of bladder/rectal wall only is FIGO stage III (Figs. 25.1, 25.2, 25.3, 25.4, 25.5, 25.6 and 25.7)

FIGO III is used for grossly or histologically evident continuous invasion beyond the myometrium into the parametrium and for "frozen pelvis" – a clinical term meaning extension to pelvic wall(s). Parametrial involvement is an indicator of poor prognosis and likely lymph node metastases. Positive peritoneal fluid is not considered in the FIGO classification.

Tumour spread: is typically to vagina, uterine corpus, parametria, lower urinary tract (ureters) and uterosacral ligaments. Involvement of regional lymph nodes relates to the stage of disease with lungs, brain and bone the commonest (5–10 %) sites of distant metastases.

25.5 Lymphovascular Invasion

Present/absent.

Intra-/extratumoural.

Lymphovascular invasion should be noted on biopsy material as it may influence the choice of

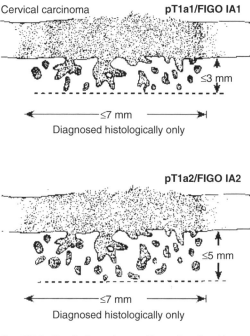

Fig. 25.1 Cervical carcinoma (Reproduced, with permission, from Wittekind et al. (2005), © 2005)

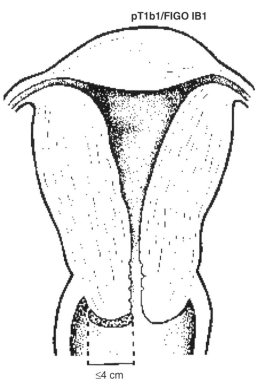

Fig. 25.2 Cervical carcinoma (Reproduced, with permission, from Wittekind et al. (2005), © 2005)

pT1b2/FIGO IB2

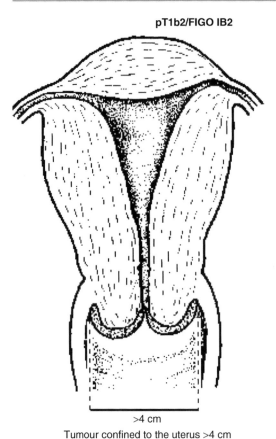

>4 cm

Tumour confined to the uterus >4 cm

Fig. 25.3 Cervical carcinoma (Reproduced, with permission, from Wittekind et al. (2005), © 2005)

more extensive surgical resection. Its presence and extent are a *strong indicator of poor prognosis* and the likelihood of lymph node metastasis and recurrence of tumour.

25.6 Lymph Nodes

Site/number/size/number involved/extracapsular spread.

Parametrial involvement increases regional lymph node metastases to about 35 % of cases.

Regional nodes: paracervical[1], parametrial[2], hypogastric[3] (internal iliac, obturator), common[5] and external iliac[4], presacral[6], lateral sacral[7]. Paraaortic lymph nodes are not regional. A regional lymphadenectomy will ordinarily include a minimum of six lymph nodes. Intraoperative frozen section examination of suspicious lymph nodes may be done as a prequel to radical surgery, and if positive, a more conservative approach adopted.

pN0	No regional lymph node metastasis.
pN1	Metastasis in regional lymph node(s) (Fig. 25.8).

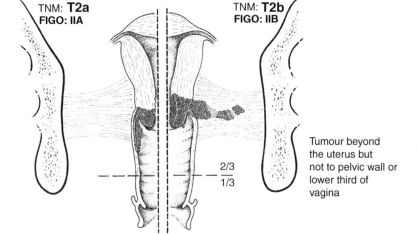

TNM: **T2a**
FIGO: **IIA**

TNM: **T2b**
FIGO: **IIB**

2/3
——
1/3

Tumour beyond the uterus but not to pelvic wall or lower third of vagina

Fig. 25.4 Cervical carcinoma (Reproduced, with permission, from Wittekind et al. (2005), © 2005

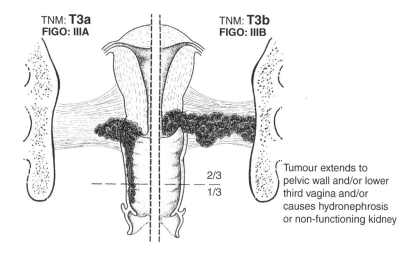

Fig. 25.5 Cervical carcinoma (Reproduced, with permission, from Wittekind et al. (2005), © 2005)

TNM: **T3a**
FIGO: **IIIA**

TNM: **T3b**
FIGO: **IIIB**

2/3
1/3

Tumour extends to pelvic wall and/or lower third vagina and/or causes hydronephrosis or non-functioning kidney

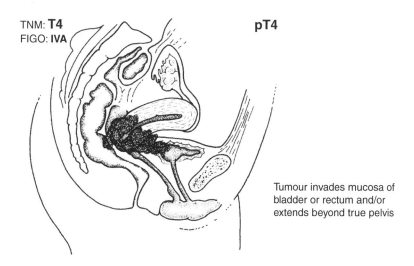

Fig. 25.6 Cervical carcinoma (Reproduced, with permission, from Wittekind et al. (2005), © 2005)

TNM: **T4**
FIGO: **IVA**

pT4

Tumour invades mucosa of bladder or rectum and/or extends beyond true pelvis

25.7 Excision Margins

Distances (mm) to the nearest deep cervical (anterior and posterior), lateral parametrial and inferior vaginal resection margins.

In a trachelectomy specimen distances (mm) to the nearest deep cervical, lateral parametrial, proximal endocervical and distal exocervical/ vaginal resection margins.

Fig. 25.7 Cervical
carcinoma (Reproduced,
with permission, from Allen
(2006), © 2006)

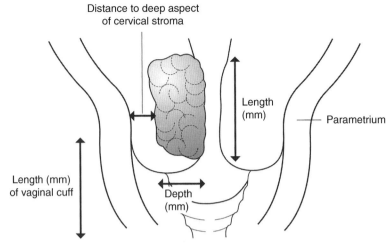

Width (mm) = sum of involved serial blocks of standard thickness
Tumour volume (mm^3) can be estimated by length × depth × width

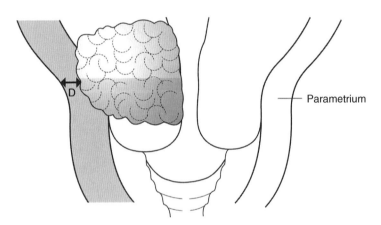

D = tumour distance (mm) to the circumferential
radial margin (CRM) of excision of
the parametrium

25.8   Other Pathology

HPV	Human papilloma virus infection causing an anogenital field change of viral lesions (flat koilocytosis/ condyloma accuminatum), intraepithelial neoplasia and carcinoma.
CIN	Cervical intraepithelial neoplasia.
SIL	Squamous intraepithelial lesion (Bethesda system).
AIS/EGD/CGIN	Adenocarcinoma in situ (AIS) and lesser changes of endocervical glandular dysplasia (EGD) corresponding to high-grade and low-grade cervical glandular intraepithelial neoplasia (CGIN), respectively.

VAIN	Vaginal intraepithelial neoplasia
VIN	Vulval intraepithelial neoplasia.
AIN	Anal intraepithelial neoplasia.
Bowenoid papulosis	A now less often used clinical term describing brown perineal patches in young women. HPV induced with histology of VIN III and a negligible risk of progression to carcinoma.

Evidence indicates that "*high-risk*" *HPV infection* results in *high-grade CIN* (*SIL*) with a higher rate of progression to carcinoma. "*Low-risk*" *HPV* and *low-grade CIN* may potentially regress. HPV infection is also an aetiological factor in cervical glandular dysplasia (CGIN), which

Fig. 25.8 Cervical carcinoma: regional lymph nodes (Reproduced, with permission, from Wittekind et al. (2005), © 2005)

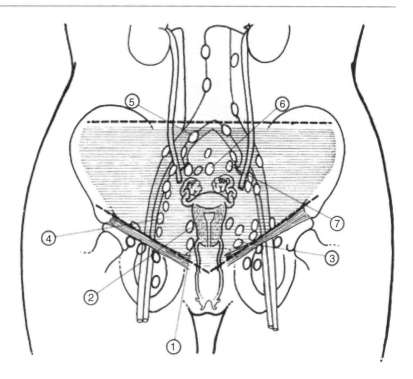

often coexists with squamous epithelial dysplasia (CIN, SIL), and occasionally SMILE (stratified mucin-producing intraepithelial lesion) of intermediate squamocolumnar character.

Low- and *high-grade CGIN* also potentially progress to invasive disease with a strong association between high-grade CGIN and invasive lesions. CGIN should also be distinguished from *benign mimics* e.g. tuboendometrial metaplasia (TEM), endometriosis, endocervical microglandular hyperplasia, mesonephric remnants and endocervical gland tunnel clusters. CGIN shows an abrupt junction with normal epithelium, nuclear atypia, mitoses and apoptosis. Ciliation is less frequent than in metaplasia. Immunohistochemistry may also be of help in that CGIN has a high Ki-67 proliferation index (>10 %), stains strongly with p16 and p53, and is focal or negative for bcl-2. Benign mimics such as TEM have a converse immunophenotype with this panel. Interobserver variation is good for high-grade CGIN but poor for low-grade. Endocervical (commonest), intestinal and endometrioid variants are described. Ki-67 positive cells in the upper two-thirds of the epithelium also reliably identifies CIN lesions in biopsy material. Retention of distinct immunophenotype may also help to distinguish neoplastic squamous or glandular epithelia from thermal cautery artifact

at diathermy loop or conisation specimen tissue margins.

"Low-risk"	HPV types 6, 11	Koilocytosis, CIN I
"High-risk"	HPV types 16, 18, 31, 33, 35, 39, 51	CIN II/III Squamous carcinoma typing by in situ hybridisation
CIN (SIL)	Low-grade	CIN I, SIL I
	High-grade	CIN II, CIN III, SIL II.

"High-risk" HPV DNA subtyping has an evolving role in primary screening, quality assurance checking, and the closer follow up of women whose cervical smears shows BNA (borderline nuclear abnormalities)/ASC-US (atypical squamous cells of uncertain significance) changes.

Immunophenotype: cervical squamous cell carcinoma is AE1/AE3, CK5/6, p63 positive, and adenocarcinoma CK7, p16 and CEA positive.

FIGO IA Carcinoma

The higher the grade and larger the CIN lesion the more likely it is to show early invasion with a *35 %*

risk of CIN III progressing to carcinoma over a10 year period. FIGO IA carcinoma is not designated on small, limited biopsy samples but rather on a large biopsy specimen e.g. cone biopsy which allows removal and assessment of the whole lesion. Five year survival rates are about 95 %. Risk factors for progression to clinically invasive carcinoma are increasing depth of invasion, increasing lateral extent (horizontal axis) of the lesion, lymphovascular invasion and incomplete removal by LLETZ/cone biopsy. Adverse factors in occult carcinoma (i.e. bigger than FIGO IA but not clinically detectable) are a depth of invasion >5 mm and lymphovascular invasion. Very occasional cases, where the CIN lesion has focal areas suspicious of penetrating the stroma but lacking definite evidence of invasion, warrant a designation of "equivocal stromal invasion". Commonly occurring tangential cutting and extension of CIN into endocervical crypts must be excluded and is supported by an intact circumscribed basement membrane. An uncommon differential is squamous cell carcinoma with a CIN III like growth pattern, for which widespread, deep expansion with luminal necrosis are useful diagnostic clues. A rare mimic of cervical cancer is buried or entrapped dysplastic epithelium in the superficial cervical stroma following a previous biopsy.

The first stage of *early invasive squamous cell carcinoma* is recognised by budding of invasive cells with morphology similar to that of the overlying CIN lesion through the basement membrane. With lesion progression the tongues of tumour become *more differentiated or "hypermature"* (*so called paradoxical maturation/differentiation*) with cytoplasmic eosinophilia and nuclear clearing. A *stromal fibro-inflammatory reaction* is also seen. The distinction between adenocarcinoma in situ and early invasive adenocarcinoma is more difficult to define and measure with features such as *depth* beyond the normal endocervical gland field, *cribriform complexity and budding* of glandular architecture, *stromal fibroinflammatory reaction* and *proximity of abnormal glands to thick walled stromal vessels* of use.

Measurement of tumour extent in cervical carcinoma is readily obtained in the longitudinal and deep axes, whereas the transverse dimension depends on summation of the number of involved adjacent blocks of known thickness. About 10 % of cervical carcinomas show multifocal stromal invasion characterised by clear separation of tumour by uninvolved tissue or an origin from different lips of the cervix. In this case the pathological stage is based on the width and depth of the largest tumour and not the combined dimensions of the various cancers.

Treatment

Treatment of cervical carcinoma is based on the tumour stage, patient age and consideration of fertility. Early invasive carcinoma may be treated with *loop or cold knife cone biopsy* ensuring a minimum 3 mm clearance of margins (note that there can be a small risk of skip or higher endocervical canal lesions), or *simple hysterectomy*. A fertility sparing procedure such as *radical trachelectomy* (removal of the upper vagina, cervix and surrounding parametria with laparoscopic lymphadenectomy) may be considered in young women with up to a FIGO IB1 tumour <2 cm in maximum dimension. *Radical hysterectomy* is indicated for larger tumours or where there is lymphovascular invasion. *Radiotherapy* produces tumour cell necrosis, degeneration, pleomorphism, maturation, inflammation and fibrosis. *Combination radio-/chemotherapy* (± brachytherapy) is used to augment radical surgery for tumours ≥ FIGO IB, or on its own for palliative control in high stage disease. Small cell neuroendocrine carcinoma is treated by chemotherapy rather than surgery.

Prognosis

Prognosis relates to tumour type and volume, invasion of endometrium, parametrium and vessels, and most importantly *stage of disease*. Overall 5 year survival rate is 55 %, with stage I carcinoma 85–90 % and 35/10 % for stages III/IV. Tumours with a glandular component, lymphovascular invasion and young age at diagnosis (<30 years) are more aggressive and more often positive for pelvic lymph node metastases. The incidence of cervical adenocarcinoma is increasing and presents on average 5 years younger than squamous cell carcinoma. Anecdotally it has a worse prognosis than squamous cell carcinoma and radical surgery is undertaken. This adverse outlook may relate to presentation with more bulky disease and greater resistance to radiotherapy. However the risk of lymph node metastasis is broadly similar for equivalent early stage cervical adenocarcinoma and squamous cell carcinoma. Therefore, early FIGO 1A1 cervical adenocarcinoma can also be treated by local excision, or small 1B1 tumours by trachelectomy if preservation of fertility is a concern. Mixed differentiation tumours, and the coexistence of CIN and CGIN particularly on the surface and in crypts respectively, are sometimes seen. High-grade CGIN or adenocarcinoma in situ is usually treated by hysterectomy although conservative conisation may be used if the patient is young (<36 years) and wishes to remain fertile.

25.9   Other Malignancy

Malignant Melanoma

- Usually metastatic.
- Primary lesion is rare: 40 % 5 year survival.

Embryonal Rhabdomyosarcoma

- Infancy/childhood.
- Syn. sarcoma botryoides.
- Cellular subepithelial cambium zone/myxoid zone/deep cellular zone.
- Small cells/rhabdomyoblasts/desmin, myogenin and myo D1 positive.
- ± heterologous elements.

Leiomyosarcoma

- 40–60 years.
- Cellular atypia, necrosis, and >5 mitoses/10 high-power fields.
- >10 mitoses/10 high power fields required if no atypia.

Adenosarcoma

- Polypoid.
- 25 % have heterologous elements (striated muscle, cartilage, fat).
- A low-grade malignancy.

Stromal sarcoma and malignant mixed mesodermal tumour are more likely to represent spread to the cervix from an endometrial lesion rather than a primary cervical tumour.

Malignant Lymphoma

- More often secondary spread from systemic/nodal disease.
- Primary: 70 % are intermediate to high-grade of large B cell type.
- Five year survival is about 75 %.

Leukaemia

- Granulocytic sarcoma as a presentation of chronic myeloid leukaemia.
- CD34/CD43/CD68/CD117/chloroacetate esterase /myeloperoxidase and neutrophil elastase positive.
- Relapse of AML, blast transformation of CML.

Bibliography

Allen DC. Histopathology reporting: guidelines for surgical cancer. 2nd ed. Springer: London; 2006.

Al-Nafussi A. Tumours of the uterine cervix that can be underdiagnosed or misinterpreted. Curr Diagn Pathol. 2003;9:56–70.

Al-Nafussi A. Histopathological challenges in assessing invasion in squamous, glandular neoplasia of the cervix. Curr Diagn Pathol. 2006;12:364–93.

Arends MJ, Buckley CH, Wells M. Aetiology, pathogenesis, and pathology of cervical neoplasia. J Clin Pathol. 1998;51:96–103.

Fox H, Wells M, editors. Haines and Taylor. Obstetrical and gynaecological pathology. 5th ed. Edinburgh: Churchill Livingstone; 2003.

Heatley MK. Dissection and reporting of the organs of the female genital tract. J Clin Pathol. 2008;61:241–57.

Herrington CS. Recent advances in molecular gynaecological pathology. Histopathology. 2009; 55:243–9.

Hirschowitz L, Nucci M, Zaino RJ. Problematic issues in the staging of endometrial, cervical and vulval carcinomas. Histopathology. 2013;62:176–202.

Histopathology Reporting in Cervical Screening. Working Party of the Royal College of Pathologists and the NHS Cervical Screening Programme. NHSCSP Publication No 10. April 1999.

Kalof AN, Cooper K. Our approach to squamous intraepithelial lesions of the uterine cervix. J Clin Pathol. 2007;60:449–55.

Kurman RJ, Amin MB. Protocol for the examination of specimens from patients with carcinoma of the cervix. Arch Pathol Lab Med. 1999;123:55–66.

Kurman RJ, Norris HJ, Wilkinson E. Tumors of the cervix, vagina and vulva. Atlas of tumor pathology. 3rd series. Fascicle 4. Washington: AFIP; 1992.

McCluggage WG. Endocervical glandular lesions: controversial aspects and ancillary techniques. J Clin Pathol. 2003;56:164–73.

McCluggage WG. Ten problematic issues identified by pathology review for multidisciplinary gynaecological oncology meetings. J Clin Pathol. 2012;65: 293–301.

McCluggage WG. New developments in endocervical glandular lesions. Histopathology. 2013; 62:138–60.

McCluggage WG, Hirschowitz L, Ganesan R, Kehoe S, Nordin A. Which staging system to use for gynaecological cancers: a survey with recommendations for practice in the UK. J Clin Pathol. 2010; 63:768–70.

Pecorelli S, FIGO Committee on Gynecologic Oncology. Revised FIGO staging for carcinoma of the vulva, cervix and endometrium. Int J Gynecol Obstet. 2009; 105:103–4.

Petignat P, Roy M. Diagnosis and management of cervical cancer. BMJ. 2007;335:765–8.

Robboy SJ, Bentley RC, Russell R, Anderson MC, Mutter GL, Prat J. Pathology of the female reproductive tract. 2nd ed. London: Churchill Livingstone Elsevier; 2009.

Scottish Intercollegiate Guidelines Network. Management of cervical cancer. Quick reference guide. Accessed at http://www.sign.ac.uk.

Scurry J, Patel K, Wells M. Gross examination of uterine specimens. J Clin Pathol. 1993;46:388–93.

Smith JHF. The future of cervical screening in the UK. Diagn Histopathol. 2009;15:330–4.

Stewart CJR, McCluggage WG. Epithelial-mesenchymal transition in carcinomas of the female genital tract. Histopathology. 2013;62:31–43.

Tavassoli F, Devilee P. WHO classification of tumours. Pathology and genetics. Tumours of the breast and female genital organs. Lyon: IARC Press; 2003.

The Royal College of Pathologists. Cancer Datasets (Vulval Neoplasms, Cervical Neoplasia, Endometrial Cancer, Uterine Sarcomas, Neoplasms of the Ovaries and Fallopian Tubes and Primary Carcinoma of the Peritoneum), and Tissue Pathways for Gynaecological Pathology. Accessed at http://www.rcpath.org/index. asp?PageID=254.

Wittekind C, International Union against Cancer, et al. TNM atlas: illustrated guide to the TNM/pTNM classification of malignant tumours. 5th ed. Berlin: Springer; 2005.

Young RH, Clements PB. Endocervical adenocarcinoma and its variants: their morphology and differential diagnosis. Histopathology. 2002;41: 185–207.

Vaginal pathology may be asymptomatic or present with bleeding, discharge, dyspareunia (pain at sexual intercourse), a feeling of discomfort or a mass. Clinical examination and direct visualisation by coloposcopy can show viral warts, dysplastic mucosal lesions (VAIN: vaginal intraepithelial neoplasia), tumour and even changes related to diethylstilboestrol exposure (DES: see below). Vaginal smear, punch or wedge biopsy allow a tissue diagnosis, and the strong associations with any previous vulval, cervical and endometrial disease must be taken into account. Pelvic MRI scan is used to stage suspected tumour including the presence of pelvic or inguinal lymphadenopathy with the latter sometimes also amenable to investigation by fine needle aspiration cytology (FNAC). Surgery in the form of either wide local excision or radical vaginectomy is used for localised, or non-responsive or recurrent tumours, respectively, otherwise chemoradiation subject to assessment and discussion at a multidisciplinary meeting. Local excision, laser ablation and topical 5-fluorouracil are additional options for superficial mucosal wart or VAIN lesions. Pelvic exenteration is sometimes used for extensive local disease or post radiotherapy necrosis if there is no evidence of extrapelvic distant metastases on CT/PET scan.

26.1 Gross Description

Specimen

- Vaginal smear/biopsy/wide local excision/partial or subtotal vaginectomy/radical vaginectomy (with hysterectomy, salpingo-oophorectomy and lymphadenectomy)/pelvic exenteration.
- Weight (g) and size (cm), number of fragments.

Tumour

Site
- Anterior/posterior/lateral (right or left)/fornices. Usually anterior or lateral and upper third (50–60 %).

Size
- Length × width × depth (cm) or maximum dimension (cm).

Appearance
- Polypoid/verrucous/papillary/sessile/ulcerated/pigmented.
- Exophytic lesions are commoner than endophytic and most are either nodular or ulcerative.

D.C. Allen, *Histopathology Reporting*,
DOI 10.1007/978-1-4471-5263-7_26, © Springer-Verlag London 2013

Edge

• Circumscribed/irregular.

26.2   Histological Type

Secondary carcinoma is more frequent than primary carcinoma in the vagina.

Squamous Cell Carcinoma

• *90–95 % of primary vaginal carcinomas.*
• Keratinising/non-keratinising.
• Large cell/small cell.
• Mainly moderately differentiated keratinising.
• variants:
• *Verrucous*: exophytic, bland cytology with deep bulbous processes and a locally invasive pushing margin.
• *Warty* (*condylomatous*): with focal invasion at the base.
• *Spindle cell*: a cytokeratin positive sarcomatoid carcinoma.

Adenocarcinoma

• *Clear cell*: PAS positive for glycogen, solid/tubules/papillae. From 1970 to 2000 most patients were 14–25 years with in utero exposure to diethylstilboestrol (DES). Following withdrawal of DES and as this cohort ages this diagnosis is decreasing. Non-DES cases in the older age group are rare comprising clear/hobnail cells ± vaginal adenosis defined as the presence of any Müllerian type glandular epithelium, often endocervical, or, tuboendometrial in character. Differential diagnosis is vaginal adenosis with microglandular hyperplasia and Arias-Stella reaction in pregnancy or hormone therapy. Prognosis is relatively good (80 % 5 year survival) if the tumour is small and superficial. Otherwise local recurrence and lymph node metastases usually occur within 3 years but sometimes late after many years.

• *Endometrioid*: possibly arising from previous endometriosis.
• *Mucinous*: endocervical or intestinal in type and the former may be associated with adenosis (endocervicosis). Note that rarely primary vaginal intestinal type adenoma of tubular/villous morphology can occur.
• *Mesonephric*: deep in the lateral vaginal walls arising from mesonephric remnants.

Adenosquamous Carcinoma

• Mixed differentiation and of worse prognosis.

Adenoid Cystic Carcinoma

• Indolent with late local recurrence and potential for metastases.

Adenoid Basal Carcinoma

• Indolent behaviour.

Small Cell Carcinoma

• Primary or secondary from cervix or lung. A poorly differentiated/high-grade neuroendocrine carcinoma. Paranuclear dot CAM5.2/synaptophysin/CD56/Ki-67 positive.

Undifferentiated Carcinoma

• No evident squamous cell or glandular differentiation.

Transitional Cell Carcinoma

• Primary (rare), or in association with concurrent bladder/urethral carcinoma.

Carcinoid Tumour

- Chromogranin/synaptophysin/CD56 positive. Low Ki-67 index (≤2 %) and a well differentiated neuroendocrine tumour of low-grade malignancy.

Endodermal Sinus Tumour

- Yolk sac spectrum of appearances and AFP/glypican 3 positive in the posterior wall and fornices of infants. It is responsive to surgery and chemotherapy.

Malignant Melanoma

- *3% of cases* and mucosal junctional activity indicates a primary lesion. It is of *poor prognosis*.
- More often represents a *metastasis* e.g. from urethra or vulva.

Metastatic Carcinoma

- *Comprises 80% of malignant vaginal tumours, far outnumbering primary lesions.*
- *Direct spread*: cervix, endometrium, rectum, vulva, bladder, urethra.
- *Distant spread*: kidney, breast, gastrointestinal tract, ovary.

  The commonest metastases (*cervix, endometrium, rectum*) are usually in the upper third of the vagina and may be submucosal. Other metastatic tumour types should also be considered e.g. vaginal recurrence of vulval or urethral malignant melanoma, or, uterine leiomyosarcoma.

26.3 Differentiation/Grade

Well/moderate/poor/undifferentiated, or, Grade 1/2/3/4.

There is no specific recommended grading system for vaginal tumours with squamous cell or glandular differentiation other than the above. Grade 4 (undifferentiated) tumours show no differentiation. Transitional cell carcinomas are designated WHOI/II/III based on cytonuclear grade.

26.4 Extent of Local Tumour Spread

Border: pushing/infiltrative.
Lymphocytic reaction: prominent/sparse.

FIGO

FIGO staging is recommended. It applies to primary carcinoma of the vagina only excluding secondary growths either by metastasis or direct extension e.g. from cervix, vulva or rectum. A vaginal carcinoma occurring 5 years after successful treatment of a carcinoma of the cervix is considered a primary vaginal carcinoma.

A category of microinvasive carcinoma is not established although superficial tumours invading ≤3 mm with no lymphovascular invasion have a low incidence of lymph node metastases.

I	Tumour confined to the vagina
II	Tumour invades paravaginal tissues (paracolpium) but does not extend to pelvic wall
III	Tumour extends to pelvic wall[a]
IV	Tumour invades mucosa of bladder or rectum, and/or extends beyond the true pelvis.

[a]The pelvic wall is defined as muscle, fascia, neurovascular structures or skeletal elements of the bony pelvis (Figs. 26.1, 26.2, 26.3 and 26.4)

"Frozen pelvis" is a clinical term meaning tumour extension to the pelvic wall(s) and is classified as FIGO III.

Spread is mainly by early direct invasion and lymph node metastases, with 50 % beyond the vagina (FIGO II) at presentation and 25 % in the rectum or bladder (FIGO IV).

M1 disease is either an upper two-thirds vaginal tumour with inguinal lymph node metastases, or, a lower third vaginal tumour with pelvic lymph node metastases. Other distant sites include lung, liver and brain.

26.5 Lymphovascular Invasion

Present/absent.
   Intra-/extratumoural.

Fig. 26.1 Vaginal carcinoma (Reproduced, with permission, from Wittekind et al. (2005), © 2005)

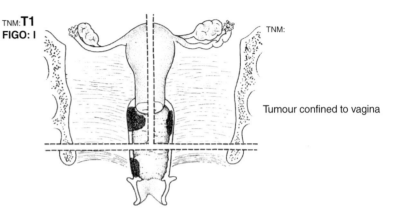

TNM:**T1**
FIGO: I

TNM:

Tumour confined to vagina

Fig. 26.2 Vaginal carcinoma (Reproduced, with permission, from Wittekind et al. (2005), © 2005)

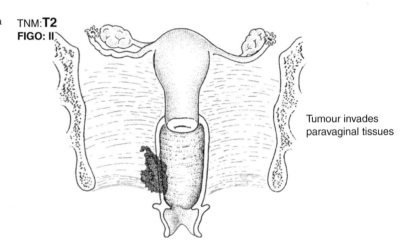

TNM:**T2**
FIGO: II

Tumour invades paravaginal tissues

TNM:**T3**
FIGO: III

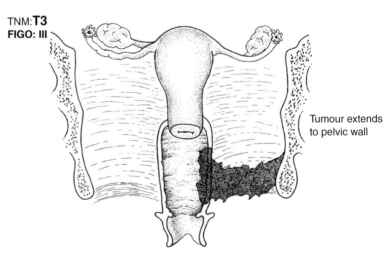

Tumour extends to pelvic wall

Fig. 26.3 Vaginal carcinoma (Reproduced, with permission, from Wittekind et al. (2005), © 2005)

Fig. 26.4 Vaginal carcinoma (Reproduced, with permission, from Wittekind et al. (2005), © 2005)

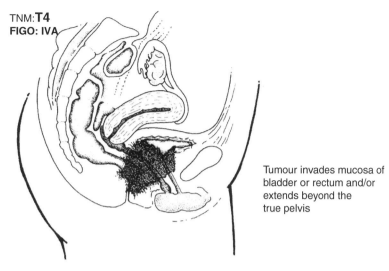

TNM:**T4**
FIGO: IVA

Tumour invades mucosa of bladder or rectum and/or extends beyond the true pelvis

26.6   Lymph Nodes

Site/number/size/number involved/extracapsular spread.

Regional nodes: upper two-thirds – obturator, internal iliac, external iliac, pelvic nodes; lower third – inguinal and femoral nodes.

A regional lymphadenectomy will ordinarily include a minimum of six lymph nodes.

26.7   Excision Margins

Distances (mm) to the nearest longitudinal resection limit and deep circumferential radial margin. The presence of epithelial (squamous or glandular) dysplasia or atypical adenosis at a mucosal resection margin may increase the frequency of recurrent tumour.

26.8   Other Pathology

Vaginal Intraepithelial Neoplasia (VAIN): Grades I/II/ III

- Rarer and less well established than the CIN or VIN – cancer sequences.

Cervical Intraepithelial Neoplasia (CIN)/Anal Intraepithelial Neoplasia (AIN)

HPV 16/18 is a common aetiology in CIN, VAIN, AIN and VIN (vulval intraepithelial neoplasia). It is instrumental in the *field change effect* of carcinogenesis in the female genital tract which results in synchronous or metachronous cancers in the vulva, cervix and vagina. The vagina is also a common site of direct spread from vulval and cervical carcinomas and it should be noted that *the commonest vaginal malignancies are secondary cervical, endometrial and rectal carcinomas.* Knowledge of a relevant past clinical history and availability of slides for comparison are, therefore, crucially important in designation of any vaginal lesion. A not uncommon differential diagnosis for adenocarcinoma on vaginal smear or vault biopsy is post-hysterectomy prolapsed fallopian tube, endometriosis or granulation tissue.

Prognosis

Initial treatment of vaginal carcinoma is by *irradiation*, with better response for squamous cell carcinoma than adenocarcinoma, malignant melanoma and sarcoma. *Surgery* is used for localized early stage disease, non-responsive cases or local recurrence. Upper vaginal lesions tend to *recur locally* while lower vaginal tumours are prone to developing *distal or pelvic side wall disease*. Prognosis relates strongly to *disease stage* e.g. 43 % 5 year survival with 70 % for stage I and 30 % for stage III. Vaginal malignant melanoma spreads early to pelvic soft tissues, lymph nodes, peritoneum, lung and bone with 5 year survival rates of 21 %.

26.9 Other Malignancy

Malignant Lymphoma/Leukaemia

* Malignant lymphoma is usually secondary to systemic disease. Rare primary lesions are intermediate to high-grade large B cell in type.

Embryonal Rhabdomyosarcoma (Sarcoma Botryoides)

* Infants/children <5 years of age, anterior vaginal wall.
* Superficial subepithelial cellular cambium layer, intermediate myxoid zone, deep cellular zone, desmin/myo D1/myogenin positive.
* *Locally aggressive* necessitating primary chemotherapy ± surgery and irradiation.

Leiomyosarcoma

* Usually >3 cm, with cell atypia and ≥5 mitoses/10 high-power fields.

* A primary lesion is rare: consider metastases e.g. uterine leiomyosarcoma.

Müllerian Stromal Sarcomas and Other Sarcomas

* e.g. alveolar soft part, malignant fibrous histiocytoma, synovial sarcoma, extragastrointestinal stromal tumours (eGISTs) of the rectosigmoid septum.

Bibliography

Fox H, Wells M, editors. Haines and Taylor. Obstetrical and gynaecological pathology. 5th ed. Edinburgh: Churchill Livingstone; 2003.

Heatley MK. Dissection and reporting of the organs of the female genital tract. J Clin Pathol. 2008;61:241–57.

Kurman RJ, Norris HJ, Wilkinson E. Tumors of the cervix, vagina and vulva. Atlas of tumor pathology. 3rd series. Fascicle 4. Washington: AFIP; 1992.

McCluggage WG. Recent developments in vulvovaginal pathology. Histopathology. 2009;54:156–73.

Nucci MR, Fletcher CDM. Vulvovaginal soft tissue tumours: update and review. Histopathology. 2000;36: 97–108.

Robboy SJ, Bentley RC, Russell R, Anderson MC, Mutter GL, Prat J. Pathology of the female reproductive tract. 2nd ed. London: Churchill Livingstone Elsevier; 2009.

Scully RE. Protocol for the examination of specimens from patients with carcinoma of the vagina. Arch Pathol Lab Med. 1999;123:62–7.

Tavassoli F, Devilee P. WHO classification of tumours. Pathology and genetics. Tumours of the breast and female genital organs. Lyon: IARC Press; 2003.

Wittekind C, International Union against Cancer, et al. TNM atlas: illustrated guide to the TNM/pTNM classification of malignant tumours. 5th ed. Berlin: Springer; 2005.

Vulval Carcinoma

Vulval cancer forms 5 % of gynaecological malignancies and occurs mainly in women aged 60–75 years. Its incidence is decreasing but that of precursor lesions (VIN: vulval intraepithelial neoplasia, lichen sclerosis) is increasing partly due to better clinical detection. Smoking and HPV (human papilloma virus) infection are known risk factors. There are two main types of vulval squamous cell carcinoma – HPV related and HPV independent.

Vulval cancer can present as itch in an area of pallor or redness (leukoplakia/erythroplakia) on a background of atrophic or hypertrophic lichen sclerosis. A nodular, verruciform or ulcerating mass may be present and a diagnostic wedge or punch biopsy taken. The former is more likely to establish the presence of any invasive disease, and the latter is sufficient for abnormalities in a flat epithelium such as VIN. CT and MRI scans are used to detect and stage local soft tissue spread and inguinal lymphadenopathy which may also be amenable to fine needle aspiration cytology (FNAC). Because of the strong association with HPV concurrent cervicovaginal and anal disease should be excluded.

Surgical treatment is geared to the patient's age, fitness, tumour site and stage with wide local excision for "early" FIGO stage IA disease. Lateral and central FIGO stage IB lesions may be treated by partial vulvectomy with ipsilateral or bilateral groin lymph node dissection, respectively. FIGO stage II cancers and above need radical vulvectomy which includes removal of the perianal skin and bilateral inguinal lymphadenectomy. Pre-operative radiotherapy may be given for tumours with extensive local invasion or involved lymph nodes in an attempt to downstage disease, facilitate surgery and avoid pelvic exenteration.

27.1 Gross Description

Specimen

- Biopsy/wide local excision/partial(hemivulvectomy)/simple/radical vulvectomy/uni-/bilateral inguinal lymphadenectomy/pelvic exenteration.
- Size (cm) and weight (g).

Tumour

Site
- Anterior/posterior.
- Lateral (right/left).
- Labia majora/labia minora/clitoris.
- Labia majora is the commonest site then labia minora and clitoris.
- Bilateral (25 %)

Size
- Length × width × depth (cm) or maximum dimension (cm).

Appearance

- Polypoid/verrucous/ulcerated/necrotic/satellite lesions/pigmented.
- 50 % are ulcerated, 30 % exophytic.

Edge

- Circumscribed/irregular.

27.2   Histological Type

Vulval carcinomas show the full range of cutaneous cancers.

Squamous Cell Carcinoma

- *90 % of malignant vulval neoplasms.*
- Keratinising or non-keratinising and of two main types
  1. 60 % of cases are in older women, independent of HPV, and a keratinising squamous cell carcinoma with a spectrum of adjacent epithelial changes viz lichen sclerosis, squamous cell hyperplasia, hyperkeratosis, or differentiated VIN
  2. 30 % of cases are in younger women, HPV 16/18 positive, of basaloid or warty histology and with adjacent VIN of classic/undifferentiated type (see Sect. 27.8).
  Variants:
- *Basaloid*: 28 % of cases occurring at a younger age (<60 years) and associated with HPV, cervical and vaginal lesions. Comprises nests of basaloid cells with peripheral palisading, central necrosis, focal keratinisation and mitoses.
- *Warty*: associated with HPV and koilocytosis. Prognosis is intermediate between that of usual squamous cell carcinoma and verrucous carcinoma. Care must be taken to distinguish from pseudoepitheliomatous hyperplasia overlying lichen sclerosis, Crohn's disease or a granular cell tumour.
- *Adenoid*: a pseudoglandular/acantholytic pattern.
- *Verrucous*: exophytic with a pushing deep margin of cytologically bland bulbous processes. Prone to local recurrence after incomplete excision or radiotherapy.

- *Spindle cell*: a cytokeratin positive sarcomatoid carcinoma.

Basal Cell Carcinoma

- *20 % local recurrence rate* and metastases are rare.
  Distinguish from basaloid squamous cell carcinoma, Merkel cell carcinoma and secondary small cell carcinoma by morphology and immunohistochemistry.

Adenocarcinoma

- Rare.
- Appendage origin/Bartholin's gland/mesonephric duct remnants, or metastatic.

Paget's Disease

- *2 % of vulval malignancy.*
- Characterized by a proliferation of *intraepithelial adenocarcinoma cells* probably arising from basal layer multipotential cells and differentiating along sweat gland lines. In *10–20 % of cases there is a locoregional or extragenital malignancy* e.g. vulval appendage tumour or bladder carcinoma, cervical carcinoma, anorectal carcinoma, breast carcinoma. Immunohistochemistry may help to indicate a possible origin from bladder (uroplakin III/CK7/20 positive) or anorectum (CK20/CDX-2, MUC2 positive). GCDFP-15 can be positive in vulval Paget's disease and metastatic breast cancer.
- *Multifocal*: check margins histologically as there is a *40 % recurrence rate.*
- *Differential diagnosis*: mucin stains and immunohistochemistry (EMA, CEA, CAM 5.2, CK7, Her-2 positive) may be necessary to distinguish from Bowenoid VIN (AE1/AE3, p63 positive, and CAM 5.2/CEA/CK7 negative) and superficial spreading malignant melanoma (S100, HMB-45, melan-A positive).
- *Prognosis*: Paget's disease without an associated neoplasm has a *very good prognosis if completely*

excised. However, it may also, per se, progress to invasive carcinoma and lymph node metastases if beyond the microinvasive stage.

Merkel Cell Carcinoma

- Exclude secondary small cell carcinoma from lung.
- A *locally aggressive* and *potentially metastasising* poorly differentiated/high-grade neuroendocrine carcinoma.
- CAM 5.2 (paranuclear), CK20, chromogranin/synapophysin/CD56 positive. High Ki-67 index. Lung small cell carcinoma is CK20 negative/TTF-1 positive.

Malignant Melanoma

- *3–10 % of malignant vulval neoplasms.*
- Usually mucosal and cutaneous involvement with Breslow depth and clinical stage the main prognostic indicators.

Metastatic Carcinoma

- *5 % of malignant vulval neoplasms.*
- *Direct spread*: cervix (50 % of cases), endometrium, vagina, urethra, bladder, anorectum.
- *Distant spread*: ovary, kidney, breast, lung, malignant melanoma, choriocarcinoma.

Secondary urethral tumours are squamous cell carcinoma, transitional cell carcinoma or malignant melanoma.

27.3   Differentiation

Well/moderate/poor/undifferentiated, or, Grade 1/2/3/4.
- Well >50 %; moderate 20–40 % of cases.
- There is no specific recommended grading system for vulval tumours other than the above which should broadly reflect that of non-melanocytic cutaneous carcinomas. Grade 4 (undifferentiated) tumours show no squamous cell or glandular differentiation.

27.4   Extent of Local Tumour Spread

Border: pushing/infiltrative. An irregular infiltrative margin has a higher incidence of lymph node metastases.

Lymphocytic reaction: prominent/sparse.

Microinvasion ≤3 mm: use of this nomenclature should be avoided as some of these carcinomas will have lymph node metastases and invasive lesions >1 mm in depth should probably have radical surgery. *Superficially invasive squamous cell carcinoma* is defined as a single lesion measuring ≤2 cm diameter and with a depth of invasion ≤1 mm i.e. FIGO IA. Over diagnosis of early invasion in VIN is avoided by a requirement in invasive disease for an irregular outline or contour of neoplastic epithelium, buds of abrupt epithelial differentiation (so called paradoxical maturation) with more plentiful eosinophilic cytoplasm compared to the overlying basaloid VIN III, and an accompanying desmoplastic stromal response. Various mimics of invasion should be discounted such as tangential sectioning of adnexal epithelium involved by VIN III, pseudoepitheliomatous hyperplasia or displaced epithelium due to previous biopsy.

Distance (mm) to the nearest painted surgical margin (lateral cutaneous, medial mucosal, deep subcutaneous).

Involvement of vagina, urethra, perineum, anus.

FIGO staging is recommended and applies to primary carcinomas of the vulva

I	Tumour confined to the vulva/perineum
(a)	≤2 cm in greatest dimension and stromal invasion ≤1 mm[a]
(b)	>2 cm in greatest dimension, or stromal invasion >1 mm
II	Tumour of any size with extension to adjacent perineal structures (lower third vagina/urethra or anus)
III	Tumour of any size with or without extension to adjacent perineal structures (lower third urethra/vagina or anus) with positive inguinofemoral lymph nodes
(a)	(i) 1–2 node metastasis(es) <5 mm
	(ii) 1 node metastasis ≥5 mm
(b)	(i) ≥2 node metastases ≥5 mm
	(ii) ≥3 node metastases <5 mm
(c)	Positive nodes with extracapsular spread

(continued)

IV   Tumour invades other regional (upper two thirds vagina/urethra) or distant structures

(a) (i) Any of upper vaginal/urethral/bladder/rectal mucosa, or fixed to pelvic bone

     (ii) Fixed or ulcerated inguinofemoral lymph nodes

(b) Any distant metastases including pelvic lymph nodes

ᵃFrom the epithelial stromal junction of the adjacent most superficial dermal papilla. Thickness is from the surface, or if there is keratinisation, from the deep aspect of the granular layer to the deepest point of invasion

Upper urethra (FIGO IV) is proximal, lower urethra (FIGO II/III) is distal. Spread is direct to the vagina, urethra, anus, inferior pubic and ischial rami and ischiorectal fossae (Figs. 27.1 and 27.2).

27.5   Lymphovascular Invasion

Present/absent.

Intra-/extratumoural.

Carcinomas invading >1 mm have a higher incidence of lymphovascular invasion and lymph node metastases. This is facilitated by the vulval subepithelial connective tissues having a particularly rich vascular network.

27.6   Lymph Nodes

Site/number/size/number involved/extracapsular spread.

Regional nodes: femoral and inguinal. A regional lymphadenectomy will ordinarily include a minimum of six lymph nodes.

Labial tumours go initially to inguinal lymph nodes whereas clitoral lesions may go directly to deep pelvic lymph nodes. Ulcerated tumours can produce *reactive regional lymphadenopathy mimicking metastatic disease* and this can be further investigated by FNAC.

27.7   Excision Margins

Distances (mm) of tumour and VIN or Paget's disease to the nearest painted lateral cutaneous, medial mucosal and deep subcutaneous excision margins, and anal, vaginal, urethral limits.

27.8   Other Pathology

Lichen Sclerosis

- Atrophic, hyperplastic with hyperkeratosis, or both (mixed dystrophy).

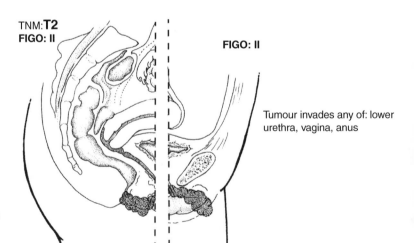

TNM:**T2**
FIGO: II

FIGO: II

Tumour invades any of: lower urethra, vagina, anus

Fig. 27.1 Vulval carcinoma (Reproduced, with permission, from Wittekind et al. (2005), © 2005)

Fig. 27.2 Vulval carcinoma (Reproduced, with permission, from Wittekind et al. (2005), © 2005)

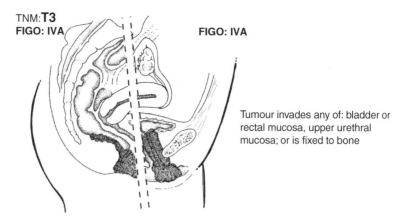

TNM:**T3**
FIGO: IVA   FIGO: IVA

Tumour invades any of: bladder or rectal mucosa, upper urethral mucosa; or is fixed to bone

- *Associated with (5–25 % of cases)* but *low risk of progression to (5 %)* carcinoma. Recurrent disease is linked to persistent VIN and lichen sclerosis.
- Can over expresses p53 and sometimes shows basal layer cytological atypia.

Condyloma

- Warty (condyloma accuminatum) or flat, and caused by HPV 6/11 with koilocytosis.

Bowenoid Papulosis

- Brown perineal patches in young women.
- HPV induced.
- Histology of VIN III.
- There is a *negligible risk of progression* to carcinoma.

Vulval Intraepithelial Neoplasia (VIN) Grades I/II/III

- Typically multifocal and present in the adjacent epithelium of 60–70 % of cases of squamous cell carcinoma.
- *Progression* to carcinoma is in the order of *10–20 %*.
- Classic, or, variant types

Classic/undifferentiated (usual) type: includes *Bowenoid/basaloid* (resembles CIN III) and *warty subtypes* (surface parakeratosis/koilocytosis), but with considerable morphological overlap and variable age presentation. Associated with HPV and multifocal genital tract cervicovaginal, perineal and anal disease. Shows diffuse positivity for p16 – a surrogate marker for HPV infection.

Variant type: *simplex or differentiated VIN* with maturation, hyperplasia, hyperkeratosis, variable parabasal cytological atypia and over expression of p53.

Prognosis

Nearly *30 % of vulval squamous cell carcinomas have metastasised* to inguinal or pelvic lymph nodes at presentation. *Prognosis relates to tumour size, an infiltrative tumour margin, depth of invasion, vascular involvement and in particular, lymph node disease*. There is no significant prognostic difference between HPV and non-HPV related cases. Stage I lesions have a 5 year survival of 90 %, stage II 80 %, stage III 60 %, stage IV 20 % and *overall 50–75 %*. Unilateral lymph node involvement (60–70 % 5 year survival) is better than bilateral lymph node disease (25 % 5 year survival). Extranodal spread may necessitate postoperative radiotherapy. *Treatment* is by *partial or total vulvectomy* with *uni-/bilateral inguinal lymph node dissection*. A *limited local excision* with wide (1 cm) surgical margins may be used in early stage (well differentiated superficially invasive) disease or medically unfit patients. VIN III may be treated by topical therapy, laser, electrocoagulation, wide local excision, partial/ total or skinning vulvectomy. *Pelvic exenteration* is reserved for locally extensive disease with no clinical or radiological evidence of extrapelvic metastases. Prognosis of *malignant melanoma* relates to tumour thickness and depth of invasion at the time of presentation, with *average 5 year survival of 30–35 %*.

27.9   Other Malignancy

Malignant Lymphoma/Leukaemia

- Secondary to systemic disease usually diffuse large B cell in type.

Adnexal/Bartholin's Gland Carcinomas

- Rare and arising from eccrine or apocrine glands when distinction from metastatic ductal carcinoma of the breast can be problematic. Bartholin's gland carcinoma forms *1–2 % of vulval neoplasms* and shows a range of differentiation: squamous cell, adenocarcinoma, mixed adenoid cystic/mucoepidermoid carcinoma. Ideally an origin from adjacent Bartholin's gland structures should be demonstrable. Five year survival rates vary from 40 to 80 % depending on the stage at presentation.

Aggressive Angiomyxoma

- Myxoid stroma, prominent vessels and spindle cells. A *locally infiltrative vulvovaginal tumour in young women* the edges of which are difficult to define surgically and therefore problematic to resect with *ischiorectal and retroperitoneal recurrence a likelihood*. Vimentin, actin positive±desmin. Nuclear

transcription factor HMGA2 positive in 50 % of cases. They are also ER and progesterone receptor positive raising a possible role for hormonal therapy.

Sarcomas

- Leiomyo-/rhabdo-/liposarcoma.
- *Leiomyosarcoma*: >5 cm diameter, infiltrating margins, >5–10 mitoses/10 high-power fields, cellular atypia.
- *Rhabdomyosarcoma*: occurs in childhood and young adults, with vaginal disease being embryonal in type, and vulval alveolar. Desmin/myo D1/myogenin positive.
- *Liposarcoma*: well differentiated adipocytic/ atypical lipoma in type.

Others

- Dermatofibrosarcoma protuberans, epithelioid sarcoma, malignant rhabdoid tumour.

Bibliography

Del Pino M, Rodriguez-Carunchio L, Ordi J. Pathways of vulvar intraepithelial neoplasia and squamous cell carcinoma. Histopathology. 2013;62:161–75.

Fox H, Wells M, editors. Haines and Taylor. Obstetrical and gynaecological pathology. 5th ed. Edinburgh: Churchill Livingstone; 2003a.

Fox H, Wells M. Recent advances in the pathology of the vulva. Histopathology. 2003b;42:209–16.

Heatley MK. Dissection and reporting of the organs of the female genital tract. J Clin Pathol. 2008;61:241–57.

Herrington CS. Recent advances in molecular gynaecological pathology. Histopathology. 2009;55:243–9.

Hirschowitz L, Nucci M, Zaino RJ. Problematic issues in the staging of endometrial, cervical and vulval carcinomas. Histopathology. 2013;62:176–202.

Kurman RJ, Norris HJ, Wilkinson E. Tumors of the cervix, vagina and vulva. Atlas of tumor pathology. 3rd series. Fascicle 4. Washington: AFIP; 1992.

McCluggage WG. Recent developments in vulvovaginal pathology. Histopathology. 2009;54:156–73.

McCluggage WG. Ten problematic issues identified by pathology review for multidisciplinary gynaecological oncology meetings. J Clin Pathol. 2012;65:293–301.

McCluggage WG, Hirschowitz L, Ganesan R, Kehoe S, Nordin A. Which staging system to use for gynaecological cancers: a survey with recommendations for practice in the UK. J Clin Pathol. 2010;63:768–70.

Nucci MR, Fletcher CDM. Vulvovaginal soft tissue tumours: update and review. Histopathology. 2000;36: 97–108.

Pecorelli S, FIGO Committee on Gynecologic Oncology. Revised FIGO staging for carcinoma of the vulva, cervix and endometrium. Int J Gynecol Obstet. 2009;105: 103–4.

Robboy SJ, Bentley RC, Russell R, Anderson MC, Mutter GL, Prat J. Pathology of the female reproductive tract. 2nd ed. London: Churchill Livingstone Elsevier; 2009.

Stewart CJR, McCluggage WG. Epithelial-mesenchymal transition in carcinomas of the female genital tract. Histopathology. 2013;62:31–43.

Tavassoli F, Devilee P. WHO classification of tumours. Pathology and genetics. Tumours of the breast and female genital organs. Lyon: IARC Press; 2003.

The Royal College of Pathologists. Cancer Datasets (Vulval Neoplasms, Cervical Neoplasia, Endometrial Cancer, Uterine Sarcomas, Neoplasms of the Ovaries and Fallopian Tubes and Primary Carcinoma of the Peritoneum), and Tissue Pathways for Gynaecological Pathology. Accessed at http://www.rcpath.org/index. asp?PageID =254.

Wittekind C, International Union against Cancer, et al. TNM atlas: illustrated guide to the TNM/pTNM classification of malignant tumours. 5th ed. Berlin: Springer; 2005.

Gestational Trophoblastic Tumours

28

Molar pregnancy affects 1–3 in every 1,000 pregnancies with women less than 16 years and more than 50 years of age at higher risk. It is characterised by an abnormal conception with excessive placental and no or minimal fetal development. It usually presents with first trimester bleeding, a uterus larger than expected for gestational dates, absence of fetal parts or a snowstorm appearance on ultrasound examination, and markedly elevated serum βHCG (β subunit human chorionic gonadotrophin). A clinical diagnosis is made in 80 % of complete moles and in 30 % of partial moles – the remainder after routine histology of evacuated products of conception. Partial moles present with spontaneous abortion. Trophoblastic disease should be considered when there is continued vaginal bleeding following delivery or an abortion.

About 10 % of hydatidiform moles result in one of the malignant forms of persistent gestational trophoblastic disease viz invasive hydatidiform mole (commonest), choriocarcinoma, placental site trophoblastic tumour or epithelioid trophoblastic tumour. In the UK persistent trophoblastic disease has a centralised system for registration, clinical monitoring and treatment. Lung is the commonest site of metastatic disease resulting in cough, haemoptysis, chest pain or dyspnoea. Curative intent chemotherapy is highly effective and delivered with minimal morbidity. It is indicated in a number of circumstances: biopsy proven choriocarcinoma, evidence of metastases (brain, lung, liver, vulva, gastrointestinal tract), heavy vaginal or gastrointestinal bleeding, serum HCG >20,000 IU/ml more than 4 weeks after evacuation, and rising or persistent serum HCG levels 6 months after evacuation. Response to treatment is assessed by falling serum HCG levels.

28.1 Gross Description

Specimen

- Curetting/hysterectomy.
- Weight (g) and size (cm), number of fragments, villous diameter.

Tumour

Site

- Endometrial/myometrial/extrauterine:
  Serosa
  Parametria
  Adnexae.
- Cavity: fundus, corpus, isthmus.

Size

- Length × width × depth (cm) or maximum dimension (cm). Size >5 cm is prognostically adverse.

Appearance

- Haemorrhagic/necrotic/vesicular/nodular/polypoid masses.

Edge

- Circumscribed/irregular.

28.2 Histological Type

Choriocarcinoma

- Suspect on curettings if there is abundant necrotic/haemorrhagic decidua, bilaminar aggregates of exuberant syncytiotrophoblast and cytotrophoblast, and no chorionic villi.
- *50 % are preceded by a molar gestation*, but also seen after normal pregnancy (20 %) or spontaneous abortion (30 %).
- *2–3 % of complete moles progress* to choriocarcinoma.
- *Destructive myometrial and vascular invasion* are common, leading to *haematogenous metastatic spread* to lung (60–80 %), vagina (30 %), pelvis (20 %), brain (17 %) and liver (11 %).
- HCG/cytokeratin/inhibin positive/HPL (human placental lactogen) focal.
- *5 year survival is >90 %* with *chemotherapy* (uterine disease >95 %, metastatic disease 83 %).

Invasive Hydatidiform Mole (Chorioadenoma Destruens)

- *16 % of complete moles.*
- Penetration into the myometrium or uterine vasculature ± adjacent structures of molar villi associated with variable degrees of trophoblast hyperplasia. Haemorrhage and perforation can occur.
- Haematogenous transport of "metastatic" nodules to vagina, lung and central nervous system. They do not affect the prognosis but may present with per vaginum bleeding or haemoptysis and respond well to chemotherapy.

Placental Site Trophoblastic Tumour (PSTT)

- Mostly following a normal term pregnancy (75 %).
- A polypoid mass composed of monomorphic intermediate trophoblast – mononuclear cytotrophoblast ± multinucleated cells,

dissecting myofibres without necrosis or haemorrhage. Peri-/intravascular growth patterns.
- HCG negative, HPL/alpha-inhibin/cytokeratin positive.
- *10–15 % are malignant* (mitoses >2/10 high-power fields, deep invasion, clear cells). Not chemoresponsive and *requires surgical removal.*

Epithelioid Trophoblastic Tumour (ETT)

- Along with choriocarcinoma and PSTT a non-villous forming potentially malignant gestational trophoblastic tumour.
- Very rare, following normal pregnancy.
- Geographical areas of necrosis with islands of uninucleate polygonal eosinophilic cells.
- Cytokeratin/alpha-inhibin positive: mostly HCG/HPL negative.
- Behaviour is similar to PSST rather than choriocarcinoma.

Differential diagnosis for choriocarcinoma, PSTT and ETT include persistent molar tissue, undifferentiated carcinoma/sarcoma and epithelioid leiomyosarcoma.

28.3 Differentiation

See above.

28.4 Extent of Local Tumour Spread

Border: pushing/infiltrative

Lymphocytic reaction: prominent/sparse. There is an improved prognosis with an intense tumour stroma interface inflammatory infiltrate in choriocarcinoma.

The TNM/FIGO classification applies to choriocarcinoma, invasive hydatidiform mole and placental site trophoblastic tumour. Histological confirmation is not required if the HCG level is abnormally elevated.

TNM (FIGO)

pT1 (I)	Tumour confined to the uterus
pT2 (II)	Tumour extends to other genital structures: vagina, ovary, broad ligament, fallopian tube by metastasis or direct extension
pM1a (III)	Metastasis to the lung(s)
pM1b (IV)	Other distant metastasis with or without lung involvement (brain, liver, kidney, gastrointestinal tract).

FIGO stages I–IV are subdivided into *A* (*low risk*) and *B* (*high risk*) categories according to a multiparameter prognostic score (Table 28.1). A more recent modification of FIGO is to qualify the stage with the prognostic score e.g. III: 4 instead of III A.

28.5   Lymphovascular Invasion

Present/absent.

Intra-/extratumoural.

Physiological trophoblast in placental site reaction is frequently endovascular with potential for myometrial invasion and this must not be over interpreted as malignancy.

Molar tissue can potentially spread to cervix, vaginal wall and vulva through a much dilated pelvic vasculature.

Choriocarcinoma typically shows *destructive myometrial and vascular invasion. Diagnostic biopsy* of metastatic deposits may be *contraindicated* due to the *risk of life threatening haemorrhage.*

28.6   Lymph Nodes

Usually tertiary metastases from a large extra-uterine lesion and of poor prognosis. Classified as metastatic MIb (FIGO IV) disease.

28.7   Excision Margins

Distances (mm) to the serosa and parametrial resection limits.

28.8   Other Pathology

Complete Hydatidiform Mole

- Androgenetic diploid 46XX.
- *Diffuse villous vesicular swelling* although this is only well developed beyond 12 weeks gestation by dates.
- *Central cistern formation.*
- *Circumferential/multifocal trophoblast.* Grading the degree of trophoblast proliferation is not of prognostic value.

Table 28.1 Prognostic score for gestational trophoblastic tumours

Prognostic score	0	1	2	3
Prognostic factor				
Age	<40	≥40		
Antecedent pregnancy	H. mole	Abortion	Term pregnancy	
Months from index pregnancy	<4	4 to <7	7–12	>12
Pretreatment serum HCG (IU/ml)	$<10^3$	10^3 to $<10^4$	10^4 to $<10^5$	$\geq10^5$
Largest tumour size including uterus	<3 cm	3 to <5 cm	≥5 cm	
Sites of metastasis	Lung	Spleen, kidney	Gastrointestinal tract	Liver, brain
Number of metastasis		1–4	5–8	>8
Previous failed chemotherapy			Single drug	2 or more drugs

Risk categories

Total prognostic score 7 or less is low risk (add "A" to FIGO Stage)

Total prognostic score 8 or more is high risk (add "B" to FIGO Stage)

- *Absence of fetal red blood cells and tissues* unless with a twin gestation.
- *Volume of placental tissue* is often abundant >100 g.
- *Early moles*: increasingly frequent with routine use of ultrasound examination. There can be a mixture of hydropic and non-hydropic villi or only lobulated villi making diagnosis problematic. Look for *branching and small sprouts* of secondary villi, some *invaginations in outline* and *trophoblast inclusions*, and a *myxoid stroma with nuclear debris*. Moderate trophoblast hyperplasia is also usually seen.

The vast majority regress but *10–15 % develop persistent trophoblastic disease* representing either incomplete removal of molar tissue, residual invasive mole within the myometrium or its vasculature, or choriocarcinoma.

Partial Hydatidiform Mole

- Biparental; triploid 69XXY, a minority are trisomy.
- ± a fetus (usually abnormal). Fetal death usually occurs around the 8th week leaving only necrotic debris or a persistent fetal circulation with open vessels and nucleated red blood cells.
- A *mixture* of focal villous vesicular swelling with central cisterns and normal sized villi.
- "Norwegian fjord" scalloped or dentate outline with *trophoblast inclusions*.
- Circumferential/multifocal *trophoblast hyperplasia*, usually syncytiotrophoblast.
- Volume of placental tissue normal.
- There is *persistent disease in up to 0.5–1 % of cases*.

In molar change vesicles of 2–3 mm diameter are usually seen grossly.

Hydropic Degeneration

- Often trisomy or triploid.
- *Villi <2–3 mm and rounded.*

- *No cisterns.*
- *Trophoblast is polar* in distribution and/or attenuated.

There is also a tendency to *over diagnose* mole in ectopic tubal pregnancy due to the exuberant trophoblast that is associated with early non-molar gestational sacs.

Other Comments

Placental site reaction: a common localised phenomenon in curettings from abortions and must not be confused with gestational trophoblastic tumours. It comprises an exaggerated response of decidua, altered myometrial smooth muscle cells and intermediate trophoblast without myometrial destruction or invasion. It is usually associated with some immature villi. Placental site nodules or plaques are characterised by small size, circumscribed margins and hyalinisation. Both are benign and do not require staging or follow up.

Trophoblast: unlikely to be neoplastic if the last known pregnancy was recent, of short duration, aborted, and characterised by a mixture of villous and placental site trophoblast. The differential diagnosis between hydropic degeneration, partial and complete moles is often difficult and *monitoring serum β subunit HCG levels* is useful to ensure that they revert to normal in time. Trophoblastic disease is associated with *persistently abnormal levels* and if this is present after 60 days with a previous diagnosis of hydatidiform mole consideration is given to use of chemotherapy. Another differential diagnosis for choriocarcinoma is non-gestational carcinoma with trophoblast metaplasia e.g. ovary, endometrium.

In curettage specimens trophoblast can be categorised as

(a) Villous trophoblast: the usual post abortion finding.
(b) Simple non-villous trophoblast: distinction between syncytio- and cytotrophoblast cannot be made and usually occurs after abortion.
(c) Suspicious non-villous trophoblast: no villi, a bilaminar arrangement of syncytio- and cytotrophoblast but no tissue invasion.

(d) Non-villous trophoblast diagnostic of choriocarcinoma: myometrial fragments with demonstrable invasion by bilaminar trophoblast.

Interpretation should be in the context of clinical, radiological and biochemical findings.

Flow cytometry: can help to distinguish between a diploid complete mole and triploid partial mole, and, between a triploid partial mole and non-molar diploid hydropic abortion. Cell proliferation markers (e.g. Ki-67) are strongly over expressed in complete moles but are of limited practical value. The product of the maternally expressed gene CDKN1C, *p57* ^{KIP2} can be stained immunohistochemically. It shows high levels of nuclear expression in the cytotrophoblast and villous mesenchyme of partial moles and hydropic abortions but is absent in complete mole and may prove a useful adjunct to the main morphological criteria in the designation of molar pregnancies. It has not been found to be of use in identifying the type of causative pregnancy in established gestational trophoblastic tumours.

Bibliography

Baergen N. Manual of pathology of the human placenta. 2nd ed. New York: Springer; 2011.

Fox H, Sebire N. Pathology of the placenta, Major problems in pathology series, vol. 7. 3rd ed. Philadelphia: Saunders; 2007.

Fox H, Wells M, editors. Haines and Taylor. Obstetrical and gynaecological pathology. 5th ed. Edinburgh: Churchill Livingstone; 2003.

Kaplan CG. Color atlas of gross placental pathology. 2nd ed. New York: Springer; 2006.

Lage JM. Protocol for the examination of specimens from patients with gestational trophoblastic malignancies. Arch Pathol Lab Med. 1999;123:50–4.

Lage JM, Minamiguchi S, Richardson MS. Gestational trophoblastic diseases: update on new immunohistochemical findings. Curr Diagn Pathol. 2003;9:1–10.

Paradinas FJ. The histological diagnosis of hydatidiform moles. Curr Diagn Pathol. 1994;1:24–31.

Paradinas FJ. The differential diagnosis of choriocarcinoma and placental site tumour. Curr Diagn Pathol. 1998;5:93–101.

Robboy SJ, Bentley RC, Russell R, Anderson MC, Mutter GL, Prat J. Pathology of the female reproductive tract. 2nd ed. London: Churchill Livingstone Elsevier; 2009.

Sebire NJ, Rees H. Diagnosis of gestational trophoblastic disease in early pregnancy. Curr Diagn Pathol. 2002;8:430–40.

Sebire NJ, Rees HC, Peston D, Seckl MJ, Newlands ES, Fisher RA. P57 ^{KIP2} immunohistochemical staining of gestational trophoblastic tumours does not identify the type of the causative pregnancy. Histopathology. 2004;45:135–41.

Silverberg SG, Kurman RJ. Tumors of the uterine corpus and gestational trophoblastic disease. Atlas of tumor pathology. 3rd series. Fascicle 3. Washington: AFIP; 1992.

The Royal College of Pathologists. Tissue Pathway for histopathological examination of the placenta. Accessed at http://www.rcpath.org/index.asp?PageID=1675.

Renal Cell and Renal Pelvis/Ureter Carcinoma

Carcinomas of the renal parenchyma and pelvis account for 2–3 % of all cancers and 7,000 cases in the UK per annum. Incidence is increasing partly due to improved diagnostic techniques and detection on radiological examination. Risk factors are smoking, obesity, exposure to carcinogenic industrial compounds through drinking water, and genetic factors e.g. von Hippel-Lindau disease, hereditary papillary renal carcinoma, and hereditary non-polyposis colorectal cancer (HNPCC). Renal pelvis/ureter carcinomas are much less common than tumours of the renal parenchyma, comprising 4–5 % of all urothelial cancers. Some 20–30 % of upper urinary tract urothelial cancers show microsatellite instability and loss of mismatch repair protein antibodies and there is an association with HNPCC.

Up to one third of renal carcinomas are asymptomatic and an incidental finding on radiological examination. Conversely about 35 % present late in their disease course with metastases. The classic triad of flank pain, mass and haematuria is infrequent and usually indicates advanced disease. Weight loss and painless haematuria are perhaps the most frequent presenting complaints. Other symptoms and signs are unexplained fever, anaemia, hypertension, hypercalcaemia and elevated ESR (erythrocyte sedimentation rate).

Investigation for renal cell carcinoma is by abdominal ultrasound and contrast enhanced CT scan which can distinguish between cystic and semi-cystic or solid lesions. They also provide staging information on lymph node, renal vein and inferior vena cava (IVC) involvement. MRI scan gives complementary information regarding the latter. Renal pelvic cancers are defined by retrograde pyelography and ureteropyeloscopy with cytological brushings and/or forceps biopsy. With increasing forceps size and improved technique and equipment, endoscopic biopsy can be diagnostic in 25–30 % of cases. However care must be taken due to the limited material produced, benign mimics of neoplasia e.g. polypoid urethritis/pyelitis, and artifact and distortion resulting in potential over diagnosis. This is particularly relevant in the absence of a clinically suspected tumour. Needle biopsy is done in a minority of renal cell cancers. This is usually when there is extensive spread for the purposes of obtaining a tissue diagnosis as a prequel to palliative adjuvant or immunotherapy, and, also to rule out a more treatable cause of the renal mass e.g. malignant lymphoma. It is also used in the investigation of an indeterminate complex, cystic renal mass, or, in tandem with local tumour destruction by cryotherapy or RFA (high radiofrequency ablation) in patients who are not medically fit for radical surgery, who have widespread disease or a solitary kidney. It is sometimes indicated prior to organ sparing partial nephrectomy, or to justify observation only management.

Otherwise most imaging proven and kidney confined mass lesions require surgical resection. Omitting an invasive needle biopsy avoids disrupting local anatomical structures and any risk of upstaging the tumour. The mainstay of surgical treatment for renal cell carcinoma is radical nephrectomy comprising removal of the kidney outside Gerota's fascia, and ipsilateral adrenalectomy with or without regional lymph-adenectomy. A laparoscopic approach is preferred with decreased patient morbidity and faster post operative recovery. Advances in preoperative imaging and staging have made partial nephrectomy an option for select patients e.g. tumour <4 cm dimension, bilateral synchronous tumours, tumour in a solitary kidney, or, with a poorly functioning contralateral kidney. Although local surgical resection for renal carcinoma is often complete (R0), haematogenous metastases are not infrequent and may occur at an early or late stage of disease. Renal pelvis/ureter carcinoma requires nephrectomy with ureterectomy. Endoscopic resection for early low-grade lesions is also now available.

29.1   Gross Description

Specimen

- Fine needle aspiration cytology (FNAC)/needle core biopsy/partial nephrectomy/nephrectomy ± ureterectomy/radical nephrectomy (kidney, pelvis, perirenal fat out to Gerota's fascia, adrenal gland, a length of ureter, ± regional lymph nodes)/segmental ureterectomy.
- Right/left: adrenal gland is superior, and the ureter lies behind the renal artery and vein and descends inferiorly.
- Weight (g) and size (cm).
- Length (cm) of attached ureter.
- Adrenal gland: present/absent.

Tumour

Site

- Upper/lower pole, midzone, hilum, medullary, cortical, subcapsular, extracapsular, pelvic/peripelvic.
- Single/multiple (satellite nodules are present in 5 % of renal cell cancers) or bilateral (1 %).

  Most renal cell carcinomas are *solitary*, randomly distributed in the renal cortex and unilateral. *Multifocality* and *bilaterality* suggests a *hereditary cancer type*.

- Most renal cell carcinomas are centred on the cortex, transitional cell carcinomas on the pelvis, or *multifocal* in the pelvicalyceal and ureteric collecting system.

Size

- Length × width × depth (cm) or maximum dimension (cm).
- Average size for renal cell carcinoma is 7 cm but there is an increasing proportion of smaller tumours with better radiological detection.

Appearance

- Cystic/solid/lobulated: renal cell carcinoma.
- Necrotic/haemorrhagic/yellow/calcification: renal cell carcinoma.
- Circumscribed/tan/central scar: oncocytoma, chromophobe and papillary carcinomas.
- White/granular/scirrhous: sarcomatoid and collecting duct carcinomas.
- Papillary/sessile/scirrhous: renal pelvis carcinoma.

Edge

- Circumscribed/irregular.

Compression/Infiltration of Structures

- Perinephric fat, capsule, cortex, medulla, pelvis, peripelvicalyceal fat (renal sinus), adrenal gland, renal vein.
- Most renal cell carcinomas have a pushing margin. Diffuse infiltration of the adjacent kidney, perirenal and renal sinus fat is uncommon in contrast to infiltrating pelvic transitional cell carcinoma.

29.2   Histological Type

Renal malignancy of childhood (nephroblastoma, clear cell sarcoma, rhabdoid tumour) is not discussed.

Renal Cell Carcinoma (WHO Classification 2004)

- Clear cell renal carcinoma, including multilocular cystic variant
- Papillary renal cell carcinoma

- Chromophobe renal cell carcinoma
- Collecting duct carcinoma
- Renal medullary carcinoma
- Tubulocystic carcinoma
- Family translocation associated carcinoma (Xp11.2, t(6;11))
- Mucinous tubular and spindle cell carcinoma
- Thyroid like follicular carcinoma of kidney
- Clear cell papillary renal cell carcinoma
- Renal cell carcinoma, unclassified
- Tumours associated with end stage kidney disease and acquired renal cystic disease

Adenocarcinoma

- *90 % of cases.*
- *Clear cell*: *70 % of cases*. Of proximal convoluted tubule origin. Solid/trabecular/alveolar/tubuloacinar/cystic patterns with a prominent sinusoidal vascular stroma and areas of haemorrhage. Glycogen and fat rich clear to eosinophilic granular cytoplasm and variable nuclear morphology.
- *Papillary*: *10–15 % of cases*. It is of better prognosis (80 % 5 year survival) than clear cell carcinoma and up to 70 % are intrarenal at diagnosis. Potentially multifocal, bilateral and familial (hereditary papillary renal carcinoma) arising on a background of precursor papillary adenoma(s). Formerly termed chromophil carcinoma. It is encapsulated, with solid and tubular patterns but at least 50–70 % of the tumour area is papillary with stromal aggregates of foam cells, focal psammomatous microcalcifications and haemorrhage. It is the commonest renal carcinoma in dialysis patients.
  Type 1 – basophilic cuboidal cell, uniform bland appearance and more often multifocal. Trisomies 7, 16, 17 are often detected.
  Type 2 – eosinophilic columnar cell with nuclear stratification. It is of worse prognosis than type 1.
- *Chromophobe*: *3–5 % of cases* arising from intercalated cells of cortical collecting ducts. It is of slightly better prognosis than clear cell carcinoma. Solid and nested patterns with a perinuclear halo, clear to flocculent cytoplasm (positive with Hale's colloidal iron and alcian blue), prominent ("koilocyte like")

cytoplasmic membranes, and "wrinkled" raisinoid hyperchromatic nuclei.
- *Collecting duct*: *1 % of cases*, located in the medulla with irregular tubules in a desmoplastic stroma, hob-nail cells and nuclear stratification. Often infiltrates perirenal/renal sinus fat. It is aggressive (50 % 2 year survival) although a rare low-grade variant exists.
- *Sarcomatoid*: *2–3 % of cases* with a pale solid/scirrhous appearance and fibrosarcomatous/malignant fibrous histiocytoma like spindle cell (± giant cell) morphology and usually with high nuclear grade. May occur either as a major or minor component with the other main subtypes, and also renal pelvic carcinoma. It is therefore regarded as *an indication of disease progression* and *a poorly differentiated or high-grade form* of them with *poor prognosis* (*median survival 19 months*) rather than a specific entity in its own right. A sarcomatoid component >50 % of the area of a renal cell carcinoma is adverse. A pale/scirrhous area within an otherwise usual renal cell carcinoma should be preferentially sampled for histology. Infiltrating transitional cell carcinoma of the renal pelvis can have a similar appearance.
- *Mixed*: about *10 % of cases* show mixed differentiation.
- *Unclassified*: *5–10 % of cases* do not fit into any distinctive category. Includes sarcomatoid carcinoma without an identifiable usual type of renal cell carcinoma, and carcinoma of undifferentiated morphology.
- *Renal medullary*: of collecting duct origin in young patients with sickle cell trait. Poorly differentiated cells in solid or cribriform clusters and intervening oedematous/collagenous stroma. Poor prognosis.
- *Translocation associated*: arise as a result of translocations in the MiTF/TFE family genes (TFE3/TFEB) on chromosome Xp11.2, constituting a higher proportion of renal cell carcinomas in children and young adults. Presentation is at an *advanced stage and is more aggressive in adults*. Alveolar and papillary patterns of clear to eosinophilic tumour cells of high nuclear grade. Psammomatous calcifications can be present. TFE3/TFEB protein and RCC antibody/CD10 positive, but only focally positive for cytokeratins and vimentin.

- *Mucinous tubular and spindle cell*: a low-grade biphasic carcinoma in females with a favourable prognosis. Macroscopically circumscribed, it comprises tubules and spindle cells in a myxoid stroma.
- *End stage/acquired cystic (haemodialysis) renal disease associated*: usual type renal clear cell carcinomas, a higher proportion of papillary renal cell carcinomas, and distinctive renal cell carcinomas with eosinophilic cytoplasm and oxalate crystals.
- *Oncocytoma*: on a spectrum with and forming a differential diagnosis for the eosinophilic variants of well differentiated (grade 1) renal cell carcinoma and chromophobe carcinoma is *benign renal oncocytoma*. A circumscribed, tan/brown lesion with a central radial scar comprising sheets, tubules and small nests of cells, with abundant eosinophilic cytoplasm and a central, small round nucleus, set in a variably oedematous stroma. It forms *3–5 % of renal neoplasms* and is usually an asymptomatic incidental finding in male patients over 50 years of age. Its cytoplasm is rich in mitochondria. It is *excluded in favour of a designation of renal cell carcinoma* by: necrosis, mitoses, clear cells, spindle cells, papillary areas, gross vascular invasion or gross extension into perirenal fat. It is occasionally multifocal and bilateral with associated microscopic oncocytomatosis.

Neuroendocrine Carcinoma

- Either well differentiated/low-grade neuroendocrine (carcinoid) tumour, or, poorly differentiated/high-grade small cell or large cell neuroendocrine carcinoma. Rare.
- Variably chromogranin/synaptophysin/CD56 and Ki-67 positive.
- Small cell carcinoma may also arise from the *pelvic mucosa* as part of a *high-grade transitional cell carcinoma* secondarily involving the kidney parenchyma. It is also important to exclude clinically and radiologically a metastasis from a lung small cell carcinoma. Both primary renal and pulmonary small cell cancers can be TTF-1 positive.

Renal Pelvis/Ureter Carcinoma

Transitional Cell (Urothelial) Carcinoma
- Generally in patients over 65 years of age and with a male to female ratio of 3:1.
- ± calculi or a history of analgaesic nephropathy with renal papillary necrosis.
- *Single/multifocal*: renal pelvis 58 %, ureter 35 %, pelvis and ureter 7 %, bilateral 2–5 %. About 30–75 % also develop synchronous or metachronous *urinary bladder tumours*.
- *10 % of renal neoplasms* and *5 % of urothelial tumours*.
- *30 % of cases are low-grade* and papillary giving hydroureter/hydronephrosis with a non-functioning kidney and a radiological filling defect in the pelvis/ureter. The other *70 % of cases are high-grade* (particularly renal pelvis) and a mixture of papillary and sessile lesions. The latter can show "cancerisation" of renal medullary tubules, and infiltrate the medulla and cortex with a scirrhous gross appearance and squamoid or spindle cell morphology. *Invasive micropapillary urothelial carcinoma* is high-grade with aggressive behaviour. Other variants include clear cell, plasmacytoid cells, rhabdoid cells and giant cells.

Squamous Cell Carcinoma
- Calculi/infection/squamous cell metaplasia of the pelvic mucosa.
- Mostly *high-grade* and *locally advanced* or *metastatic* at presentation. Prognosis is poor.
- Mixed: as part of a high-grade transitional cell carcinoma (*20–40 % of WHO III TCCs*).

Adenocarcinoma
- Pure: tubulovillous/mucinous/signet ring cell/papillary non-mucinous. Adjacent pyelitis cystica/glandularis secondary to chronic inflammation, e.g. calculi.
- Mixed: as part of a high-grade transitional cell carcinoma (*2–5 % of WHO III TCCs*).

Sarcomatoid Carcinoma
- Spindle cell carcinoma with high nuclear grade and cytokeratin positive. It may be combined with foci of usual transitional cell carcinoma, or show carcinosarcomatous homologous

or heterologous components. Usually at an *advanced stage at diagnosis* and pursues an *aggressive course*.

Metastatic Carcinoma

- Often small and bilateral (50 %).
- *Direct spread*: cervix, prostate, bladder (distal ureter), gastrointestinal tract, retroperitoneal metastases e.g. lung and breast.
- *Distant spread*: lung, malignant melanoma (skin), breast, stomach, pancreas, ovary, testis.

29.3 Differentiation/Grade

Renal Cell Carcinoma

Well/moderate/poor/undifferentiated, or, Fuhrman nuclear grade 1/2/3/4.

Differentiation and nuclear grade are not infrequently *heterogeneous* within a lesion. Tumour size does not consistently relate to tumour grade i.e. small tumours can be of high nuclear grade. The renal carcinoma cell typically has abundant cytoplasm with a low nuclear/cytoplasmic ratio.

Nuclear Grade (Fuhrman)

1. Round, uniform, 10 μm, nucleoli absent
2. Slightly irregular, 15 μm, nucleoli visible
3. Moderately to markedly irregular, 20 μm, large nucleoli
4. Bizarre multinucleated forms, ≥20 μm, prominent nucleoli, clumped chromatin.

Grades 2 (35 %) and 3 (35 %) account for the majority of cases. Prognostic significance of nuclear grade also varies according to tumour type e.g. metastatic papillary renal carcinoma is usually high-grade whereas metastatic clear cell renal carcinoma can be variably low to high nuclear grade.

Tumour Cell Necrosis

Coagulative tumour cell necrosis is an *adverse prognostic indicator*. It should be distinguished from the more usual degenerative changes such as hyalinization, haemorrhage and fibrosis. Any history of preoperative embolisation to reduce the risk of intraoperative haemorrhage should be borne in mind.

Transitional Cell Carcinoma

WHO I/II/III.

Low-grade (WHO I) or high-grade (WHO II/III).

For further discussion of classification of urothelial neoplasms see Chap. 30.

For non-transitional pelviureteric cancers: well/moderate/poor/undifferentiated, or, Grade 1/2/3/4.

29.4 Extent of Local Tumour Spread

Border: pushing/infiltrative.

Lymphocytic reaction: prominent/sparse.

Capsule, Perirenal Fat, Medulla

The capsule is often elevated and compressed by the pushing and lobulated margin of renal cell adenocarcinoma and this must be distinguished from actual histologically proven invasion of perirenal fat by tumour cells (pT3a). In this respect the capsule and fat should not be stripped from the kidney prior to sectioning perpendicular to it otherwise the cortex/capsule/fat interface is lost. *Extension to the renal sinus* (peripelvicalyceal fat) should be actively examined for as it is particularly susceptible to *small vessel vascular invasion*. Invasion of the medullary collecting system is infrequent but is thought to confer a worse prognosis in low stage disease.

Adrenal Gland

Involvement of the ipsilateral adrenal gland (5 % of cases) is either by direct spread or metastasis. Risk is related to tumour grade, size and location with upper pole tumours particularly prone.

Renal Vein

Renal cell adenocarcinoma has a propensity for *venous invasion*, and involvement of the *renal* vein or its segmental (muscle containing) branches should be identified grossly at specimen dissection with subsequent histological confirmation. In partial nephrectomy specimens presumptive absence of renal vein involvement is dependent on clinical imaging studies as it is usually not submitted in these specimens.

Pelvis, Ureter

Renal pelvic transitional cell carcinoma is not infrequently multifocal (40%) with concurrent ureteric lesions±bladder tumour. The adjacent urothelium is often abnormal ranging from hyperplasia through dysplasia to carcinoma in situ.

The TNM7 classifications apply to renal cell, renal pelvis and ureter carcinomas.

Renal Cell Carcinoma

pT1	Tumour ≤7 cm in greatest dimension, limited to the kidney
	(a) ≤4 cm.
	(b) 4 cm < tumour ≤7 cm.
pT2	Tumour >7 cm in greatest dimension, limited to the kidney
	(a) 7 cm < tumour ≤10 cm.
	(b) Tumour>10 cm.
pT3	Tumour invades:
	(a) Perinephric fat[a] or grossly extends into the renal vein or its segmental (muscle containing) branches
	(b) Tumour extends into IVC below the diaphragm
	(c) Tumour extends into IVC above the diaphragm or invades IVC wall
pT4	Tumour invades beyond Gerota's fascia, including contiguous extension into the ipsilateral adrenal gland.

[a]Includes renal sinus (peripelvicalyceal fat)
See Fig. 29.1

Contralateral adrenal gland involvement is rare (pM1). Gerota's (renal) fascia is retrorenal and prerenal with invasion beyond the latter sometimes resulting in peritoneal involvement (pT4). Renal sinus involvement has been noted to be the commonest site of extrarenal extension (pT3) and

vascular involvement, and, correlates with tumour type, grade and size. Its evaluation which has been frequently omitted in the past can upstage disease if involved. Careful scrutiny is required.

Involvement of renal vein and ipsilateral adrenal gland is seen in 10 and 5% of cases respectively. Extrarenal tumour is present in up to 30–45% of cases at presentation its frequency varying with tumour type e.g. 85 % of chromophobe carcinomas are organ confined at diagnosis. Metastases occur in the lung, pleura, skeleton, soft tissues and skin, and to almost any site where they can mimic primary clear cell tumour in the involved organ e.g. kidney, thyroid, ovary. Preferential metastatic sites are seen with various subtypes of carcinoma e.g. papillary carcinoma has fewer lung metastases and more lymph node deposits than clear cell carcinoma, and chromophobe carcinoma tends to spread to liver.

Pelvis/Ureter Carcinoma

pTis	Carcinoma in situ
pTa	Papillary non-invasive
pT1	Tumour invades subepithelial connective tissue
pT2	Tumour invades muscularis propria
pT3	Tumour invades beyond muscularis into peripelvic fat or renal parenchyma (pelvis)
	Tumour invades beyond muscularis into periureteric fat (ureter)
pT4	Tumour invades adjacent organs, or through the kidney into perinephric fat.

See Fig. 29.2

For ureter adjacent organs include parietal peritoneum. Ureteric pT3 disease is prognostically equivalent to pT4 renal pelvis tumour.

Pelvis/ureter carcinoma: single/multifocal lesion(s); hydroureter/hydronephrosis.

For the purposes of TNM7 the pelviureteric system is considered as a single organ and synchronous pelviureteric lesions are classified according to the highest pT category e.g. pT2 (m). In contrast synchronous renal pelvis and bladder cancers are classified independently.

50 % present as superficial disease and 50 % are deeply invasive (pT2 or beyond).

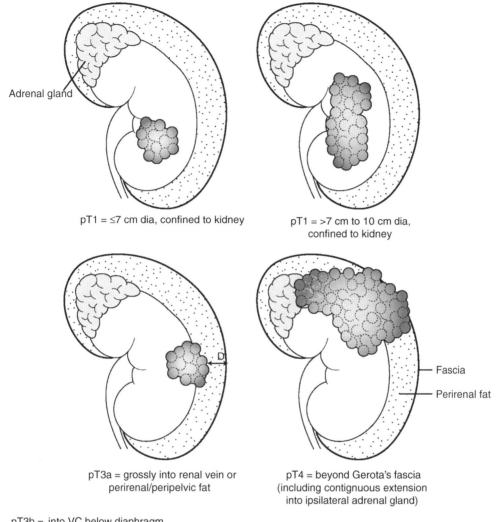

pT1 = ≤7 cm dia, confined to kidney

pT1 = >7 cm to 10 cm dia,
confined to kidney

pT3a = grossly into renal vein or
perirenal/peripelvic fat

pT4 = beyond Gerota's fascia
(including contiguous extension
into ipsilateral adrenal gland)

pT3b = into VC below diaphragm
pT3c = into VC above diaphragm
D = Tumour distance (mm) to the circumferential radial
margin (CRM) of excision of perinephric fat

Fig. 29.1   Renal cell carcinoma (Reproduced, with permission, from Allen (2006), © 2006)

29.5   Lymphovascular Invasion

Present/absent.

Intra-/extratumoural.

Renal cell carcinoma has a tendency to *involve the main renal vein* while infiltrating pelvic transitional cell carcinoma often shows invasion of *small lymphovascular channels* in the medulla and cortex. However, it can also subsequently involve the renal vein. In renal cell carcinoma prognostically adverse *renal sinus (peripelvical-yceal) fat macro- and microvascular invasion* should also be sought and identified.

29.6   Lymph Nodes

Site/number/size/number involved/limit node/extracapsular spread.

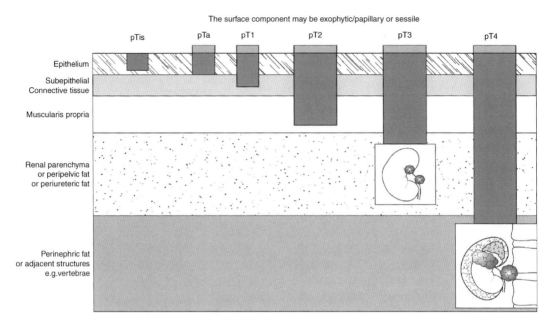

The surface component may be exophytic/papillary or sessile

Fig. 29.2 Renal pelvis and ureter carcinoma (Reproduced, with permission, from Allen (2006), © 2006)

Regional nodes: hilar, abdominal para-aortic, paracaval (ureter-intrapelvic). A regional lymphadenectomy will ordinarily include a minimum of eight lymph nodes although in UK surgical practice lymph nodes are found in <5 % of nephrectomy specimens with an overall positive metastasis rate of 4 %. A few lymph nodes may be found at the renal hilum and occasionally individual operatively suspicious nodes will be submitted. Sometimes coincidental pathology e.g. sarcoidosis is found as a basis for the lymphadenopathy. Separate dissection of the paraaortic and paracaval lymph nodes gives optimal staging information in that a pNX specimen has worse 5 year survival (61 %) than a pN0 nephrectomy (74 %) implying inaccurate downstaging.

Renal Cell Carcinoma

pN0	No regional lymph node metastasis
pN1	Metastasis in a single regional node
pN2	Metastasis in more than one regional node.

Regional lymph node metastases occur in *10–15 % of cases* and are associated with an adverse prognosis.

Pelvis/Ureter Carcinoma

pN0	No regional lymph node metastasis
pN1	Single regional node metastasis ≤2 cm
pN2	Single regional node metastasis >2–5 cm, multiple ≤5 cm
pN3	Regional node metastasis >5 cm.

Regional lymph node metastases occur in *5–10 %* of renal pelvic urothelial carcinomas.

29.7 Excision Margins

Distances (mm) to the distal ureteric limit, renal vein limit, perirenal fat and periureteric resection margins. Also the renal parenchyma resection limit in partial nephrectomy specimens.

29.8 Other Pathology

Macro-/micro morphology of renal carcinoma: there is a degree of correlation between gross morphology, cell type and architectural patterns in renal cell carcinoma e.g. clear cell is lobulated, yellow with areas of haemorrhage and non-papillary. Chromophobe and papillary tumours are circumscribed and tan in colour. Sarcomatoid carcinoma is usually pale and scirrhous in appearance with a differential diagnosis of invasive pelvic transitional cell carcinoma. Renal clear cell adenocarcinoma may become totally cystic with only residual mural nodules of viable tumour. *Multilocular cystic renal cell carcinoma* has a very good prognosis with no evidence of progression. It comprises numerous cysts with fibrous septa lined by clear cells with grade 1 nuclei.

Chromosomal analysis: characterises various morphological subtypes, e.g. *papillary* versus *non-papillary renal carcinoma*. Cytogenetically papillary tumours show a trisomic gain on chromosomes 7, 16 and 17 rather than the 3p13 deletion of usual renal clear cell carcinoma. Chromophobe carcinomas can be hypodiploid with multiple monosomies. Renal cell carcinoma with familial Xp11 translocations are identified by fluorescent in situ hybridization (FISH). Primary pelviureteric carcinoma is associated with HNPCC.

Von Hippel-Lindau (VHL) disease: has an increased incidence (*40–50% overall and a 70% risk by 70 years of age*) of renal cell carcinoma, as do *acquired cystic disease* (e.g. long term dialysis) and *autosomal dominant polycystic kidney disease (ADPKD: 5–10%)*. VHL has cysts with variable single cell, hyperplastic or solid clear cell epithelial lining. The renal clear cell carcinoma tends to be multiple and there are cysts elsewhere in kidney, liver and pancreas, phaeochromocytoma and cerebellar haemangioblastoma. ADPKD shows similar precancerous and established clear cell foci.

Miscellaneous renal and systemic features: occasionally renal cell carcinoma can spontaneously *regress* and also be host to *cancer metastasis to within cancer*, particularly from lung carcinoma. Other associated characteristics are *fever, hepatic dysfunction, hypercalcaemia, hypertension* (*secretion of renin*), *polycythaemia* (*secretion of erythropoietin*) and *hormonal effects* (*secretion of ACTH like substance*). *Amyloid* can be present in the renal interstitium adjacent to renal cell carcinoma and systemic in distribution. *Glomerulonephritis* is also an association. Examination of adjacent non-neoplastic parenchyma, beyond the usual compressed zone, shows pathological abnormalities in 60 % of nephrectomies for renal tumour, commonly related to *coincidental vascular disease* (*arteriosclerosis, atherosclerosis, hypertension*) or *diabetes*. Severe changes can be associated with progressive deterioration in postoperative renal function.

Xanthogranulomatous pyelonephritis (XGP), malakoplakia: both can mimic pelvic and renal cell carcinoma grossly and on needle biopsy. XGP comprises CD68 positive macrophages lacking cytokeratin positive epithelial cells, while malakoplakia shows eosinophilic macrophages with von Kossa or PAS stainable Michaelis-Gutmann bodies. Other differential diagnoses of a renal nodule or mass can be

- *Renal papillary adenoma*: circumscribed, <0.5 cm, papillae with fine fibrovascular cores ± tubules and a single layer of uniform cuboidal, eosinophilic or basophilic cells. Associated with renal cell carcinoma, papillary renal cell carcinoma, oncocytoma, long term haemodialysis and acquired renal cystic disease, and may be multiple.
- *Metanephric adenoma/adenofibroma*: circumscribed, small uniform cells in crowded tubules and papillae forming glomeruloid bodies. Scanty intervening stroma with psammoma bodies but areas of fibrosis in the adenofibroma variant. It is EMA/CK7 negative unlike its differential diagnosis papillary renal carcinoma.
- *Oncocytoma*: see above.
- *Angiomyolipoma*: epithelioid variant (HMB-45 positive). See Sect. 29.9.
- *Multicystic nephroma*: simple cysts lined by flat cuboidal to columnar hob-nail cells and intervening fibrous stroma ± muscle, cartilage and focal blastematous elements (cystic partially differentiated nephroblastoma).

Clear cell morphology: a solid clear cell lesion of any size should be regarded as a renal carcinoma with a 3 cm dimension considered a threshold for metastatic potential. Adenoma is reserved for small papillary, or, metanephric lesions as defined above.

Percutaneous FNAC: usually avoided but can give a diagnosis of simple renal cysts versus cystic or solid renal cell carcinoma. Carcinoma is cellular, shows nuclear atypia with a low nuclear/cytoplasmic ratio, nucleolar enlargement and variable fat/glycogen positive cytoplasmic vacuolation. Pelvic carcinoma also shows cytological features of malignancy. *FNAC* has a more defined role in the *investigation of suspected metastatic disease*.

Immunophenotype

Renal clear cell carcinoma: typically cytokeratin (AE1/AE3, CK8, CK18)/EMA/vimentin/CD10/N-cadherin positive, variable for RCC antibody/PAX-2/PAX-8, and negative for CK7/E-cadherin/Ber EP4/MOC 31 and CD117.

Papillary renal cell carcinoma: CK7/RCC antibody/Ber EP4/EMA positive, and variable for CD 10/MOC 31/PAX-2/PAX-8, and CD117 negative.

Chromophobe carcinoma: CK7/EMA/E--cadherin/MOC 31/BerEP4 and CD117 positive, and CD10/RCC antibody/vimentin/N-cadherin negative.

Collecting duct carcinoma: CK7, EMA, CEA, 34βE12 positive.

Sarcomatoid carcinoma: retains vimentin and focal keratin positivity.

Oncocytoma: CD117 positive, CK7 focal, and CD10/MOC 31 negative.

Thus the various combinations of immunophenotype can aid morphology in distinguishing the histological subtypes although there can be a marked overlap of expression between categories. A recent survey of European uropathologists showed that the most commonly used antibodies in nephrectomy surgical pathology are:

CK7 (95 %), CD10 (93 %), vimentin (86 %), HMB-45 (68 %) and CD117 (61 %).

A useful limited diagnostic panel is:

Oncocytoma	CD117/CK7(focal) positive
Chromophobe carcinoma	CD117/CK7 positive
Papillary carcinoma	CK7 positive and CD117 negative
Clear cell carcinoma	CK7/CD117 negative and EMA/CD10 positive.

Renal clear cell carcinoma (CD10 positive, melan-A/inhibin negative) may also be discriminated from *adrenal gland carcinoma* which has a converse immunophenotype. Immunoprofile is of use in determining a renal origin for clear cell carcinoma metastatic to various body sites e.g. skin, liver, lung, pleura. RCC antibody and CD10 mark proximal tubules, MOC 31 and BerEP4 distal tubules. CD10 is also positive in renal pelvic transitional cell carcinoma particularly high-grade and stage tumours but its expression is inversely related to tumour grade in renal clear cell carcinoma. *High-grade urothelial cancer* invading the medulla may mimic renal parenchymal cancers of various types. Use of p63, 34βE12 (positive in urothelial carcinoma) and PAX-8 (variably positive in renal carcinomas) may help make the distinction.

Treatment

Renal cell carcinoma: is treated by *surgical excision*, either partial or heminephrectomy (nephron sparing surgery), or radical nephrectomy depending on the size and location of the tumour. *Partial nephrectomy* ranges from tumour enucleation to heminephrectomy with part of the pelvicalyceal system and related overlying perirenal fat. *Radical nephrectomy* removes an entire kidney, en bloc adrenal gland, perirenal fat out to Gerota's fascia, and variable lengths of hilar vessels and ureter. Indications for nephron sparing surgery are: tumour <4 cm diameter, location at a renal pole and of non-papillary type, and compromised function in the contralateral kidney.

Renal pelvis/ureter carcinoma: requires *laparoscopic nephrectomy with ureterectomy*, often including resection of the *ureteric orifice* because of multifocality and involvement of its *terminal, vesical* (*intramural*) *portion*. Solitary distal ureteric lesions may be treated by *segmental ureterectomy with ureteral reimplantation. Ureterectomy with endoscopic resection* of small low-grade, superficial pelvic lesions may be used as a renal sparing procedure when there is solitary kidney or poor renal function. Occasionally a pelvic carcinoma may be found in a radical nephrectomy supposedly removed for a diagnosis of renal cell carcinoma. This leaves the issue of potential metachronous disease in the residual ureter and secondary ureterectomy may be considered. *Resection of solitary pulmonary metastases* can be of benefit for renal cell and renal pelvic cancers.

Prognosis

Renal cell carcinoma: *up to 35% of cases* present with *spread beyond the kidney* and *10% involve renal vein* with a tendency to solitary *distant haematogenous metastases* e.g. lung, skin and bone with pathological fracture e.g. neck of femur. *Recurrence develops in 40% of patients* treated for localized tumour. Recurrence is an end point, the likelihood of which is risk stratified in clinical algorithms (Memorial Sloan Kettering or Mayo Clinic) based on clinical presentation, performance status and various pathological factors. Chromophobe (mortality <10 %) and papillary carcinomas have a better prognosis than equivalent grade and stage renal clear cell carcinoma while sarcomatoid and unclassified cancers are worse (94, 86, 76, 35 and 24 % 5 year survivals, respectively). *Overall 5 year survival is 70%* relating to *tumour grade*, *type* (*e.g. grade III/IV and sarcomatoid lesions are aggressive*), *necrosis*, *vascular invasion* and *stage* (particularly extrarenal disease), although cure is possible even with main vessel involvement. *Chemotherapy* is largely ineffective although when combined with immunotherapy it may have a role to play in lymph node positive or widespread disease. 5 year survival figures are:

pT1	60–80 %
pT2	40–70 %
pT3	10–40 %
pT4	5 %.

Carcinoma of the renal pelvis/ureter: is predominantly *transitional cell or urothelial* in type with occasional squamous cell, adenocarcinoma and sarcomatoid carcinomas. Typically there are *multifocal*, synchronous pelviureteric (25 %) and bladder (15 %) lesions with a *50% risk of* *subsequent metachronous tumours* at these sites. About *30% are low-grade* and *70% high-grade* with *50% representing superficial disease* and *50% deeply invasive* (pT2 or beyond). The latter can form poorly differentiated nests, sheets and cords of tumour in a desmoplastic stroma often assuming a squamoid appearance. Retrograde involvement of medullary collecting ducts (mimicking adenocarcinoma) and lymphovascular invasion are not uncommon. *Low-grade superficial lesions are of good prognosis but critical invasion of or beyond ureteric muscle coat, renal pelvic wall or parenchyma results in 5 year survival rates of 35% (pT1: 91%, pT2: 23%)*. Chemotherapy and targeted therapies have an evolving role to play.

29.9 Other Malignancy

Malignant Lymphoma/Leukaemia

- Usually *secondary to systemic/nodal disease* and present in up to 50% of cases, and potentially bilateral. If established on clinical and radiological grounds as a primary lymphoma it is usually *diffuse large B cell* in type. Diffuse parenchymal tumour cell permeation or discrete tumour masses.
- Malignant lymphoma is occasionally associated with renal cell carcinoma.
- Post-transplant lymphoproliferative disorder.

Leiomyosarcoma, Liposarcoma, Malignant Fibrous Histiocytoma, Rhabdomyosarcoma, Synovial Sarcoma, Ewing's Sarcoma/Peripheral Neuroectodermal Tumour (PNET)

- *All are rare*, and important to exclude more common diagnoses i.e. sarcomatoid renal cell carcinoma, or, primary retroperitoneal sarcoma with secondary renal involvement.
- *Leiomyosarcoma*: is the commonest primary sarcoma (50–60% of cases) arising from the renal capsule, parenchyma, pelvic muscularis or renal vein. It is *aggressive* with a majority of patients dead from disease within 1 year of diagnosis.

Angiomyolipoma with Malignant Transformation

- A perivascular epithelioid cell tumour (PEComa) forming 1% of surgically resected renal tumours and is *usually benign*.
- There is an association with *tuberous sclerosis in 30% of cases* (more frequent in the epithelioid variant), and PEComa may be *multifocal (30%)* or *bilateral (15%)*.
- *Classic triphasic histology* comprising: HMB-45/melan-A/CD117/desmin positive *spindle cells* with variable cellularity and pleomorphism (giant/epithelioid cells)±mitoses, *mature fat*, and *dystrophic thick walled vessels* in varying proportions. This gives a distinctive radiological appearance on CT scan due to its fat content.
- Capsular invasion and lymph node disease may be seen and often regarded as multicentricity rather than malignancy. *Rarely true malignant change can occur* (epithelioid variant) with a 30% risk of metastases.
- Prone to *catastrophic/potentially fatal retroperitoneal haemorrhage* particularly if>4 cm.
- Rarely associated with concurrent renal cell carcinoma.

Bibliography

Algaba F, Delahunt B, Berney DM, Camparo P, Comperat E, Griffiths D, Kristiansen G, Lopez-Beltran A, Martignoni G, Moch H, Montironi R, Varma M, Egevad L. Handling and reporting of nephrectomy specimens for adult renal tumours: a survey by the European network of uropathology. J Clin Pathol. 2012;65:106–13.

Allen DC. Histopathology reporting: guidelines for surgical cancer. 2nd ed. Springer: London; 2006.

Amin MB, Amin MB, Tamboli P, Javidan J, Stricker H, Venturina MD-P, Deshpande A, Menon M. Prognostic impact of histologic subtyping of adult renal epithelial neoplasms. An experience of 405 cases. Am J Surg Pathol. 2002;26:281–91.

Association of Directors of Anatomic and Surgical Pathology. Recommendations for the reporting of surgically resected specimens of renal cell carcinoma. Am J Clin Pathol. 2009;131:623–30.

Bijol V, Mendez GP, Hurwitz S, Rennke HG, Nose V. Evaluation of the nonneoplastic pathology in tumor nephrectomy specimens. Predicting the risk of progressive renal failure. Am J Surg Pathol. 2006;30:575–84.

Bonsib SM. Macroscopic assessment, dissection protocols and histologic sampling strategy for renal cell carcinomas. Diagn Histopathol. 2008;14(4):151–6.

Bostwick DG, Cheng L. Urologic surgical pathology. 2nd ed. St. Louis: Mosby/Elsevier; 2008.

Carvalho JC, Wasco MJ, Kunju LP, Thomas DG, Shah RB. Cluster analysis of immunohistochemical profiles delineates CK7, vimentin, S100A1 and C-kit (CD117) as an optimal panel in the differential diagnosis of renal oncocytoma from its mimics. Histopathology. 2011;58:169–79.

Carvalho JC, Thomas DG, McHugh JB, Shah RB, Kunju LP. p63, CK7, PAX8 and INI-1: an optimal immunohistochemical panel to distinguish poorly differentiated urothelial cell carcinoma from high-grade tumours of the renal collecting system. Histopathology. 2012;60:597–608.

Commentary FS. Renal cell carcinoma in acquired cystic kidney disease. Histopathology. 2010;56:395–400.

D' Agati VD, Jennette JC, Silva FG. Non-neoplastic kidney diseases, Atlas of nontumor pathology. Washington: AFIP; 2005.

Eble JN, Sauter G, Epstein JI, Sesterhenn IA. WHO classification of tumours. Pathology and genetics. Tumours of the urinary system and male genital organs. Lyon: IARC Press; 2004.

Fleming S. Recently recognized epithelial tumours of the kidney. Curr Diagn Pathol. 2005;11:162–9.

Fleming S, Griffiths DFR. Nephrectomy for renal tumour; dissection guide and dataset. ACP best practice no 180. J Clin Pathol. 2005;58:7–14.

Fuhrman SA, Lasky LC, Limas C. Prognostic significance of morphologic parameters in renal cell carcinoma. Am J Surg Pathol. 1982;6:655–63.

Griffiths DFR, Vujanic GM. Cystic lesions of the kidney-selected topics. Curr Diagn Pathol. 2002; 8:94–101.

Griffiths DFR, Nind N, O'Brien CJ, Rashid M, Verghese A. Evaluation of a protocol for examining nephrectomy specimens with renal cell carcinoma. J Clin Pathol. 2003;56:374–7.

Kovacs G, Akhtar M. The Heidelberg classification of renal cell tumours. J Pathol. 1997;183:131–3.

Langner C, Ratschek M, Rehak P, Schips L, Zigeuner R. CD10 is a diagnostic and prognostic marker in renal malignancies. Histopathology. 2004;40:460–7.

Mathers C, Pollock AM, Marsh C, O'Donnell M. Cytokeratin 7: a useful adjunct in the diagnosis of chromophobe renal cell carcinoma. Histopathology. 2002;40:563–7.

Murphy WM, Grignon DJ, Perlman EJ. Tumors of the kidney, bladder and related urinary structures. Atlas of tumor pathology. 4th series. Fascicle. Washington: AFIP; 2004.

Olgae S, Mazumdar M, Dalbagni G, Reuter VE. Urothelial carcinoma of the renal pelvis. A clinicopathologic study of 130 cases. Am J Surg Pathol. 2004;28:1545–52.

Pan C-C, Chen PC-H, Ho DM-T. The diagnostic utility of MOC31, BerEP4, RCC marker and CD10 in the classification of renal cell carcinoma and renal oncocytoma: an immunohistochemical analysis of 328 cases. Histopathology. 2004;45:452–9.

Perez-Montiel D, Suster S. Upper urinary tract carcinomas: histological types and unusual morphological variants. Diagn Histopathol. 2007;14:48–54.

Renshaw AA. Subclassification of renal cell neoplasms: an update for the practising pathologist. Histopathology. 2002;41:283–300.

Sebire NJ, Vujanic VM. Paediatric renal tumours: recent developments, new entities and pathological features. Histopathology. 2009;54:516–28.

Shah RB, Bakshi N, Hafez K, Wood DP, Kunju LP. Image-guided biopsy in the evaluation of renal mass lesions in contemporary urological practice: indications, adequacy, clinical impact and limitations of the pathological diagnosis. Hum Pathol. 2005;36:1309–15.

Tavora F, Fajardo DA, Lee TK, Lotan T, Miller JS, Miyamoto H, Epstein JI. Small endoscopic biopsies in the ureter and renal pelvis. Pathologic pitfalls. Am J Surg Pathol. 2009;33:1540–6.

The Royal College of Pathologists. Cancer Datasets (Adult Renal Parenchymal Cancer, Renal Tumours in Childhood, Penile Cancer, Prostatic Carcinoma, Testicular Tumours and Post-Chemotherapy Residual Masses, Tumours of the Urinary Collecting System) and Tissue Pathways (Medical Renal Biopsies, Urological Pathology). Accessed at http://www.rcpath.org/index.asp?PageID=254.

Thomas JO, Tawfik OW. Recent advances in the diagnosis of renal cell carcinoma. Diagn Histopathol. 2008;14(4):157–63.

Thomas DH, Verghese A, Kynaston HG, Griffiths DFR. Analysis of the prognostic implications of different tumour margin types in renal cell carcinoma. Histopathology. 2003;43:374–80.

Tickoo SK, de Peralta-Venturina MN, Harik LR, Worcester HD, Salama ME, Young AN, Moch H, Amin MB. Spectrum of epithelial neoplasms in end-stage renal disease. Am J Surg Pathol. 2006;30:141–53.

Trpkov K, Yilmaz A, Uzer D, Dishongh KM, Quick CM, Bismar TA, Gokden N. Renal oncocytoma revisited: a clinicopathological study of 109 cases with emphasis on problematic diagnostic features. Histopathology. 2010;57:892–906.

Veeratterapillay R, Simren R, El-Sherif A, Johnson MI, Soomro N, Heer R. Accuracy of the revised 2010 TNM classification in predicting the prognosis of patients treated for renal cell cancer in the north east of England. J Clin Pathol. 2012;65:367–71.

Venturina MD-P, Moch H, Amin M, Tamboli P, Hailemarian S, Mitatsch M, Javidan J, Stricker H, Ro JY, Amin MB. Sarcomatoid differentiation in renal cell carcinoma. A study of 101 cases. Am J Surg Pathol. 2001;25:275–84.

Bladder cancer is the seventh commonest cancer worldwide (3.2 % of cases) with a male to female ratio of 3.5:1 and geographical variation with highest incidence in the Western hemisphere. Predisposing factors to bladder cancer are smoking, exposure to industrial aniline dyes (aromatic amines), petrochemicals, cyclophosphamide, and the analgaesic phenacetin. A minority of cases have a positive family history. Advances in early detection and treatment have improved prognosis with 5 year survival rates of 60–80 %. In terms of local recurrence rates, disease free survival and mortality, bladder cancer comprises two distinct groups: either genetically stable low-grade, non-invasive papillary tumours, or, genetically unstable high-grade and invasive cancers (including pTaG3 lesions and CIS (carcinoma in situ)).

Bladder cancer commonly presents as an exophytic papillary, solid, or ulcerated endophytic mass at cystoscopy with symptoms of painless haematuria. Terminal haematuria at the end of micturition points to bladder neck pathology. Rarely, advanced bladder cancer may present with a pelvic mass, lower limb oedema due to lymphatic obstruction, or distant metastases. Investigation is by urinary cytology, cystoscopy and biopsy. Cytology is good at designating high-grade papillary, in situ and invasive urothelial neoplasia but poor at separating low-grade papillary lesions from reactive atypia and cellular changes associated with calculi, in-dwelling catheters, recent instrumentation and post therapy changes. Other roles for cytology are in the clinical follow up and surveillance of high-grade

urothelial carcinoma and CIS. Biopsy is with "cold" cup forceps or a small diathermy loop, the advantage of the former being good preservation of histological detail. Flexible cystoscopy is easier for the patient and allows a wide field of vision but rigid cystoscopy with a larger lumen allows instrument access for transurethral resection of superficial bladder tumours (TURBT) and diathermy to the base. However, this can be associated with extensive distorting diathermy artifact that compounds accurate histological assessment of tumour grade and stage. Deep biopsy of the muscularis propria is important staging information in invasive tumours and may be submitted separately by the urologist. Further staging is by a combination of endoluminal ultrasound, CT and MRI scans. Diagnostic accuracy for PET scan in invasive disease is poor. CIS can present with irritative bladder symptoms and appears as multifocal red patches on cystoscopy, although it can be endoscopically inapparent and require multiple random biopsies. It can occur in isolation (primary CIS) but more usually in association with prior (secondary CIS), synchronous (concomitant CIS) or subsequent bladder cancer.

CIS is usually treated by intravesical topical chemotherapy (mitomycin) or immunotherapy (Bacille Calmette Guerin (BCG) therapy), or if localized in extent resected by TURB. Widespread disease determined by multiple site biopsy of the urothelium (bladder, ureters, urethra, prostatic ducts, seminal vesicles) may necessitate radical surgery. Superficial urothelial cancer (i.e. that confined to the mucous membrane) is resected

D.C. Allen, *Histopathology Reporting*,
DOI 10.1007/978-1-4471-5263-7_30, © Springer-Verlag London 2013

transurethrally with submission of multiple fragments and follow up by cystoscopy. Adjuvant intravesical chemo-/immunotherapy and/or radiotherapy are used for high-grade or recurrent disease. Recurrent superficial cancer refractory to local resection and adjuvant therapy, and muscle invasive tumours, require radical surgery with cystectomy ± in continuity prostatectomy/urethrectomy and regional lymphadenectomy. In the female this entails cystourethrectomy or an anterior exenteration. Partial cystectomy is reserved for solitary, dome or urachal tumours with no previous bladder tumour, CIS, bladder neck or trigone involvement. Pelvic lymph node dissection imparts staging information and is of potential therapeutic benefit. Neoadjuvant chemoradiation has a role to play. Radiotherapy is also used as a palliative measure. Cystoscopy requires alternative urinary drainage. Options include: urinary diversion and intestinal ileal conduit, continent cutaneous diversion, continent orthotopic reservoir ('neobladder'), or, ureterosigmoidostomy.

30.1 Gross Description

Specimen

- Urine cytology/bladder washings/cystoscopic biopsy/transurethral resection bladder (TURB)/cystectomy/cystourethrectomy/cystoprostatectomy (including seminal vesicles)/cystoprostatourethrectomy/anterior or total exenteration (including uterus and adnexae ± rectum).
- Weight (g) and size (cm).
- Length (cm) of ureters and urethra.

Tumour

Site
- Fundus/body/trigone/neck/ureteric orifices.
- Anterior/posterior/lateral (right or left).
- Single/multifocal.
- Diverticulum.

Size
- Length × width × depth (cm) or maximum dimension (cm).

Appearance
- Papillary/sessile/ulcerated/mucoid/keratotic/calcification.
- Bladder mucosa: erythematous/oedematous (CIS).

Edge
- Circumscribed/irregular.

30.2 Histological Type

Transitional Cell (Urothelial) Carcinoma

- *90% of cases.*
- Usual type: papillary or sessile (solid).
- Urothelial carcinoma has a propensity for *divergent differentiation* (squamous cell and glandular are the commonest) usually in association with high-grade, high stage disease. Variants with deceptively benign features:
- *Microcystic*: intraurothelial microcysts containing protein secretions mimicking cystitis cystica and adenocarcinoma. It is of no particular prognostic significance.
- *Inverted*: architecturally similar to inverted papilloma but has WHO II/III cytology. Look for stromal and muscle invasion. It is of relatively indolent behaviour.
- *Nested*: uniform cell nests in the lamina propria mimicking florid von Brunn's nests/cystitis glandularis/cystica, or paraganglioma. The cell nests are crowded with an irregular margin and look for muscle and lymphovascular invasion. It is *potentially aggressive* with bladder wall invasion disproportionate to its histological grade.
- *Micropapillary*: resembles ovarian serous papillary carcinoma. It comprises fine papillary, filiform epithelial processes, sometimes with a central core and a surrounding clear space. This stromal retraction artifact mimics lymphovascular invasion. It also often shows true *lymphovascular invasion* and is a *high-grade tumour* with frequent presentation at an *advanced stage*. Early cystectomy should be considered even if only superficially invasive disease is apparent.

- *Others*: variants include clear cell, tubular, plasmacytoid, lipoid cell, rhabdoid cell (aggressive), with pseudosarcomatous stroma (see below), giant cell, trophoblastic cells (HCG positive), or prominent lymphoid infiltrate (lymphoepithelioma: EBV negative).

Squamous Cell Carcinoma

- *2–5% of cases*.
- *Keratinising squamous cell metaplasia* of the urothelium (to be distinguished from physiological trigonal vaginal type squamous epithelium) due to chronic irritation (catheter, calculi, parasitic infection) is a *risk factor for the development of carcinoma*. It is present adjacent to 20–60 % of squamous cell cancers and potentially progresses to dysplasia and carcinoma. Its presence is also a predictor for local tumour recurrence post radical cystectomy.
- *Classical/verrucous/basaloid/sarcomatoid* i.e. the same range of tumours as encountered in the upper aerodigestive tract.
- Old age and associated with calculi, schistosomiasis (prevalent in Egypt and Africa forming 75 % of bladder cancers in endemic areas), diverticulum, non-functioning bladders, renal transplantation, chronic infection and long term cyclophosphamide treatment. *Prognosis is poor* with a *13–35% 5 year survival* and two thirds are stage pT3/pT4 at presentation.
- Designated as a primary lesion only after exclusion of high-grade urothelial carcinoma with squamous cell differentiation, and secondary squamous cell carcinoma from e.g. cervix.

Adenocarcinoma

- The common cloacal embryological origin of bladder and rectum highlights the *range of glandular differentiation* that can be seen in the bladder mucosa.
- *2% of bladder malignancy*. A gland forming carcinoma devoid of urothelial or squamous cell carcinoma components. *Direct spread or metastasis from elsewhere is commoner* and should always be excluded clinically particularly in the absence of mucosal glandular intestinal metaplasia, dysplasia or in situ changes. Usually secondary adenocarcinoma is from a *colorectal (35%), prostatic (19%) or cervical (11%) primary*. Distinction must also be made from various *benign mimics* of adenocarcinoma: nephrogenic adenoma, endometriosis, endocervicosis, Mullerian inclusions, or, urachal remnants.

- *Enteric, mucinous (colloid), signet ring cell, clear cell (mesonephroid), hepatoid, ex villous adenoma, or, adenocarcinoma of no special type (NST)*, enteric, mucinous and NST each comprising 20–30 % of cases.
- *Urachal or non-urachal in origin, bladder adenocarcinoma* can arise out of chronic irritation associated with intestinal metaplasia/cystitis glandularis (60 %), neurogenic bladder, extrophy, diverticulum, endometriosis or bladder dome wall urachal remnants (30 %). Usually muscle invasive and of poor prognosis (particularly signet ring cell carcinoma) due to *advanced stage at presentation* and an *18–47% 5 year survival*.
- Infrequently there is adjacent adenocarcinoma in situ. Histology cannot reliably distinguish between a urachal or non-urachal origin and this is more determined by the anatomical site of origin, urachal lesions arising either in the bladder dome or high anterior aspect with an epicentre in the bladder wall. Adenocarcinoma complicating extrophy tends to be localised in the anterior abdominal wall.
- Immunophenotype is often enteric (CK20, CDX-2, CK7±) in character.

Transitional Cell (Urothelial) Carcinoma with Mixed Differentiation

- *Squamous cell carcinoma or adenocarcinoma* components are seen in *20–30%* and *5–10%*, respectively, of *high-grade invasive transitional cell carcinomas* emphasising a capacity for *divergent differentiation* and carrying *a worse prognosis*. An adenocarcinoma component is reported to confer an increased resistance to chemotherapy, presentation at a more advanced stage and likelihood of progression.

Spindle Cell Carcinoma

- "*Sarcomatoid carcinoma*" or *carcinosarcoma*.
- Old age. Large and polypoid with a *poor prognosis (50 % dead within 1 year)*. There may be a recognisable in situ or invasive epithelial component (transitional cell, glandular, squamous cell or undifferentiated), and cytokeratin/vimentin positive spindle cells (34βE12, CK5/6 in 25 % of cases, usually only focal) with varying stromal differentiation. This ranges from non-specific fibrosarcoma/MFH like to specific heterologous, mesenchymal differentiation e.g. rhabdomyosarcoma, chondrosarcoma, osteosarcoma.

Small Cell Carcinoma

- A poorly differentiated/high-grade neuroendocrine carcinoma either primary or secondary from lung. Tumours presenting with predominantly urological symptoms and signs are usually primary in nature. It is CAM 5.2/synaptophysin/CD56 positive with a high Ki-67 index, and, *aggressive with early metastases at presentation in 56 % of cases* to lymph nodes, liver, bone and peritoneum. *Five year survival is <10 %*. It is treated with 'small cell type' chemoradiotherapy. Small cell carcinoma may be *pure or mixed* with other in situ or invasive bladder cancer subtypes and coexistent prostatic disease, both in up to 50 % of cases.
- Large cell neuroendocrine carcinoma also occurs rarely.

Undifferentiated Carcinoma

- No specific differentiation and an *aggressive high-grade* tumour.

Malignant Melanoma

- Primary or secondary (commoner).
- Note there can be spread to bladder from a primary urethral lesion.

Metastatic Carcinoma

- *Metastases should be considered in any bladder tumour with unusual histology* e.g. adenocarcinoma or squamous cell carcinoma. Knowledge of a *previous positive history* and *comparison of morphology* are crucial. Metastatic disease in the bladder is usually solitary.
- *Direct spread*: from adjacent pelvic organs (>70 % of cases) – prostate, cervix, uterus, anus, rectum, colon. To distinguish primary adenocarcinoma from secondary colorectal carcinoma look for an origin at the dome from urachal remnants, or areas of adjacent mucosal intestinal metaplasia/cystitis glandularis in a primary lesion. Bladder adenocarcinoma can be of enteric morphology and immunophenotype and this is not necessarily indicative of the organ of origin. Strong nuclear staining for βcatenin may indicate a colorectal primary. Knowledge of a prior positive colorectal biopsy or resection is helpful. A previous positive history on cervical smear/biopsy or endometrial sampling raises the possibility of a primary gynaecological tract malignancy. Oestrogen receptor positivity may also help.
- Prostatic cancer is PSA/PSAP positive but CK7/CK20/34βE12 negative which is the converse of bladder neck urothelial cancer. Note that some poorly differentiated or metastatic prostate cancers stain more strongly with polyclonal rather than monoclonal PSA with the potential for a false negative result using only the latter.
- *Distant spread*: breast, malignant melanoma, lung, stomach.

30.3   Differentiation/Cytological Grade

Flat, papillary and invasive urothelial neoplasia are graded separately. There are several classification options although in the UK the *WHO 1973* scheme remains in favour. This is preferred over the WHO/ISUP 1998 consensus and WHO 2004 classification due to concerns about their reproducibility. A European uropathology network survey has shown an even split in the use of these classifications. In

Table 30.1 Classification of papillary urothelial neoplasms

	Transitional cell papilloma	Transitional cell carcinoma		
WHO 1973	WHO 0/G0	WHO I/G1[a]	WHO II/G2[a]	WHO III/G3[b]
WHO/ISUP 1998	Urothelial papilloma	Papillary urothelial neoplasm of low malignant potential (PUNLMP)	Low-grade urothelial carcinoma	High-grade urothelial carcinoma
WHO 2004	Urothelial papilloma	Papillary urothelial neoplasm of low malignant potential (PUNLMP)	Urothelial carcinoma WHO I/G1	WHO II/G2 WHO III/G3

Note that the columns are not discrete categories or directly transferable but represent a spectrum of cytoarchitectural abnormalities

Transitional cell (urothelial) papilloma can be exophytic or inverted in type

[a]Low-grade disease. Includes most (but not all) WHO II/G2 tumours

[b]High-grade disease

the UK the Royal College of Pathologists has recommended use of both systems in parallel pending prospective audit of comparative patient outcomes. In general, these classification schemes are based on the *degree of cytoarchitectural abnormality* characterised by increasing nuclear atypia, hyperchromasia and crowding with upregulated proliferative and mitotic activity.

Flat urothelial neoplasia: comprises *urothelial dysplasia* (mild/moderate/severe) on a spectrum with, and severe dysplasia equating to, *carcinoma in situ* (*CIS*). Urologists will follow up and not treat a diagnosis of dysplasia, but, *initiate treatment for CIS* which may entail BCG immunotherapy, intravesical chemotherapy or surgery. Dysplasia and CIS (syn: *low-* and *high-grade intraurothelial neoplasia* respectively) are to be distinguished from *urothelial hyperplasia* (thickening of the urothelium without cytological atypia), and *regenerative atypia* which can be encountered in a range of conditions e.g. cystitis, calculi, an indwelling urinary catheter or post chemo-/radiotherapy. In addition to morphological clues dysplasia/CIS over expresses *p53* and *Ki-67* with strong, diffuse *panepithelial CK20 staining*. Non-neoplastic urothelium tends to show only basal layer proliferative activity, CK20 staining of surface umbrella cells and increased staining for *CD44 and CK5/6*. A Ki-67 index ≥16 % in flat mucosa favours a diagnosis of CIS over non-CIS conditions. Nuclear inclusions due to Polyoma virus infection are another diagnostic pitfall. A further consideration is atypical urothelium adjacent to a carcinoma i.e. non-representative sampling of the lesion, or, residual papillary carcinoma post treatment.

Papillary urothelial neoplasia: papillary urothelial lesions with a spectrum of minimal to marked cytoarchitectural abnormalities. This ranges from the very rare benign transitional cell papilloma covered by normal urothelium to the common place transitional cell carcinomas cytological grades WHO I/II/III (G1/G2/G3). A *WHO I/G1 carcinoma* is the least disordered being a *low-grade* lesion with <5 % *risk of progression* to invasion. A *WHO III/G3 tumour* is the most anaplastic being *high-grade* with a *30–60 % risk of progression*. Thus a papillary neoplasm is *typed, graded and staged* by assessing the degree of cytoarchitectural changes and the presence of underlying connective tissue invasion. Comment is also made on the absence or presence of dysplasia or CIS in the represented flat mucosa in the rest of the sample. A comparison of the classifications is given in Table 30.1.

Invasive urothelial neoplasia: well/moderate/poor, or, *WHO I/II/III* (*G1/2/3*). Note that WHO III invasive urothelial carcinoma often assumes a squamoid appearance in addition to actual mixed squamous cell or glandular differentiation (20–30 % of cases). High-grade often correlates with advanced stage of disease.

Non-urothelial invasive neoplasia: well/moderate/poor/undifferentiated, or, Grade 1/2/3/4. For squamous cell carcinoma based on keratinisation, cellular atypia and intercellular bridges, and, for adenocarcinoma on the tumour percentage gland formation (well/G1: >95 %, moderate/G2: 50–95 %, poor/G3: <50 %). Signet ring cell adenocarcinoma is high-grade (G3).

30.4 Extent of Local Tumour Spread

Border: pushing/infiltrative.

Lymphocytic reaction: prominent/sparse.

The TNM7 classification applies to urinary bladder carcinomas (non-invasive and invasive) and also papillary urothelial (transitional cell) neoplasm of low malignant potential (PUNLMP).

pTis	Flat carcinoma in situ: potential multifocal urinary tract field change
pTa	Papillary non-invasive
pT1	Invasion of subepithelial connective tissue
pT2a	Invasion of superficial muscle (inner half)
pT2b	Invasion of deep muscle (outer half)
pT3	Invasion of perivesical fat:
	(a) Microscopically
	(b) Extravesical mass (macroscopically)
pT4	Invasion of:
	(a) Prostatic stroma, seminal vesicles, uterus, vagina
	(b) Pelvic wall, abdominal wall.

See Fig. 30.1

Direct invasion of distal ureter is classified by the depth of greatest invasion in any of the involved organs.

Invasive bladder cancer with associated CIS extending into prostatic urethra or duct epithelium is classified according to the depth of bladder wall invasion and comment on the CIS changes noted by use of a suffix e.g. pT2b (ispu) for prostatic urethral involvement.

Involvement of prostatic stroma by invasive bladder disease is pT4a, as is small or large intestine, peritoneum covering the bladder and seminal vesicles.

Superficial tumours: are regarded as either pTa or pT1 and are often histological grade WHO I or II. Formal substaging of pT1 bladder tumours is not usually done but if feasible comment is made on the degree of invasion e.g. focal or extensive, above/at/below muscularis mucosae (pT1a: cores of papillae, pT1b: lamina propria, pT1c: below muscularis mucosae). Notably, the *extent of invasion* (≤ or >1 high power field) *stratifies risk for local recurrence*.

Deep (muscle invasive) tumours: are pT2 or pT3 and more often non-papillary and histological grade WHO III. They have an adverse prognosis requiring more radical treatment and assessment of *invasion of the detrusor layer of the muscularis propria* is of crucial importance in their designation. Unless submitted separately by the urologist, superficial and deep muscle cannot be distinguished on TURBT samples and the stage is reported as at least pT2a. As well as invasion of the bladder wall urothelial cancer can extend into the bladder neck, prostate, urethra and seminal vesicles. Because of this urethral biopsy is done in staging patients with CIS or high-grade invasive disease and if positive, en bloc prostatourethrectomy is favoured at the time of cystectomy.

30.5 Lymphovascular Invasion

Present/absent.

Intra-/extratumoural.

Invasion into the lamina propria may result in prominent *retraction artifact* spaces around tumour cells and nests *mimicking lymphovascular invasion*. This phenomenon is particularly prominent in invasive micropapillary carcinoma which also does show a propensity for lymphovascular and lymph node disease. For true vascular involvement identify an endothelial lining with adherent tumour and red blood cells. Endothelial markers (CD31, CD34) may be of use. *Vascular invasion* is associated with an *increased rate of recurrence*.

30.6 Lymph Nodes

Site/number/size/number involved/limit node/extracapsular spread.

Regional lymph nodes: pelvic lymph nodes below the bifurcation of the common iliac arteries – hypogastric, obturator, external iliac, presacral

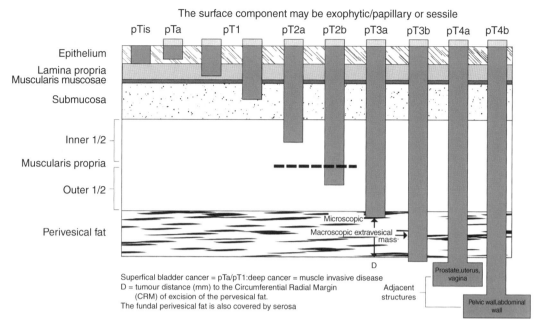

The surface component may be exophytic/papillary or sessile

pTis pTa pT1 pT2a pT2b pT3a pT3b pT4a pT4b

Epithelium
Lamina propria
Muscularis muscosae
Submucosa

Inner 1/2
Muscularis propria
Outer 1/2

Perivesical fat

Microscopic
Macroscopic extravesical
mass

D

Prostate,uterus,
vagina

Pelvic wall,abdominal
wall

Adjacent
structures

Superfical bladder cancer = pTa/pT1:deep cancer = muscle invasive disease
D = tumour distance (mm) to the Circumferential Radial Margin
(CRM) of excision of the pervesical fat.
The fundal perivesical fat is also covered by serosa

Fig. 30.1 Urinary bladder carcinoma (Reproduced, with permission, from Allen (2006), © 2006)

pN0	No regional lymph nodes metastasis
pN1	Metastasis in a single regional pelvic lymph node
pN2	Metastasis in multiple regional pelvic lymph nodes
pN3	Metastasis in a common iliac lymph node

Lymph node metastases are present in *25 % of invasive transitional cell carcinomas*. The total number and proportion of involved lymph nodes, and the presence of extracapsular spread are prognostic indicators. Common sites of *distant metastases* are lungs, liver, bone and central nervous system.

30.7 Excision Margins

Distances (mm) to the limits of the urethra, ureters, circumferential perivesical fat margin and the inferior resection limit of the bladder wall in a partial cystectomy. Note also the presence of any dysplasia/CIS at the ureteric and urethral limits. Intraoperative frozen section is sometimes required to assess tumour clearance of the urethra and ureters during cystectomy. A *positive margin*

post cystectomy is an *adverse indicator*. Great care must be taken not to miss a subtle pattern of invasion in the muscle coat or external connective tissue adventitia.

30.8 Other Pathology

Diagnostic Criteria for Transitional Cell Carcinoma (TCC)

Carcinoma in Situ (CIS)

- Flat urothelium of variable thickness (3–20 layers).
- *Marked cytological abnormality of usually (but not always) the whole epithelial thickness of either large cell (± pleomorphism) or small cell types.*
- Note unusual patterns such as the Pagetoid variant, undermining (lepidic) growth, or clinging ('denuding') CIS resulting from dyscohesion and shedding of cells.
- CIS equates to severe dysplasia and is by its nature a *high-grade lesion*.
- CIS comprises *1–3 % of urothelial neoplasms* and is present adjacent to invasive carcinoma

in *50–60% of cases*. It is a strong marker for subsequent tumour relapse, disease progression, decreased survival and increased risk of developing upper urothelial tract cancer.

- *CIS shows strong, diffuse panepithelial positivity for CK20, Ki-67 and p53 but is negative for CD44 and CK5/6. There is progression to invasive malignancy in up to 30% of cases.*
- Beware of overcalling dysplasia or in situ change, as normal urothelium often partially denudes on biopsy leaving a thin covering of basal cells which can then appear hyperchromatic.
- Note that a biopsy diagnosis of *dysplasia* with no previous history may *progress* to CIS or invasive malignancy in up to *19%* of cases over the course of several years.

Papillary TCC

- >7 cell layers thick.
- *Papillae with fine stromal cores* which are not true lamina propria (a distinguishing feature from the broad oedematous cores of polypoid cystitis).
- Variable grade of *nuclear atypia*.

Growth Pattern

Papillary, Exophytic

- The vast majority of cases.

Sessile/Solid

- Tends to be associated with high-grade lesions.

Endophytic and Non-invasive, or Invasive

- Differentiate from *inverted papilloma* which occurs at a younger age and at the bladder trigone. It is characterized by a covering of normal urothelium, no atypia or mitoses, inversion of the epithelial layers, and an endophytic nested and anastomosing jig-saw like pattern.
- Non-invasive lesions have an intact, round basement membrane and no desmoplastic or inflammatory stromal response. They often represent a complex crypt pattern to the lesion

base or extension of malignant epithelium into Brunn's nests. Invasive endophytic lesions can have a rounded deep border with no inflammatory reaction making assessment of invasion difficult – look for atypical urothelium present in relation to surrounding fibres of muscularis propria.

Microinvasion

- Characterised by *single cells, irregular spicules or nests of atypical urothelium budding into or lying separately in the superficial lamina propria*. They are often associated with stromal oedema, retraction artifact mimicking lymphovascular invasion, or a loose fibroblastic response. Its *extent is defined as ≤5 mm* from the nearest basement membrane or *<20 cells* in number. Its identification can be facilitated by use of cytokeratin immunohistochemistry. It is to be distinguished from CIS inhabiting von Brunn's nests. *Extent of CIS >25%* of the bladder is strongly associated with the presence of *microinvasion (34%)* and *progression (5.8%)* to lymph node metastases and death. *Deeper invasion* comprises irregular cell nests separated by variably desmoplastic submucosa or detrusor muscle bundles. Histological interpretation can be partially compromised by TURBT diathermy distortion.

Pathological Predictors of Prognosis

- *Number of tumours/multifocality*: both within the bladder and extravesical e.g. ureters and renal pelvis is a strong marker for subsequent *tumour recurrence*.
- *Size* of tumour.
- *Depth* of invasion.
- Histological *grade*.
- *Coexistent CIS/dysplasia* adjacent to or away from the tumour are markers of higher risk for recurrence and progression.
- *Progression* of grade and stage with time is more likely if the index histology shows: high-grade, CIS, pT1 disease, lymphovascular invasion and a micropapillary pattern.
- *Poor initial response* to chemo-/radiotherapy

- Current international research is focusing on the search for biomarkers predictive for tumour BCG response, recurrence, disease progression and survival. Some of these include over expression of ezrin, p53, FGFR3 and methylated myopodin and PMF1. The commercial Urovysion system for the detection of tumour recurrence is based on the FISH identification of aneuploidy in chromosomes 3, 7 and 17, and, loss of the 9p21 locus.

Additional Comments

Biopsies

Stage and field change: assess material from the *base* (*for pT stage*), and *adjacent and distant mucosa* (*for pTis*). Clear distinction between superficial and deep muscle coat cannot be made on biopsy material (unless submitted separately by the clinician), so that muscle invasive carcinoma should be reported as *at least pT2a in depth*. The muscle bundles should be coarse indicating the detrusor layer or muscularis propria rather than the fine fibres of the poorly defined lamina propria. Strong smoothelin antibody positivity of muscularis propria fibres may be of help in this regard as staining is reported as negative or weak/focal in the muscularis mucosae, although the effectiveness of this needs further assessment. Note that fat may also be present in the lamina propria and between muscle coat bundles and does not necessarily mean invasion of perivesical tissue. This designation is reserved for complete assessment of the cystectomy specimen. A European uropathologist network survey has shown that there is an educational and training need for standardization of various reporting parameters with regard to pathological staging in relation to invasion of muscle, perivesical fat and prostate.

Mimics of bladder cancer: biopsies from other lesions that can *mimic a papillary neoplasm* are polypoid cystitis, nephrogenic adenoma/metaplasia, follicular cystitis, cystitis cystica, malakoplakia, prostatic adenocarcinoma, villous adenoma and inverted transitional cell papilloma. Although *inverted papilloma* is benign a small minority can be multifocal and recurrent and difficult to distinguish from urothelial carcinoma with an inverted pattern. *Polypoid cystitis* has broad oedematous connective tissue cores covered by reactive urothelium and there may be a history of an indwelling urinary catheter. *Nephrogenic adenoma* is often associated with prior instrumentation, treatment, calculi, cystitis or in 8 % of cases renal transplantation. Its distinctive tubulo-papillary, polypoid and sometimes cystic pattern of cuboidal to variably atypical epithelial cells (CK7, AMACR, PAX-2, PAX-8 positive) is distinguished from adenocarcinoma and clear cell adenocarcinoma by its low mitotic and proliferative (Ki-67, p53) activity. It is considered either metaplastic or in transplant patients of renal tubular stem cell origin. *Villous adenoma* is analogous to its intestinal counterpart and can be benign, associated with urachal adenocarcinoma, or progress (20–30 %) to non-urachal adenocarcinoma. *Prostatic adenocarcinoma* (PSA/PSAP positive) is a consideration in material derived from the bladder base or prostatic urethra. *Mimics of a solid urinary neoplasm* are previous biopsy or local ablation site reaction, myofibroblastic proliferations, amyloid, endometriosis, sarcoma, extrinsic and metastatic carcinoma.

Resection Specimen Blocks

- Urethral limit: transverse section.
- Ureteric limits: transverse section.
- Prostate, seminal vesicles: in *30–50 % of radical cystoprostatectomy specimens for urothelial cancer systematic sampling shows that there is concurrent, undiagnosed prostatic adenocarcinoma* which requires separate typing, Gleason score, TNM staging and assessment of margin status.
- Normal bladder: lateral walls, dome, trigone.
- Tumour and wall: one section per cm of tumour diameter to show the deepest point of mural invasion.

Post-operative Necrobiotic Granuloma

- *Post-TURP fibrinoid necrosis with palisading histiocytes*. Biopsy site reaction to previous TURB often shows prominent neofibrotic granulation tissue, focal dystrophic calcification and a foreign body giant cell response which may be associated with diathermy coagulum. The giant cells can be epithelioid and "pseudocarcinomatous" in appearance and cytokeratin/CD68 staining may be necessary to help distinguish from residual invasive urothelial carcinoma.

Myofibroblastic Proliferations: Post-operative Spindle Cell Nodule (PSCN), Inflammatory Myofibroblastic Tumour (IMFT/Pseudosarcomatous Fibromyxoid Tumour/Inflammatory Pseudotumour)

A range of myofibroproliferative processes histologically resembling sarcoma. PSCN is small (5–9 mm) and has a history of recent genitourinary tract instrumentation. It comprises a proliferation of cytologically bland spindle cells in which normal mitoses are readily seen and it occurs at the operative site. *IMFT* occurs de novo, can be several centimetres in diameter and forms a polypoid mass. The atypical myofibroblastic proliferation is associated with prominent inflammation and granulation tissue type vasculature. Mitoses can be seen, but are not prominent or abnormal. *Both lesions are usually benign* and must be distinguished from sarcoma although some cases of IMFT have been reported to recur and even progress with local infiltration of muscularis propria. Cytokeratin is positive in PSCN but can be negative in IMFT (a useful discriminator from spindle cell carcinoma); actin and desmin/h-caldesmon are variably positive (40–80 %). IMFT can be ALK 1 positive but is p53 negative in contradistinction to sarcoma.

Immunophenotype

Transitional cell carcinoma is positive for cytokeratins 7, 8, 18 and 20, CEA, uroplakin III, CK5/6, 34βE12, p63, CA19-9, Leu M1 and Lewis X antigen. Over expression of p53 correlates with the likelihood of progression in superficial disease. A useful panel is 34βE12/CK7/CK20/p53 positive: PSA/PSAP negative with the converse for poorly differentiated prostatic carcinoma which helps to clarify the nature of poorly differentiated carcinoma at the bladder base. Positive marking with uroplakin III or GATA-3 can be of help in assessing metastatic carcinoma of unknown primary site particularly in pelvic and retroperitoneal lymph nodes.

Treatment

Treatment of bladder transitional cell carcinoma is usually by *transurethral resection* and *cystoscopic follow up*. High-grade or refractory superficial disease (pT1G3 i.e. confined to the mucosa or submucosa) may also need *radiotherapy* and/or *intravesical chemotherapy/BCG*. The latter are also useful for transitional cell CIS. Nonresponsive superficial or deep (muscle invasive) cancer necessitates *radical surgical resection*. In follow up *intravesical agents* such as cyclophosphamide or mitomycin can result in *urothelial atypia* which must not be confused with dysplasia or CIS. Due to the slow turnover of urothelial cells these changes can persist for long periods of time. The nuclei are focally enlarged and have a "smudged" chromatin appearance rather than the angular, ink blank hyperchromasia of CIS. Post radio-/chemotherapy pseudocarcinomatous and atypical stromal cells are also encountered. BCG often results in inflammation and superficial noncaseating granulomas but tubercle are usually not seen. A range of other post therapy changes can be seen with systemic chemotherapy, radiotherapy, laser and photodynamic therapy. Urachal related adenocarcinoma at the bladder dome may be considered for a *partial cystectomy* with resultant preservation of urinary function.

Prognosis

Muscle invasive cancer often starts as CIS or a flat/sessile rather than a papillary lesion and relates strongly to histological grade (WHO I=2 % invasive; WHO III=40 % invasive). Invasive cancer will develop in up to 30–50 % (or more) of patients with untreated CIS but 85–90 % 5 year survival rates can be achieved by radical surgery which is also targeted at multifocal field change in the urothelium (bladder, prostatic ducts, urethra, ureters, seminal vesicles). Up to *80% of urothelial carcinomas are non-invasive at the time of presentation* and although *tumour recurrence* is common (single lesion 30–45 %, multiple 60–90 %, <5 % risk after a disease free interval of 5 years), *tumour progression (10%)* relates strongly to histological grade, tumour size, multifocality, short disease free interval between local recurrences, non-tumour dysplasia/CIS of bladder mucosa, and depth of invasion. Over expression (>20 % of tumour cells) of Ki-67, p53 and Her-2 may also be another indicator. *Five year survival rates* also vary according to these parameters:

Transitional cell carcinoma	Superficial invasion	
	Grade I	70 %
	Grade III	60 %
	Deep muscle invasion	40–55 %
Squamous cell carcinoma		15 %
Adenocarcinoma		15–35 %

As can be seen, *squamous cell carcinoma* and *adenocarcinoma* are of *worse prognosis*. Other *adverse histological types* are: nested and invasive micropapillary transitional cell carcinoma, urothelial carcinoma with rhabdoid or plasmacytoid features, sarcomatoid carcinoma, undifferentiated carcinoma and small cell carcinoma.

30.9   Other Malignancy

Malignant Lymphoma/Leukaemia

- *Usually secondary* to advanced stage systemic disease.
- *Primary malignant lymphoma* comprises *<1% of bladder neoplasms* and varies from low-grade MALToma with indolent behavior,

to *diffuse large B cell malignant lymphoma* (*commoner*). It can be a solitary mass (70 %), multifocal (20 %) or diffuse in distribution. Leukaemic involvement is seen in 15–30 % of cases especially chronic lymphocytic leukaemia (CLL).

Carcinoid Tumour

- Rare. A well differentiated/low-grade neuroendocrine tumour: 25 % have regional lymph node or distant metastases but most are treated adequately by local excision. Chromogranin/synaptophysin/CD56 positive with a low Ki-67 index (≤2 %).

Phaeochromocytoma

- Young women, classically with paroxysmal hypertension, intermittent haematuria, and 'micturition attacks' due to spasmodic increased catecholamine levels in the blood. It forms a paragangliomatous nested pattern of cells with eosinophilic cytoplasm and variable nuclear features. Chromogranin/synaptophysin positive with S100 positive sustentacular cells.
- *Local recurrence* and *metastases* can occur in about *10% of cases*. Histology does not reliably predict behaviour, although higher stage tumours are more prone to metastases which can occur up to many years later.

Leiomyosarcoma

- Commonest sarcoma but *<1% of bladder malignancy*. In adults, at the bladder dome and infiltrates muscle. It is an *aggressive tumour* with 70 % developing metastases, recurrent or fatal disease.
- Nuclear atypia, mitoses and tumour necrosis: some are extensively myxoid.
- Desmin/h-caldesmon positive.
- Mucosal leiomyoma is small, cytologically bland and lacks mitotic activity.

Other Sarcomas

- Rhabdomyosarcoma, malignant fibrous histiocytoma, angiosarcoma, osteosarcoma: all
rare and must exclude bladder sarcomatoid
carcinoma (carcinosarcoma). Other rarely
occurring sarcomas are Ewing's/PNET, malignant peripheral nerve sheath tumour and alveolar soft part sarcoma.

Rhabdomyosarcoma

- Embryonal variant in children, sarcoma botryoides. There are also low-grade spindle
cell, and aggressive alveolar subtypes. Rare
in adults and must exclude bladder sarcomatoid carcinoma with rhabdomyoblastic
differentiation.
- Cellular subepithelial cambium layer with a
loose myxoid zone and cellular deep zone ±
rhabdomyoblasts. Desmin/myo D1/myogenin
positive.

Choriocarcinoma and Yolk Sac Tumour

- Choriocarcinoma: exclude urothelial carcinoma with trophoblastic differentiation.
- Yolk sac tumour: rare; childhood (<2 years of
age).

Bibliography

Allen DC. Histopathology reporting: guidelines for surgical cancer. 2nd ed. London: Springer; 2006.

Bates AW, Baithun SI. Secondary neoplasms of the bladder are histological mimics of nontransitional cell
primary tumours: clinicopathological and histological
features of 282 cases. Histopathology. 2000;36:32–40.

Bates AW, Norton AJ, Baithun SI. Malignant lymphoma
of the urinary bladder: a clinicopathological study of
11 cases. J Clin Pathol. 2000;53:458–61.

Bertz S, Denzinger S, Otto W, Wieland WF, Stoehr R,
Hofstaedter F, et al. Substaging by estimating the
size of invasive tumour can improve risk stratification in pT1 bladder cancer – evaluation of a large
hospital-based single-centre series. Histopathology.
2011;59:722–32.

Bostwick DG, Cheng L. Urologic surgical pathology. 2nd
ed. Philadelphia: Mosby/Elsevier; 2008.

Bovio IM, Al-Quran SZ, Rosser CJ, Algood CB, Drew
PA, Allan RW. Smoothelin immunohistochemistry is a useful adjunct for assessing muscularis propria invasion in bladder carcinoma. Histopathology.
2010;56:951–6.

Chandra A, Griffiths D, McWilliam LJ. Best practice:
gross examination and sampling of surgical specimens
from the urinary bladder. J Clin Pathol. 2010;63:475–9.

Eble JN, Sauter G, Epstein JI, Sesterhenn IA. WHO classification of tumours. Pathology and genetics.
Tumours of the urinary system and male genital
organs. Lyon: IARC Press; 2004.

Epstein JI, Amin MB, Reuter VR, Mostofi FH and the
Bladder Consensus Conference Committee. The
World Health Organization/International Society of
Urological Pathology consensus classification of uro-
thelial (transitional cell) neoplasms of the urinary
bladder. Am J Surg Pathol. 1998;22:1435–48.

Fleischmann A, Thalmann GN, Markwalder R, Studer UE.
Prognostic implications of extracapsular extension of
pelvic lymph node metastases in urothelial carcinoma
of the bladder. Am J Surg Pathol. 2005;29:89–95.

Gunia S, Kakies C, Erbersdobler A, Koch S, May M.
Scoring the percentage of Ki67 positive nuclei is
superior to mitotic count and the mitosis marker
phosphohistone H3 (PHH3) in terms of differentiating flat lesions of the bladder mucosa. J Clin Pathol.
2012;65:715–20.

Harik LR, Merino M, Coindre J-M, Amin MB, Pedeutour
F, Weiss SW. Pseudosarcomatous myofibroblastic proliferations of the bladder. A clinicopathological study
of 42 cases. Am J Surg Pathol. 2006;30:787–94.

Harnden P. Transitional cell tumours of the bladder: classification and diagnostic pitfalls. Curr Diagn Pathol.
2002;8:76–82.

Hirsch MS, Cin PD, Fletcher CD. ALK expression in pseudosarcomatous myofibroblastic proliferations of the
genitourinary tract. Histopathology. 2006;48:569–78.

Lopez-Beltran A, Luque RJ, Mazzucchelli R, Scarpelli M,
Montironi R. Changes produced in the urothelium by
traditional and newer therapeutic procedures for bladder cancer. J Clin Pathol. 2002;55:641–7.

Lott S, Lopez-Beltran A, Montironi R, MacLennan GT,
Cheng L. Soft tissue tumors of the urinary bladder part
II: malignant neoplasms. Hum Pathol. 2007;38:963–77.

Magi-Galluzzi C, Epstein JI. Urothelial papilloma of the
bladder. A review of 34 de novo cases. Am J Surg
Pathol. 2004;28:1615–20.

McKenney JK, Gomez JA, Desai S, Lee MW, Amin MB.
Morphologic expressions of urothelial carcinoma in-
situ. A detailed evaluation of its patterns with emphasis on carcinoma in-situ with microinvasion. Am J
Surg Pathol. 2001;25:356–62.

Montironi R, Lopez-Beltran A, Scarpelli M, Mazzucchelli
R, Cheng L. Morphological classification and definition of benign, preneoplastic and non-invasive neoplastic lesions of the urinary bladder. Histopathology.
2008a;53:621–33.

Montironi R, Mazzucchelli R, Scarpelli M, Lopez-Beltran A, Cheng L. Morphological diagnosis of urothelial neoplasms. J Clin Pathol. 2008b;61:3–10.

Paner GP et al. Diagnostic utility of antibody to smoothelin in the distinction of muscularis propria from muscularis mucosae of the urinary bladder: a potential ancillary tool in the pathologic staging of invasive urothelial carcinoma. Am J Surg Pathol. 2009; 33:91–8.

Procter I, Stoeber K, Williams GH. Biomarkers in bladder cancer. Histopathology. 2010;57:1–13.

Ramos D, López-Guerrero JA, Navarro S, Llombart-Bosch A. Prognostic markers in low-grade papillary urothelial neoplasms of the urinary bladder. Curr Diagn Pathol. 2005;11:141–50.

Shanks JH, Iczkowski KA. Divergent differentiation in urothelial carcinoma and other bladder cancer subtypes with selected mimics. Histopathology. 2009a;54:885–900.

Shanks JH, Iczkowski KA. Spindle cell lesions of the bladder and urinary tract. Histopathology. 2009b;55:491–504.

The Royal College of Pathologists. Cancer Datasets (Adult Renal Parenchymal Cancer, Renal Tumours in Childhood, Penile Cancer, Prostatic Carcinoma, Testicular Tumours and Post-Chemotherapy Residual Masses, Tumours of the Urinary Collecting System) and Tissue Pathways (Medical Renal Biopsies, Urological Pathology). Accessed at http://www.rcpath.org/index.asp?PageID=254.

Varma M, Morgan M, Amin MB, Wozniak S, Jasani B. High molecular weight cytokeratin antibody (clone 34βE12): a sensitive marker for differentiation of high-grade invasive urothelial carcinoma from prostate cancer. Histopathology. 2003;42:167–72.

Westfall DE, Folpe AL, Paner GP, Oliva E, Goldstein L, Alsabeh R, et al. Utility of a comprehensive immunohistochemical panel in the differential diagnosis of spindle cell lesions of the urinary bladder. Am J Surg Pathol. 2009;33:99–105.

Williamson SR, Lopez-Beltran A, Montironi R, Cheng L. Glandular lesions of the urinary bladder: clinical significance and differential diagnosis. Histopathology. 2011;58:811–34.

Prostatic adenocarcinoma is a common visceral malignancy with a 1 in 6 lifetime risk and crude mortality figures of 22 %. It is androgen dependent its incidence increasing with age and is present in 80 % of men by the age of 80 years. Some 5–10 % have a strong family history. Racial (black) ethnicity, a high calorie diet and lack of physical exercise are contributory. Many men die with their disease due to its indolent behaviour rather than because of it, although a significant minority show aggressive behaviour with metastases. It is the second commonest cause of cancer related death in men after lung cancer.

Prostatic cancer is symptomatic in 25 % of cases and this is often indicative of widespread disease with lumbar pain as a result of bone metastases. It may also present with symptoms of prostatism (nocturia, urinary frequency, hesitancy and dribbling). However it is often asymptomatic and detected because of an elevated serum PSA (Prostate Specific Antigen) with digital rectal examination (DRE), either as part of a screening programme or a family practitioner's well man check up clinic. Further investigation comprises transrectal ultrasound (TRUS) to identify classical tumour related hypoechoic areas. Because 70 % of prostatic cancer is present posteriorly and peripherally this is coupled to per rectum clinical or TRUS directed needle core biopsies. Clinical samples provide multiple random cores from each lobe. TRUS biopsies are targeted with sextant core samples (3 each side) aimed at the apex, midzone and base regions of the gland. Recent evidence shows that 25–30 % of cancers are isoechoic and a minority anterior dominant. Because of this an extended 12 core (saturation/template) biopsy regime has been advised with a reported increased detection rate of up to 35 %. The resultant fine biopsy cores need careful handling, wrapping and painting with alcian blue prior to processing to allow their visualisation at the block cutting stage. Otherwise initial block trimming may result in loss of diagnostic tissue. Blocks are cut through at least 3 histological levels and the intervening ribbons kept pending any subsequent need for immunohistochemistry. This is required for diagnosis in 3 % of cases and reduces diagnostic uncertainty from 6 to 2 % of cases. Microscopic assessment is at low power looking for abnormalities of glandular architecture and medium to high power to confirm cytological features of malignancy. The biopsy report should indicate which biopsy site(s) is/are positive, the Gleason tumour grade, the number of positive cores and percentage of involved tissue, and the maximum linear dimension of carcinoma. It may be possible to comment on other features such as perineural or lymphovascular invasion, and, staging information e.g. spread into extracapsular fat or neurovascular bundles, or, involvement of seminal vesicles. Another indication for prostatic biopsy is a rising serum PSA after radiotherapy or brachytherapy for a previously proven cancer. Reasons for a repeat biopsy are an insufficient index biopsy, features suspicious but not diagnostic of malignancy, high-grade PIN (Prostatic Intraepithelial Neoplasia), and a rising serum PSA after a negative biopsy.

D.C. Allen, *Histopathology Reporting*,
DOI 10.1007/978-1-4471-5263-7_31, © Springer-Verlag London 2013

Treatment of prostatic cancer is age, fitness, Gleason grade and tumour stage dependent. This ranges from watchful waiting, to radiotherapy and hormonal therapy (androgen deprivation) for focal, and, locally advanced or metastatic disease, respectively. Androgen deprivation is effected by use of LHRH (luteinizing hormone releasing hormone) agonists or oestrogen preparations. Metastatic disease is assessed by radioisotope bone scan. CT scan and MRI scan have limited sensitivity for local spread although MRI scan can be helpful in detection of biopsy negative central or anteriorly sited tumours (20–25 % of cases). Radical prostatectomy is aimed at younger patients (age 56–60 years) with low to modest elevations in serum PSA who are more likely to have gland confined disease and negative surgical margins. It is an operation with significant morbidity and side effects e.g. incontinence, impotence. Some of these may be avoided by a selective nerve sparing procedure, although this can have implications for the completeness of excision and tumour clearance of the margins. An equivalent alternative with fewer complications is radical radiotherapy, and there is also increasing use of brachytherapy (radioactive seed implants), or cryotherapy of the tumour and its bed. Preoperative combination therapy can downsize tumour while use of post-operative radiotherapy and/or chemotherapy are based on the Gleason component and sum scores, margin status and the presence of extracapsular disease. Prostatic chippings piece-meal resect the periurethral and central zones and transurethral resection of the prostate (TURP) is performed in two main situations

(a) In patients with benign hypertophy of the medial aspect of the gland who have persistent troublesome prostatism that is refractory to medical therapy, or who develop acute urinary retention

(b) TURP channel re-do in a patient with known cancer and significant prostatic symptoms.

In the former incidental cancer may be detected by microscopy in up to 8 % of cases, and the significance of this is then interpreted in light of the patient's serum PSA and clinical staging. It may either be an incidental low volume, low-grade cancer arising from the transitional zone, or, contiguous spread from a larger, often high-grade, peripherally sited tumour.

31.1   Gross Description

Specimen

- Fine needle aspirate cytology (FNAC)/needle core biopsy (18 gauge)/transurethral resection (TUR) chippings/radical prostatectomy (including seminal vesicles) and regional lymphadenectomy.
- Weight (g) and size (cm).
- Number and length of cores (mm).

Tumour

Site

- Inner (transitional)/outer (central and peripheral) zones. The transitional zone surrounds the proximal urethra and the central zone is posterior to it. The peripheral zone occupies 70 % of the gland in a horseshoe shape around its posterior and lateral aspects.
- Medial/lateral (right or left) lobes. These are not defined anatomical structures but relate to clinically palpable masses on per rectum examination. For the purposes of TNM staging the gland is notionally divided into right and left lobes about a mid-point sagittal plane.
- Posterior/subcapsular.
- The majority of carcinomas are *posterior* and *peripheral* with *multicentricity present in up to 75 % of cases.*

Size

- Length × width × depth (cm) or maximum dimension (cm).
- *Tumour volume (cm³)*. Derived by outlining and calculating the area of tumour in each slide and then multiplying by the mean block thickness (the anteroposterior (AP) diameter divided by the number of coronal slices). The volume is the sum total for all the blocks/slides. Alternatively a quicker method is to

outline the tumour in each slide, lay them out on the bench and estimate the total percentage area involved e.g. 60 %. Knowing the gland volume (AP × width × depth) the tumour volume is presumed to be 60 % of it assuming even tumour distribution throughout each block. The ratio of positive to negative blocks on microscopy is an alternative time efficient index of tumour volume. Clinicians vary in the use of these data but pragmatically they give an indication of low or high volume tumour and the consequent *risk of extracapsular disease* being present. It is also useful for correlation with serum PSA and TRUS assessment (maximum dimension of any dominant tumour nodule) along with tumour site location. However, its importance is far outweighed by that of consistent Gleason scoring, and assessment of the capsule and margin status, as even small volume cancers (<10 mm maximum dimension) can show extraprostatic extension and margin positivity depending on their location within the gland. Given the heterogeneity of tumour distribution within the prostate, the inapparent macroscopic features of prostate cancer, and increasingly early stage detection, volume estimates are more accurate based on whole gland serial slices and processing. This can mean 40–50 slides for a small gland using routine blocks. Two alternatives are

(a) Whole mount sections that reduce the block numbers and allow easier assessment of anatomical tumour distribution, or,

(b) A sampling strategy to include the base and apical margins, seminal vesicles, all posterior sections and a mid-slice of the anterior prostate on either side.

The latter may result in a loss of prognostic data e.g. extraprostatic extension or positive margins, the significance of which varies in the literature. A European uropathologist network survey found that 71.6 % of respondents embedded the entire prostate, with variation in other parameters such as specimen inking, Gleason grading, stratifying the degree of extraprostatic extension, reporting TNM stage and the location of positive margins. Whole mounts and standard blocks were used in 37.5 and 55.5 % of laboratories respectively. In needle biopsy and TURP specimens the number of cores, linear millimeters of carcinoma and percentage of chippings involved are routinely given in the surgical histopathology report. A combination of *millimeters of cancer* and *Gleason sum score* in a core biopsy is a *predictor* of the *presence of extraprostatic disease*.

Appearance
- Soft/firm
- Pale/yellow/granular

Similar changes are seen in tuberculosis, infarction, granulomatous prostatitis and acute and chronic prostatitis, i.e. tumour is difficult to define macroscopically and histological assessment is necessary.

Edge
- Circumscribed/irregular.

31.2 Histological Type

The *vast majority of prostate cancers* are of *acinar origin* including and coexisting with a minority of variants, namely, atrophic, pseudohyperplastic, foamy cell, mucinous (colloid), signet ring cell, oncocytic, and lymphoepithelioma like.

About *5–10 % of prostate cancers* are of *non-acinar origin* – sarcomatoid, periurethral ductal, squamous cell, adenosquamous, urothelial, small cell, basal cell and clear cell carcinomas.

Peripheral Acinar Origin

Adenocarcinoma of Usual Type
- >90–95 % *of cases* with a range of acinar, papillary, cribriform, comedo and single cell patterns of infiltration.
- Acini are usually small to medium in size and can be rounded or angular in contour. The cell cytoplasm is amphophilic (clear to light eosinophilia) in character. Diagnosis is made at low power magnification on the basis of a *gland rich haphazard infiltrative pattern* in comparison to, and between adjacent benign prostatic

ducts and acini. Medium to high power can then confirm the *lack of an epithelial bilayer* and *nuclear characteristics of malignancy* (enlargement/angularity/membrane folds/nucleolar prominence). Luminal crystalloids, glomerulations, mucinous fibroplasia or mucin extrusion may also be present. Cribriform and comedo patterns resemble intraductal carcinoma and can be difficult to distinguish from high-grade PIN, but again are architecturally too ductal rich compared to adjacent tissues.

• *Diagnostic pitfalls* are large gland, atrophic and pseudohyperplastic variants of carcinoma which can resemble post atrophic or benign hyperplastic prostate. Occasionally foamy gland adenocarcinoma is encountered to be distinguished from cytokeratin negative/CD68 positive aggregates of xanthomatous histiocytes. Notably these well differentiated carcinoma variants are negative for the *basal layer cytokeratin markers 34βE12 and p63*, and, are variably positive for *AMACR*. In radical prostatectomy specimens they are often admixed with usual acinar pattern adenocarcinoma. Patient outcomes for these variants are not significantly different from usual prostate cancer.

Mucinous (Colloid) Adenocarcinoma

• Distinguish from *secondary colorectal or bladder cancer* by a relevant past history, and also usually CK7/CK20 negative with variable PSA/PSAP expression. Indicators to a bladder/urethral origin are CK7/CK20 positivity, and for colorectum CK20/CDX-2/βcatenin positivity.

• ≥25 % of the tumour area is intra-/extracellular mucin.

• More frequent bone metastases and *less hormone/radioresponsive* than usual prostatic carcinoma, although a difference in biological behaviour and outcome from usual prostate cancer is uncertain.

Signet Ring Cell Adenocarcinoma

• Rare; distinguish from secondary gastric or colorectal cancer by a relevant past history, and also usually CK7/CK20 negative with variable PSA/PSAP expression.

• ≥25 % of the tumour area is signet ring cells, usually coexisting with other poorly differentiated carcinoma and of *poor prognosis* presenting at an *advanced stage*.

Lymphoepithelial Carcinoma

• Analagous to nasopharyngeal carcinoma but EBV (Epstein Barr virus) negative. Of *poor prognosis* and presentation is with obstructive symptoms, elevated PSA and locally advanced disease.

Non-acinar Origin

Sarcomatoid/Spindle Cell Carcinoma

• Syn. carcinosarcoma or metaplastic carcinoma.

• Cytokeratin positive spindle cells with variable malignant stromal mesenchymal differentiation which is usually homologous ± heterologous elements (bone, cartilage, striated muscle).

• It presents in older men with obstructive symptoms, variable serum PSA levels, an enlarged hard gland, and sometimes a prior acinar adenocarcinoma treated by hormones or radiation. It is of *poor prognosis* with a *3 year median survival*.

Periurethral Duct Adenocarcinoma

• Old age with haematuria or obstructive symptoms and polypoid/villous or infiltrative on cystoscopy. Has a higher volume and more *advanced stage at presentation* (12–20 % have distant metastases to testis, penis, lung or bone) and is *aggressive*. May be associated with a diverticulum and can also be sited in the gland periphery. Serum PSA may not be elevated.

• Variable papillary, cribriform and endometrioid patterns (uterine carcinoma analogue), and may coexist with usual pattern prostate adenocarcinoma. PSA/PSAP positive, ± androgen deprivation/oestrogen sensitive. AMACR can be reduced in intensity and 34βE12 focally present.

• There may be associated Paget's disease of the prostatic urethra.

• Exclude secondary renal clear cell carcinoma if mesonephroid or hob-nail clear cell in type.

Adenosquamous/Squamous Cell Carcinoma

- Rare and *poor prognosis*. Exclude squamous cell metaplasia due to infarction or hormone therapy, or, spread from an anal cancer.
- Up to 50 % may arise *in patients with previous usual prostate cancer treated by endocrine or radiotherapy* at an interval of several months to years. Squamous cell carcinoma is also associated with schistosomiasis.
- *Mean survival of 6–24 months*, direct pelvic spread and metastases to lymph nodes and bone (osteolytic rather than the usual osteosclerotic prostate cancer deposits).

Transitional Cell (Urothelial) Carcinoma

- *2 % of prostatic cancers.*
- Arises from the transitional cell lining of the prostatic urethra or proximal periurethral ducts.
- Usually *high-grade* with extension into ducts, central comedonecrosis ± adjacent *stromal invasion* the presence of which is the *strongest prognostic indicator*. Survival for urothelial CIS (carcinoma in situ) is good but for invasive carcinoma 17–29 months.
- Rarely primary, and usually represents spread from a bladder/urethral transitional cell carcinoma, or, multifocal urothelial field change. This association is *present in up to 40 % of locally extensive high-grade bladder cancer cases.*
- CK7, CK20, 34βE12 positive: PSA/PSAP negative.

Undifferentiated, Small Cell Type Carcinoma

- A poorly differentiated/high-grade neuroendocrine carcinoma which is CAM5.2/synaptophysin/CD56 positive ± TTF-1 with a high Ki-67 index. Immunonegative cases are classified as poorly/undifferentiated prostatic carcinoma. Usually PSA/PSAP negative.
- Lung small cell carcinoma analogue.
- In the vast majority of cases primary, either pure or mixed (25–50 %) with usual prostatic carcinoma ± an associated bladder component. The usual prostate cancer may precede it or have received prior hormonal therapy. Rarely, secondary from lung.
- *Aggressive* often *presenting with disseminated disease*, typically low volume osseous involvement in the presence of visceral metastases. It is sometimes associated with inappropriate ACTH/ADH secretion. *Survival is 9–17 months* and it requires different chemotherapy to usual prostate cancer. It cannot be followed up clinically by serum PSA levels.
- *Carcinoid* (*well differentiated/low-grade neuroendocrine*) *tumour* is rare. Up to 33 % of usual prostatic carcinomas can show neuroendocrine differentiation on immunohistochemistry and this is usually of no prognostic significance.
- *Large cell neuroendocrine carcinoma* is rare with a mean survival of 7 months.

Basal Cell Carcinoma and Clear Cell Carcinoma

- A morphological continuum from typical through florid basal cell hyperplasia/adenoma to carcinoma with infiltrative edges, stromal desmoplasia, comedonecrosis and adenoid cystic like differentiation. 34βE12 positive and a tumour of variable malignant potential, *mostly indolent*, but 14 % show local recurrence and distant metastases.
- Clear cell carcinoma typically arises from the anterior or transitional zone of the prostate.

Mixed Acinar/Non-acinar Types

Metastatic Carcinoma

- *Direct spread*: bladder (present in 40 % of radical cystoprostatectomies for bladder cancer), colorectum, anus, retroperitoneal sarcoma.
- *Distant spread*: kidney, lung (squamous cell carcinoma), malignant melanoma.

31.3 Differentiation/Grade

Well/moderate/poor/undifferentiated, or, Grade 1/2/3/4.

- Well/G1 = Gleason sum score 2–4: moderate/G2 = Gleason sum score 5–6: poor/G3 = Gleason sum score 7–10.

- *Heterogeneity of tumour grade*: single grade; 16 % of cases, 2 grades; >70 %, and, 3 grades; >50 % of cases.
- Signet ring cell carcinoma is poorly differentiated (grade 3) and small cell carcinoma undifferentiated (grade 4).
- Although scoring is more applicable to usual prostatic adenocarcinoma, *specific carcinoma variants* can be allocated a Gleason score as follows
    - Pattern 3: atrophic, pseudohyperplastic
    - Pattern 4: foamy gland, ductal, mucinous
    - Pattern 5: sarcomatoid, squamous cell/adenosquamous (usually high-grade), lymphoepithelioma like, ductal (with necrosis), small cell and signet ring cell carcinomas (Fig. 31.1).

Gleason Score for Usual Prostatic Adenocarcinoma

The Gleason system proposes that any given prostate carcinoma may show one or several of five histological glandular architectural patterns ranging from the lowest grade (grade 1) to the highest grade (grade 5). Taking the two predominant patterns one can arrive at a *sum score* (e.g. 2+3=5; 3+4=7) which has *prognostic significance correlating with biochemical evidence of treatment failure, development of distant metastases, survival post radiotherapy, progression free survival and overall survival.* The following rules apply:

(a) Choose the two predominant patterns where more than two are present. The primary pattern must be ≥50 %, and the secondary pattern >5 % but <50 % of the total. The minor pattern is often of a higher grade.

(b) When there is only one pattern, double it, e.g. 3+3=6.

(c) In limited samples (e.g. needle biopsy, TURP chippings) where there are more than two patterns and the worst grade is neither the predominant nor the second most predominant pattern, choose the main pattern and the highest grade. For example, if grade 3 is 60 %, grade 2 is 30 % and grade 4 is 10 %, the score is 3+4=7. An alternative description is Gleason 3+2=5 with tertiary grade 4. Incorporation of *higher grade tertiary patterns* into the Gleason sum score correlates with biochemical failure post treatment, tumour volume and mortality. Note that due to sampling error and crush artifact needle

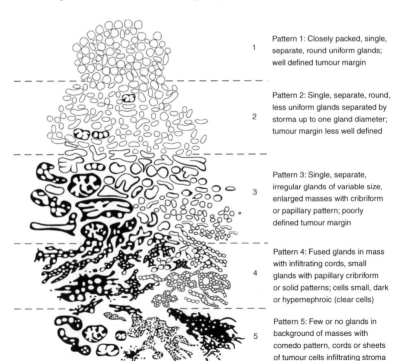

Fig. 31.1 Gleason score in prostatic carcinoma (Gleason 1977).

Pattern 1: Closely packed, single, separate, round uniform glands; well defined tumour margin

Pattern 2: Single, separate, round, less uniform glands separated by storma up to one gland diameter; tumour margin less well defined

Pattern 3: Single, separate, irregular glands of variable size, enlarged masses with cribriform or papillary pattern; poorly defined tumour margin

Pattern 4: Fused glands in mass with infiltrating cords, small glands with papillary cribriform or solid patterns; cells small, dark or hypernephroic (clear cells)

Pattern 5: Few or no glands in background of masses with comedo pattern, cords or sheets of tumour cells infiltrating stroma biopsy samples can *underestimate the Gleason score* compared with the subsequent resection specimen in 25–50 % of cases, and scoring is subject to observer variability and underscoring. *Grading is undertaken at low power magnification with no contribution from the cytological details.* A useful tip when assessing Gleason score is: *f for fusion and 4* i.e. packed glands with elimination of intervening stroma. *Cribriform, glomeruloid (patterns 4)* and *comedo (pattern 5)* areas may also be present. Where there are multiple needle biopsies or foci in a prostatectomy with different Gleason scores the score of the least differentiated areas should be recorded. Urological oncologists also like to know the *component parts of the sum score* (i.e. $3 + 4 = 7$) as management is often based on the worst element. By convention a $3 + 4 = 7$ score is a lower grade than a $4 + 3 = 7$ cancer as the primary grade is notified first in the sequence. *Gleason sum score 7 cancer* also has distinct therapeutic implications as it has a prognosis between Gleason sum scores 5–6 and 8–10 cancers. Evidence for grade progression remains uncertain – larger tumours tend to be of higher grade, but some small cancers may be high-grade from the outset.

Note that a needle biopsy positive for prostatic adenocarcinoma is, in the vast majority of cases, of at least *Gleason pattern 3* i.e. small, angular individual glands infiltrating stroma, and this is regarded as the *'default' grade*. Gleason pattern 1 or 2 cancers comprise larger, uniform glands (round, regular size, regular spacing) in circumscribed nodules more easily appreciated in TURP specimens and rarely attributed in peripheral needle core biopsies. Useful guides to Gleason scoring of prostatic adenocarcinoma are found at http://www.bostwicklaboratories.com and from the 2005 ISUP Consensus Conference (Epstein et al. 2005; Delahunt et al. 2012).

31.4   Extent of Local Tumour Spread

Border: pushing/infiltrative.
Lymphocytic reaction: prominent/sparse.

Weight of chippings or length of cores, and the *proportion (%) of the chippings*, or, *number of cores involved*. Give a *maximum linear dimension (mm)* of carcinoma.

Apex of gland, urethral limit, proximal bladder limit, capsule and margins, seminal vesicles.

The TNM7 classification applies only to prostatic adenocarcinomas. Transitional cell carcinoma of the prostate is classified as a urethral tumour.

pT1	Clinically inapparent tumour not palpable or visible by imaging
T1a	Incidental histological finding in ≤5 % of tissue resected
T1b	Incidental histological finding in >5 % of tissue resected
T1c	Identified by needle biopsy (e.g. because of elevated PSA)
pT2	Tumour confined within the prostate
T2a	Involves one half of one lobe or less
T2b	Involves more than one half of one lobe but not both
T2c	Involves both lobes
pT3	Tumour extends through the prostatic capsule
T3a	Extracapsular extension (unilateral or bilateral) including microscopic bladder neck involvement
T3b	Invades seminal vesicle(s)
pT4	Tumour is fixed or invades neighbouring structures other than seminal vesicles: external sphincter, rectum, levator muscles, and/or pelvic wall.

(Figs. 31.2, 31.3 and 31.4)

The subdivision of pT2 based on lobar distribution is somewhat subjective and non-anatomical. It has been suggested that stratification of pT2 by tumour size with dimension thresholds of 5 and 16 mm would give more clarity. Invasion into but not beyond prostatic apex or capsule is pT2.

The capsule: is a condensation of smooth muscle and collagen rich soft tissue around the prostate but with no clear fascia. It can be difficult to define in a prostatectomy specimen for the purposes of assessing *extracapsular disease* (tumour in fat or neurovascular bundles beyond the contour of the prostate). It sometimes has to be visually extrapolated from more obvious adjacent areas in any given slide. Completeness of the capsule also depends on patient anatomy, surgical

Fig. 31.2 Prostatic
carcinoma (Reproduced, with
permission, from Allen
(2006), © 2006)

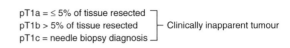

pT1a = ≤ 5% of tissue resected ⌉
pT1b > 5% of tissue resected   ⎬ Clinically inapparent tumour
pT1c = needle biopsy diagnosis ⌋

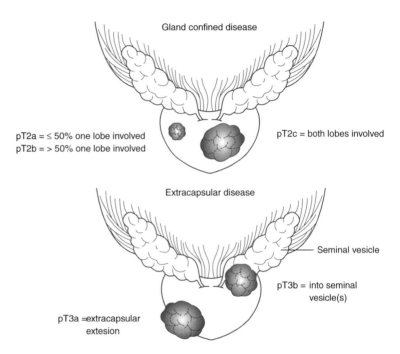

Gland confined disease

pT2a = ≤ 50% one lobe involved
pT2b = > 50% one lobe involved

pT2c = both lobes involved

Extracapsular disease

Seminal vesicle

pT3b = into seminal
        vesicle(s)

pT3a =extracapsular
        extesion

Fig. 31.3 Prostatic carcinoma
(Reproduced, with permis-
sion, from Wittekind et al.
(2005), © 2005)

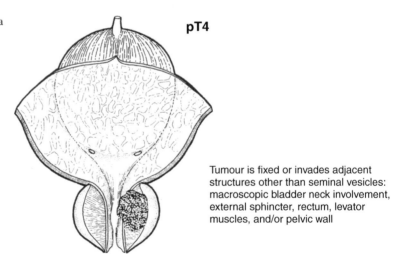

pT4

Tumour is fixed or invades adjacent
structures other than seminal vesicles:
macroscopic bladder neck involvement,
external sphincter, rectum, levator
muscles, and/or pelvic wall

expertise and choice of operative technique e.g. a
nerve sparing procedure. *Extracapsular extension* can be described as *focal (<1 high power
field in no more than 2 sections)* or *extensive* with
an adverse prognosis. Its quantitation is a predictor for *biochemical recurrence* after radical prostatectomy and of potential *disease progression*.

Due to the inferoposterior approach of per rectal needle biopsy there may be representation of
extracapsular and *seminal vesicle tissues* which
should be assessed for invasion (= pT3). Note
that fat and muscle can also be, albeit rarely,
intraprostatic, and involvement on its own in a
needle biopsy, while suspicious of, does not

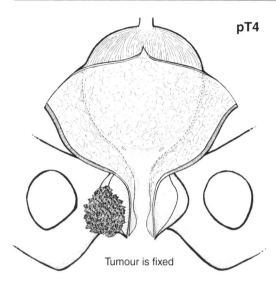

pT4

Tumour is fixed

Fig. 31.4 Prostatic carcinoma (Reproduced, with permission, from Wittekind et al. (2005), © 2005)

necessarily imply extracapsular disease. However, *tumour in perineural spaces in neurovascular bundles in fat is an indicator of extracapsular spread*, as is *infiltration around ganglion cells*. Tumour in fibrous tissue in the same anatomical plane as fat is another helpful clue. These features are most commonly encountered at the posterolateral aspect of the gland. Occasionally benign acini may be present in perineural spaces but they do not show the circumferential or intraneural disposition of malignancy. Seminal vesicle involvement (pT3b) occurs in 4 % of cases indicative of high stage disease and adverse prognosis. It is defined as invasion of the seminal vesicle smooth muscle wall and not just the surrounding connective tissue between it and the prostate. Seminal vesicle must not be confused with similar looking intraprostatic ejaculatory duct type epithelium which is orientated to loose, vascular connective tissue and surrounded by prostate gland.

Advanced disease: manifests spread into seminal vesicle, prostatic urethra and bladder. Presentation can be by an anterior rectal mass or stricture and PSA staining of rectal biopsy material is diagnostically useful. "*Frozen pelvis*" is a clinical term meaning tumour extension to the pelvic wall(s) with fixation and is designated pT4. Optional descriptors are pT4a (external

sphincter, rectum) and pT4b (levator muscles, fixed to pelvic wall). Note that the normal prostatic apex may incorporate some striated muscle fibres and cancer lying in relation to these does not necessarily imply extraprostatic disease.

Histological cancer in TURPs performed within 2 months of each other should have a pT1a or pT1b designation based on the sum total of carcinoma over both specimens. In a prostatectomy specimen where part of the capsule is missing the pT designation can only be accurately assigned if the tumour is clearly surrounded by non-malignant prostatic tissue.

31.5 Lymphovascular Invasion

Perineural and lymphovascular space: present in *75–90 % of radical prostatectomy specimens*. While its positive predictive value is low, *perineural invasion* is an indicator of *potential extraprostatic extension*, and is associated with prostatic carcinoma of higher Gleason score and volume. Microvascular invasion is also a potential predictor of biochemical recurrence after radical prostatectomy and tumour progression.

Present/absent.

Intra-/extratumoural.

31.6 Lymph Nodes

Site/number/size/number involved/limit node/extracapsular spread.

Regional nodes: pelvic lymph nodes below the bifurcation of the common iliac arteries. These are present in <5 % of radical prostatectomy specimens but may be submitted as separate pelvic lymph node specimens.

pN0	No regional lymph node metastasis
pN1	Metastasis in regional lymph node(s).

Lymph node metastases are present in up to *10–30 % of prostate cancer patients* relating to tumour stage (in 50 % of pT3 patients at diagnosis), volume, differentiation or grade, and serum

PSA levels. However they are only present in some *1–2% of radical prostatectomy specimens*. This is related to preferred surgical practice, PSA screening and better clinical imaging with patient selection for surgery. Some patients with high risk disease defined by serum PSA level and biopsy tumour grade may have frozen section assessment of regional lymph nodes prior to carrying out radical surgery. Even with positive pelvic lymph nodes, radical prostatectomy with regional lymphadenectomy followed by adjuvant therapy is a treatment option. *The presence of lymph node metastasis, the proportion of involved nodes, and nodal tumour volume or maximum diameter, are indices of disease free survival and metastatic potential.* The commonest sites of *distant metastases* are bone (osteoblastic in character), lung, and occasionally testis. Visceral metastases often represent end stage disease. Occult primary disease can present with metastases to unusual sites e.g. pleura, bronchus, mediastinal and supraclavicular lymph nodes. Bronchial biopsy and aspiration cytology coupled with PSA immunoreactivity can be useful in these circumstances particularly as the pattern can mimic other cancers e.g. secondary colonic adenocarcinoma. Lymph node metastases of prostate cancer can also be encountered incidentally in other contexts e.g. anterior resection with total mesorectal excision for a rectal cancer. If not recognized as such the rectal cancer may be erroneously over staged and receive inappropriate adjuvant therapy.

31.7 Excision Margins

Distances (mm) to the circumferential surgical resection margins, proximal bladder and distal urethral limits.

A margin is involved or positive (+SM: focal or extensive) if *tumour is present histologically at the covering of ink*. If close to but not touching the ink it is negative. Occasionally assessment is not clear cut and margin status is deemed to be equivocal. Interpretation of the benign or malignant nature of crushed or diathermied glands at a margin is in the context of adjacent preserved

glands, and can be helped with use of the standard immunohistochemical panel (34βE12, p63, AMACR). A positive margin does not necessarily alter the stage or mean pT3a disease as the gland may have been excised at or internal to the capsule at this particular point. The apex and posterolateral margins are unduly susceptible to positive margins, and proximally a pT4 designation generally requires gross tumour rather than just microscopic involvement (pT3a) of the bladder neck. The proximal and distal limits are transverse sectioned and then serially sliced perpendicular to this to satisfactorily demonstrate their actual outer surfaces.

Capsular and *marginal invasion* are strong *indicators of extraprostatic disease* and *potential progression*. Note that the prostatic capsule is poorly defined particularly at the base and apex of the gland where there is a paucity of fat and extraprostatic extension is hard to ascertain. *A positive margin* may be designated R1 by TNM i.e. incomplete resection with residual microscopic disease (e.g. pT3 (R1)) and its *linear extent (< or >3 mm or 10 mm)* is significantly associated with PSA relapse (see below).

31.8 Other Pathology

High-grade prostatic intraepithelial neoplasia (HGPIN): extent and location which is usually peripheral and multifocal as in carcinoma. HGPIN is a *precancerous condition* and has *malignant cytology* (i.e. nuclear/nucleolar enlargement) within *preserved ducts* and *acini*. It can show focal disruption of the basal cell layer with high molecular weight 34βE12 cytokeratin and p63 stains. Its intraductal architectural patterns are tufting, micropapillary, cribriform and flat. Other rare patterns are signet ring, small cell, foamy gland and hob-nail. *It is present in 5–10% of needle core biopsies and about 40–50% are associated with either concurrent, or subsequent adenocarcinoma developing within 10 years.* It is most strongly linked to intermediate grade cancer many of which are diagnosed on rebiopsy following a core biopsy finding of PIN. Its extent correlates with cancer stage, Gleason grade, margin involvement and perineural invasion. *Its presence in biopsy cores or chippings indicates the need to process more tissue and for clinical reassessment and follow up.* One focus requires rebiopsy within a year, and multiple foci short to intermediate term rebiopsy. *PIN present in 1, 3 or more than 3 cores has a 30, 40 and 75% cancer risk, respectively.* HGPIN does not cause a significant rise in serum PSA or form a palpable mass. *It is a histological finding* and is not detected by ultrasound. Its prevalence and extent are decreased by androgen deprivation and radiation therapy. A differential diagnosis is with invasive ductal cribriform adenocarcinoma. Low-grade PIN is not reported due to variation in its observer reproducibility and uncertainty as to its significance as a precursor lesion.

Ancillary immunohistochemistry and differential diagnoses: may be used in up to 20–25 % of diagnostic prostatic specimens according to local pathological practice, although this decreases considerably with acquired morphological experience. *High molecular weight cytokeratin antibody 34βE12* and *p63* antibodies react with the *basal cells* of prostatic glands in *benign conditions*, but are *negative in adenocarcinoma.* Important *morphological markers of adenocarcinoma* are: nuclear/nucleolar enlargement, cytoplasmic amphophilia, absence of the basal cell layer, perineural invasion (especially if circumferential and intraneural) and loss of gland architecture. This comprises small, crowded round to angular, amphophilic glands infiltrating between benign glands. A stromal desmoplastic reaction is usually not present. Luminal crystalloids, mucinous fibroplasia (collagenous micronodules), glomerulations and extracellular mucin extension may also be seen. A putatively *positive immunomarker* for *prostatic adenocarcinoma* is *alpha-methylacyl co-enzyme A racemase (AMACR/P504S)*. The basal layer can be difficult to identify on morphology and is best identified by 34βE12 and p63 staining.

A *34βE12, p63, AMACR/P504S panel* is of use in *difficult differential diagnoses of low-grade prostatic adenocarcinoma.* These conditions include: HGPIN, atrophy/partial atrophy, post-atrophic hyperplasia, sclerosing adenosis, atypical adenomatous hyperplasia (benign cytology within an abnormal glandular architecture at the edge of hyperplastic nodules), nephrogenic adenoma, verumontanum mucosal gland hyperplasia, central zone epithelium, mesonephric remnants, various hyperplasias (transitional/squamous cell/cribriform), and Cowper's glands. *Overdiagnosis* of entrapped distorted rectal glands, seminal vesicle and ejaculatory duct epithelium as malignant should also be borne in mind: look for cytoplasmic lipofuscin pigment and characteristic cytoarchitectural appearances in the latter two contexts. Basal cell hyperplasia/adenoma are also strongly 34βE12/p63 positive, and, can *mimic high-grade prostatic carcinoma* as can other benign pathology such as: florid clear cell cribriform hyperplasia, healed infarcts, reactive epithelial atypia (e.g. radiation induced), granulomatous prostatitis, malakoplakia and prostatic xanthoma. *False positive diagnoses* can be avoided by an awareness of these various benign mimics, and other local malignancy e.g. bladder neck urothelial cancer. *False negative diagnosis* should also be borne in mind due to focal distribution of cancer within the gland and individual specimens, the deceptively bland appearances of some adenocarcinoma variants, and prior effects of adjuvant treatments. About 3 % of needle biopsy specimens show *atypical small acinar proliferation (ASAP) suspicious but not diagnostic of malignancy.* This can be due either to the presence of small atypical glands without fully developed cytoarchitectural features of malignancy, or, a very limited number (e.g. <2–3) of glands with overtly malignant features i.e. quality and quantity (the "Q^2 of positive diagnosis"). There may be associated adjacent PIN. Interpretation must be viewed in light of the clinical findings e.g. a rising serum PSA. Further biopsy may be necessary.

Effects of non-surgical therapies: *radiotherapy* (external beam or interstitial brachytherapy seeds) and *hormonal treatment* (androgen deprivation therapy) produce a range of changes. This includes glandular atrophy with nuclear apoptosis and smudging, cytoplasmic vacuolation, mucinous change, squamous cell metaplasia and stromal fibrosis. These may lead to underestimation of tumour volume in post-treatment resection specimens and difficulty in deriving and in validating the Gleason score. Other modalities include high intensity focused ultrasound (HIFU), photodynamic and interstitial laser thermotherapy, and gamma knife radiosurgery. These treatment related changes along with better diagnosis of early disease can result, in 0.5 % of cases, in the *minimal residual* or *"vanishing cancer" phenomenon* in prostatectomy specimens. In such cases the needle biopsy material should be reviewed to verify the primary diagnosis and future management based on its prognostic indicators. Conversely, lack of morphological response to neoadjuvant therapy has adverse prognosis. Note that treatment related changes may persist for up to several years, and may be complicated by secondary cancer e.g. squamous cell carcinoma.

Secondary carcinoma: mucinous and signet ring cell carcinoma have to be distinguished from *secondary colorectal carcinoma*. Immune markers PSA and PSAP will be positive in 95 % of primary prostatic carcinomas but may be negative in mucinous prostatic cancers. If immune markers are negative absence of any obvious primary elsewhere is important in designation as a primary prostate lesion. Note that PSAP can also be positive in rectal carcinoid tumours and anal carcinoma. PSA can also stain some ovarian, salivary gland, skin and breast cancers.

Periurethral duct carcinoma: has a worse prognosis than prostatic carcinoma of usual type but may also be androgen deprivation/oestrogen sensitive. It has cribriform or papillary patterns and is PSA positive. Many coexist with typical acinar prostatic carcinoma and may be related to it.

Cancer distribution and extent: prostatic carcinoma has a tendency to be *peripheral and posterior in distribution* allowing a diagnosis to be made in a significant number of cases by *multiple per rectal needle biopsies*. Multiple sextant biopsies can also act as a guide to the distribution and extent of the lesion. Biopsies should be examined histologically through multiple levels (at least 3) to detect focal lesions. Measurement of the *maximum tumour dimension (mm)* should be given.

Small foci (<3 mm) in one core may represent true focal cancer, or, a sampling issue and not representative of the whole lesion. Small areas of tumour in a biopsy may indicate small volume disease in the radical prostatectomy but the considerable overlap that exists in individual patients poses considerable limitations on this as a predictor. Conversely *high percentage tumour involvement and measurable linear dimension in needle core biopsies generally correlate with high volume, potentially advanced stage disease*. The weight of prostatic chippings determines the number of blocks processed for histology but it is estimated that with selection 5–8 blocks will detect 90–98 % of the prostatic carcinomas that are represented in a specimen.

Postoperative necrobiotic granuloma: post-TURP ductocentric fibrinoid necrosis with palisading histiocytes. Also granulomatous prostatitis (idiopathic, BCG).

Myofibroblastic proliferations: postoperative spindle cell nodule/inflammatory myofibroblastic tumour (IMFT/pseudosarcomatous fibromyxoid tumour).

See Chap. 30.

Prognosis

Prognosis in prostate cancer is related to the *volume of tumour, Gleason score and presence of extracapsular extension*. Tumour volume can only really be derived by systematic measurement of serial slices of prostatectomy specimens. However, *the proportion or percentage of TURP chippings or needle biopsy cores involved, and the maximum linear dimension of cancer, give a reasonable estimate of disease extent. Overall 10 year survival is 50%* and up to *30% can be regarded as cured*. Gland-confined disease (pT1/pT2) shows 80–95 % 10 year survival depending on tumour volume whereas *extraprostatic extension (pT3/pT4)* decreases 10 year survival to 60 % and a "cure" rate of only 25 %. *Other prognostic factors* are positive surgical margins, perineural and lymphovascular invasion and serum PSA levels (an indirect indicator of tumour volume and extension). The *risk of tumour recurrence* can be stratified on the basis of stage, Gleason score and serum PSA at diagnosis as:

(a) Low risk: pT1–pT2a, Gleason ≤6, PSA <10 ng/ml

(b) Intermediate risk: pT2b–pT2c, Gleason 7, PSA 10–20 ng/ml, or,

(c) High risk: pT3–pT4, Gleason 8–10, PSA >20 ng/ml.

Treatment (surveillance only for localised disease, radical prostatectomy, radiotherapy, hormonal manipulation) is tailored to the patient's *age, general level of health, grade* and *clinicopathological stage of disease. Non-surgical modalities* are of use in localised disease and as palliation in locally advanced (pT3/pT4) or metastatic disease. Indications for *radical prostatectomy* are a younger patient (up to the sixth/seventh decade) with persistent but modestly elevated serum PSA (less than 10–15 ng/ml), needle biopsy proven adenocarcinoma, and an absence of extraprostatic spread on bone scan. Serum PSA >15 ng/ml is associated with a greater likelihood of the tumour not being gland confined and subsequent positive surgical margins. *Gleason score ≥4 + 3 = 7, extracapsular disease or positive surgical margins* necessitate *post operative radiotherapy* as they are predictors of poor prognosis and treatment failure.

Serum PSA Level

Serum PSA is a biochemical marker used as a screening, diagnostic, prognostic and clinical follow up tool. High levels in relation to the patient's age (>4–5 ng/ml at ≥50 years: >2.8 ng/ml at <50 years: free to total ratio <15 %), and *changing levels over time* (velocity >0.75 ng/ml per year) of PSA should prompt processing of further tissue and/or multiple levels as there is a strong correlation with the presence of adenocarcinoma (elevated in 64 % of cases). Levels above 4 and 10 ng/ml confer *cancer risks of 25 and 50 %* respectively. There is also a significant positive correlation with Gleason grade as poorly differentiated tumours are usually of high volume. Serum levels >0.2 ng/ml post radical prostatectomy can represent biochemical failure or relapse,

local recurrence or metastatic disease. Elevated levels in inflammatory conditions (prostatitis, infarct, benign hypertrophy, post catheterisation) are usually of lesser magnitude, transitory and resolve with time and treatment. Screening is based on digital rectal examination (DRE), transrectal ultrasound (TRUS) and serum PSA levels. Tissue expression of PSA/PSAP is useful in identifying a prostatic origin for metastatic carcinoma and distinguishing it from poorly differentiated transitional cell carcinoma (PSA/PSAP negative, CK7/CK20/34βE12/p53 positive) particularly in TURP specimens derived from the bladder neck, or, in prostatic needle biopsies.

Immunophenotype

The vast majority of prostatic adenocarcinomas are strongly *PSA* and *PSAP* positive although a small minority of poorly differentiated tumours may show only focal staining for monoclonal PSA and are serum PSA negative. This is strengthened by use of polyclonal PSA with PSAP, the caveat being the cross reaction of rectal carcinoid and anal tumours with the latter. Loss of the basal layer and *lack of 34βE12* has become a standard tool in diagnosing prostatic adenocarcinoma. This can be equally well demonstrated with other basal layer markers such as *CK5/6* or *p63. AMACR/P504S* has emerged as a good diagnostic counterpart to *34βE12/p63* showing cytoplasmic granular positivity in up to 80 % of malignant prostatic glands or atypical glands suspicious of malignancy. It arose as a product of high throughput microarray technology and although it has sensitivity and specificity limitations it is now routinely used in tandem with 34βE12/p63 in the assessment of atypical glandular foci. Note that it can also be positive in PIN, atypical adenomatous hyperplasia, nephrogenic adenoma and prostatic periurethral ducts emphasising the importance of using these *markers in the context of appropriate morphology.* A combination of PSA/PSAP with AMACR/P504S and basal layer immunohistochemistry also remains relatively robust for the identification of residual tumour after radiotherapy, hormonal treatment or HIFU. The role of negative CK7/ CK20/p53/34βE12 staining in prostatic carcinoma versus urothelial cancer has already been mentioned. A potential marker for prostatic malignancy and prostatic tissue of origin is over expression of ERG protein – a product of the TMPRSS2-ERG gene fusion present in 50 % of prostatic carcinomas.

31.9   Other Malignancy

Malignant Lymphoma/Leukaemia

- Especially chronic lymphocytic leukaemia (20 % of cases at autopsy).
- Primary MALToma (rare), diffuse large B cell malignant lymphoma, or secondary to systemic/nodal lymphoma; prognosis is poor; 33 % 5 year survival.

Leiomyosarcoma

- Rare, with *local recurrence* and *metastases common* and a survival of 3–4 years.

Other rare sarcomas e.g. prostatic stromal sarcoma or synovial sarcoma, must be distinguished from sarcomatoid carcinoma with homologous or heterologous differentiation, GIST or solitary fibrous tumour. Direct spread from a retroperitoneal or pelvic primary sarcoma must also be considered

Embryonal Rhabdomyosarcoma

- <20 years age with an averge age of 5 years.
- Second commonest site after head and neck.
- Usually extensive tumour of prostate, bladder and surrounding soft tissues with a botryoid (grape-like) appearance.
- Cellular subepithelial cambium layer, loose myxoid zone, cellular deep zone ± rhabdomyoblasts.
- Vimentin, desmin, myo D1, myogenin positive. Many are cured or remain disease free for long periods of time. About 15–20 % die from presentation with high stage disease.

A minority are alveolar and more aggressive. Adult rhabdomyosarcoma does not respond to multimodal therapy and has a poor prognosis.

Bibliography

Ali TZ, Epstein JI. Perineural involvement by benign prostatic glands on needle biopsy. Am J Surg Pathol. 2005;29:1159–63.

Allen DC. Histopathology reporting: guidelines for surgical cancer. 2nd ed. London: Springer; 2006.

Association of Directors of Anatomic and Surgical Pathology. Recommendations for the reporting of prostate carcinoma. Am J Clin Pathol. 2008;129: 24–30.

Bennett VS, Varma M, Bailey DM. Guidelines for the macroscopic processing of radical prostatectomy and pelvic lymphadenectomy specimens. J Clin Pathol. 2008;61:713–21.

Berney DM, Fisher G, Kattan MW, Oliver RTD, Moller H, Fearn P, Eastham J, Scardino P, Cuzick J, Reuter VE, Foster CS for the Trans-Atlantic prostate group. Pitfalls in the diagnosis of prostate cancer: retrospective review of 1791 cases with clinical outcome. Histopathology. 2007;51:452–7.

Bostwick DG, Cheng L. Urologic surgical pathology. 2nd ed. Philadelphia: Mosby/Elsevier; 2008.

Bostwick DG, Cheng L. Precursors of prostate cancer. Histopathology. 2012;60:4–27.

Cheng L, Montironi R, Bostwick DG, Lopez-Beltran A, Berney DM. Staging of prostate cancer. Histopathology. 2012;60:87–117.

Delahunt B, Miller RJ, Srigley JR, Evans AJ, Samaratunga H. Gleason grading: past, present and future. Histopathology. 2012;60:75–86.

Deng F-M, Mendrinos SE, Das K, Melamed J. Periprostatic lymph node metastasis in prostate cancer and its clinical significance. Histopathology. 2012;60: 1004–8.

Doud N, Li G, Evans AJ, van der Kwast TH. The value of triple antibody (34βE12 + p63 + AMACR) cocktail stain in radical prostatectomy specimens with crushed surgical margins. J Clin Pathol. 2012;65:437–40.

Eble JN, Sauter G, Epstein JI, Sesterhenn IA. WHO classification of tumours. Pathology and genetics. Tumours of the urinary system and male genital organs. Lyon: IARC Press; 2004.

Egevad L, Algaba F, Berney DM, Boccon-Gibod L, Griffiths DF, Lopez-Beltran A, Mikuz G, Varma M, Montironi R. Handling and reporting of radical prostatectomy specimens in Europe: a web-based survey by the European Network of Uropathology (ENUP). Histopathology. 2008;53:333–9.

Egevad L, Ahmad AS, Algaba F, Berney DM, Boccon-Gibod L, Comperat E, Evans AJ, Griffiths D, Grobholz R, Kristiansen G, Langer C, Lopez-Beltran A, Montironi

R, Moss S, Oliveira P, Vainer B, Varma M, Camparo P. Standardization of Gleason grading among 337 European pathologists. Histopathology. 2013;62:247–56.

Epstein JI. Diagnosis of limited adenocarcinoma of the prostate. Histopathology. 2012;60:28–40.

Epstein JI, Allsbrook WC, Amin MB, Egevad LL and the ISUP Grading Committee. The 2005 International Society of Urological Pathology (ISUP) Consensus Conference on Gleason grading of prostatic carcinoma. Am J Surg Pathol. 2005;29:1228–42.

Epstein JI, Srigley J, Grignon D, Humphrey P. Recommendations for the reporting of prostate carcinoma. Hum Pathol. 2007;38:1305–9.

Evans AJ. α - Methylacyl Co A racemase (P504S): overview and potential in diagnostic pathology as applied to prostate needle biopsies. J Clin Pathol. 2003;56:892–7.

Gleason D. Histologic grading and clinical staging of prostatic carcinoma. In: Tannenbaum M, editor. Urologic pathology. The prostate. Philadelphia: Lea and Febiger; 1977. p. 171–98.

Gleason DF. Histologic grading of prostate cancer; a perspective. Hum Pathol. 1992;23:273–9.

Herawi M, Epstein JI. Specialized stromal tumors of the prostate: a clinicopathologic study of 50 cases. Am J Surg Pathol. 2006;30:694–704.

Humphrey PA. Diagnosis of adenocarcinoma in prostate needle core biopsy tissue. J Clin Pathol. 2007;60:35–42.

Humphrey PA. Histological variants of prostatic carcinoma and their significance. Histopathology. 2012;60:59–74.

Kench JG, Delahunt B, Griffiths DF, Humphrey PA, McGowan T, Trpkov K, Varma M, Wheeler TM, Srigley JR. Dataset for reporting of prostate carcinoma in radical prostatectomy specimens: recommendations from the International Collaboration on Cancer Reporting. Histopathology. 2013;62:203–18.

Kristiansen G. Diagnostic and prognostic molecular biomarkers for prostate cancer. Histopathology. 2012;60:125–41.

Lopez JI, Etxezarraga C. The combination of millimetres of cancer and Gleason index in core biopsy is a predictor of extraprostatic disease. Histopathology. 2006;48:663–7.

Marks RA, Lin H, Koch MO, Cheng L. Positive-block ratio in radical prostatectomy specimens is an independent predictor of prostate-specific antigen recurrence. Am J Surg Pathol. 2007;31:877–81.

McNeal JE. Normal histology of the prostate. Am J Surg Pathol. 1998;12:619–33.

Montironi R, Mazzucchelli R, Algaba F, Lopez-Beltram A. Morphologic identification of the patterns of prostatic intraepithelial neoplasia and their importance. J Clin Pathol. 2000;53:655–65.

Montironi R, Scarpelli M, Mazzucchelli R, Cheng L, Lopez-Beltran A. The spectrum of morphology in non-neoplastic prostate including cancer mimics. Histopathology. 2012;60:41–58.

Oliai BR, Kahane H, Epstein JI. A clinicopathologic analysis of urothelial carcinomas diagnosed on prostate needle biopsy. Am J Surg Pathol. 2001;25:794–801.

Osunkoya A, Netto GJ, Epstein JI. Colorectal adenocarcinoma involving the prostate: report of 9 cases. Hum Pathol. 2007;38:1836–41.

Paner GP, Aron M, Hansel DE, Amin AB. Non-epithelial neoplasms of the prostate. Histopathology. 2012;60:166–86.

Pickup M, van der Kwast TH. My approach to intraductal lesions of the prostate gland. J Clin Pathol. 2007;60:856–65.

Ryan P, Finelli A, Lawrentschuk N, Fleshner N, Sweet J, Cheung C, van der Kwast T, Evans A. Prostatic needle biopsies following primary high intensity focused ultrasound (HIFU) therapy for prostatic adenocarcinoma: histopathological features in tumour and non-tumour tissue. J Clin Pathol. 2012;65:729–34.

Schowinsky JT, Epstein JI. Distorted rectal tissue on prostate needle biopsy. A mimicker of prostate cancer. Am J Surg Pathol. 2006;30:866–70.

Srigley JR, et al. Protocol for the examination of specimens from patients with carcinoma of the prostate gland. Arch Pathol Lab Med. 2009;133:1568–76.

Srigley JR, Delahunt B, Evans AJ. Therapy-associated effects in the prostate gland. Histopathology. 2012;60:153–65.

Sung M-T, Davidson DD, Montironi R, Lopez-Beltran A, Cheng L. Radical prostatectomy specimen processing: a critical appraisal of sampling methods. Curr Diagn Pathol. 2007;13:490–8.

The Royal College of Pathologists. Cancer Datasets (Adult Renal Parenchymal Cancer, Renal Tumours in Childhood, Penile Cancer, Prostatic Carcinoma, Testicular Tumours and Post-Chemotherapy Residual Masses, Tumours of the Urinary Collecting System) and Tissue Pathways (Medical Renal Biopsies, Urological Pathology). Accessed at http://www.rcpath.org/index.asp?PageID=254.

Vainer B, Toft BG, Olsen KE, Jacobsen GK, Marcussen N. Handling of radical prostatectomy specimens: total or partial embedding? Histopathology. 2011;58:211–6.

Van der Kwast TH, Lopes C, Santonja C, Pihl C-G, Neetens I, Martikainen P, Di Lollo S, Bubendorf L, Hoedemaeker RF. Members of the pathology committee of the European Randomised Study of Screening for Prostate Cancer (ERSPC). Guidelines for processing and reporting of prostatic needle biopsies. J Clin Pathol. 2003;56:336–40.

Van Oort IM, Bruins HM, Kiemeney LA, Knipscheer BC, Witjes JA, Hulsbergen-van de Kaa CA. The length of positive surgical margins correlates with biochemical recurrence after radical prostatectomy. Histopathology. 2010;56:464–71.

Vargas SO, Jiroutek M, Welch WR, Nucci MR, D'Amico AV, Renshaw AA. Perineural invasion in prostate needle biopsy specimens. Correlation with extraprostatic extension at resection. Am J Clin Pathol. 1999;111:223–8.

Varma M, Jasani S. Diagnostic utility of immunohistochemistry in morphologically difficult prostate cancer: review
of current literature. Histopathology. 2005;47:1–16.

Varma M, Morgan M, Amin MB, Wozniak S, Jasani B.
High molecular weight cytokeratin antibody (clone
34βE12): a sensitive marker for differentiation of
high-grade invasive urothelial carcinoma from prostate cancer. Histopathology. 2003;42:167–72.

Wittekind CF, Greene FL, Hutter RVP, Klimpfinger M,
Sobib LH. TNM atlas: illustrated guide to the TNM/
pTNM classification of malignant tumours. 5th ed.
Berlin: Springer; 2005.

Wolters TK, van der Kwast TH, Vissers CJ, Bangma CH,
Roobol M, Schroder FH, van Leenders GJ. False-
negative prostate needle biopsies: frequency, histo-
pathologic features, and follow-up. Am J Surg Pathol.
2010;34:35–43.

Yao JL, Huang J, di Sant'Agnese PA. Small cell carcinoma of the prostate. Diagn Histopathol. 2008;14:
117–21.

Young RH, Srigley JR, Amin MB, Ulbright TM, Cubilla
A. Tumors of the prostate gland, seminal vesicle, male
urethra and penis. Altas of tumour pathology. Series 3.
Fascicle 28. Washington DC: AFIP; 2000.

Urethral Carcinoma

32

Primary urethral cancer is relatively rare compared to secondary involvement of the urethra by high-grade bladder cancer, in which there is a reported incidence of up to 10–20 %. Urethral cancer occurs more commonly in females, with chronic irritation and HPV (Human Papilloma Virus) infection having aetiological roles. Proximal lesions are transitional cell in type and distal lesions squamous cell in character. A small minority are adenocarcinoma associated with a diverticulum, periurethral glands, or, the prostate gland in men.

Urethral cancers can present with haematuria, urinary hesitancy or retention mimicking benign prostatism. Proximal lesions can be relatively asymptomatic and present at a late stage. Investigation is by urethroscopy and biopsy, often combined with cystoscopy. CT/MRI scans determine tumour stage and spread into local soft tissues that might require en bloc resection. CT/PET scan has a role in detecting distant metastatic disease.

Treatment is by surgical excision, the extent of which depends on the location and stage of disease e.g. local excision for cancer of the distal or meatal male urethra, with or without partial or radical penectomy. Radiotherapy can preserve the penis but results in troublesome strictures and higher local recurrence rates. Advanced proximal tumours may require a combination of radical surgery and radiotherapy for palliative control. Surgery may comprise radical cystoprostatectomy, penectomy and pelvic lymph node dissection. Brachytherapy and radiosensitising chemotherapy are other options. Secondary urethral cancers from the penis or bladder are excised as part of a penectomy (see Chap. 34) or cysto(prostato)urethrectomy, respectively. In women urethrectomy is usually in continuity as part of a radical cystectomy, although with careful preoperative biopsy staging it may be preserved for orthotopic functional reconstruction using a neobladder. In men preoperative biopsies are carried out to determine the presence of urethral disease (either in situ or invasive). If positive, the procedure is then carried out in two stages viz cystoprostatectomy down to the level of the urogenital diaphragm and then a perineal urethrectomy for the residual urethra. Follow up may require cytological washings or biopsy from the urethral stump. Recurrent disease may necessitate secondary urethrectomy. Intraoperative frozen section may be required to confirm negative surgical margins.

32.1 Gross Description

Specimen

- Biopsy/urethrectomy or as part of cysto-(prostato)urethrectomy.
- Weight (g) and size/length (cm), number of fragments.

Tumour

Site

- Prostatic/bulbomembranous/pendulous ure-thras/meatus.

Size

- Length × width × depth (cm) or maximum dimension (cm).

Appearance

- Polypoid/verrucous/papillary/sessile/ulcer-ated/pigmented.

Edge

- Circumscribed/irregular.

32.2 Histological Type

Primary urethral carcinoma is rare and a urethral cancer is much more likely to represent *secondary involvement* from adjacent structures e.g. penis or urinary bladder.

Squamous Cell Carcinoma

- *60–70 % of cases.*
- *Distal in location.*
- Keratinising/non-keratinising, well to moderately differentiated.
- Large cell/small cell.
- *Verrucous*: exophytic, pushing deep margin of cytologically bland bulbous processes. It may coexist with usual squamous cell carcinoma.

Transitional Cell Carcinoma

- *20–30 % of cases.*
- *Proximal in location*: either high-grade in situ or invasive disease.

Adenocarcinoma

- *10 % of cases.*
- Female > male; arising in strictures, diverticula or fistulae.

- Either *non-clear cell* (60 %: glandular, enteric, mucinous, signet ring cell, papillary), or *clear cell* (40 %) patterns, with or without urethritis cystica/glandularis. Of variable low to high cytological grades.
- Prostatic urethra: 'endometrioid' carcinoma (PSA positive), also known as carcinoma of the prostatic periurethral ducts. See Chap. 31.

Adenosquamous Carcinoma

- Rare.

Small Cell Carcinoma

- A poorly differentiated/high-grade neuroendocrine carcinoma either primary, or secondary from lung.
- CAM 5.2/synaptophysin/CD56 positive with a high Ki-67 index.

Malignant Melanoma

- *4 % of urethral malignancy.*
- Extensive radial growth is usual leading to *local recurrence. Metastatic spread is common* to regional lymph nodes, liver, lungs and brain. The *poor prognosis*, relates to the tumour thickness. Mucosal junctional activity indicates a primary lesion.

Metastatic Carcinoma

- *Multifocal/direct spread*: urothelial cancer from bladder is commoner than a primary lesion. Other cancers that spread directly are penis, rectum, vagina, cervix and endometrium.
- *Distant spread*: ovary, kidney (distinguish from primary clear cell carcinoma).

32.3 Differentiation/Grade

Well/moderate/poor/undifferentiated, or, Grade 1/2/3/4.

• For squamous cell carcinoma based on cellular atypia, keratinisation and intercellular bridges, and, for adenocarcinoma on the tumour percentage gland formation (well/G1: > 95 %, moderate/G2: 50–95 %, poor/G3: <50 %). WHO I/II/III for transitional cell carcinoma (see Chap. 30).

32.4   Extent of Local Tumour Spread

Border: pushing/infiltrative.

Lymphocytic reaction: prominent/sparse.

The TNM7 classification applies to carcinomas of the urethra and transitional cell carcinoma of the prostate and prostatic urethra.

Urethra (Male and Female)

pTa	Non-invasive papillary, polypoid or verrucous carcinoma
pTis	Carcinoma in situ
pT1	Tumour invades subepithelial connective tissue
pT2	Tumour invades any of: corpus spongiosum, prostate, periurethral muscle
pT3	Tumour invades any of: corpus cavernosum, beyond prostatic capsule, anterior vagina, bladder neck
pT4	Tumour invades other adjacent organs.

Transitional Cell Carcinoma of Prostatic Urethra

pTis	pu: carcinoma in situ, involvement of prostatic urethra
pTis	pd: carcinoma in situ, involvement of prostatic ducts
pT1	Tumour invades subepithelial connective tissue
pT2	Tumour invades any of: prostatic stroma, corpus spongiosum, periurethral muscle
pT3	Tumour invades any of: corpus cavernosum, beyond prostatic capsule, bladder neck (extraprostatic extension)
pT4	Tumour invades other adjacent organs (invasion of the bladder).

Distinction must be made between periurethral duct involvement by tumour (pTis pd) and *invasion into periurethral or prostatic stroma* (pT2) as the latter worsens the prognosis.

In urethral diverticular carcinoma, a differentiation between T2 and T3 is not possible and it is classified as T2.

32.5   Lymphovascular Invasion

Present/absent.

Intra-/extratumoural.

32.6   Lymph Nodes

Site/number/size/number involved/limit node/extracapsular spread.

Regional lymph nodes: inguinal, pelvic.

pN0	No regional lymph node metastasis
pN1	Metastasis in a single regional lymph node ≤2 cm maximum dimension
pN2	Metastasis in a single regional lymph node >2 cm maximum dimension or multiple regional lymph nodes.

32.7   Excision Margins

Distances (mm) to the proximal and distal longitudinal and deep circumferential resection limits.

32.8   Other Pathology

Bladder cancer: urethral *involvement by bladder carcinoma* is much commoner than primary urethral carcinoma which is a relatively rare disease. In the female the urethra is short (4 cm) and removed by cystectomy, which involves total urethrectomy. However, there is potential for local recurrence in the residual male urethra. The histological status of the prostatic urethra is therefore assessed by biopsy prior to definitive surgical resection and consideration of cystoprostatourethrectomy.

Urinary tract field change: multifocal transitional cell carcinoma of urethra, bladder, ureter, and renal pelvis can occur either as papillary carcinoma, carcinoma in situ or Pagetoid urethral spread from a bladder lesion.

Gender and site disposition: the female to male ratio is 3:1 for urethral carcinoma. Carcinomas arising *proximally* (proximal one third in women; prostatic, bulbomembranous urethra in men) are generally *transitional cell carcinoma* while *distal* lesions (distal two thirds in women; penile urethra in men) are usually *squamous cell carcinoma*. In the distal one third they are often well differentiated squamous cell or verrucous in type. *Clear cell* (*mesonephroid*) *adenocarcinoma* is rare, arising in either the female or prostatic urethra where it may be associated with a stricture or diverticulum. It should be distinguished from similar lesions arising in the female genital tract and metastatic renal cell adenocarcinoma by clinical history and anatomical distribution of disease. Another differential diagnosis is nephrogenic adenoma, which is usually small and lacks significant cellular atypia and mitoses. *Prostatic duct* ('*endometrioid*') *adenocarcinoma* arises from periurethral prostatic ducts (PSA, PSAP positive) and may be oestrogen sensitive.

Benign mimics of carcinoma: *nephrogenic adenoma* is a reactive (probably metaplastic) proliferative lesion associated with recent instrumentation, calculi, trauma and cystitis. It is benign and does not predispose to but rarely may be associated with concurrent carcinoma e.g. with adenocarcinoma in a urethral diverticulum. It usually has a distinctive exophytic, polypoid or papillary growth pattern with a covering tubulopapillary proliferation of cuboidal epithelium also present in the underlying lamina propria. The cells may show tubule formation and cystic change with degenerative atypia but are not mitotically active. The cells are CK7, AMACR/P504S, PAX2, PAX8 positive, and an origin from renal tubular stem cells in renal transplant patients has been postulated. Other *protuberant urethral lesions that can mimic carcinoma* at cystoscopy are benign prostatic urethral polyp, prominent verumontanum, fibrovascular polyp, villous adenoma and inverted transitional cell papilloma. Condyloma accuminatum associated with "high-risk" HPV types (16, 18, 31, 33, 35) may rarely undergo malignant transformation to verrucous or infiltrating squamous cell carcinoma.

Prognosis

Distal urethral carcinoma (well differentiated squamous cell/verrucous) presents early with a reasonable prognosis. *Overall prognosis of urethral carcinoma (40 % 5 year survival)* relates to the *anatomical site and stage of disease*, e.g. pendulous urethral carcinomas have *60–70 % 5 year survival* while the figure for bulbomembranous/prostatic lesions is *20 %*. Proximal cancers also present at a more advanced stage and with high-grade (poorly differentiated) histology in which it may be difficult to distinguish squamous cell from transitional cell carcinoma.

32.9 Other Malignancy

Malignant Lymphoma/Leukaemia

- As a manifestation of systemic disease.

Embryonal Rhabdomyosarcoma

- Sarcoma botryoides in children.
- Superficial subepithelial cambium layer, intermediate myxoid zone, deep cellular zone, desmin/myo D1/myogenin positive.

Aggressive Angiomyxoma

- Myxoid stroma/thick vessels with HMGA2 positive stellate/spindle mesenchmyal cells.
- Locally recurrent/infiltrative.

Bibliography

Bostwick DG, Cheng L. Urologic surgical pathology. 2nd ed. Philadelphia: Mosby/Elsevier; 2008.

Eble JN, Sauter G, Epstein JI, Sesterhenn IA. WHO classification of tumours. Pathology and genetics. Tumours of the urinary system and male genital organs. Lyon: IARC Press; 2004.

Young RH, Srigley JR, Amin MB, Ulbright TM, Cubilla A. Tumors of the prostate gland, seminal vesicle, male urethra and penis. Altas of tumour pathology. Series 3. Fascicle 28. Washington D.C.: AFIP; 2000.

Testicular Cancer

Testicular cancer represents less than 1 % of malignancy in men although it is the commonest cancer in those under 45 years of age, and its incidence is increasing by 2–3 % per annum. About 95 % are germ cell tumours and predisposing factors include cryptorchidism, infertility, genetic factors, testicular dysgenesis, prior testicular tumour and intratubular germ cell neoplasia (ITGCN). Patient age and a testicular or paratesticular location are important indicators to likely tumour type (Table 33.1).

Testicular cancer usually presents with a painless unilateral lump or swelling of some duration, and any non-resolving lump lasting more than 2–3 weeks should be referred to a urologist. Occasionally there is scrotal pain, backache or endocrine effects such as gynaecomastia. Torsion or incidental trauma to a fully descended or undescended testis may draw attention to underlying tumour. Delay in presentation correlates with the development of metastases. Some cases may present with malignant axial or cervical lymphadenopathy of unknown primary site, and up to 10–30 % of patients have metastatic disease at diagnosis. Investigation involves careful clinical examination, serum tumour markers (AFP: alphafetoprotein, HCG: human chorionic gonadotrophin, LDH: lactate dehydrogenase), and ultrasound assessment to detect hypoechoic areas of tumour. Ultrasound scan is 95–100 % sensitive for detecting a scrotal abnormality and determining an intra- or extratesticular location. Tumour staging is by chest x-ray and CT scan for pulmonary involvement, and CT/PET scan for abdominopelvic and mediastinal lymph node disease. FNAC (fine needle aspiration cytology) and needle biopsy are avoided due to the potential risk of iatrogenic tumour dissemination, and because a testis should always be excised if there is a suspicion of tumour. Exceptions to this would be patients with known disseminated leukaemia, malignant

Table 33.1 Testicular cancer diagnosis by age and site

Age	Testis	Paratesticular
Neonate	Juvenile granulosa cell tumour	
Infant	Yolk sac tumour	Rhabdomyosarcoma
Young adult	Germ cell tumours – non-seminoma (second/third decade) or seminoma (third/fourth decade)	Rhabdomyosarcoma
		Adenomatoid tumour
		Desmoplastic small blue cell tumour
	Sex cord stromal tumours	
Older adult (>60 years)	Spermatocytic seminoma	Adenomatoid tumour
	Sex cord stromal tumours	Malignant lymphoma
	Malignant lymphoma	Metastatic cancer
	Metastatic cancer	Liposarcoma, and other sarcomas

lymphoma or carcinoma in whom FNAC/core biopsy would provide a relatively accessible and non-invasive tissue diagnosis of relapse as a basis for further systemic treatment.

Serum AFP and HCG are significantly raised in >80 % of non-seminomatous germ cell tumours, specifically embryonal carcinoma, yolk sac tumour and choriocarcinoma. HCG may be modestly elevated in pure seminoma, and LDH is an indicator of bulky advanced or metastatic germ cell tumour.

In the radical orchidectomy specimen the pathologist must determine

(a) The extent or stage of tumour spread
(b) Distinguish between seminoma (radiosensitive), teratoma (chemosensitive) and sex cord stromal tumours (surgery alone), and
(c) Establish if blood or lymphatic vascular invasion is present as this is an indicator for chemotherapy in stage I malignant germ cell tumours.

Resection is by radical inguinal orchidectomy as a scrotal approach would then in addition incorporate pelvic lymph nodes as regional. The patient is offered a testicular prosthesis and sperm storage if chemoradiation is anticipated. For patients with proven metastases and high serum tumour marker levels orchidectomy may be delayed until after chemotherapy is completed or other surgery is being performed e.g. excision of residual retroperitoneal masses. Some specialist centres occasionally offer partial orchidectomy for a tumour <2 cm in size, where there are bilateral tumours, a metachronous tumour or tumour in a solitary testis. The residual testis is treated with radiotherapy. Overall, oncological therapeutic options and prognosis are based on histological tumour type (seminoma versus non-seminoma), the presence or absence of lymphovascular invasion, levels of serum tumour markers, and radiological determination of the clinical stage of disease. Management should be by a specialist multidisciplinary testicular cancer team and cure rates of 95 % are achieved. Central review of pathology has noted discrepancy rates of up to 4 and 10 % in tumour type (seminoma changed to non-seminoma) and presence of vascular invasion, respectively, both of which are important criteria for treatment decisions.

33.1   Gross Description

Specimen

- FNAC/biopsy (open or needle)/radical orchidectomy (testis, tunica vaginalis, coverings and spermatic cord).
- Weight (g) and size (cm): overall and testicular.
- Length of spermatic cord (cm).

Tumour

Site
- Testicular/paratesticular.
- Bilateral: 1–3 % of cases, synchronous or metachronous, similar or dissimilar types. The commonest bilateral tumours are seminoma or spermatocytic seminoma but beware malignant lymphoma in the older age group.

Size
- Length × width × depth (cm) or maximum dimension (cm).
- Embryonal carcinoma tends to present at a smaller size than seminoma.

Appearance
- Pale/fleshy/nodular ± necrosis: seminoma/malignant lymphoma.
- Cysts/cartilage ± necrosis: teratoma.
- Haemorrhage: choriocarcinoma, yolk sac tumour.
- Fibrous/calcific scar: regression.
- Pale or tan/lobulated, often small and circumscribed: Leydig cell/stromal tumours.
- Note that some inflammatory conditions e.g. granulomatous orchitis or malakoplakia can mimic germ cell tumour clinically and macroscopically.

Edge
- Circumscribed/irregular.

33.2   Histological Type

Germ cell tumours comprise 95 % of testicular neoplasms (of which 40–50 % are seminoma), and *sex cord stromal lesions* 4 % of cases.

Therapeutic distinction is drawn between *seminomatous* and *non-seminomatous germ cell tumours* due to adjunctive radiotherapy and chemotherapy approaches, respectively. List and semi-quantify the *percentage of tumour types* present in a mixed germ cell tumour. Histopathological grading is not applicable, biological behaviour being determined by the constituent tumour types present.

Seminoma

- *40–50% of testicular tumours* occurring in patients of mean age 40 years and 70 % present with stage I disease.
- *Classical (93% of cases)*, or, anaplastic with the same behaviour despite different mitotic rates and the term anaplastic is not justified. Note that this remains uncertain as some studies have noted higher stage at presentation and worse prognosis with high mitotic count, aneuploid seminomas.
- Seminoma typically comprises large, polygonal cells with clear to eosinophilic cytoplasm and an intervening stroma with aggregates of lymphocytes. Granulomas and HCG positive syncytiotrophoblastic giant cells (7 % of cases) may also be present.
- Usually sheets of cells but trabecular, diffuse single cell interstitial, pseudoglandular and tubular patterns also occur. There can also be "cystic" spaces due to oedema, sclerotic stroma, and Pagetoid spread into the rete.
- Seminoma cells are: PLAP, CD117, OCT3/4, SALL4, D2-40 (podoplanin) positive, cytokeratin focal or negative.
- *Spermatocytic*: benign with three cell types and PLAP negative presenting usually in old age (see Sect. 33.8).

Non-seminomatous Germ Cell Tumours

- A range of tumours showing either
  - (a) Embryonic differentiation: *teratoma –* mature, immature, ± a malignant somatic component,

  - (b) *Embryonal carcinoma*, or,
  - (c) Extraembryonic differentiation: *yolk sac (endodermal sinus) tumour, choriocarcinoma (malignant teratoma trophoblastic)*.

They are generally *more aggressive*, metastasise earlier, and have a greater tendency for *haematogenous spread* than seminomas with a cure rate of 95 % dropping to 40–95 % if metastases are present. *Extensive pulmonary disease* is an *adverse prognostic indicator*. Metastases may also *change differentiation* and are *radioresistant*.

Note that there are terminological differences between the British Testicular Tumour Panel (BTTP) and the WHO systems interpreted as follows (optional):

BTTP	WHO
Malignant teratoma differentiated, MTD	Teratoma mature
MTD (with immature elements)	Teratoma immature
MTD (with malignant transformation)	Teratoma with an overtly malignant somatic component
Malignant teratoma intermediate, MTI	Embryonal carcinoma or yolk sac tumour mixed with mature or immature teratoma ("teratocarcinoma")
Malignant teratoma trophoblastic, MTT	Choriocarcinoma
Malignant teratoma undifferentiated, MTU	Embryonal carcinoma.

The BTTP classification is based on the presumption that all testicular teratomas arise from pluripotent stem cells and show variable type and differentiation rather than representing distinct entities. However there is justification for the WHO approach because of the distinctive morphological features and prognostic associations of the various prototypical germ cell tumours e.g. yolk sac tumour and embryonal carcinoma. The *WHO classification is recommended* with reporting of the BTTP equivalent in parallel.

Teratoma
- *5–10% of cases* with cellular components from 2 or 3 germ cell layers (endoderm, mesoderm, ectoderm).

- *Mature teratoma*: benign in childhood (usually <4 years of age) but potentially malignant in the postpubertal patient with metastases in up to 25 % of cases (*MTD*: *malignant teratoma differentiated*). Serum AFP is useful in distinguishing from yolk sac tumour. Mature somatic tissues commonly represented are: cartilage, muscle, neuroglia, enteric glands, squamous/respiratory and urothelial epithelia. Ovarian type cystic teratoma with sebum and hair is rare. Distinguish also from a benign testicular epidermoid cyst containing laminated keratin and lined by mature stratified squamous epithelium but no mural appendage structures or adjacent ITGCN.
- *Immature teratoma*: immature/fetal type tissues e.g. cartilage, variably cellular mesenchymal stroma arranged concentrically around glandular epithelium, neuroectoderm, blastema and embryonic tubules. It is uncertain as to whether grading is of prognostic significance but a semi-quantitative and qualitative assessment of the amount (rare, focal, diffuse) and degree of immaturity (low/high-grade) should be made.
- *Malignant somatic transformation*: in 3–6 % of patients. Adenocarcinoma, squamous cell carcinoma, but more than 50 % are sarcoma of no specific type, or, showing distinct differentiation features e.g. leiomyosarcoma, rhabdomyosarcoma, PNET (peripheral neuroectodermal tumour). A designation of sarcoma requires at least one low power field of atypical mesenchyme. A lack of organoid pattern and atypical mitoses are also helpful. Poor prognosis is not a consequence if the tumour is testis confined, but is an *adverse finding in metastases* e.g. in the retroperitoneum, as they are *non-responsive to germ cell chemotherapy and require surgical resection*.

Embryonal Carcinoma (EC/MTU: Malignant Teratoma Undifferentiated)

- Present in *87%* of non-seminomatous germ cell tumours but usually as part of a mixed germ cell tumour, and rarely in 2 % of cases in pure form. With the *poorest prognosis* of the germ cell tumours it comprises primitive anaplastic epithelial cells in solid, glandular or tubulopapillary patterns. *Vascular invasion* in the adjacent testicular parenchyma and overlying tunica is relatively common. EC is CAM5.2, CD30, OCT3/4, SALL4, SOX2, D2-40 positive, PLAP±.

Yolk Sac Tumour (YST)

- The commonest prepubertal testicular germ cell tumour (75–90 % of cases) requiring orchidectomy with follow up. It is present as a component in up to *40–50%* of adult lesions and is treated as for other non-seminomatous germ cell tumours. It is histologically heterogeneous assuming a spectrum of patterns, the commonest being microcystic/reticular, honeycomb and vacuolated, in addition to papillary, endodermal sinus (perivascular Duvall-Schiller bodies), parietal, hepatoid, solid, myxomatous and glandular (enteric or endometrioid). Other characteristics are PAS positive diastase-resistant, intra- and extracellular hyaline globules and deposition of extracellular basement membrane. AFP is present in 55–75 % of cases but can be patchy in expression and is in the tumour cell cytoplasm rather than the globules. YST is also SALL4, glypican 3 positive, PLAP±, and negative for CD30, OCT3/4, D2-40 and HCG. CD117 can be focal in expression.

Choriocarcinoma (MTT: Malignant Teratoma Trophoblastic)

- MTT (*1% of cases*) requires *biphasic syncytiotrophoblastic and cytotrophoblastic differentiation* for diagnosis, although the "syncytio" element may be inconspicuous. *Angioinvasion* with *tumour haemorrhage* is common. Designation is dependent on the morphology and not the serum hormone levels. The syncytiotrophoblast is HCG positive capping the cytokeratin 7 positive cytotrophoblast and may also show positive staining for HPL, EMA, cytokeratins, inhibin, PLAP and CEA. OCT3/4 and SALL4 are negative. Given its propensity for *angioinvasion* it can present with advanced stage disease and *early haematogenous metastases* to liver, lung, mediastinum and retroperitoneum. This produces diverse symptomatology: dyspnoea, haemoptysis, haematemesis, central nervous system dysfunction, with potential *haemorrhage* at multiple visceral sites. Serum HCG correlates with tumour extent and can produce endocrine effects such as gynaecomastia or thyrotoxicosis. *Radical orchidectomy* and *systemic chemotherapy* are required. A favourable indicator is post chemotherapy cystic change in retroperitoneal metastases.

Mixed Germ Cell Tumour

More than one germ cell type in any combination occurs in *30–40% of cases overall* and *70%* of non-seminomatous tumours e.g. seminoma and EC, EC and teratoma, EC with YST and teratoma (*MTI: malignant teratoma intermediate*). Sample extensively (1 block/cm tumour diameter) and target block any unusual gross appearance, e.g. the association of choriocarcinoma with haemorrhage, to allow for this tumour heterogeneity particularly if there are significantly elevated serum AFP and HCG levels.

Anaplastic Germ Cell Tumour

- Morphologically and immunohistochemically intermediate between seminoma and EC. Rarely, a tumour with admixed features may be encountered but with careful scrutiny separation into either seminoma, EC, or mixed germ cell tumour can usually be made.

Mixed Germ Cell and Sex Cord Stromal Tumour

- *Gonadoblastoma*: a mixture of seminoma type cells and sex cord (Sertoli/granulosa) cells in a nested arrangement progressing, in 30 % of cases, to invasive germ cell tumour, usually seminoma. Mostly found in dysgenetic gonads of intersex patients with a Y chromosome.

Sex Cord Stromal Tumours

- *4 % of testicular tumours in adults* and *30 % in infants and children* containing sex cord epithelial cells (Sertoli/granulosa) mixed with mesenchymal elements (Leydig/theca lutein cells) in varying combinations, proportions and states of differentiation. There is no adjacent ITGCN. These tumours are serum marker negative but may be associated with a clinical syndrome.
- *Leydig cell tumour*: 1–3 % of testicular neoplasms and 30 % bilateral or hormonally active with gynaecomastia or precocious puberty. Well circumscribed, yellow to tan in colour with eosinophilic or clear cells and Reinke's crystalloids (25 %). Inhibin (40 %), calretinin positive, melan-A, cytokeratin ±, and EMA/AFP/PLAP/OCT3/4 negative.
- *Sertoli cell tumour*: <1 % of testicular neoplasms. Not otherwise specified (including sclerosing variant) and large cell calcifying types. Sheets, nests, tubules and cords of Sertoli cells with a hyaline stroma. Cytokeratin, inhibin, calretinin positive, melan-A±, and EMA, PLAP, OCT3/4 negative. Often non-functional but can be associated with gynaecomastia, testicular feminization syndrome, Peutz-Jeghers and Carney's (large cell variant) syndromes.
- *Granulosa cell tumour*:
  Adult – microfollicular (Call-Exner bodies), nuclear grooves with a range of morphology similar to that seen in the ovary. Rare, usually non-functional and 10–20 % are malignant. Cytokeratin ± but EMA negative. Inhibin, calretinin and variably melan-A positive. Also SF-1, FOXL2 and WT1.
  Juvenile – <1 year old presenting as a scrotal or abdominal mass in an undescended testis, 20 % have ambiguous external genitalia. Cystic follicular structures, and benign. The commonest neonatal testicular cancer. Distinguish from YST by morphology and immunohistochemistry.
- *Undifferentiated or mixed types*: thecoma/fibroma and other gonadal stromal tumours are rare.

Malignancy (10% of adult sex cord stromal tumours): cannot be reliably predicted but relates to size (>5–7 cm), cellular atypia, mitoses (>3/10 high-power fields), infiltrative margins, vascular invasion and a high Ki-67 proliferation index.

A diagnostic pitfall is sex cord stromal tumour positivity for S100 and melan-A mimicking metastatic malignant melanoma. However, they are usually HMB-45 negative.

Other Tumours

- *Adenocarcinoma of the rete* (rare, poor prognosis).
- *Cystadenocarcinoma of the epididymis* (very rare). Papillary cystadenoma is associated with von Hippel-Lindau syndrome.
- *Metastatic carcinoma*

   2–3% of testicular neoplasms with a mean age of 50 years. Prostate, lung, malignant melanoma, Merkel cell carcinoma, colon, kidney, stomach, pancreas.

   Bilaterality, vascular involvement and absence of ITGCN favour metastatic disease. Malignant melanoma, renal cell carcinoma and malignant lymphoma are particular mimics of germ cell tumour.
- *Carcinoid tumour*

   Good prognosis, a well differentiated/low-grade neuroendocrine tumour or monodermal teratoma, but 20 % have other teratomatous elements. Exclude metastatic carcinoid e.g. from ileum (vascular invasion, extratesticular extension, bilateral).
- *Primitive neuroectodermal tumour*

   Can be primary but more frequently arises within a testicular teratoma.

   Particularly look for its presence with adverse prognosis in retroperitoneal metastases.

33.3 Extent of Local Tumour Spread

Border: pushing/infiltrative.

Lymphocytic reaction: prominent/sparse.

Lymphocytic reaction: a consistent (80 %) feature of seminoma, and *granulomas* can also be present in up to 50 % of cases. Sometimes the inflammatory infiltrate can be so intense that it partially obscures the germ cells and immunohistochemical markers are necessary. The intensity of inflammation and presence of granulomas are not prognostically significant.

ITGCN/carcinoma in situ: sample the adjacent testis.

Intratubular spread: seminoma/EC.

It can be difficult to distinguish between ITGCN and intratubular spread although in EC ITGCN will be PLAP/CD117 positive, and intratubular spread PLAP negative/CD30 positive. Intratubular EC has been suggested as an intermediate step between ITGCN and established EC. Intratubular spread of seminoma and ITGCN into the rete can also mimic EC or carcinoma of the rete.

Rete testis: Pagetoid or luminal spread of seminoma/EC. Distinguish from true *invasion of the rete stroma* which is an indicator for *postoperative adjuvant therapy*. Extratesticular extension of germ cell tumours is commoner at the rete/hilum.

The TNM7 classification applies to germ cell tumours of the testis.

pTis	ITGCN (carcinoma in situ)
pT1	Tumour involves testis and epididymis or tunica albuginea, no lymphovascular invasion or involvement of tunica vaginalis
pT2	Tumour involves testis and epididymis with lymphovascular invasion, or, extends through tunica albuginea to involve tunica vaginalis
pT3	Tumour involves spermatic cord ± lymphovascular invasion
pT4	Tumour involves scrotum ± lymphovascular invasion.

In mixed germ cell tumours the pT classification is determined by the highest stage of its components. Synchronous bilateral tumours are staged as independent primary tumours.

Invasion beyond tunica albuginea involves scrotal structures except scrotal skin or subcutaneous tissues (both pT4).

Invasion of the spermatic cord refers to direct extension beyond the rete or epididymis. It is recognized by solid nodules of tumour within the cord not contiguous with the testis, and is rare (Fig. 33.1).

Fig. 33.1 Testicular germ cell tumours (Reproduced, with permission, from Allen (2006), © 2006)

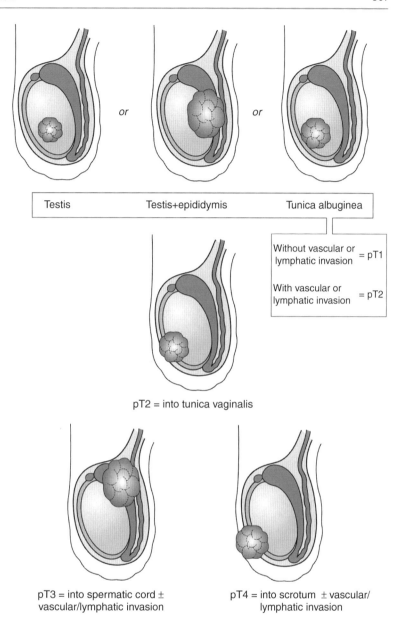

Testis | Testis+epididymis | Tunica albuginea

Without vascular or lymphatic invasion = pT1

With vascular or lymphatic invasion = pT2

pT2 = into tunica vaginalis

pT3 = into spermatic cord ± vascular/lymphatic invasion

pT4 = into scrotum ± vascular/lymphatic invasion

33.4 Lymphovascular Invasion

Present/absent.

Intra-/extratumoural.

Lymphovascular invasion correlates with a significantly elevated *risk of distant metastasis* (40–50 % versus 15 % if absent) and is an *indication for chemotherapy*. Consequently strict criteria for its identification are necessary i.e. an endothelial lined space with tumour conformed to its shape ± thrombosis or a point of attachment to the endothelium. Sample particularly the tumour/parenchyma interface and the overlying tunica looking for vasculocentric nodular deposits. As testicular cancers are cellular tumours with delayed fixation due to the relatively impervious tunica, beware of knife carry-in misinterpreted as vascular invasion and characterized as loose floating tumour cells in vascular spaces. This can be particularly prominent in seminomas.

33.5 Lymph Nodes

Site/number/size/number involved/limit node/ extracapsular spread.

Regional nodes: abdominal periaortic and pericaval, those located along the spermatic veins. The intrapelvic and inguinal nodes are considered regional after scrotal or inguinal surgery.

pN0	No regional lymph node metastasis
pN1	Regional lymph node metastasis ≤2 cm and ≤5 positive nodes
pN2	Regional lymph node metastasis >2 cm but ≤5 cm, or >5 positive nodes, or extranodal extension
pN3	Regional lymph node metastasis >5 cm.

Seminoma tends to metastasise through lymphatics while *choriocarcinoma shows haematogenous spread* with presentation from metastatic disease to lung, liver, brain, bone and gastrointestinal tract. *EC spreads by a combination of these mechanisms.* Lymph node involvement depends on the stage of disease and laterality of the primary tumour. Initial spread is periaortic but external iliac and inguinal node involvement may be seen if the tumour spreads to the epididymis and scrotal skin respectively. Mediastinal and left supraclavicular lymph node metastases occur late in the disease course. YST spreads in a similar manner to other non-seminomatous germ cell tumours, although it can present with haematogenous deposits, e.g. lungs (Fig. 33.2).

33.6 Clinical Stage

Modified Royal Marsden Staging System

I	Tumour confined to the testis
II	Lymph nodes involved below the diaphragm
III	Lymph nodes involved above the diaphragm – supraclavicular or mediastinal
IV	Extranodal metastases – lung or brain.

Up to 10–15 % of patients with seminoma have *metastases at the time of diagnosis*, 30–60 % with EC, and the majority with choriocarcinoma.

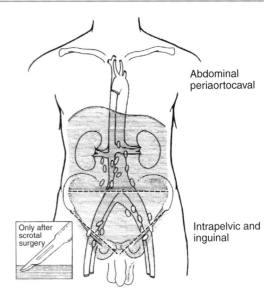

Fig. 33.2 Testicular germ cell tumours: regional lymph nodes (Reproduced, with permission, from Wittekind et al. (2005), © 2005)

Clinical staging: is based on the radiological determination of the anatomical extent of disease and the assessment of postorchidectomy serum markers LDH, ßsubunit HCG and AFP. *High levels* (AFP > 10,000 ng/ml, HCG > 50,000 IU/l, LDH > 10× normal) indicate *worse prognosis* and usually a diagnosis of *non-seminomatous germ cell tumour*.

Metastatic germ cell tumour: is an important diagnostic consideration in a *young male with evidence of extensive visceral disease but no known primary somatic site carcinoma*. This is particularly so if there is cervical, mediastinal or retroperitoneal lymphadenopathy or lung metastases. Ultrasound may show a small or scarred testicular lesion. Tumour regression is characterized by an irregular or nodular scar with adjacent ghosted tubules showing ITGCN or intratubular microcalcifications. Immunohistochemistry can be relatively robust in the presence of tumour necrosis and helpful in subtyping residual tumour – particularly cytokeratins, OCT3/4, CD117 and CD30. Biopsy of metastases may only show undifferentiated tumour and chemotherapy is instigated empirically on the basis of elevated serum markers. Occasionally poorly differentiated carcinoma of stomach, lung, breast or bladder may cause a modest elevation in serum HCG. AFP is raised in hepatocellular carcinomas and some gastrointestinal cancers. Crucially the pathologist has to think of the possibility of germ cell tumour and look for the distinctive morphological and immunohistochemical clues with a panel of germ cell tumour markers (SALL4, PLAP, CD117, OCT3/4, CD30, SOX2).

33.7   Excision Margins

Distances (mm) to the proximal limit of the spermatic cord.

33.8   Other Pathology

ITGCN: the *precursor lesion* of all germ cell tumours except spermatocytic seminoma, infantile teratoma differentiated and YSTs. It is usually seen in a patchy distribution within the testicular tubules away from and adjacent to the tumour in up to 90 % of seminomas and malignant teratomas. It may also be detected by needle biopsy as a *risk factor* for tumour development in the *contralateral testis* particularly if the testis is soft, atrophic or of low volume. It can be treated by *surveillance*, *orchidectomy* or *low-dose irradiation* as *50–90 % of untreated ITGCN will progress to germ cell tumour over a 5 year period*. Chemotherapeutic agents do not cross the blood/testis barrier. It comprises a proliferation of seminoma like cells (clear cytoplasm, PAS/PLAP/CD117(c-kit)/p53/OCT3/4/D2-40/SALL4 positive) at the base of the tubules which often have a hyalinised and thickened basement membrane and absence of spermatogenesis. Tubular microcalcifications may be present. It can be associated with intratubular or extratubular (microinvasive) interstitial extension as either seminoma or EC and usually accompanied by a herald lymphocytic infiltrate.

Predisposing conditions: *prior testicular tumour* on the contralateral side confers an increased malignancy risk ×5–10. *Maldescent/cryptorchidism* and *infertility* confer an increased malignancy risk ×3–5 and 1 % incidence respectively, correlating with ITGCN rates of 2–4 % and 1 %. Various *genetic conditions* may be associated with testicular tumours e.g. mediastinal and testicular germ cell tumours in Klinefelter's syndrome, Sertoli cell proliferation and tumour in Peutz-Jeghers syndrome, and Carney complex (cardiac myxomas, Cushing's syndrome, hyperpigmentation).

Tumour regression: "scar" cancer (fibrosis, haemosiderin-laden macrophages, intratubular calcification) with retroperitoneal secondaries is regression of the primary and *presentation with metastatic disease*, especially EC or choriocarcinoma.

Age incidence: age is also a helpful indicator in that malignant germ cell tumours and sex cord stromal tumours present in the *third and fourth decades* but malignant lymphoma and spermatocytic seminoma occur in old age. Seminoma is usually in patients 10 years older than those with non-seminomatous germ cell tumours. YST is the commonest testicular neoplasm in children but also a common component of adult germ cell tumours.

Clinical mimics: other scrotal swellings mimicking testicular cancer include epididymoorchitis, granulomatous orchitis, malakoplakia and peritesticular hydrocoele. Ultrasound examination is useful in delineating the latter and intratesticular lesions. This, coupled with increased male health awareness, has led to an increasing proportion of small and unusual tumours being detected e.g. sex cord stromal lesions, epidermoid inclusion cyst.

FNAC: can be of use in those patients suspected of having *metastatic carcinoma* in the testes, or *testicular relapse in malignant lymphoma and leukaemia*. It is usually limited in germ cell tumours to those patients who are medically unfit for orchidectomy but in whom a tissue diagnosis is necessary for further management. Due to the considerable heterogeneity of germ cell tumours it can be subject to marked sampling error. Abdominal and thoracic FNAC (± core biopsy) are useful for the assessment of germ cell tumour metastases which should be categorised as seminomatous (requiring radiotherapy ± chemotherapy depending on the bulk of disease) or non-seminomatous. The latter is either pure tera-tomatous (requiring surgery) or other, e.g. EC or YST (requiring chemotherapy). Serum HCG and AFP levels are also useful in making these management decisions.

Spermatocytic seminoma: 1–2 % of germ cell tumours, *indolent behaviour* and treated by *orchidectomy alone*. It presents in the *older age group* (50–70 years) and shows *no evidence of adjacent ITGCN*. It is lobulated ± microcystic with stromal oedema and comprises a *tripartite population* of small, intermediate and large glycogen negative cells with indistinct cell boundaries, a "spireme" chromatin pattern and scattered mitoses. It lacks a stromal lymphocytic component, is *germ cell marker negative* (PLAP/OCT3/4/CD117/D2-40/HCG/EMA/CD30), and variably CAM 5.2 positive. Differential diagnosis is seminoma of usual type (distinct cell boundaries, uniform polygonal cells with clear cytoplasm, an enlarged nucleus with nucleoli and clumped nuclear chromatin, lymphocytic stroma, PLAP/OCT3/4/CD 117/SALL4/D2-40 positive), and malignant lymphoma (CD 45, CD 20, κ/λ light chain restriction, interstitial/peritubular infiltration, can be bilateral). Rarely spermatocytic seminoma undergoes highly malignant (rhabdomyo-) sarcomatous change.

Immunophenotype

The reactions of different tumour types with immunohistochemical markers are summarised as follows

CIS/ITGCN	SALL4, OCT3/4, CD117, PLAP+, and CAM5.2±
Seminoma	SALL4,OCT3/4,CD117,PLAP+,andCAM5.2–
YST	AFP, CAM5.2, glypican3+, CD117±, and SALL4, OCT3/4–
EC	SALL4, OCT3/4, CAM5.2, CD30, SOX2+, and CD117, PLAP, HCG, AFP±
MTT	HCG+, CAM5.2±, and SALL4, OCT3/4, CD117, PLAP–

A simple algorithm for the use immunohistochemistry in subtyping testicular germ cell tumours is given in Table 33.2.

Table 33.2 Germ cell tumour immunohistochemistry

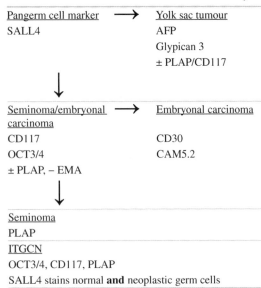

Pangerm cell marker ⟶	Yolk sac tumour
SALL4	AFP
	Glypican 3
	± PLAP/CD117
↓	
Seminoma/embryonal carcinoma ⟶	Embryonal carcinoma
CD117	CD30
OCT3/4	CAM5.2
± PLAP, – EMA	
↓	
Seminoma	
PLAP	
ITGCN	
OCT3/4, CD117, PLAP	

SALL4 stains normal **and** neoplastic germ cells

PLAP positivity in seminoma/ITGCN is membranous and not cytoplasmic as seen in some non-small cell lung carcinomas and malignant melanomas. OCT3/4, SALL4 and SOX2 are nuclear epitopes. Markers may also help distinguish metastatic EC (CAM+, CD30+, SALL4+, OCT3/4+, SOX2, PLAP±, EMA–) from metastatic carcinoma (CAM+, CD30–, SALL4–, OCT3/4–, SOX2–, EMA+). Seminoma is generally CAM 5.2– , CD30– and EMA– but can show focal positivity for these markers as well as CK7 and AE1/AE3. EC is strongly positive for various cytokeratin markers, CD30, SALL4, OCT3/4 and SOX2 but variable (often only focal) for CD117. YST is AFP+, glypican3+, CD117± but SALL4–, OCT3/4–. SALL4 is a robust pluripotential pan germ cell marker staining tumour and normal germ cells. Due to the latter careful correlation with morphology is required in designation of ITGCN.

Serum markers: often do not show good correlation with their tumour tissue expression but are good for *monitoring disease treatment response and relapse* as they are raised in >80 % of patients with non-seminomatous germ cell tumours. Seminoma may have mildly elevated high HCG levels (15 %) and increased serum PLAP levels (40 % of cases). Seminoma and teratoma rarely give elevated AFP levels. If present, other elements e.g. YST or EC are identified by taking extra blocks to confirm their presence.

Apparently aberrant tissue expression is acceptable without changing the diagnosis or prognosis e.g. seminoma with HCG positive syncytiotrophoblastic cells (10–20 % of cases) or EC with elevated serum HCG.

Prognosis

With modern oncological treatment regimes the prognosis of even metastatic germ cell tumour is excellent with *more than 90% cure*. It relates to *serum tumour marker levels, stage of disease, histological type and lymphovascular invasion*. Stage I disease and stage II with non-bulky (<5–10 cm) retroperitoneal secondaries have 5 year survival rates of 90–95 % for both seminoma and EC, whereas the rate for bulky stage II tumour is 70–80 %. YST presents as stage I (90 %) in childhood with >90 % 5 year survivals however it can exhibit chemoresistance in adults with metastatic disease. The presence of YST elements in an immature teratoma of childhood is also an indicator for potential recurrence of disease. *Extensive pulmonary disease in EC is a poor prognostic indicator*.

Prognosis of seminoma worsens with:
1. Tumour diameter ≥4 cm.
2. Age <34 years.
3. Vascular invasion.
4. Rete testis invasion.
   Prognosis of teratoma worsens with:
1. Increasing stage.
2. Presence of EC.
3. Absence of YST.
4. Lymphovascular invasion.

The Medical Research Council scheme scores 1 for each of: presence of EC, absence of YST, lymphatic invasion, blood vessel invasion.

Tumour score:

0–2	Surgery with follow-up only
3–4	Surgery with adjuvant chemotherapy.

Low volume/percentage tumour area of EC and a low Ki-67 index are beneficial. *Relapse*

rates are 15–20% for seminoma (80 % in the retroperitoneum) and *30–35% for teratoma* (66 % in the retroperitoneum, 33 % in the lung or mediastinum). *Vascular invasion* is a strong determinant of *postoperative chemotherapy* in stage I disease. Stage I *seminoma* is treated by *orchidectomy* and then either *surveillance* (serum tumour markers, chest x-ray, CT scan) for low risk tumour (<4 cm dimension, no rete invasion), *single dose carboplatin chemotherapy*, or *radiation* to regional lymph node sites. Stage II and more advanced disease require more extensive radiotherapy, and in addition chemotherapy. *Non-seminomatous germ cell tumours* require *orchidectomy* alone with *surveillance* for stage I disease with no high risk factors (particularly lymphovascular invasion). Otherwise this is combined with *platinum based chemotherapy*. This is supplemented by *retroperitoneal lymph node dissection (RPLND)* for post-treatment residual disease or recurrent disease refractory to chemotherapy. Postchemotherapy cytoreduction of metastases results in necrosis, xanthomatous inflammation, fibrosis and variably viable tumour tissue. *Ominously, carcinomatous* or *sarcomatous (e.g. rhabdomyosarcoma, primitive neuroectodermal tumour) differentiation* may occasionally occur. Metastatic disease not infrequently *changes differentiation* with treatment leaving residual masses of cystic, mature tissues in the lung or para-aortic lymph nodes. They can be insensitive to adjuvant therapy, press on local structures (the growing teratoma syndrome), and may require surgical resection. Alternatively they can be monitored by serum tumour marker levels and CT scan and further investigated for malignant change if growth recurs. *Prognosis of metastatic disease* relates to the size, site and number of metastases, the extent of tumour mass shrinkage during chemotherapy, completeness of excision, nature of the resected masses and serum HCG and AFP levels. Metastases comprising total necrosis or fully mature tissue correlate with better prognosis. Fibrosis, necrosis and differentiated teratoma are present in 20–70 % of RPLNDs; EC, choriocarcinoma and YST in 5–25 % of cases. A minority of seminomas may develop non-seminomatous germ cell tumour metastases. This may relate either to true transformation of seminoma, or a focus of non-seminomatous germ cell tumour in the primary lesion which was not sampled. In orchidectomy and RPLND specimens sufficient numbers of blocks should be sampled to establish the presence of any malignant components as a basis for further chemotherapy e.g. germ cell, carcinomatous, sarcomatous or primitive neuroectodermal elements.

The number of chemotherapy cycles is minimised by titrating against normalisation of the serum tumour marker levels. This is done to *decrease the risk of developing a second malignancy* in later life e.g. sarcoma or malignant lymphoma, predisposition to which is greatest in those treated before the age of 30 years. *Relapse* following complete remission after chemotherapy for metastatic testicular cancer is only seen in *10 % of patients* and is more likely if there has been advanced disease.

33.9   Other Malignancy

Malignant Lymphoma

- *Diffuse large B cell non-Hodgkin's malignant lymphoma* (70–80 % of cases) in older men (60–80 years of age). Uni-/bilateral (20 %), comprising *2 % of testicular neoplasms*, and 5 % of extranodal malignant lymphomas in men. Primary (60 % of cases) or secondary to systemic/nodal disease, and often associated with disease elsewhere e.g. central nervous system, skin, soft tissues, liver, kidney, lung, bone, orbit and Waldeyer's ring. Classically shows an interstitial/peritubular pattern of infiltration. Prognosis is stage dependent with a *70–80 % overall survival.*

  In children: *Burkitt's lymphoma* ("starry sky" pattern, CD10/Ki-67 positive), *lymphoblastic lymphoma* or diffuse large B cell lymphoma.

Leukaemia

ALL: children, site of relapse in 5–10 % and predictive of systemic relapse.

CLL: the testis is involved in 20–35 % of patients.

Leukaemia can be bilateral and testicular disease the presenting feature in a minority of cases. Granulocytic or myeloid sarcoma is CD34, CD43, CD68, CD117, myeloperoxidase and chloroacetate esterase positive.

Plasmacytoma

- Rare, usually secondary to an established myeloma. Differential diagnosis is spermatocytic seminoma. Plasmacytoma expresses CD79a, CD38 and CD138.

Paratesticular Tumours: Sarcomas (Liposarcoma, Rhabdomyosarcoma, Leiomyosarcoma), Mesothelioma of the Tunica Vaginalis, Desmoplastic Small Round Cell Tumour, Mullerian Tumours

- Treatment of sarcomas is orchidectomy with high ligation of the cord and post operative radiation therapy. Presentation is with a large rapidly growing inguinoscrotal mass.
- *Liposarcoma*: adults and well differentiated adipocytic/sclerotic with variation in adipocyte size and scattered lipoblasts. Local excision and a 23 % local recurrence rate. Occasionally represents an extension from a retroperitoneal neoplasm.
- *Rhabdomyosarcoma*: in children (peak age 7 years) of embryonal round cell (± spindle cells) type with mitoses and necrosis. Desmin and myogenin/myo D1 positive. Excision and adjuvant therapy give *80 % long term survival* with localized and disseminated tumours having 95 and 60 % 5 year survival rates, respectively. There is also a low-grade fascicular spindle cell variant of good prognosis, but alveolar rhabdomyosarcoma (6 %) has an adverse outlook.
- *Leiomyosarcoma*: adults with atypia, necrosis, mitoses.
- *Mesothelioma*: cystic/solid/nodular masses lining a hydrocoele/hernia sac and a variably aggressive clinical course. There may be

associated asbestos exposure. Epithelial (75 %), sarcomatoid or biphasic patterns. Distinguish from *benign cystic adenomatoid tumour* of mesothelial origin forming >30 % of testicular adnexal tumours: circumscribed, glands, cysts, cords of CK5/6, calretinin, WT1 positive cells. Excision is curative. Sites of occurrence are spermatic cord, epididymis, tunica, rete.

- *Desmoplastic small round cell tumour*: lower abdomen, pelvi-inguinal and scrotal area of young men. It comprises nests of small cells in a fibrous stroma, and is polyimmunopheno-typic – cytokeratin, desmin (dot reactivity), synaptophysin, WT1 positive. Most develop peritoneal or retroperitoneal disease within 2 years and die in 3–4 years with metastases to liver and lungs.

- *Papillary serous carcinoma, Mullerian subtype*: rare, ovarian tumour analogue.

- *Malignant lymphoma*: usually represents secondary spread from the adjacent testis, diffuse large B cell in type.

Bibliography

Allen DC. Histopathology reporting: guidelines for surgical reporting. 2nd ed. London: Springer; 2006.

Berney DM. A practical approach to the reporting of germ cell tumours of the testis. Curr Diagn Pathol. 2005; 11:151–61.

Berney DM. Staging and classification of testicular tumours: pitfalls from macroscopy to diagnosis. ACP best practice. J Clin Pathol. 2008;61:20–4.

Berney DM, Lee A, Randle SJ, Jordans S, Shamash J, Oliver RTD. The frequency of intratubular embryonal carcinoma: implications of the pathogenesis of germ cell tumours. Histopathology. 2004;45:155–61.

Bostwick DG, Cheng L. Urologic surgical pathology. 2nd ed. Philadelphia: Mosby/Elsevier; 2008.

Cullen MH, Stenning SP, Parkinson MC, Fossa SD, Kaye SB, Horwich AH. Short-course adjuvant chemotherapy in high-risk stage I nonseminomatous germ cell tumours of the testis. A Medical Research Council report. J Clin Oncol. 1996;14:1106–13.

Delaney RJ, Sayers CD, Walker MA, Mead GM, Theaker JM. The continued value of central histopathological review of testicular tumours. Histopathology. 2005;47:166–9.

Eble JN, Sauter G, Epstein JI, Sesterhenn IA. WHO classification of tumours. Pathology and genetics. Tumours of the urinary system and male genital organs. Lyon: IARC Press; 2004.

Emerson RE, Ulbright TM. Morphological approach to tumours of the testis and paratestis. J Clin Pathol. 2007;60:866–80.

Howard GCW, Nairn M on behalf of the Guideline Development Group. Management of adult testicular germ cell tumours: summary of updated SIGN guideline. BMJ. 2011;342:919–21.

Miller JS, Lee TK, Epstein JI, Ulbright TM. The utility of microscopic findings and immunohistochemistry in the classification of necrotic testicular tumors. A study of 11 cases. Am J Surg Pathol. 2009;33:1293–8.

Nogales FF, Preda O, Nicolae A. Yolk sac tumours revisited. A review of their many faces and names. Histopathology. 2012;60:1023–33.

Rajab R, Berney DM. Ten testicular trapdoors. Histopathology. 2008;53:728–39.

Shanks JH, Iczkowski KA. Non-germ cell tumours of the testis. Curr Diagn Pathol. 2002;8:83–93.

Stenning SP, Parkinson MC, Fisher C, Mead GM, Cook PA, Fossa SD, et al. Post-chemotherapy residual masses in germ cell tumour patients; content, clinical features and prognosis. Medical Research Council Testicular Tumour Working Party. Cancer. 1998;83:1409–19.

The Royal College of Pathologists. Cancer Datasets (Adult Renal Parenchymal Cancer, Renal Tumours in Childhood, Penile Cancer, Prostatic Carcinoma, Testicular Tumours and Post-Chemotherapy Residual Masses, Tumours of the Urinary Collecting System) and Tissue Pathways (Medical Renal Biopsies, Urological Pathology). Accessed at http://www.rcpath.org/index.asp?PageID=254.

Theaker JM, Mead GM. Diagnostic pitfalls in the histological diagnosis of testicular germ cell tumours. Curr Diagn Pathol. 2004;10:220–8.

Ulbright TM. The most common, clinically significant misdiagnoses in testicular tumor pathology, and how to avoid them. Adv Anat Pathol. 2008;15:18–27.

Ulbright TM, Amin MB, Young RH. Tumors of the testis, adnexa, spermatic cord, and scrotum. Atlas of tumor pathology. 3rd series. Fascicle 25. Washington: AFIP; 1999.

Von der Maase H, Rorth M, Walbom-Jorgensen S, Sorensen BL, Christophersen IS, Hald T, Jacobsen GK, Berthelsen JG, Skakkebaek NE. Carcinoma in situ of contralateral testis in patients with germ cell cancer: study of 27 cases in 500 patients. BMJ. 1986;293:1398–401.

Wittekind CF, Greene FL, Hutter RVP, Klimpfinger M, Sobib LH. TNM atlas: illustrated guide to the TNM/pTNM classification of malignant tumours. 5th ed. Berlin: Springer; 2005.

Young RH, Talerman A. Testicular tumours other than germ cell tumours. Semin Diagn Pathol. 1987;4:342–60.

Penile cancer is relatively uncommon in the UK representing less than 1 % of all cancers in men indicating the need for clinical assessment and treatment by supra-regional specialist teams. There is worldwide variation in incidence being highest in South America, Asia and Africa. Predisposing factors are human papilloma virus (HPV) infection, phimosis, psoriasis, smoking, and chronic non-viral infection associated with poor hygiene and lack of circumcision.

Penile cancer can present as a warty/nodular lesion (47 %), erythematous plaque (17 %) or bleeding ulcer (35 %) commonly on the foreskin (21 %), glans penis (48 %) or in the coronal sulcus. Investigation is by diagnostic punch or wedge biopsy, although in well differentiated exophytic lesions definite invasive malignancy may be hard to demonstrate in a limited sample and difficult to distinguish from wart virus infection or pseudoepitheliomatous hyperplasia. The clinical impression is then important in designation and planning of management. Fine needle aspiration cytology (FNAC) of inguinal lymphadenopathy may demonstrate metastases (10–15 % of cases at diagnosis) as a prequel to radical surgery and regional ilioinguinal lymphadenectomy. Alternatively lymph node enlargement may be solely on the basis of inflammation or infection. CT scan can demonstrate the presence of any ilioinguinal lymphadenopathy that is subclinical in extent. CT/PET scan can help to detect distant metastases.

A majority of penile cancers are superficial and well to moderately differentiated with metastases uncommon. They can be treated by penile sparing limited resection (wedge resection, wide local excision with circumcision, glansectomy) with reconstruction of the glans rather than amputation or primary radiotherapy. Accurate assessment of the proximal extent and depth of invasion (e.g. corporal or urethral involvement) by MRI scan is important to avoid incomplete excision or unnecessarily extensive resection. In some specialist centres this may be determined intraoperatively by frozen section. The treatment goal is complete local excision with adequate margins and choice of therapy is related to tumour size, extent of infiltration and destruction of normal tissues. Radiotherapy is reserved for high stage tumours, recurrences, metastatic disease and patients unfit for surgery. It may be followed by salvage surgery. Localised tumours of the prepuce are treated by circumcision. Glansectomy removes the foreskin and glans for carcinoma in situ or localised cancer, but there is a higher risk of incomplete removal and local recurrence. Partial penectomy relies on transection of the penis 2 cm proximal to the gross tumour edge but may be precluded in favour of total penectomy because of tumour size, site and destruction. Ilioinguinal lymphadenectomy is for known metastases, or clinically negative nodes but poorly differentiated high risk carcinomas. In some specialist centres sentinel lymph node biopsy is used as a guide to whether inguinal lymph node block dissection is necessary. In medically unfit patients radiotherapy to the groin is an option, and it may also decrease inguinal recurrences in the adjuvant setting.

D.C. Allen, *Histopathology Reporting*,
DOI 10.1007/978-1-4471-5263-7_34, © Springer-Verlag London 2013

34.1   Gross Description

Specimen

- Wedge biopsy/wide local excision with circumcision/penile sparing resection (glansectomy/partial penectomy)/total penile amputation/radical penectomy (including scrotum, testes, spermatic cords, groin lymph node dissection).
- Size (cm) and weight (g).

Tumour

Site
- Urethral meatus/glans/prepuce/coronal sulcus/penile urethra/shaft (dorsal/ventral/lateral).
- Multicentric: particularly foreskin.

Size
- Length × width × depth (cm) or maximum dimension (cm).
- Tumour thickness (mm) is a gauge of depth of invasion and prognosis.

Appearance
- Exophytic (warty, verrucous, papillary, fungating)
- Superficial spreading (plaque)
- Endophytic (sessile, ulcerated, infiltrative)
- Pale/pigmented.

Edge
- Circumscribed/irregular.

34.2   Histological Type

Squamous Cell Carcinoma

- *95 % of penile malignancies*, 60–80 years of age.
- *Usual type (70 % of cases)*:
- Exophytic or endophytic.
- Large cell/small cell.
- Keratinising/non-keratinising.
  Variants (in order of frequency):
- *Warty* and *papillary*: exophytic and well differentiated, the former with HPV related surface koilocytic atypia, and the latter irregular, complex papillae and stromal cores.

- *Basaloid*: comprises *5–10 % of cases* and is a poorly differentiated *aggressive high-grade tumour* 50 % of which present with lymph node metastases. It is usually ulcerated and endophytic with nests of basaloid cells showing abrupt central keratinisation or comedone-crosis. It is HPV related.
- *Verrucous*: on the glans and foreskin, *5–16 % of cases* and exophytic with a deep pushing margin of cytologically bland bulbous processes. Prone to multifocality and local recurrence if incompletely excised, and may dedifferentiate with radiotherapy. It generally has a good prognosis. It can coexist with usual squamous cell carcinoma.
- *Spindle cell (sarcomatoid)*: arises de novo or post radiotherapy. It comprises cytokeratin (34βE12) positive spindle cells associated with a surface epithelial origin or more recognisable in situ or invasive squamous cell component. It is a high-grade endophytic cancer with *poor prognosis* and a *high rate of local recurrence*.
- *Pseudohyperplastic*: rare, foreskin, associated with lichen sclerosis, good prognosis.
- *Mixed types*: *25 % of cases*. Adequate tumour sampling is necessary to find less differentiated components.

Basal Cell Carcinoma

- A local carcinoma of penile shaft skin.

Transitional Cell Carcinoma

- Either as a primary lesion of the proximal urethra, or secondary to bladder cancer, both of which can show Pagetoid urethral spread

Malignant Melanoma

- <1 % of cases and primary or secondary situated on the glans penis. Fifty percent have lymph node metastases at presentation and *poor prognosis*, being related to tumour thickness and stage with 2 and 5 year survivals of 61 and 20 %, respectively.

Metastatic Carcinoma

- Characteristic multinodular growth pattern in the corpora cavernosa.
- Rare; originating in prostate, bladder, kidney, gut, testis.
- Usually as a late manifestation of systemic disease and *poor prognosis* with a *71% 6 month mortality*. Can present with priapism, or as extramammary Paget's disease from an underlying adnexal tumour or distant spread e.g. bladder.

34.3 Differentiation

Well/moderate/poor/undifferentiated, or, Grade 1/2/3/4.

Many are exophytic and well to moderately differentiated with variable keratinisation. Ulcerated, infiltrating cancers of the glans penis tend to be moderately to poorly differentiated and non-keratinising. About 50 % of shaft cancers are poorly differentiated and only 10 % of prepuce tumours. *Grading* based on the degree of keratinisation, intercellular bridges, mitoses, cellular atypia and inflammatory infiltrate *correlates with prognosis*. Grading is based on the worst component. Sarcomatoid change is regarded as undifferentiated (G4). Over expression of p53 and Ki-67 correlate with tumour grade but not cancer specific and overall survivals.

34.4 Extent of Local Tumour Spread

Border: pushing/infiltrative.

Lymphocytic reaction: prominent/sparse.

Microscopic growth patterns are: verruciform, superficial spreading (horizontal with superficial invasion), vertical with deep penetration, or multicentric. Superficial spreading and vertical growth patterns have 10 and 67 % mortality rates, respectively.

Anatomical levels are: epithelium (1 mm thick), lamina propria (2 mm thick), corpus spongiosum (periurethral and limited inferiorly by tunica albuginea), and corpus cavernosum (surrounded by tunica albuginea with its distal tapered end within the glans). A suggested *threshold value for metastatic potential is 4–6 mm invasion into the corpus spongiosum.*

pTis	Carcinoma in situ
pTa	Noninvasive verrucous carcinoma
pT1	Tumour in subepithelial connective tissue
1a	No lymphovascular invasion, not poorly differentiated or undifferentiated
1b	With lymphovascular invasion, or poorly differentiated or undifferentiated
pT2	Tumour in corpus spongiosum or cavernosum[a]
pT3	Tumour in urethra
pT4	Tumour in other adjacent structures

[a]Optional descriptors are (a) corpus spongiosum and (b) corpus cavernosum

Initial spread is local and intercompartmental into the prepuce, coronal sulcus, glans and penile shaft. The *depth or extent and the pattern of infiltrative spread* correlate with the incidence of *lymph node metastases*. Satellite nodules are not unusual and occasionally there is Pagetoid spread along the urethra to involve its proximal margin. Despite the vascularity of the structures *haematogenous spread* to the liver, heart, lung and bone is *rare* (2 %) (Figs. 34.1, 34.2, 34.3 and 34.4).

34.5 Lymphovascular Invasion

Present/absent.

Intra-/extratumoural.

Vascular invasion is an important adverse factor and predictor of lymph node metastases. Perineural invasion should also be noted.

34.6 Lymph Nodes

Site/number/size/number involved/limit node/extracapsular spread.

Regional nodes: superficial and deep inguinal and pelvic.

pN0	No regional lymph node metastasis
pN1	Metastasis in one inguinal lymph node
pN2	Metastasis in multiple or bilateral inguinal lymph nodes
pN3	Metastasis in pelvic lymph node(s), unilateral or bilateral or extranodal extension of regional lymph node metastasis.

Fig. 34.1 Penile carcinoma (Reproduced, with permission, from Wittekind et al. (2005), © 2005)

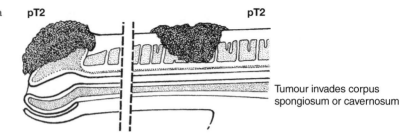

Tumour invades corpus spongiosum or cavernosum

Fig. 34.2 Penile carcinoma (Reproduced, with permission, from Wittekind et al. (2005), © 2005)

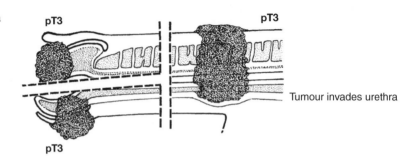

Tumour invades urethra

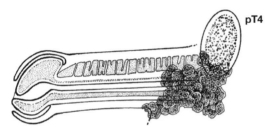

Fig. 34.3 Penile carcinoma: tumour invades other adjacent structures (Reproduced, with permission, from Wittekind et al. (2005), © 2005)

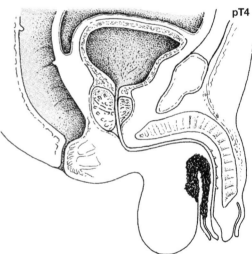

Fig. 34.4 Penile carcinoma: tumour invades other adjacent structures (Reproduced, with permission, from Wittekind et al. (2005), © 2005)

The incidence of lymph node metastases is greater (>80%) in deeply invasive than superficially spreading carcinomas (30%). Pattern of spread is initially to superficial then deep inguinal lymph nodes, pelvic and lastly retroperitoneal lymph nodes. Rarely, skip metastases can occur e.g. direct to deep inguinal lymph nodes. *Survival is influenced by the number of positive lymph nodes, the presence of extracapsular invasion, and the level of lymph node involvement (inguinal versus pelvic).* Lymphadenectomy improves prognosis but is only carried out when there are known metastases, lymphovascular invasion, or in high-grade disease e.g. basaloid, sarcomatoid or undifferentiated carcinoma. Low-grade tumours such as verrucous carcinoma seldom result in lymph node disease although there may be lymphadenopathy due to inflammation or infection.

34.7   Excision Margins

Distance (mm) to the proximal limit of excision in a penectomy specimen.

Distances (mm) to the deep corporal and lateral glans or cutaneous margins in a local resection specimen.

Local recurrence is rare if margins are tumour free. Traditionally a margin clearance of 15–25 mm was required but this has been reduced with the use of organ sparing surgery in an effort to achieve better cosmetic and functional outcomes. Margin clearance may require checking by intraoperative frozen section examination.

34.8   Other Pathology

Predisposing factors and lesions: *predisposing factors* for penile carcinoma are old age (rare <40 years of age), lack of circumcision, poor hygiene and phimosis. Cases can be non-HPV or HPV related. *Predisposing lesions* are *squamous hyperplasia* (leukoplakia), *balanoposthitis xerotica obliterans* (lichen sclerosis equivalent), and *penile intraepithelial neoplasia (PeIN)/squamous intraepithelial lesion (SIL)*. PeIN is of two types, either *differentiated* (simplex: non-HPV related) or *classical* (basaloid/warty: HPV related). These precursor lesions can be multifocal. Treatments are local excision, Moh's surgery with reconstruction, laser therapy, electrodessication and curettage, cryosurgery and topical 5-fluorouracil.

Squamous hyperplasia (leukoplakia)
- Hyperkeratosis, epithelial hyperplasia ± dysplasia. The squamous epithelial basal layers can be p53 positive overlapping with differentiated PeIN.

Balanoposthitis xerotica obliterans
- Similar to lichen sclerosis in the vulva it may be associated with penile carcinoma.
- Present in up to 30–50 % of penile cancers, particularly warty and verrucous carcinomas.

PeIN/SIL (erythroplasia de Queyrat/Bowen's disease/Bowenoid papulosis)
- There is variable use of these traditional clinical terms with progression to carcinoma estimated as 10–30 %/5–10 %/0 % respectively. All show features of carcinoma in situ or high-grade PeIN. Erythroplasia is a velvety plaque lesion of the glans penis, whereas Bowen's disease and Bowenoid papulosis are abnormalities of the penile/perineal skin. The latter is caused by HPV infection in young men and is often self limiting. A minority of Bowen's disease are associated with a visceral malignancy e.g. lung, gastrointestinal or urinary tract.

Condyloma accuminatum
- Coronal sulcus, inner foreskin.
- *HPV 16, 18* (60 %/13 % of cases respectively) are particularly associated with warty and basaloid PeIN and their respective cancer types, but not typical keratinizing squamous cell carcinoma.
- HPV 6, 11 are not associated with PeIN and penile cancer.

Extramammary Paget's disease
- *Secondary* to concurrent urothelial neoplasia ± Pagetoid spread of transitional cell carcinoma into the penile urethra (CK7/CK20 positive), or, *primary* and limited to the glans penis (CK7 positive, CK20 negative).

Clinical mimics of penile cancer
- Beware Zoon's plasma cell balanitis, nicorandil (an anti-angina drug) induced penile ulceration, sexually transmitted diseases (e.g. syphilis), Wegener's granulomatosis.

Prognosis

More than 95 % of penile carcinomas are squamous cell carcinoma. At presentation about 40 % are exophytic and superficially invasive with extensive in situ change, 30 % endophytic and deeply invasive, 10–20 % verrucous and 5–10 % multifocal. *Inguinal lymph node metastases are present in 15–45 % of cases*. Prognosis relates to the tumour site, size, infiltrative growth pattern, depth of invasion, stage, histological grade, and vascular invasion with on average *70–80 % 5 year survival rates*. Adverse factors are lymphovascular invasion, vertical growth pattern, and, basaloid, sarcomatoid, solid, undifferentiated and pseudoglandular subtypes.

34.9   Other Malignancy

Sarcoma

- More often affecting the penile shaft than the distal or glans penis and forming *<5 % of penile malignancy*, especially:

Kaposi's sarcoma: about 20 % of HIV/AIDS male patients on the skin of the shaft or glans and usually associated with other systemic lesions. It is HHV8 positive.

Leiomyosarcoma: 50–70 years of age. Superficial and subcutaneous has a good prognosis, whereas corporal and deep in location with early metastases has a poor prognosis.

Epithelioid haemangioendothelioma: varying grade and outlook (CD 31/CD34 positive epithelioid cells with intracytoplasmic vacuoles).

Others: angiosarcoma, rhabdomyosarcoma, fibrosarcoma, epithelioid sarcoma.

Malignant Lymphoma

- Primary lesions are very rare and malignant lymphoma is usually secondary to systemic disease.

Bibliography

Arya M, Kalsi J, Kelly J, Muneer A. Malignant and premaligant lesions of the penis. BMJ 2013;346:30–34.

Bostwick DG, Cheng L. Urologic surgical pathology. 2nd ed. Philadelphia: Mosby/Elsevier; 2008.

Chaux A, Soares F, Guimaraes GC, Cunha IW, Reuter V, Barreto J, Rodriguez I, Cubilla AL. The Prognostic index: a useful pathologic guide for prediction of nodal metastases and survival in penile squamous cell carcinoma. Am J Surg Pathol. 2009;33:1049–57.

Cubilla AL. The role of pathologic prognostic factors in squamous cell carcinoma of the penis. World J Urol. 2009;27:169–77.

Cubilla AL, Piris A, Pfannl R, Rodriguez I, Aguero F, Young RH. Anatomic levels: important landmarks in penectomy specimens. A detailed anatomic and histologic study based in examination of 44 cases. Am J Surg Pathol. 2001;25:1091–4.

Eble JN, Sauter G, Epstein JI, Sesterhenn IA. WHO classification of tumours. Pathology and genetics. Tumours of the urinary system and male genital organs. Lyon: IARC Press; 2004.

Gunia S, Kakies C, Erbersdobler A, Hakenberg OW, Koch S, May M. Expression of p53, p21 and cyclin D1 in penile cancer: p53 predicts poor prognosis. J Clin Pathol. 2012;65:232–6.

Oertell J, Caballero C, Iglesias M, Chaux A, Amat L, Ayala E, Rodriguez I, Velazwuez EF, Barreto JE, Ayala G, Cubilla AL. Differentiated precursor lesions and low-grade variants of squamous cell carcinoma are frequent findings in foreskins of patients from a region of high penile cancer incidence. Histopathology. 2011;58:925–33.

Oxley JD, Corbishley C, Down L, Watkin N, Dickerson D, Wong NA. Clinicopathological and molecular study of penile melanoma. J Clin Pathol. 2012;65: 228–31.

Stankiewicz E, Ng M, Cuzick J, Mesher D, Watkin M, Lam W, Corbishley C, Berney DM. The prognostic value of Ki-67 expression in penile squamous cell carcinoma. J Clin Pathol. 2012;65:534–7.

The Royal College of Pathologists. Cancer Datasets (Adult Renal Parenchymal Cancer, Renal Tumours in Childhood, Penile Cancer, Prostatic Carcinoma, Testicular Tumours and Post-Chemotherapy Residual Masses, Tumours of the Urinary Collecting System) and Tissue Pathways (Medical Renal Biopsies, Urological Pathology). Accessed at http://www.rcpath.org/index.asp?PageID=254.

Wittekind CF, Greene FL, Hutter RVP, Klimpfinger M, Sobib LH. TNM atlas: illustrated guide to the TNM/pTNM classification of malignant tumours. 5th ed. Berlin: Springer; 2005.

- Nodal Malignant Lymphoma (with Comments on Extranodal Malignant Lymphoma and Metastatic Cancer)

Nodal Malignant Lymphoma (with Comments on Extranodal Malignant Lymphoma and Metastatic Cancer)

35

Representing 5–7 % of all cancers and 55 % of haematological malignancies with an increasing incidence, malignant lymphoma presents as persistent, mobile, rubbery and non-tender lymphadenopathy with or without associated systemic symptoms such as weight loss, itch or night sweats. Investigation is by full blood picture (infections/leukaemias), serology (infections/autoimmune diseases), fine needle aspiration cytology (FNAC: to exclude metastatic cancer) and biopsy. Clinical staging is by CT/PET/MRI scans appropriate to the clinical context, bone marrow aspirate and trephine biopsy.

In the UK contemporary guidance from the Royal College of Pathologists and the NHS National Cancer Action Team indicates concordance of diagnosis for malignant lymphomas of less than 85 %. It is advised that diagnosis should be the remit of a specialist integrated haematological malignancy diagnostic service covering a catchment population of at least two million. There should be a single integrated report encompassing the requisite specialist morphological expertise, immunohistochemistry, flow cytometry, cytogenetics, in situ hybridization and molecular diagnostics. Local arrangements will require at least prompt referral through the cancer network to the appropriate haematological malignancy diagnostic team. Underpinning this will be the ongoing need for general diagnostic pathologists to competently recognize the wide range of haematolymphoid pathology so that relevant and expeditious clinicopathological referrals are made.

35.1 Gross Description and Morphological Recognition

Specimen

- FNAC/needle biopsy core/excisional biopsy/regional lymphadenectomy.
- Regional lymphadenectomy comprises part of a formal cancer resection operation. This can either be for removal of a primary malignant lymphoma e.g. gastrectomy, or, where malignant lymphoma is found incidentally in a resection for a primary carcinoma e.g. in the mesorectal nodes of an anterior resection for rectal cancer.
- Size (cm) and weight (g)
- Colour, consistency, necrosis.

The *preferred specimen* for *diagnosis, subtyping and grading of nodal malignant lymphoma* is an *excisional lymph node biopsy* carefully taken by an experienced surgeon to ensure representation of disease and avoidance of traumatic artifact. Submission of the specimen fresh to the laboratory allows material to be collected for flow cytometry, or imprints to be made, to which a wide panel of immunohistochemical antibodies can be applied some of which are more effective than on formalin fixed paraffin processed tissue sections e.g. the demonstration of light chain restriction. Tissue can also be harvested for molecular and genetic techniques. *Morphological classification* is generally based on well fixed, thin slices, processed through to paraffin with high quality 4 μm H&E sections. *Core biopsy* may be the only option if the patient is unwell or the lesion is relatively inaccessible e.g. mediastinal or para-aortic lymphadenopathy. Allowances must be made in interpretation for underestimation of nuclear size, sampling error and artifact. Confirmation of lymphomatous (or other) malignancy is the prime objective and further comments on subtyping and grading given with care and only if definitely demonstrable. Despite these considerations a positive diagnosis can be given in a significant percentage of cases. Importantly, interpretation should be in light of the clinical context i.e. the presence of palpable or radiologically proven significant regional or systemic lymphadenopathy, and the absence of any obvious carcinoma primary site. Tumour heterogeneity must also be borne in mind. The same principles apply to *FNAC*, which is excellent at excluding inflammatory lymphadenopathy e.g. abscess or sarcoidosis, and non-lymphomatous cancer (e.g. metastatic squamous cell carcinoma, breast carcinoma or malignant melanoma). It is also reasonably robust at designating Hodgkin's and high-grade non-Hodgkin's malignant lymphoma. *Morphology is the principal diagnostic criterion* when assessing excisional lymph node biopsies, core biopsies and FNAC but is supplemented by *immunohistochemical antibody panels* targeted at the various diagnostic options e.g. a small lymphoid cell proliferation (lymphocytic lymphoma versus mantle cell lymphoma etc). In addition, *flow cytometry* and *molecular gene rearrangements* can be important in determining a *diagnosis* and its attendant *treatment* and *prognosis*. Limited needle sampling techniques can also be used in patients with a previous biopsy proven tissue diagnosis of malignant lymphoma and in whom recurrence is suspected. However, possible *transformation* of grade must be considered and even change of malignant lymphoma type e.g. small lymphocytic lymphoma to Hodgkin's malignant lymphoma, or Richter's transformation to diffuse large B cell malignant lymphoma. A range of inflammatory and neoplastic lymph node pathology may also be encountered secondary to chemotherapy and *immunosuppression* e.g. tuberculosis, EBV (Epstein Barr Virus) driven lymphoproliferation, and various malignant lymphomas.

A systematic approach to excisional lymph node biopsies will allow the majority to be categorised as specific inflammatory pathology, benign or malignant, and the latter as haematolymphoid or non-haematolymphoid in character. *Diagnostic morphological clues* to malignant lymphoma are *architectural* and *cytological*.

Architectural descriptors are: diffuse, follicular, nodular, marginal zone, sinusoidal, paracortical, and angiocentric distributions.

Cytological descriptors are: cell size (small, medium (the size of a histiocyte nucleus), large), the relative proportions of the cell populations, specific cytomorphological features, and cellular proliferative activity (mitoses, apoptosis, Ki-67 index). Various malignant lymphomas are also characterized by a typical host connective tissue and/or cellular inflammatory response.

Low Power Magnification
- Capsular/extracapsular spillage of lymphoid tissue
- Capsular thickening and banded septal fibrosis or hyaline sclerosis
- Loss of sinusoids with either compression or filling due to a cellular infiltrate
- Alteration in follicular architecture with changes in
  (a) Distribution: proliferation in the medulla
  (b) Size and shape: relative uniformity of appearance
  (c) Definition: loss of the mantle zone- germinal centre interface/"filling up" of the germinal centre/loss of tingible body macrophages
  (d) Absence: the architecture may be completely effaced by a diffuse infiltrate
- Prominent post capillary venules.

High Power Magnification
- Presence of a background polymorphous inflammatory cellular infiltrate e.g. eosinophils, plasma cells and histiocytes (epithelioid in character ± granulomas)
- Alterations in the proportions of the normal cellular constituents
- Dominance of any mono- or dual cell populations
- Presence of atypical lymphoid cells
  (a) Nuclei: enlargement/irregularity/hyperchromasia/bi- or polylobation/mummification/apoptosis
  (b) Nucleoli: single/multiple/central/peripheral/eosinophilic/basophilic/Dutcher inclusions

(c) Cytoplasm: clear/vacuolar/eosinophilic/scant/plentiful/paranuclear hof.

A *morphological diagnostic short list* should be created e.g. mixed cellularity Hodgkin's lymphoma versus T cell malignant lymphoma versus T cell rich large B cell malignant lymphoma, and a *targeted immunohistochemical antibody panel* used. The determination of *cell lineage* is a prerequisite for diagnosis. In the majority of cases immunohistochemistry will confirm the preliminary diagnosis, but will in a minority lead to its modification and either a refinement within or revision of diagnostic category. A pitfall for the unwary is *aberrant expression* of T cell antigens by a B cell malignant lymphoma and vice versa e.g. expression of CD5 in chronic lymphocytic lymphoma/leukaemia. *Clonality* and *gene rearrangement studies*, either by immunohistochemistry, flow cytometry or molecular techniques can be important in confirming the neoplastic character of the B and T cell populations. Another relevant ancillary technique in various clinical settings is in situ hybridization for *EBERs* (Epstein Barr Encoded RNAs). *Patient age*, *disease site and distribution* also contribute to making a correct diagnosis e.g. nodular lymphocyte predominant Hodgkin's malignant lymphoma usually presents in younger patients and as solitary or localized lymphadenopathy rather than extensive disease.

35.2 Histological Type and Differentiation/Grade

Therapeutic and prognostic distinction is made between *Hodgkin's* and *non-Hodgkin's malignant lymphomas* (*HL/NHLs*), with a significant proportion of the former being reclassified as variants of the latter on the basis of improved immunophenotyping. Within classical Hodgkin's malignant lymphoma there is a differentiation spectrum from nodular sclerosis and lymphocyte rich through mixed cellularity to lymphocyte depleted, with nodular sclerosis divided into two subtypes that are of prognostic significance in limited stage disease. In non-Hodgkin's malignant lymphoma better differentiated tumours are of a follicular pattern and small cell type, and less differentiated lesions diffuse and large cell in character. This differentiation spectrum can predict the likelihood of untreated disease progression from indolence to aggressive behaviour, but paradoxically often does not correlate with extent of disease stage, chemoresponsiveness, long term disease free survival and potential for cure. For example, grade 1/2 follicular lymphoma is often of extensive distribution (stage IV), indolent in behaviour, yet incurable and ultimately fatal at 5–10 years after diagnosis. Thus, morphology with corroborative immunophenotyping (e.g. a Ki-67 proliferation index >90 %) can identify those high-grade diagnoses requiring curative intent high dose multi-agent chemotherapy e.g. Burkitt's malignant lymphoma, mediastinal large B cell malignant lymphoma, lymphoblastic lymphoma. As can be seen size matters in grading, but not always as cell maturation (Burkitt's, lymphoblastic lymphoma) and aggressive behaviour linked to specific underlying chromosomal alterations (e.g. mantle cell lymphoma) must be taken into account. Thus the prognostic information used to determine treatment of malignant lymphoma is provided by the *histological subtyping* and *grading*, supported by *immunohistochemistry* the diagnostic importance of which varies with the malignant lymphoma subtype e.g. a significant contributor to diagnoses such as T cell malignant lymphoma and anaplastic large cell malignant lymphoma. Compatible *molecular analysis* is also of importance in defining these characteristic malignant lymphoma types, treatment response and behaviour.

Non-Hodgkin's Malignant Lymphoma

Non-Hodgkin's malignant lymphoma (NHL) is classified according to the WHO system (Table 35.1) which defines each disease by its *morphology*, *immunophenotype*, *genetic characteristics, proposed normal counterpart* and *clinical features*. It is *reproducible*, with *prognostic* and *therapeutic implications*. Broad categories are malignant lymphomas of B, T or NK (natural killer) cell types. Malignant lymphomas and leukaemias are

Table 35.1 WHO classification of lymphoid neoplasms

B cell neoplasms

Precursor B cell neoplasms

  Precursor B lymphoblastic lymphoma/leukaemia

Mature B cell neoplasms

  Chronic lymphocytic leukaemia/small lymphocytic lymphoma

  B cell prolymphocytic leukaemia

  Lymphoplasmacytic lymphoma/Waldenströms macroglobulinaemia

  Heavy chain disease (α, γ, μ)

  Splenic marginal zone lymphoma

  Hairy cell leukaemia

  Plasma cell myeloma

  Solitary plasmacytoma of bone

  Extra osseous plasmacytoma

  Extranodal marginal zone B cell lymphoma of mucosa associated lymphoid tissue (MALT lymphoma)

  Nodal marginal zone B cell lymphoma

  Follicular lymphoma

    Grading:

      Grade 1: 0 to 5 centroblasts per high power field#

      Grade 2: 6 to 15 centroblasts per high power field#

      Grade 3: greater than 15 centroblasts per high power field#

      Grade 3a: centrocytes are still present

      Grade 3b: centroblasts form solid sheets with no residual centrocytes

      #average over 10 high power fields

    Reporting of pattern:

      Follicular: greater than 75 % follicular

      Follicular and diffuse: 25–75 % follicular

      Focally follicular: less than 25 % follicular

      Diffuse

    Variant:

    Cutaneous follicle centre lymphoma

  Mantle cell lymphoma

    Variants: Blastoid (classic or pleomorphic), others

  Diffuse large B cell lymphoma (DLBCL)

    Variants: T cell/histiocyte rich, DLBCL of CNS, cutaneous leg type

  Mediastinal (thymic) B cell lymphoma

  Intravascular large B cell lymphoma

  ALK positive large B cell lymphoma

Plasmablastic lymphoma

  Primary effusion lymphoma

  Burkitt's lymphoma

    Variants: intermediate between BL and DLBCL, or, BL and HL

Table 35.1 (continued)

B cell proliferations of variable malignant potential

Lymphomatoid granulomatosis

Post-transplant lymphoproliferative disorders (PTLD): early (plasmacytic hyperplasia, infectious mononucleosis like), polymorphic, or monomorphic (B, T, NK types), and classic HL

T cell neoplasms

Precursor T cell lymphomas

  Precursor T lymphoblastic lymphoma/leukaemia

  Blastic NK cell lymphoma

Mature T cell and NK cell neoplasms

  T cell prolymphocytic leukaemia

  Variants: small cell, cerebriform cell (Sézary cell-like)

  Large granular cell lymphocyte leukaemia

  Aggressive NK cell leukaemia/lymphoma

  Adult T cell lymphoma/leukaemia

  Extranodal NK/T cell lymphoma, nasal type

  Enteropathy type T cell lymphoma

  Hepatosplenic T cell lymphoma

  Subcutaneous panniculitis like T cell lymphoma

  Mycosis fungoides (MF) and Sézary syndrome

    Variants:

      Pagetoid reticulosis

      MF associated follicular mucinous

      Granulomatous slack skin disease

  Primary cutaneous anaplastic large cell lymphoma (C-ALCL)

  Primary cutaneous γδ T cell lymphoma

  Peripheral T cell lymphoma, unspecified

  Angioimmunoblastic T cell lymphoma

  Anaplastic large cell lymphoma, ALK positive, ALK negative

T cell proliferation of uncertain malignant potential

Lymphomatoid papulosis

CD30 positive T cell lymphoproliferations

Histiocytic and dendritic cell neoplasms

Histiocytic sarcoma

Langerhans cell histiocytosis

Interdigitating dendritic cell sarcoma

Follicular dendritic cell sarcoma

Fibroblastic reticulum cell sarcoma

Intermediate dendritic cell tumour

both included as many haematolymphoid neoplasms have both solid and fluid circulatory phases. *Prognosis* relates to *stage of disease*, *treatment protocols* and *individual disease biology*.

Hodgkin's Malignant Lymphoma

WHO Classification

Comprising *nodular lymphocyte predominant Hodgkin's malignant lymphoma* (NLPHL – a B cell malignant lymphoma), and *classic Hodgkin's malignant lymphomas* encompassing nodular sclerosis, lymphocytic rich, mixed cellularity and lymphocyte depleted variants. Hodgkin's malignant lymphoma is *a tumour of abnormal B lymphocyte cell lineage*.

Lymphocyte and Histiocyte (L and H) Predominant: Multilobated "Popcorn" Cell

- Nodular: a B cell lymphoma of early stage (cervical, axilla, groin) in young men and low-grade indolent behaviour (80 % 10 year survival) with a 4 % risk of diffuse large B cell change. Some arise from progressive transformation of germinal centres.
- Diffuse: a controversial category with overlap between lymphocyte rich classic Hodgkin's malignant lymphoma, vaguely nodular lymphocyte predominant Hodgkin's, and exclusion of other entities such as T cell/histiocyte rich large B cell NHL.

Classic Hodgkin's lymphoma includes nodular sclerosis, lymphocyte rich classical, mixed cellularity and lymphocyte depleted categories. They vary in their clinical features, growth pattern, degree of fibrosis, background cells, tumour cell numbers and atypia, and, frequency of EBV infection.

Nodular Sclerosis: Lacunar Cell

- Female adolescents, young adults. Mediastinal or cervical involvement and either localised disease or high stage at presentation. Moderately aggressive but curable.
- Birefringent fibrous bands (capsular and intranodal septa) with mixed inflammatory cell nodules containing lacunar cells, or, cellular phase (rich in lacunar cells, scant fibrosis)
- Type 1.[1]

---

[1] Grade 1/grade 2 British National Lymphoma Investigation (BNLI).

- Type 2:[2] lymphocyte depletion or pleomorphism of R-S (Reed Sternberg) cells in more than 25 % of nodules. An alternative descriptor is syncytial variant (sheets/clusters of R-S cells with central necrosis and a polymorph infiltrate).

Mixed Cellularity: Reed Sternberg Cell

- Male adults, high stage disease at presentation: lymph nodes, spleen, liver±bone marrow. Moderately aggressive but curable.
- R-S cells of classic type in a mixed inflammatory background. A category of exclusion in that no specific features of other subtypes are present.

Lymphocyte Rich Classic

- Scattered R-S cells against a nodular or diffuse background of small lymphocytes but no polymorphs.

Lymphocyte Depleted

- Older patients, high stage disease at presentation, aggressive, association with HIV.
- R-S cells±pleomorphism; diffuse fibrosis (fibroblasts obscure scattered R-S cells) and reticular variants (cellular, pleomorphic R-S cells).

Other Features

- Follicular and interfollicular Hodgkin's, Hodgkin's with a high epithelioid cell content (granulomas).
- R-S cells: classic mirror image, binucleated cell with prominent eosinophilic nucleolus ("owl's eye" appearance) characteristic of the mixed cellularity and lymphocyte depleted categories. Mononuclear, polylobated and necrobiotic (mummified) forms are also common. Lacunar cells (nodular sclerosis) can be mono-, bi- or polylobated (± necrobiotic), with characteristic perinuclear artifactual cytoplasmic retraction and clarity. Mononuclear cells tend to be termed Hodgkin's cells. Hodgkin/R-S cells are derived from germinal centre B cells with monoclonal, non-functional immunoglobulin gene rearrangements.

---

[2] See footnote 1.

Immunophenotype

Lymphocyte Predominant Hodgkin's Lymphoma

- Popcorn cells: CD45/CD20/CD79a/EMA/J chain/bcl-6 positive, CD30 weak or negative, CD15 negative, EBV negative. Nuclear transcription factors Oct2/BoB1 positive.
- Small lymphocytes: nodules of B cells (CD20) and intervening T cells (CD3).
- Rosettes: CD57/CD4 positive T cell rosettes around the popcorn cells.

Classic Hodgkin's Lymphoma

- R-S cells: CD15/CD30 in 75 %/90 % of cases respectively, EBV (60–70 % of cases), CD20/ 79a±, CD45/ALK negative. MUM1/PAX5 positive. CD15 positivity can be weak and focal limited to the Golgi apparatus in 15 % of cases.
- Small lymphocytes: T cells (CD3/CD4).

In Hodgkin's lymphoma the *heterogeneous cellular background (comprising 90 % of the tissue) is an important part of the diagnosis*: small lymphocytes, eosinophils, neutrophils, fibroblasts, histiocytes and follicular dendritic cells. Note that this cytokinetic diathesis is also seen in T cell NHLs and T cell rich B cell NHLs. Another differential diagnosis with which there can be overlap is anaplastic large cell lymphoma. Other features are progressive transformation of germinal centres (particularly associated with NLPHL), granulomas, necrosis, interfollicular plasma cells and reactive follicular hyperplasia, all of which should prompt a careful search for R-S cells.

Differential Diagnoses in Haematolymphoid Pathology

Relatively common diagnostic difficulties in lymph node assessment are:

- Follicular hyperplasia vs. follicular lymphoma
- Follicular hyperplasia vs. partial nodal involvement by in situ follicular lymphoma
- Progressive transformation of germinal centres vs. NLPHL
- T cell hyperplasia vs. dermatopathic lymphadenopathy vs. T cell lymphoma
- Underestimation of grade in small lymphocytic infiltrates e.g. mantle cell or lymphoblastic lymphomas

- Burkitt's lymphoma vs. Burkitt's like diffuse large B cell lymphoma
- Hodgkin's lymphoma vs. anaplastic large cell lymphoma, and subtle infiltration of sinusoids by the latter
- Interfollicular Hodgkin's lymphoma
- Anaplastic large cell lymphoma vs. metastatic carcinoma, malignant melanoma or germ cell tumour
- Post immunosuppression lymphoproliferative disorders.

Important *non-malignant differential diagnoses* for malignant lymphoma are Castleman's disease (hyaline vascular and plasma cell variants), drug induced (e.g. phenytoin) and viral reactive hyperplasia with paracortical transformation (e.g. herpesvirus, infectious mononucleosis), and necrotising and granulomatous lymphadenitis (Kikuchi's, toxoplasmosis, tuberculosis, sarcoidosis). A clinical history of immunosuppression and subsequent EBV driven lymphoproliferation must always be borne in mind.

35.3 Extent of Local Tumour Spread

Part of node or whole node.

Extracapsular into adjacent soft tissues or organ parenchyma.

A TNM classification is not used as the primary site of origin is often uncertain and attribution of N and M stages would therefore be arbitrary.

Stage: Ann Arbor Classification

I	Single lymph node region or localised extralymphatic site/organ
II	Two or more lymph node regions on same side of the diaphragm or single localised extralymphatic site/organ and its regional lymph nodes ± other lymph node regions on the same side of the diaphragm
III	Lymph node regions on both sides of the diaphragm ± a localised extralymphatic site/organ or spleen

IV	Disseminated (multifocal) involvement of one or more extralymphatic organs ± regional lymph node involvement, or single extralymphatic organ and non-regional nodes. Includes any involvement of liver, bone marrow, lungs or cerebrospinal fluid
	(a) Without weight loss/fever/sweats
	(b) With weight loss/fever/sweats:
	Fever >38 °C
	Night sweats
	Weight loss >10 % of body weight within the previous 6 months.
Subscripts e.g.	III$_E$ denotes stage III with Extranodal disease
	III$_S$ denotes stage III with splenic involvement
	III$_3$ denotes stage III with involvement of 3 lymph node regions: >2 is prognostically adverse.
Lymph node regions	Head, neck, face
	Intrathoracic
	Intraabdominal
	Axilla/arm
	Groin/leg
	Pelvis.

Other major structures of the lymphatic system are the spleen, thymus, Waldeyer's ring (palatine, lingual and pharyngeal tonsils), vermiform appendix and ileal Peyer's patches. Minor sites include bone marrow, liver, skin, lung, pleura and gonads.

Bilateral involvement of axilla/arm or inguinal/leg regions is considered as involvement of two separate regions.

Direct spread of lymphoma into adjacent tissues or organs does not alter the classification e.g. gastric lymphoma into pancreas and with involved perigastric lymph nodes is stage II$_E$.

Involvement of two or more discontinuous segments of gastrointestinal tract is multifocal and classified as stage IV e.g. stomach and ileum. However multifocal involvement of a single extralymphatic organ is I$_E$.

Involvement of both organs of a paired site e.g. lungs is also I$_E$. Regional nodes for an extranodal lymphoma are those relevant to that particular site e.g. gastric lymphoma – perigastric, left gastric, common hepatic, splenic and coeliac nodes (Figs. 35.1, 35.2, 35.3, 35.4 and 35.5)

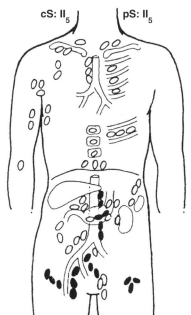

cS: II$_5$ pS: II$_5$

Two or more lymph node regions on the same side of the diaphragm

Fig. 35.1 Malignant lymphoma (Reproduced, with permission, from Wittekind et al. (2005), © 2005)

Fig. 35.2 Malignant
lymphoma (Reproduced,
with permission, from
Wittekind et al. (2005),
© 2005)

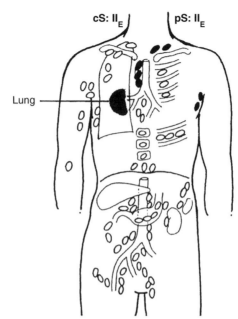

A single extralymphatic organ or
site and its regional node(s)
± other lymph node regions on
the same side of the diaphragm

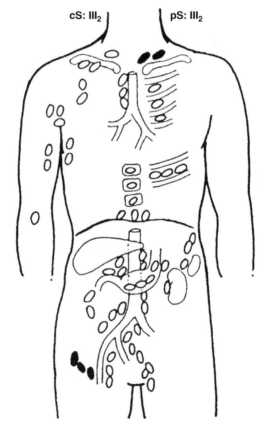

Involvement of lymph node
regions on both sides of the
diaphragm (III) (Fig. 35.3),
which may also be
accompanied by localized
involvement of an
asscociated extralymphatic
organ or site (III$_E$) (Fig. 35.4),
or by involvement of the
spleen (III$_S$), or both (III$_{E+S}$)
(Fig. 35.5)

Fig. 35.3 Malignant
lymphoma (Reproduced,
with permission, from
Wittekind et al. (2005),
© 2005)

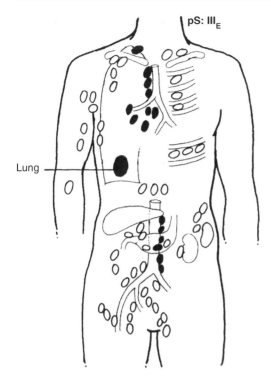

Fig. 35.4 Malignant lymphoma (Reproduced, with permission, from Wittekind et al. (2005), © 2005)

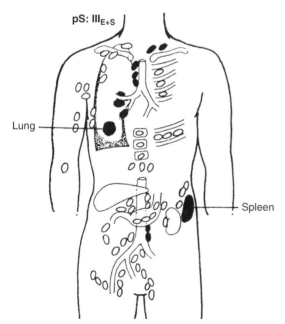

Fig. 35.5 Malignant lymphoma (Reproduced, with permission, from Wittekind et al. (2005), © 2005)

Once the primary tissue diagnosis has been made staging laparotomy has been replaced by assessment of *clinical* and *radiological parameters* e.g. peripheral blood differential cell counts, abnormal liver function tests, and imaging for hepatosplenomegaly and lymphadenopathy. Bone marrow biopsy remains part of normal staging which is otherwise mostly clinical. Bone marrow or nodal granulomas per se are not sufficient for a positive diagnosis of involvement and diagnostic Hodgkin's cells are needed. Bone marrow involvement by NHL can be diffuse, nodular or focal, and paratrabecular infiltration is a characteristic site of distribution.

35.4 Lymphovascular Invasion

Present/absent.

Intra-/extratumoural.

Vessel wall invasion and destructive angiocentricity can be a useful indicator of malignancy in NHL and in specific subtypes e.g. nasal angiocentric T/NK cell lymphoma.

35.5 Immunophenotype

In general an *antibody panel* is used with both expected positive and negative antibodies, and, *two antibodies per lineage. Select combinations* are targeted at determining the nature of the various lymphoid proliferations e.g. *follicular* (follicular lymphoma vs reactive hyperplasia), *small cell* (CLL/SLL vs. mantle cell lymphoma), and *large cell* (HL vs. NHL vs. ALCL). Interpretation must take into account artifacts such as *poor fixation* or lymph node *necrosis* following FNAC. In the latter expression of nuclear antigens is affected first and T cell stains can give false positive results in inflammatory debris. Some antigens such as CD20 retain remarkably robust expression. *Expression must also be appropriate* to the antibody concerned e.g. localization to the nucleus, cytoplasm or cell membrane. Suitable in built positive, and, external positive and negative *controls* are used. Interpretation must also account for expression in physiological cell populations in the test tissue. Commonly used antibodies available for formalin fixed, paraffin embedded sections are

CD45	Pan lymphoid marker (Leucocyte Common Antigen) and excellent in the characterisation of a poorly differentiated malignant tumour e.g. malignant lymphoma vs. carcinoma vs. malignant melanoma.
CD20	Mature B cell marker (and some cases of plasma cell myeloma). Lymphoma cell positivity is a marker for specific rituximab monoclonal antibody therapy.
CD79a	As for CD20 but also less mature (pre B: lymphoblastic) cells and plasma cell tumours.
CD3	Pan T cell marker.
CD5	T cell marker and aberrant expression in some variants of B cell lymphoma (lymphocytic, mantle cell and splenic marginal zone lymphomas).
CD4, CD8	T cell subsets of use in some T cell proliferations e.g. mycosis fungoides. CD7, AML and granzyme C may also be useful in extranodal cases. Other T cell markers include CD45R0 (UCHL1), CD43 (MT1) and TIA-1.
CD10	Lymphoblastic lymphoma (CALLA), Burkitt's lymphoma and follicle centre lymphoma. Also with CD5 and CD23 in the differential diagnosis of small B cell lymphomas (lymphocytic CD5/CD23+: mantle cell CD5+: follicle centre cell CD10+). Forty percent of DLBCL are CD10 positive.
CD15, CD30	Classic Hodgkin's lymphoma R-S cells. CD30 is also positive in ALCL, a proportion of DLBCLs, embryonal carcinoma and malignant melanoma. CD15 is positive in some large T cell lymphomas.
CD56, CD57	Natural killer (NK) cells e.g. angiocentric sinonasal lymphoma. Also T cells and plasma cell myeloma/AML (CD56).
CD68	Macrophages, cells of granulocytic lineage.
CD 38/138	Plasma cells and multiple myeloma (usually CD45/20 negative; CD79a±). Other low grade B cell lymphomas (CD38+ CLL has a worse prognosis).
CD123	Hairy cell leukaemia, AML.
κ, λ light chains	Immunoglobulin light chain restriction is difficult to demonstrate satisfactorily in paraffin sections but more easily shown on fresh imprint preparations or by in situ hybridisation.
CD21, CD23	Follicular dendritic cells. CD23 also stains most B cell lymphocytic lymphomas, some follicular and DLBCLs.
bcl-1/cyclin D1	Mantle cell lymphoma with the t(11:14) translocation. A nuclear epitope. Also some hairy cell leukaemia and plasma cell myeloma cases. $p27^{kip1}$ is positive in cyclin D1 negative mantle cell lymphoma.
bcl-2	An apoptosis regulator: many B cell lymphomas including follicular t(14:18) and others. Also normal B, T cells and negative in reactive germinal centres. Strong expression is adverse in DLBCLs.
bcl-6	Follicle centre lymphoma, Burkitt's lymphoma and a large proportion of DLBCLs. A transcription factor in the nuclei of germinal centre cells.
Ki-67/MIB-1	Nuclear proliferation marker useful for identifying high-grade lymphomas e.g. Burkitt's (98–100 %), lymphoblastic lymphoma (also tdt positive), and DLBCL with a high proliferation fraction. Its distribution in the follicle centre is helpful in distinguishing reactive lymphoid hyperplasia from low-grade lymphoma.
EBV	LMP-1 (latent membrane protein) antibody is positive in a proportion of R-S cells in HL. In situ hybridisation is more sensitive with a higher rate (60–70 %) of positivity.
Tdt	Terminal deoxynucleotidyltransferase is positive in precursor B and T cell lymphoblastic lymphomas. A nuclear epitope.
CD1a	Langerhans cell histiocytosis, cortical thymic T cells.

ALK-1/(CD246)	Nucleophosmin-anaplastic lymphoma kinase fusion protein associated with the ALK-1 gene t(2:5) translocation and good prognosis ALCLs.
MYC	Identifies an aggressive subset of DLBCLs that are less responsive to usual chemotherapy agents.
MUM1	A nuclear proliferation/differentiation epitope positive in post germinal centre B cells. It is of prognostic value in DLBCLs and stains classic R-S cells.
PAX5	A nuclear gene expression/differentiation transcription factor in B lymphoctyes and R-S cells.
Oct2/BoB1	B cell transcription factors positive in the nuclei of NLPHL L and H popcorn cells. Also in DLBCL.
EMA	Plasma cells, ALCL, NLPHL L and H cells.
Lysozyme	(muramidase/myeloperoxidase) – granulocytic and myeloid cell lineages.
AML	Also CD34, CD43, CD68, CD117, neutrophil elastase and chloroacetate esterase.
p53	A prognostic marker in various lymphoid neoplasms.
p21	A prognostic marker in multiple myeloma.
S100	Interdigitating reticulum cells, Langerhans cells.
Factor VIII/CD61	Markers of megakaryocytes.

Molecular Techniques

Immunoglobulin clonal heavy and light chain restriction and *T cell receptor (TCR) gene rearrangements* using polymerase chain reaction are of use in difficult diagnostic cases e.g. follicular hyperplasia vs. follicular lymphoma, or T zone reactive hyperplasia vs. malignant lymphoma. Also, where immunohistochemistry has been equivocal (e.g. dubious cyclin D1 staining in mantle cell lymphoma) chromosomal studies for specific translocations have a role to play. These techniques vary in their applicability to fresh tissue and routine paraffin sections and suitable arrangements for prompt tissue transportation and *referral on a regional network basis* should be put in place. A majority of malignant lymphomas can be provisionally diagnosed without these techniques but their role is rapidly evolving in importance with respect to diagnostic confirmation, prognostication and therapy.

The evolution of new generation robust antibodies applicable to paraffin sections with unmasking of antigenic sites by antigen retrieval methods and more sensitive visualization techniques has led to considerable reclassification of malignant lymphomas and emergence of new entities. For example lymphocyte depleted and mixed cellularity Hodgkin's lymphoma are diminishing as the full spectrum of NHL widens viz. T cell NHL, anaplastic large cell NHL, T cell rich B cell lymphoma (<10 % CD20 positive large cells on a background of CD3 small lymphocytes). Unusually composite (HL/NHL) and borderline (HL/ALCL) cases also occur. It is important that a panel of antibodies is used and markers assessed in combination. An example of this is in the sometimes difficult differential diagnosis of florid reactive hyperplasia versus follicular lymphoma. Benign follicle centres are bcl-2 negative, contain CD 68 positive macrophages, and show strong polar zonation of Ki-67 positivity. Conversely malignant follicles are diffusely bcl-2 positive with a low and evenly distributed Ki-67 proliferation index (unless predominantly centroblastic) and an absence of CD 68 positive macrophages. Thus *morphology and immunohistochemistry are used in tandem supplemented by molecular immunoglobulin and gene rearrangement studies*. It should also be noted that clonality does not always correlate with progression to malignant lymphoma as has been demonstrated in some inflammatory skin, salivary and gastric biopsies.

Formalin fixation and high quality, thin (4 μm) paraffin sections are adequate for morphological characterisation in most cases. Fixation should be sufficient (24–36 h) but not excessive as this may mask antigenic sites.

Progressive transformation of germinal centres will sometimes subsequently develop nodular lymphocyte predominant Hodgkin's disease characterised by the emergence of diagnostic popcorn or R-S cells.

The majority (60–70%) of NHLs are diffuse large B cell lymphomas and follicular lymphoma.

35.6 Characteristic Lymphomas

Precursor B Cell Lymphoblastic Lymphoma/Leukaemia

- Presents as childhood leukaemia or occasionally solid tumour (skin, bone, lymph node) and relapses in the central nervous system or testis.
- 75 % survival in childhood but <50 % in adults. Aggressive but potentially curable by multiagent chemotherapy.
- Medium sized round lymphoid cells with small nucleolus, mitoses.
- CD79a, CD10, tdt, CD99±, Ki-67 >95 %, CD20±.

B Cell Lymphocytic Lymphoma/ Chronic Lymphoctic Leukaemia (CLL)

- *5–10% of lymphomas* occurring in older adults with diffuse lymph node, bone marrow and blood involvement, and hepatosplenomegaly.
- Indolent and incurable with 5–10 year survival even without treatment but ultimately fatal.
- Small lymphocytes with pale proliferation centres (immunoblasts/prolymphocytes)
- CD45, CD20, CD5, CD23, bcl-2, Ki-67 <20 %. Cyclin D1 and CD10 negative.
- Richter's transformation to large cell lymphoma in 3–5 % of cases. Worse prognosis cases are CD38 positive.
- Occasional cases have Hodgkin's like cells (CD30/15) and <1 % develop classic HL.

Lymphoplasmacytic Lymphoma

- *1–2% of cases* and in the elderly involving bone marrow, nodes and spleen. Indolent course with a median survival of 5–10 years.
- Monoclonal IgM serum paraprotein with hyperviscosity symptoms and autoimmune/ cryoglobulin phenomena.
- Small lymphocytes, plasmacytoid and plasma cells.

- Intranuclear Dutcher and cytoplasmic Russell bodies.
- CD45, CD20, VS38 positive and CD5/CD10/ CD23 negative.

Marginal Zone Lymphoma of MALT (Mucosa Associated Lymphoid Tissue)

- *8% of NHLs*, stomach 50 % of cases, also salivary gland, lung, thyroid, orbit and skin. Multiple extranodal sites in 25–45 % of cases. Eighty percent are stage I or II disease and indolent. Many are cured by local excision, or antibiotic therapy in gastric MALToma.
- Usually extranodal associated with chronic autoimmune or antigenic stimulation.
- Centrocyte like cells, lymphocytes, plasma cells (scattered immunoblast and centroblast like cells).
- Destructive lymphoepithelial lesions, reactive germinal centres and follicular colonisation by the lymphoma cells.
- CD45, CD20 positive but CD5/10/23 negative.
- Lymph node variant is monocytoid B cell lymphoma: indolent (60–80 % 5 year survival) but has potential for large cell transformation.
- Gastric MALT with t(11:18) confers resistance to anti-helicobacter treatment.
- Splenic marginal zone lymphoma: splenomegaly, lymphocytosis, stage III/IV disease.

Hairy Cell Leukaemia

- Rare, elderly in the bone marrow, spleen and lymph nodes. Typically marked splenomegaly with pancytopaenia. Ten year survival >90 %.
- "Fried egg" perinuclear cytoplasmic clarity with prominent cell boundaries.
- CD45, CD20, CD72(DBA44), CD123, tartrate resistant acid phosphatase (TRAP) positive, cyclin D1 ±.

Mantle Cell Lymphoma

- *6% of NHLs* predominantly in older adult males (75 %).
- Extensive disease including spleen, bone marrow, Waldeyer's ring ± bowel involvement (multiple lymphomatous polyposis).

- Monomorphic small to medium sized irregular nuclei (centrocytic). Rare blastoid and pleomorphic variants.
- Diffuse with vague architectural nodularity.
- CD45, CD20, and typically CD5/cyclin D1 (t 11:14) /CD43 positive.
- CD10, CD23, bcl-6 negative. Cyclin D1 negative cases can be p27^{kip1} positive.
- Aggressive with mean survival of 3–5 years. A high Ki-67 index (>40–60 %) is prognostically adverse.

Follicular (Follicle Centre) Lymphoma

- *30 % of adult NHLs* and transformation to DLBCL is relatively common.
- Patterns: follicular, follicular and diffuse, diffuse (see Table 35.1)
- Cell types: centroblasts with large open nuclei, multiple small peripheral basophilic nucleoli and variable cytoplasm.
  - Centrocytes with medium sized irregular nuclei.
- Grade: 1/2/3 according to the number of centroblasts per high power field (see Table 35.1). Grade 3 has a high Ki-67 and 50 % may be bcl-2 negative – it is high-grade requiring R-CHOP chemotherapy and is to be distinguished from low-grade (grade 1/2) disease.
- CD45, CD20, CD10 (60 %), bcl-2 (t 14:18; 70–95 %), bcl-6.
- Usually CD21/23 positive and CD5 negative (20 % positive).
- High stage disease at presentation (splenomegaly and bone marrow involvement in 40 % of cases), and indolent time course, but late relapse (5–10 years) with large cell transformation in 25–35 % of cases to DLBCL.
- Pattern and grade can vary within a lymph node necessitating adequate sampling.

Diffuse Large B Cell Lymphoma (DLBCL)

- *30 % of adult NHLs, 40 % are extranodal* (especially stomach, skin, central nervous system, bone, testis etc). Forms a rapidly growing mass in older patients which usually arises de-novo, or, occasionally from low-grade B cell NHL. Aggressive but potentially curable – rituximab therapy has improved outlook considerably.
- Centroblasts, immunoblasts (prominent central nucleolus), bi-/polylobated, cleaved, anaplastic large cell (ALK+), plasmablastic (HIV+) forms, basophilic cytoplasm.
- Aggressive variants: T cell/histocyte rich, mediastinal/thymic, intravascular, primary effusion (chronic inflammation associated), primary central nervous system.
- CD45, CD20, CD79a, Ki-67 40–90 %, CD10 (30–60 %), bcl-2 (30 %), bcl-6 (60–90 %), CD5/23/CD30/CD43±. MUM1(35–65 %).
- Strong bcl-2 expression is adverse.
- *Hans clinical algorithm*: DLBCLs of germinal centre origin (CD10+, or, CD10-/bcl-6 +/ MUM1−) are of better prognosis (76 % 5 year survival) than those of non-germinal centre origin (CD10-/bcl-6– or, CD10-/bcl-6+/MUM1+: 34 % 5 year survival). "Germinal centre markers" include CD10, bcl-6, CD21 and CD23 while MUM-1 (Interferon Regulating Factor 4: IRF4) is expressed by post germinal centre destined B cells.
- MYC protein overexpression correlates with MYC gene translocation and identifies DLBCLs that are more aggressive, of worse prognosis and show a good response to R-CHOP (rituximab – cyclophosphamide, doxorubicin, vincristine, prednisolone) therapy.

Burkitt's Lymphoma

- *1–2.5 % of NHLs.*
- Childhood or young adult: endemic/sporadic/ HIV related (EBV: 95 %/15–20 %/30–40 % of cases respectively).
- Jaw and orbit (early childhood/endemic), or abdomen (ileocaecal/late childhood or ovaries/young adult/sporadic) and breasts with risk of central nervous system involvement.
- Monomorphic, medium-sized lymphoid cells, multiple small central nucleoli, basophilic cytoplasm.
- Mitoses, apoptosis, "starry-sky" pattern.
- CD79a, CD20, CD10, bcl-6, Ki-67 98–100 %, and bcl-2/tdt/CD5/23 negative.

- t(8:14) and t(2:8)/t (8:22) variants. Demonstration of t(8:14) requires fresh tissue. Has a characteristic MYC translocation on in situ hybridization.
- Requires aggressive polychemotherapy and is potentially curable: 90 % in low stage disease, 60–80 % with advanced disease, children better than adults. It can be difficult to distinguish from Burkitts like DLBCL.

Peripheral T Cell Lymphoma, Unspecified

- *10 % of NHLs and 30 % of T cell NHLs*. Adults. Generalised lymph node or extranodal disease at presentation with involvement of skin, subcutaneous tissue, viscera and spleen. Aggressive with relapses but potentially curable.
- Interfollicular/paracortical or diffuse infiltrate.
- Variable nuclear morphology from medium sized centrocyte like to blast cells, "crows-feet" appearance with irregular nuclear contours.
- Cytoplasmic clearing.
- Accompanying eosinophils, histiocytes and vascularity with prominent post capillary venules.
- Lymphoepithelioid variant (Lennert lymphoma).
- Usually CD3, CD4, CD5 and TCR gene rearrangement positive, sometimes CD7/CD8/CD15/CD30/CD56/TIA-1.
- *Of worse prognosis than B cell lymphomas*.
- Variants:
  - Angioimmunoblastic T cell lymphoma (CD3, CD4, CD8, TCR (75 %), high endothelial venules, prominent dendritic cells). In adults with fever, skin rash and generalized lymphadenopathy. Moderately aggressive.
  - Mycosis fungoides/Sézary syndrome (usually CD3, CD5, TCR and CD4+/CD8−). Cutaneous patch, plaque and tumour stages with or without lymph node involvement. Indolent but stage related and can transform to high-grade NHL of large cell type. Sézary syndrome is more aggressive with peripheral blood involvement.
  - Enteropathy type T cell lymphoma (pleomorphic, CD3, associated gluten enteropathy or ulcerative jejunitis). Aggressive and

in adults with abdominal pain, mass, ulceration or perforation, or a change in responsiveness to a gluten free diet.
  - Subcutaneous panniculitis like T cell lymphoma (nodules trunk/extremities, CD3, CD8, TCR). An 80 % 5 year survival but sometimes haemophagocytic syndrome supervenes with poor prognosis.
  - γδ hepatosplenic T cell lymphoma. Male adolescents and young adults. Aggressive and relapses despite treatment with survival <2 years. Liver, spleen and lymph node sinus involvement. CD3+, CD4/8−, γδ TCR.

Extranodal NK/T Cell Lymphoma, Nasal Type

- Necrotising lethal midline granuloma. Also seen in skin and soft tissues. Aggressive with 30–40 % survival.
- Polymorphic inflammatory infiltrate of eosinophils and histiocytes which may obscure the tumour cells.
- Variably sized atypical lymphoid cells, EBV positive on in situ hybridisation.
- Angiocentric and destructive.
- Variably CD2, CD56, CD45R0, TCR−. Cytoplasmic but not surface CD3. Also ±CD57, perforin, granzyme B, TIA-1.

Anaplastic Large Cell Lymphoma (ALCL)

- *2.5 % of NHLs* in adults and *10–20 % of childhood malignant lymphomas*.
- Elderly and young (25 % <20 years): ALK negative and ALK positive/males, respectively.
- May also follow mycosis fungoides, lymphomatoid papulosis or HL.
- Cohesive, sinusoidal growth pattern of "epithelioid" cells mimicking carcinoma, malignant melanoma and germ cell tumour.
- Large pleomorphic nuclei, multiple nucleoli, polylobated forms, "hallmark cells" with

horseshoe or reniform nucleus; rarely small cell variant.

- CD30, and, EMA/CD45/CD3±.
- Mainly T (60–70 % TCR), B (0–5 %) and null (20–30 %) cell types. Ninety percent have clonal TCR rearrangements.
- 12–50 % of adult cases are t(2:5) and ALK-1 positivity confers a good prognosis (80 % 5 year survival) despite presentation with stage III/IV disease. ALK-1 negative cases have 40 % 5 year survival. Relapses are common (30 %) but treatable.

Precursor T Lymphoblastic Lymphoma/Leukaemia

- CD3, CD4, CD8, CD43, Ki-67 >95 %, tdt. Presents in childhood/adolescence as leukaemia or a mediastinal mass (also lymph nodes, skin, liver, spleen, central nervous system, gonads). Aggressive with 20–30 % 5 year survival but potentially curable.

Granulocytic (Myeloid) Sarcoma

- Myelomonocytic markers are CD68, myeloperoxidase, chloroactetate esterase, neutrophil elastase, lysozmye, CD15, CD34, CD43, CD117.
- Megakaryocytic component: CD61, factor VIII.
- If a tumour looks like a malignant lymphoma but does not show appropriate immunohistochemical marking, think of granulocytic (myeloid) sarcoma or plasma cell myeloma.

35.7 Extranodal Lymphoma

Of *NHLs, 25–40% are extranodal*, defined as when a NHL presents with the main bulk of disease at an extranodal site usually necessitating the direction of treatment primarily to that site. In order of decreasing frequency sites of occurrence are

- Gastrointestinal tract (especially stomach then small intestine)
- Skin
- Waldeyer's ring
- Salivary gland
- Thymus
- Orbit
- Thyroid
- Lung
- Testis
- Breast
- Bone.

A majority are *aggressive large B cell lymphomas* although *T cell lesions* also occur (cutaneous T cell lymphoma, enteropathy associated T cell lymphoma, subcutaneous panniculitis like T cell lymphoma, NK/T cell sinonasal lymphoma). Their incidence is rising partly due to increased recognition and abandonment of terms such as pseudolymphoma, but also because of aetiological factors e.g. HIV, immunosuppression after transplantation or chemotherapy, autoimmune diseases (e.g. systemic lupus erythematosis), and chronic infections (*H. pylorii*, EBV, hepatitis C virus).

Many are *low-grade in character with indolent behaviour*, remaining localised to the site of origin. However a significant proportion present as or undergo high-grade transformation and when they metastasise typically do so to other extranodal sites. This site homing can be explained by the embryological development and circulation of mucosa associated lymphoid tissue (MALT). The *low-grade MALTomas* often arise from a background of chronic antigenic stimulation:

Gastric lymphoma	*H. pylorii* gastritis
Thyroid lymphoma	Hashimoto's thyroiditis
Salivary gland lymphoma	Lympho(myo-)epithelial sialadenitis/Sjögren's syndrome.

Their classification does not strictly parallel that of nodal lymphoma but mirrors marginal zone or monocytoid B cell lymphoma. They normally comprise a sheeted or nodular infiltrate of centrocyte like cells, destructive lymphoepithelial lesions and monotypic plasma cell immunoglobulin expression. Interfollicular infiltration or follicular colonisation of reactive follicles by the neoplastic cells is characteristic. There is often a component of blast cells and the *immunophenotype is one of exclusion* in that they are CD 5 and cyclin-D1 negative ruling out mantle cell lymphoma and other small B lymphocyte lymphoproliferative disorders. Other extranodal lymphomas have diverse morphology and immunophenotype correlating with the full spectrum of the WHO classification, although the lymph node based categories are not consistently transferable to extranodal sites.

Immunosuppressed post transplant (solid organs or bone marrow) patients are prone to a wide spectrum of nodal/extranodal *EBV associated* polyclonal and monoclonal B cell *lymphoproliferative disorders (PTLD)*. Three main categories exist: plasmacytic hyperplasia/infectious mononucleosis like (low-grade PTLD), polymorphic B cell hyperplasia/polymorphic B cell lymphoma (intermediate-grade PTLD) and monomorphic immunoblastic or centroblastic lymphoma/ multiple myeloma (high-grade PTLD). There is considerable overlap between the categories but in general monomorphic/ monoclonal lesions are worse than polymorphic/ polyclonal lesions. However even what appears to be high-grade lymphoma *may potentially regress if immunosuppressant therapy is decreased*. Serum titres and/or tissue expression of EBV are ascertained and clinical response to alteration of immunotherapy and anti-viral therapy assessed prior to use of chemotherapy. Similar findings can also be present in patients receiving chronic immunosuppression therapy for autoimmune and rheumatological disorders.

35.8   Prognosis

For some malignant lymphomas *watchful waiting* is the initial course of action and treatment is only instigated once the patient is symptomatic. Otherwise, *chemotherapy* and *radiotherapy* are the two principal treatment modalities for malignant lymphoma. However, *surgical excision* is often involved for definitive subtyping in primary lymph node disease, or, for removal of a bleeding or obstructing tumour mass and primary diagnosis of extranodal malignant lymphoma e.g. gastric lymphoma. *Prognosis* relates to *lymphoma*

type/grade (small cell and nodular are better than large cell and diffuse), and *stage of disease. Low-grade or indolent nodal malignant lymphomas* have a high frequency (>80 % at presentation) of bone marrow and peripheral blood involvement. They are incurable pursuing a protracted time course and relapse at a late date (5–10 years) with potentially blast transformation (e.g. CLL: 23 % risk at 8 years). *High-grade or aggressive lymphomas* develop bone marrow or peripheral involvement as an indication of advanced disease and are fatal within 1–2 years if left untreated. Prior to this the majority show good chemoresponsiveness with complete remission in 80 % and potential cure in 60 %. Overall, four broad prognostic categories are identified in NHL, although outlook does vary within individual types e.g. grades 1/2 or 3 follicle centre (follicular) lymphoma:

NHL type	5 year survival (%)
1. Anaplastic large cell/MALT/ follicular	>80
2. Nodal marginal zone/small lymphocytic/lymphoplasmacytoid	60–80
3. Mediastinal B cell/large B cell/ Burkitt's	30–70
4. T lymphoblastic/peripheral T cell/mantle cell	<50

Hodgkin's malignant lymphoma is relatively *radiotherapy and chemotherapy responsive. Prognosis* relates to *histological category* (e.g. type 2 nodular sclerosis is worse than type 1), but more importantly, *stage of disease* which is also an important factor in treatment selection. Average 5 year survival and cure rates for HL are 75 % with worse outcome for older patients (> 40–50 years), disease of advanced stage (i.e. more than one anatomical site), involvement of the mediastinum by a large mass (>1/3 of the widest thoracic diameter), spleen or extranodal sites. Lymphocyte-depleted HL is least favourable with the mixed cellularity category being of intermediate outlook. Both usually present with high stage disease involving spleen, retroperitoneal nodes and abdominal organs. However, histological type is usually regarded as having prognostic value only in limited disease (stage I or II). HL has a *bimodal age presentation* (15–40 years, 60–70 years) with nodular sclerosis type in the head and neck of young people being the commonest (75 % of cases). About 25 % of patients have *prognostically adverse B cell symptoms* at presentation but the commonest complaint is painless cervical lymphadenopathy ± mediastinal disease. Disease usually involves contiguous, axial lymph node groups (neck, axilla, mediastinum, retroperitoneum, groin) with occasional extranodal involvement.

There is evidence that early (confined to the mucosa), *low-grade gastric MALToma* is potentially reversible on removal of the ongoing antigenic stimulus i.e. *antibiotic treatment of H. pylorii*. However, high-grade disease or low-grade lesions with deep submucosal or muscle invasion require *chemotherapy supplemented by surgery* if there are local mass effects e.g. bleeding or pyloric outlet stenosis. Prognosis of MALT derived NHL relates to the histological grade and stage of disease.

T cell lymphomas form a minority of NHL (10–15%) and tend to have a *worse prognosis* than B cell lesions. Their cytological features are not particularly reliable at defining disease entities or clinical course, which is more dependent on tumour site and clinical setting. *Involvement of extranodal sites* and *relapse* there is not infrequent with typically an *aggressive disease course* e.g. enteropathy type T cell lymphoma and T/NK (angiocentric) sinonasal lymphoma. Cutaneous ALCL has a favourable prognosis while that of systemic ALCL with skin involvement is poor: 50 % present with stage III/IV disease and there is a 65–85 % 5 year survival rate but relapse is high (30–60 %).

Similarly some B cell lymphomas have site specific characteristics and clinical features e.g. *mantle cell lymphoma* in the gut (lymphomatous polyposis) or *diffuse mediastinal large B cell lymphoma* – young females with a rapidly enlarging mediastinal mass associated with superior vena cava syndrome. A large (>10 cm) mass and extramediastinal spread indicate poor prognosis. *Generally adverse prognostic factors in NHLs are*:

- Age >60 years.
- Male gender.
- Systemic symptoms (fever >38 °C, weight loss >10 %, night sweats).
- Poor performance status.
- Anaemia
- Elevated serum LDH.
- Tumour bulk:
  - 5–10 cm (stage I/II); > 10 cm (stage III/IV)
  - Large mediastinal mass
  - Palpable abdominal mass
  - Combined paraortic and pelvic nodal disease.
  - Combinations of these parameters can be scored in a clinical prognostic index to give risk and 5 year survival figures.

35.9 Other Malignancy

Carcinoma, germ cell tumours and *malignant melanoma* frequently *metastasise to lymph nodes* and are seen either in diagnostic biopsies (or FNAC) in patients with lymphadenopathy, or in regional lymph node resections in patients with known cancer. Spread of *malignant mesothelioma* or *sarcoma* to lymph nodes is *unusual* although it does occur e.g. alveolar rhabdomyosarcoma, epithelioid sarcoma, synovial sarcoma. Assessment is by *routine morphology supplemented by ancillary techniques e.g. immunohistochemistry* and *molecular methods*, although it should be noted that the significance of nodal micrometastases in a number of cancers is still not resolved. Metastases are initially in the subcapsular sinus network expanding to partial or complete nodal effacement with potential for extracapsular spread. *Anatomical site of involvement* can be a clue as to the *origin of the cancer* e.g. neck (cancer of the upper aerodigestive tract, lung, breast, salivary glands or thyroid gland), supraclavicular fossa (lung, stomach, prostate, testis, ovary or breast cancer), axilla (breast, lung cancer or malignant melanoma), groin (cancer of the perineum or perianal area, cutaneous melanoma and rarely the pelvis) and retroperitoneum (germ cell tumour, genitourinary cancers). The metastatic deposit may be necrotic or cystic (e.g. squamous cell carcinoma of the head and neck, germ cell tumour in the retroperitoneum), resemble the primary lesion or be more or less well differentiated. Cell cohesion with nesting, necrosis, focal or sinusoidal distribution, solid lymphatic plugs of tumour and plentiful cytoplasm favour non-lymphomatous neoplasia although this is not always the case e.g. ALCL, or, DLBCL. In this respect a *broad but basic panel of antibodies* is crucial for accurate designation (e.g. cytokeratins, CD 45, CD 30, OCT3/4, S100, melan-A, chromogranin) occasionally supplemented by histochemistry (e.g. PAS diastase resistant mucin positivity, an organoid pattern of reticulin fibres). Some metastases also induce characteristic inflammatory responses e.g. squamous cell carcinoma of head and neck, large cell lung cancer and nasopharyngeal carcinoma (lymphocytes, leukaemoid reaction, eosinophils, granulomas) even mimicking HL. Some diagnostic clues are:

Malignant melanoma	Cell nests, eosinophilic nucleolus, spindle/epithelioid cells, melanin pigment, S100, HMB-45, melan-A.
Germ cell tumour	Midline (mediastinum or retroperitoneum), elevated serum βHCG or AFP (± tissue expression), PLAP/CD117 (seminoma), cytokeratins/CD30 (embryonal carcinoma). Also SALL4 and OCT3/4 (except yolk sac tumour).
Lobular breast cancer	Sinusoidal infiltrate of sheeted, non-cohesive small cells, intracytoplasmic lumina, cytokeratins (CAM 5.2, AE1/AE3, CK7), GCDFP-15 and ER positive. Metastatic ductal cancer often has a nested pattern of larger cells with variable ER/Her-2 positivity (Grade 1 or 2 tumours will have a tubular component).
Small cell carcinoma	Small (×2–3 the size of a lymphocyte), round to fusiform cells, granular chromatin, inconspicuous nucleolus, moulding, crush and DNA artifact, ± paranuclear dot CAM 5.2, and, chromogranin/synaptophysin/CD56/TTF-1 (Merkel cell carcinoma is CK 20 positive). In addition to positivity with the above markers other metastatic neuroendocrine tumours (e.g. carcinoid, large cell neuroendocrine carcinoma) show stronger chromogranin and cytokeratin expression than small cell carcinoma.

Lung adenocarcinoma	Variably glandular or tubulopapillary, CK7/TTF-1/napsin-A/CEA/BerEP4/MOC31.
Thyroid carcinoma	Papillae, characteristic nuclei (overlapping, optically clear, grooves), psammoma bodies, CK7/TTF-1 and thyroglobulin/CK19.
Colorectal adenocarcinoma	Glandular with segmental and dirty necrosis, CK20/CEA/CDX-2/βcatenin.
Upper gastrointestinal and pancreaticobiliary adenocarcinoma	Tubuloacinar, tall columnar cells with clear cytoplasm, CK7/CEA/CA19-9/± CK20/CDX-2.
Ovarian carcinoma	Serous (tubulopapillary, psammoma bodies, CK7/CA125/WT-1/p16), or mucinous (glandular, CK7, ±CK20/CA125).
Uterine adenocarcinoma	Endometrioid (CK7/vimentin/ER) or serous (CK7/p53/Ki-67/HMGA2/PTEN).
Prostate adenocarcinoma	Acinar or cribriform, PSA m/p, PSAP/AMACR.
Bladder carcinoma	Nested (squamoid) or micropapillary, CK7/CK20/34βE12/CK5/6/uroplakin III/GATA-3.
m = monoclonal	p = polyclonal

The reader is referred to the Introduction for further discussion of the use of immunohistochemistry.

Bibliography

Alizadeh AA, Eisen MB, Davis RE. Distinct types of large B-cell lymphoma identified by gene expression profiling. Nature. 2000;403:503–11.

Banerjee SS, Verma S, Shanks JH. Morphological variants of plasma cell tumours. Histopathology. 2004;44:2–8.

Brady G, MacArthur GJ, Farrell PJ. Epstein-Barr virus and Burkitt lymphoma. J Clin Pathol. 2007;60:1397–402.

Brown D, Gatter K, Natkunam Y. Bone marrow diagnosis: an illustrated guide. Oxford: Wiley Blackwell; 2006.

Brunning RD, Arber DA. Chapter 23. Bone marrow. In: Rosai J, editor. Rosai and Ackerman's surgical pathology. 10th ed. Edinburgh: Elsevier; 2011.

Bryant RJ, Banks PM, O'Malley DP. Ki-67 staining as a diagnostic tool in the evaluation of lymphoproliferative disorders. Histopathology. 2006;48:505–15.

Campo E, Chott A, Kinney MC, Leoncini L, Meijer CJLM, Papadimitriou CS, Piris MA, Stein H, Swerdlow SH. Update on extranodal lymphomas. Conclusions of the workshop held by the EAHP and the SH in Thessaloniki, Greece. Histopathology. 2006;48:481–504.

Chan JKC. Tumours of the lymphoreticular system, including spleen and thymus. In: Fletcher CDM, editor. Diagnostic histopathology of tumours, vol. 3. 3rd ed. London: Harcourt; 2007. p. 1139–310.

Chan JKC, Banks PM, Cleary ML, Delsol G, de Wolf-Peters C, Falini B, Gatter KC, Grogan TM, Harris NL, Isaacson PG, Jaffe ES, Knowles DM, Mason DY, Müller-Hermelink HK, Pileri SA, Piris MA, Ralfkiaer E, Stein H, Warnke RA. A proposal for classification of lymphoid neoplasms (by the International Lymphoma Study Group). Histopathology. 1994;25: 517–36.

De Kerviler E, Guermazi A, Zagdanski AM, et al. Image-guided core-needle biopsy in patients with suspected or recurrent lymphoma. Cancer. 2000;89: 647–52.

Delecluse H-J, Feederle R, O'Sullivan B, Taniere P. Epstein-Barr virus-associated tumours: an update for the attention of the working pathologist. J Clin Pathol. 2007;60:1358–64.

DeLeval L, Harris NL. Variability in immunophenotype in diffuse large B-cell lymphoma and its significance. Histopathology. 2003;43:509–28.

Du M-Q, Bacon CM, Isaacson PG. Kaposi sarcoma-associated herpesvirus/human herpesvirus 8 and lymphoproliferative disorders. J Clin Pathol. 2007;60: 1350–7.

Grogg KL, Miller RF, Dogan A. HIV infection and lymphoma. J Clin Pathol. 2007;60:1365–72.

Hall JG. The functional anatomy of lymph nodes. In: Stansfield AG, d'Ardenne AJ, editors. Lymph node biopsy interpretation. 2nd ed. Edinburgh: Churchill Livingstone; 1992. p. 3–28.

Hans CP, Weisenburger DD, Greiner TC, Gascoyne RD, Delabie J, Ott G, Müller-Hermelink HK, Campo E, Braziel RM, Jaffe ES, Pan Z, Farinha P, Smith LM, Falini B, Banham AH, Rosenwald A, Staudt LM, Connors JM, Armitage JO, Chan WC. Confirmation of the molecular classification of diffuse large B-cell lymphoma immunohistochemistry using a tissue microarray. Blood. 2004;103:275–82.

Harris NL, Jaffe ES, Stein H, et al. A revised European-American classification of lymphoid neoplasms: a proposal from the International Lymphoma Study Group. Blood. 1994;84:1361–92.

Harris NL, Jaffe ES, Diebold J, Flandrin G, Müller-Hermelink HK, Vardiman J, Lister TA, Bloomfield CD. The World Health Organization classification of neoplastic diseases of the haemopoietic and lymphoid tissues: report of the clinical advisory committee meeting, Airlie House, Virginia, November 1997. Histopathology. 2000;36:69–87.

Hermans J, Krol AD, van Groningen K, et al. International Prognostic Index for aggressive non-Hodgkin's lymphoma is valid for all malignancy grades. Blood. 1995;86:1460–3.

Isaacson PG. Haematopathology practice: the commonest problems encountered in a consultation practice. Histopathology. 2007;50:821–34.

Kapatai G, Murray P. Contribution of the Epstein-Barr virus to the molecular pathogenesis of Hodgkin lymphoma. J Clin Pathol. 2007;60:1342–9.

Kluin PM, Feller A, Gaulard P, Jaffe ES, Meijer CJ, Müller-Hermelink HK, Pileri S. Peripheral T/NK-cell lymphoma: a report of the IXth workshop of the European Association for haematopathology. Histopathology. 2001;38:250–70.

Kocjan C. Cytological and molecular diagnosis of lymphoma. ACP Best Practice No 185. J Clin Pathol. 2005;58:561–7.

Leoncini L, Delsol G, Gascoyne RD, Harris NL, Pileri SA, Piris MA, Stein H. Aggressive B-cell lymphomas: a review based on the workshop of the XI meeting of the European Association for Haematopathology. Histopathology. 2005;46:241–55.

Maes B, De Wolf-Peeters C. Marginal zone cell lymphoma – an update on recent advances. Histopathology. 2002;40:117–26.

Matutes E. Adult T-cell leukaemia/lymphoma. J Clin Pathol. 2007;60:1373–7.

Müller-Hermelink HK, Zettl A, Pfeifer W, Ott G. Pathology of lymphoma progression. Histopathology. 2001;38:285–306.

O'Malley DP, George TI, Orazi A, editors. Benign and reactive conditions of lymph node and spleen. Washington D.C.: ARP Press; 2009.

Oudejans JJ, van der Walk P. Diagnostic brief. Immunohistochemical classification of B cell neoplasms. J Clin Pathol. 2003;56:193.

Prakash S, Swerdlow SH. Nodal aggressive B-cell lymphomas: a diagnostic approach. J Clin Pathol. 2007;60: 1076–85.

Rosai J. Chapter 22. Lymph nodes, spleen. In: Rosai J, editor. Rosai and Ackerman's surgical pathology. 10th ed. Edinburgh: Elsevier; 2011.

Sagaert X, De Wolf-Peeters C. Anaplastic large cell lymphoma. Curr Diagn Pathol. 2003;9:252–8.

Swerdlow SH, Campo E, Harris NL, Jaffe ES, Pileri SA, Stein H, Thiele J, Vardiman JW. WHO classification of tumours. Pathology and genetics. Tumours of haemopoietic and lymphoid tissues. Lyon: IARC Press; 2008.

Tapia G, Lopez R, Munoz-Marmol AM, Mate JL, Sanz C, Marginet R, Navarro J-T, Ribera J-M, Ariza A. Immunohistochemical detection of MYC protein correlates with *MYC* gene status in aggressive B cell lymphomas. Histopathology. 2011;59:672–8.

Taylor CR. Hodgkin's disease is a non-Hodgkin's lymphoma. Hum Pathol. 2005;36:1–4.

The National Cancer Action Team and The Royal College of Pathologists. Additional Best Practice Commissioning Guidance for developing Haematology Diagnostic Services. In line with the NICE Improving Outcomes Guidance for Haemato-oncology 2003. Accessed at http://www.ncat.nhs.uk.

The Royal College of Pathologists and The British Committee for Standards in Haematology. Best Practice in Lymphoma Diagnosis and Reporting – Specific Disease Appendix. Accessed at http://www. rcpath.org/index.asp?PageID=254.

Viswanatha DS, Dogan A. Hepatitis C virus and lymphoma. J Clin Pathol. 2007;60:1378–83.

Warnke RA, Weiss LM, Chan JKC, Cleary ML, Dorfman RF. Tumors of the lymph nodes and spleen. Atlas of tumor pathology. 3rd series. Fascicle 14. Washington: AFIP; 1995.

Wilkins BS. Pitfalls in lymphoma pathology: avoiding errors in diagnosis of lymphoid tissues. J Clin Pathol. 2011;64:466–76.

Wilkins BS, Wright DH. Illustrated pathology of the spleen. Cambridge: Cambridge University Press; 2000. p. 1–31.

Wittekind CF, Greene FL, Hutter RVP, Klimpfinger M, Sobib LH. TNM atlas: illustrated guide to the TNM/pTNM classification of malignant tumours. 5th ed. Berlin: Springer; 2005.

Part IX

Bone and Soft Tissue Cancer

- Bone and Soft Tissue Sarcomas (with Comments on Retroperitoneum and Adrenal Gland)

Bone and Soft Tissue Sarcomas (with Comments on Retroperitoneum and Adrenal Gland)

36

Bone and soft tissue sarcomas are relatively uncommon and more appropriately managed by a regional multidisciplinary clinical team inclusive of specialist pathology review. Histological tumour type is a strong indicator of likely biological behaviour and prognosis, and, along with tumour grade, size, depth, stage and completeness of surgical excision helps determine selection of patients for neoadjuvant, adjuvant and targeted therapies.

Bone tumours often present as severe continuous pain unrelieved by anti-inflammatory agents, swelling, or sometimes as a pathological fracture following low impact trauma. Investigation is by plain x-ray and CT scan looking particularly for signs of periosteal reaction. A tissue diagnosis is obtained by needle core biopsy under radiological control. Osteosarcoma and Ewing's sarcoma are treated by a combination of chemotherapy and surgery, chondrosarcoma by surgery. Where feasible, surgery is limb salvage and curative in intent. Most primary bone tumours arise de-novo but a minority occur in association with recognisable precursors e.g. Paget's disease, or a history of radiation. Metastatic bone disease due to secondary carcinomatosis can cause hypercalcaemia and is detected by isotope bone, CT or MRI scans. A past medical history of cancer is important in raising awareness of this possibility. Typical primary sites are breast, lung, thyroid, kidney and prostate.

Benign soft tissue tumours far outnumber malignant cases by a ratio of 50–100:1. Clinical ultrasound examination can rapidly triage benign from more suspicious lesions. Soft tissue sarcomas form 1 to 2 % of cancers with an incidence of 25 per million in the UK, and, occur mainly in the extremities (often thigh) but also the retroperitoneum and trunk wall. They are usually deep seated and progressively increase in size causing a lump or swelling, and sometimes pain with a loss of function in the limb or adjacent organs. Plain x-ray may show focal calcification (e.g. synovial sarcoma), but MRI is the investigation of choice in defining the nature of the mass, its extent and involvement of adjacent structures. CT scan is used for lesions of the trunk, for detection of bone involvement, and as for bone sarcomas, for pretreatment staging of pulmonary metastases. After full clinical and radiological assessment most centres use needle core biopsy to obtain a tissue diagnosis and open biopsy only when needle core biopsy has proven inconclusive (in 5–10 % of cases only). Fine needle aspiration cytology (FNAC) also has a diagnostic role, particularly in confirming recurrence or metastasis in a patient with a previously diagnosed sarcoma. Surgery is the mainstay of treatment with the aim of complete excision, limb salvage and retention of function. Postoperative radiotherapy is indicated for deep seated tumours, intermediate to high-grade tumours, or those with a close or involved surgical margin. Large pelvic or retroperitoneal sarcomas impacting on several organ systems may require a specialist multidisciplinary surgical team e.g. gynaecological, urological, gastrointestinal and vascular surgeons as appropriate. Chemotherapy is indicated for Ewing's sarcoma and rhabdomyosarcoma.

D.C. Allen, *Histopathology Reporting*,
DOI 10.1007/978-1-4471-5263-7_36, © Springer-Verlag London 2013

A small minority of bone and soft tissue sarcomas (osteosarcoma/angiosarcoma) can arise in the vicinity and several years after use of a metallic orthopaedic or Dacron smooth surface vascular surgical implant. Immunosuppression after cancer therapy or organ transplantation can result in a range of cutaneous and soft tissue lesions e.g. squamous cell carcinoma, lymphoproliferative disorders, low-grade smooth muscle proliferations and vascular endothelial tumours.

36.1   Gross Description

Specimen

- FNAC/needle core biopsy/open biopsy (incisional/curettings/reamings)/enucleation (marginal excision)/wide local excision/compartmentectomy/segmental resection/en bloc resection/pelvic exenteration/amputation (limb (below/above knee, etc))/complex resection (forequarter/hindquarter/hemipelvectomy).
- Right or left.
- Size (cm) and weight (g).

Tumour

Site

- Osseous: paracortical (paraosteal/periosteal); cortical; medullary (epiphysis/metaphysis/diaphysis); soft tissue extension.
- Soft tissues: dermis/subcutaneous tissue/deep fascia/peripheral nerve/muscle/osseous extension/retroperitoneal/pelvic/mediastinal/paratesticular.
- Satellite nodules: size (cm) and distance (cm) from the main tumour.
- Location: may be indicative e.g. pelvis – Ewing's sarcoma or chondrosarcoma; chest wall – Askin (thoracopulmonary neuroectodermal) tumour, alveolar rhabdomyosarcoma.

Size

- Length × width × depth (cm) or maximum dimension (cm).
- It is generally recommended that 1 block per 1 cm diameter (up to a maximum of 12) be sampled to account for the variation in grade and differentiation that is encountered in some

sarcomas. Tumour regression after neoadjuvant therapy must also be accounted for.

Appearance

- Solid/cystic/necrotic/lobulated/fatty/myxoid/cartilaginous/osseous.
- The percentage tumour necrosis after neoadjuvant therapy is a prognostic indicator.

Edge

- Circumscribed/irregular.

Vessels

- Relationship of tumour to vessels.

36.2   Histological Type

Prior to histological evaluation of any bone or soft tissue sarcoma the pathologist must be aware of the patient's age, anatomical site of the lesion, subsite (eg epiphysis, metaphysis or diaphysis of bone) and crucially, the radiological appearances. For example, a rapidly growing chest wall lesion in a young male may be nodular fasciitis rather than a sarcoma, peripheral chondroid lesions are benign whereas proximal/axial lesions are more likely to be malignant, and an epiphyseal lesion is likely to be a giant cell tumour (adult) or chondroblastoma (child) rather than an osteosarcoma (young/metaphysis). Age also closely correlates with the type of soft tissue sarcoma: embryonal rhabdomyosarcoma (infants), synovial sarcoma (young adult), liposarcoma (middle aged to elderly) and malignant fibrous histiocytoma (elderly). *Close clinicopathological correlation* is therefore fundamental to the diagnosis.

Osteosarcoma, chondrosarcoma, Ewing's/PNET (peripheral neuroectodermal tumour), liposarcoma, synovial sarcoma, fibrosarcoma, rhabdomyosarcoma, leiomyosarcoma, angiosarcoma, malignant peripheral nerve sheath tumours, malignant fibrous histiocytoma and variants are amongst the main categories of sarcoma and each comprises variable numbers of subtypes (Tables 36.1 and 36.2).

Morphology is the mainstay of diagnosis but a panel of *immunohistochemical antibodies*, other markers (e.g. alkaline phosphatase on fresh tissue touch imprints for osteosarcoma), and *cytogenetic analysis* should be used as appropriate. This

Table 36.1 Bone neoplasms

Adamantinoma
  Conventional
  Osteofibrous-dysplasia like (well differentiated)

Angiosarcoma

Chondrosarcoma
  Conventional
  Clear cell
  Dedifferentiated
  Mesenchymal
  Peripheral juxtacortical (periosteal)
  Myxoid
  Arising in association with osteochondroma
  Other

Chordoma
  Conventional
  Chondroid
  Dedifferentiated

Ewing's sarcoma/Peripheral Neuroectodermal Tumour (PNET)

Fibrosarcoma
  Conventional
  Periosteal

Giant cell tumour of bone (specify: conventional, malignant)

Haemangioendothelioma
  Epithelioid

Haemangiopericytoma/solitary fibrous tumour

Haemopoietic tumours (plasma cell myeloma, malignant lymphoma)

Leiomyosarcoma

Liposarcoma

Malignant fibrous histiocytoma

Malignant mesenchymoma

Malignant peripheral nerve sheath tumour

Osteosarcoma
  Conventional
  Chondroblastic
  Fibroblastic
  Osteoblastic
  Mixed (specify cell types)
  Low grade central
  Intraosseous, well differentiated
  Giant cell rich
  Small cell
  Telangiectatic
  Epithelioid
  Osteoblastoma like
  Chondroblastoma like
  Associated with (specify fibrous dysplasia, Paget's disease of bone)
  Post-radiation

Table 36.1 (continued)

Surface
  Parosteal
  Dedifferentiated parosteal
  Periosteal
  High grade surface

Rhabdomyosarcoma

Table 36.2 Soft tissue sarcomas

Adipocytic tumours
  Atypical lipomatous tumour/well differentiated liposarcoma

(a) Lipoma like

(b) Sclerosing

(c) Inflammatory

(d) Spindle cell

Dedifferentiated liposarcoma

Myxoid liposarcoma

Round cell liposarcoma

Pleomorphic liposarcoma

Fibrous/myofibroblastic tumours
  Solitary fibrous tumour (includes haemangiopericytoma)
  Inflammatory myofibroblastic tumour
  Dermatofibrosarcoma protuberans
  Low-grade myofibroblastic sarcoma
  Myxoinflammatory fibroblastic sarcoma
  Infantile fibrosaroma
  Adult fibrosarcoma
  Myxofibrosarcoma
  Low-grade fibromyxoid sarcoma
  Sclerosing epithelioid fibrosarcoma

Fibrohistiocytic tumours

Plexiform fibrohistiocytic tumour

Giant cell tumour of soft tissue

Undifferentiated pleomorphic sarcoma/pleomorphic "MFH"

Undifferentiated pleomorphic sarcoma with giant cells/giant cell "MFH"

Undifferentiated pleomorphic sarcoma with prominent inflammation/inflammatory "MFH"

Malignant tenosynovial giant cell tumour

Smooth muscle tumours
  Leiomyosarcoma

Perivascular tumours
  Malignant Glomus Tumour

Skeletal muscle tumours
  Rhabdomyosarcoma

(a) Embryonal, including botryoid and spindle cell

(b) Alveolar

(c) Pleomorphic

(continued)

Table 36.2 (continued)

Vascular tumours
Kaposi sarcoma
Epithelioid haemangioendothelioma
Angiosarcoma (includes lymphangiosarcoma)
Neuroectodermal tumours
Malignant peripheral nerve sheath tumour
With heterologous rhabdomyosarcoma (Triton tumour)
With (specify other mesenchymal heterology)
Epithelioid variant
Malignant granular cell tumour
Malignant melanotic schwannoma
Malignant peripheral primitive neuroectodermal tumour (PNET, extraskeletal Ewing's sarcoma)
Extraskeletal chondro-osseous tumours
Extraskeletal mesenchymal chondrosarcoma
Extraskeletal osteosarcoma
Tumours of uncertain differentiation
Angiomatoid "MFH"
Ossifying fibromyxoid tumour
Myoepithelioma/mixed tumour
Alveolar soft part sarcoma
Epithelioid sarcoma
Synovial sarcoma
Extraskeletal myxoid chondrosarcoma
Clear cell sarcoma (malignant melanoma of soft parts)
Desmoplastic small round cell tumour
Extrarenal rhabdoid tumour
Intimal sarcoma
PEComa
Malignant mesenchymoma

allows *subclassification as to histogenetic type in the majority of lesions* with, by exclusion, a minority of undifferentiated/pleomorphic sarcomas traditionally designated as malignant fibrous histiocytoma (MFH). Electron microscopy has a limited role to play in the diagnosis of some peripheral nerve sheath tumours, marker negative synovial sarcomas and pleomorphic sarcomas. Most soft tissue sarcomas arise from primitive multipotential mesenchymal cells which can differentiate along one of several lines resulting in histological overlap. One morphological approach is to categorise lesions based on their çell type (pleomorphic/spindle cell/round cell/rhabdoid) and/or pattern (fascicular/storiform/myxoid), or a combination e.g.

(a) Predominantly spindle cell with various patterns: e.g. monomorphic fibrosarcomatous

(synovial sarcoma) or pleomorphic MFH like (pleomorphic liposarcoma).

(b) Spindle cells mixed with other mesenchymal elements: e.g. liposarcoma (fat), synovial sarcoma (epithelial component) or myxoid liposarcoma (myxoid material, plexiform vasculature).

(c) Round cell morphology: e.g. PNET and rhabdomyosarcoma (small cells), clear cell sarcoma (large cells) or desmoplastic small round cell tumour (rhabdoid cells).

Diagnostic pointers to sarcoma: can be *general or distinctive*. The former include deep seated anatomical location, progressive increase in size with compression of adjacent structures, irregularity of margins, cellularity, cytological atypia, necrosis, mitotic activity and vascular invasion. Some distinctive features are

Liposarcoma

Forms a majority of deep limb, retroperitoneal and pelvic sarcomas and is prone to *local soft tissue recurrence.*

Well differentiated	Variation in adipocyte size and shape, multivacuolar lipoblasts, atypical mesenchymal nuclei in broad connective tissue septa.
Myxoid	Myxoid stroma with signet ring lipoblasts, plexiform capillary network ± a high-grade round cell component (epithelioid cells/cords/trabeculae).
Dedifferentiated	Abrupt transition from well differentiated liposarcoma to non-lipogenic sarcoma with spindle cell or MFH patterns overlapping with pleomorphic liposarcoma. Associated with a *15–20 % metastasis rate.*

Liposarcoma can be MDM2, CDK4 positive.

Leiomyosarcoma

Usually a monomorphic spindle cell tumour and a fibrosarcomatous pattern of cells with tapering eosinophilic cytoplasm and blunt ended nuclei. Mitoses, atypia and necrosis may not be prominent so anatomical location and radiological findings are important. Forms a significant proportion of *retroperitoneal sarcomas* some of which arise from large blood vessels e.g. inferior vena cava. Epithelioid and myxoid variants occur. Also primary cutaneous, peripheral soft tissue and visceral (e.g. uterine, vulvovaginal, pelvic, gastrointestinal) lesions. *Site of origin is a strong predictor of subsequent biological behaviour* – in general a deep seated lesion with any mitotic activity is considered to have metastatic potential. A proportion of retroperitoneal smooth muscle tumours are oestrogen receptor positive and potentially hormone responsive.

Synovial Sarcoma

Either *classical biphasic* with a glandular epithelial component and background spindle cells, or *monophasic* with a fibrosarcomatous spindle cell pattern. Focal microcalcification may be present. Can be small and peripheral (e.g. tendons of the hand or foot), or large and central (e.g. head and neck area).

Malignant Fibrous Histiocytoma (MFH)/Undifferentiated Pleomorphic Sarcoma

Elderly, lower limbs. Storiform (cartwheel/whorls) or fascicular spindle cell patterns. Mononuclear, osteoclast type and bizarre pleomorphic giant cells are not uncommon. *Excluded by histological identification of a more specific line of differentiation* e.g. lipoblasts. Many retroperitoneal MFH lesions are now considered to be dedifferentiated liposarcomas. Tumours with *myogenic differentiation* have a *worse prognosis*.

Pleomorphic rhabdomyosarcoma is a rare high-grade sarcoma in the deep soft tissues of the lower extremities of adults, or, a primary visceral lesion e.g. uterus, which can be pure, or more commonly a component of a carcinosarcoma (malignant mixed Mullerian tumour), or testicular germ cell tumour.

Dermatofibrosarcoma Protuberans (DFSP)

Uniform, moderately cellular dermal plaque of spindle cells in a storiform pattern with lace like honeycomb infiltration of subcutaneous fat. There is an uninvolved Grenz zone between overlying non-hyperplastic epidermis, elimination of dermal collagen and appendage structures, with diffuse CD34 positivity. These features help to distinguish it from usual dermatofibroma or benign fibrous histiocytoma. There is a *40% local recurrence rate* within 3 years if incompletely excised.

Malignant Peripheral Nerve Sheath Tumour (MPNST)

Monophasic fibrosarcomatous pattern with prominent nodularity and entrapped nerves at the tumour periphery. Can be epithelioid in character or include a biphasic glandular epithelial component or rhabdomyogenic foci (malignant Triton tumour). *Fifty percent arise in von Recklinghausen's disease.* Shows only focal S100 positivity.

Angiosarcoma

Primary (e.g. scalp in the elderly) or secondary (e.g. post radiotherapy for breast carcinoma). It comprises a branching vasoformative network dissecting collagen and lined by abnormal endothelial cells which are CD31/CD34 positive. Intracytoplasmic vacuoles containing red blood cells. Epithelioid variants are INI 1 positive.

Epithelioid haemangioendothelioma (retroperitoneum/liver/skin/lung) is of intermediate-grade malignancy with a tendency for local recurrence. It forms cords of small epithelioid cells with paranuclear intracytoplasmic lumina.

Kaposi's Sarcoma

Cutaneous or visceral mucosal lesions with patch, plaque and tumour stages. Nodules of spindle cells (± hyaline globules) and slit like spaces containing red blood cells. Primary or immunosuppression related (e.g. HIV), and HHV8 positive.

Epithelioid Sarcoma

Nodular dermal/subcutaneous lesion in the hand/wrist of young adults with a "pseudonecrobiotic granulomatous" pattern of CAM 5.2/EMA/CD34 positive spindle/epithelioid cells. It can mimic granuloma annulare/rheumatoid nodule and squamous cell carcinoma.

Clear Cell Sarcoma of Tendon Sheath

Nests of S100 positive polygonal/fusiform cells in dense collagen septate stroma. Often in the foot or ankle of young adults.

Alveolar Soft Part Sarcoma

Organoid nests of large eosinophilic cells with central dyscohesion giving an alveolar pattern. Cytoplasmic PAS-diastase positive rhomboidal crystals. Found in the extremities in adults, and head and neck in children.

Fibrosarcoma

Relatively rare and only after excluding other sarcomas with a fibrosarcomatous pattern. Fibroblast bundles in a herring bone pattern with variable collagen content. Biological behaviour relates to mitotic activity, infiltrating margins and adequacy of excision.

Pecomas

A family of tumours showing *Perivascular Epithelioid Cell differentiation*. It includes renal and hepatic angiomyolipomas (associated with tuberous sclerosis complex), pulmonary lymphangioleiomyomatosis and clear cell "sugar" tumour, visceral (gastrointestinal/uterine), and soft tissue (retroperitoneal/abdominopelvic) lesions. Predominantly in females comprising nests of epithelioid and/or spindle cells with clear to granular cytoplasm and associated with a proliferation of thick walled

dystrophic vessels and fat. The tumour cells are HMB-45 and melan-A positive. A minority (size >7 cm, cytological atypia, mitotically active, necrosis) behave in a malignant fashion. PEComas can be prone to *spontaneous life threatening retroperitoneal haemorrhage*.

Small Round Cell Tumours

More often in children and young adults including *Ewing's sarcoma/PNET* (pelvis, long bones, ribs), *rhabdomyosarcoma* (alveolar/chest wall, and, embryonal/bladder, biliary tract, head and neck subtypes) and *desmoplastic small round cell tumour* (abdominopelvic area/peritoneum with nests of cells in a prominent collagenous stroma). To be distinguished by characteristic anatomical locations and immunophenotype from other small cell malignancy e.g. neuroblastoma, malignant lymphoma/leukaemia, small cell malignant melanoma or osteosarcoma, and small cell carcinoma.

Chondrosarcoma

Axial location in older adults and hypercellular hyaline cartilage with atypical chondrocyte nests and nuclei. It shows an infiltrative, lobulated and pushing margin into bone medulla, cortex or soft tissues. Grading is prognostically important. There are also clear cell, myxoid, mesenchymal and dedifferentiated variants. Chondrosarcoma tends to be *low-grade* and prone to *local recurrence*. Dedifferentiated lesions are *high-grade* and *metastasise early*.

Osteosarcoma

Metaphysis/diaphysis in long bones of children or young adults. Infiltrative and destructive with elevation of the periosteum. Variably pleomorphic spindle cells associated with formation of osteoid matrix. There are a number of variants including osteoblastic, chondroblastic, fibroblastic, giant cell, small cell and telangiectatic. Also low-grade central (medullary) and parosteal forms, and, intermediate periosteal and high-grade surface osteosarcomas.

Differential Diagnosis

A monomorphic or pleomorphic spindle cell tumour in breast, bowel, lung, kidney or other viscera is usually a sarcomatoid carcinoma, and, in skin or lymph node metastatic malignant melanoma. A similar soft tissue lesion is usually a sarcoma but *metastatic malignant melanoma, carcinoma and malignant lymphoma must be considered and excluded.* Also consider soft tissue chloroma or *myeloid sarcoma*, particularly if the tumour looks like it is a malignant lymphoma but does not show positive expression with the usual panel of lymphoid immunohistochemical markers.

Metastatic carcinoma: is the commonest malignant tumour of bone typical primary sites being lung, kidney, breast, prostate and thyroid. It can be single or multiple, 70 % affect the axial skeleton, and metaphysis is the preferred site. Metastatic carcinomatosis is rare distal to the elbow or knee.

Multiple myeloma: must always be borne in mind. In the elderly, multiple lytic bone lesions, serum monoclonal gammopathy, Bence Jones proteinuria with renal dysfunction, CD138 positive plasma cells with κ/λ light chain restriction.

36.3 Differentiation/Grade

Well/moderate/poor, or, Grade 1/2/3.
- Based on the degree of resemblance to adult mesenchymal tissues, cytological atypia, necrosis and mitotic activity with grade 1/well differentiated equating to low-grade, and, grade 2/moderate and grade 3/poor differentiation to high-grade.

Low-grade/high-grade. Some lesions define their own grade by way of their inherent clinical behaviour:
- *Low-grade*: well differentiated liposarcoma, dermatofibrosarcoma protuberans, well differ-

entiated chondrosarcoma, angiomatoid malignant fibrous histiocytoma.
- *High-grade*: Ewing's sarcoma/PNET, rhabdomyosarcoma (except spindle cell and botryoid types), angiosarcoma, pleomorphic liposarcoma, osteosarcoma (medullary and soft tissue), mesenchymal chondrosarcoma, desmoplastic small round cell tumour, malignant fibrous histiocytoma.

Others are allocated a grading score (synovial sarcoma (3), extraskeletal myxoid chondrosarcoma (2)), or, are not graded but are potentially metastatic and usually regarded as high-grade: clear cell sarcoma, alveolar soft part sarcoma, epithelioid sarcoma.

Grading can be prognostically useful in adult soft tissue spindle cell sarcomas: leiomyosarcoma, fibrosarcoma.

Grading (Fédération Nationale des Centres de Lutte Contre le Cancer (FNCLCC)).

Scores		
Differentiation		
Well	1	Sarcoma closely resembling adult mesenchymal tissue e.g. well differentiated liposarcoma.
Moderate	2	Sarcoma of certain histological type e.g. myxoid liposaroma.
Poor	3	Embryonal and undifferentiated sarcomas and sarcomas of uncertain type e.g. synovial sarcoma.
Necrosis		
None	1	
≤50 %	2	
>50 %	3	
Mitoses/10HPFs		
0–9	1	
10–19	2	
≥20	3	

HPF, high power field (×40 objective in the most proliferative area of the tumour).

Grade 1 = ≤3
Grade 2 = 4 or 5
Grade 3 = ≥6

A *Ki-67 index* can give complementary information to the mitotic count and may have some predictive value in grade 2/3 tumours. *Up to 75 % of sarcomas are high-grade histological type and malignancy.*

Histological differentiation or grade can be heterogeneous within a tumour e.g. juxtaposition of well differentiated and dedifferentiated chondrosarcoma or liposarcoma. The less differentiated component is chosen for grading purposes.

Preoperative adjuvant therapy can lead to quite extensive necrosis and changes in morphology potentially *invalidating grading criteria* on the resection specimen. In sarcomas the degree of *histological tumour response* can be graded from I (no effect identified) to IV (no viable tumour noted). A *90–97 % response (III)* is a target standard of *favourable prognostic significance* e.g. in osteosarcoma chemotherapy induced necrosis of >90 or <90 % can result in disease free survival figures of >90 and <50 % respectively. Note that treatment effects (necrosis or fibrosis) cannot be reliably distinguished from spontaneous tumour necrosis or degeneration. A majority of paediatric soft tissue sarcomas are treated chemotherapeutically while surgical excision is used in most adolescent and adult patients. High-grade tumours benefit from a combination of *local surgical control and systemic therapy.*

36.4 Extent of Local Tumour Spread

Border: pushing/infiltrative.

Lymphocytic reaction: prominent/sparse.

Lymphatics/vessels/nerves including the proximal limit.

Single/more than one anatomical compartment e.g. skin/subcutaneous tissue, fascial/subfascial tissue, or more than one anatomical plane.

Soft Tissue Sarcoma

The TNM7 classification applies to alveolar soft part sarcoma, epithelioid sarcoma, extraskeletal chondrosarcoma/osteosarcoma/Ewing's/PNET, fibrosarcoma, leiomyosarcoma, liposarcoma, malignant fibrous histiocytoma, malignant

haemangiopericytoma, malignant mesenchymoma, malignant peripheral nerve sheath tumour, rhabdomyosarcoma, synovial sarcoma and sarcoma, not otherwise specified. The following are excluded: angiosarcoma, Kaposi's sarcoma, dermatofibrosarcoma protuberans, fibromatosis and sarcomas arising from dura mater, brain, hollow viscera or parenchymatous organs except breast. Uterine sarcoma has a separate specific FIGO staging scheme.

pT1	Tumour ≤5 cm in greatest dimension
	(a) Superficial
	(b) Deep
pT2	Tumour >5 cm in greatest dimension
	(a) Superficial
	(b) Deep

Superficial tumour is located exclusively above the superficial fascia. *Deep tumour* is located either exclusively beneath the superficial fascia (Fig. 36.1) or superficial to the fascia with invasion of or through the fascia. Retroperitoneal, intraperitoneal, visceral, paratesticular, noncutaneous major head and neck, mediastinal and pelvic sarcomas are deep.

Stage grouping also incorporates histological grade: localised non-metastatic lesions are stage I (low-grade) or II (high-grade). Stage III is localised, high-grade pT2b cancers, and stage IV metastatic disease of any pT or histological grade.

Bone Sarcoma

The TNM7 classification applies to all primary malignant bone tumours except malignant lymphomas, multiple myeloma, surface/juxtacortical osteosarcoma, and juxtacortical chondrosarcoma

pT1	Tumour ≤8 cm in greatest dimension
pT2	Tumour >8 cm in greatest dimension
pT3	Discontinuous tumours in the primary bone site
pM1a	Lung metastasis
pM1b	Other distant sites

See Fig. 36.1

Metastasis in another bone is classified as distant metastasis.

Fig. 36.1 Sarcoma (Reproduced, with permission, from Allen (2006), © 2006)

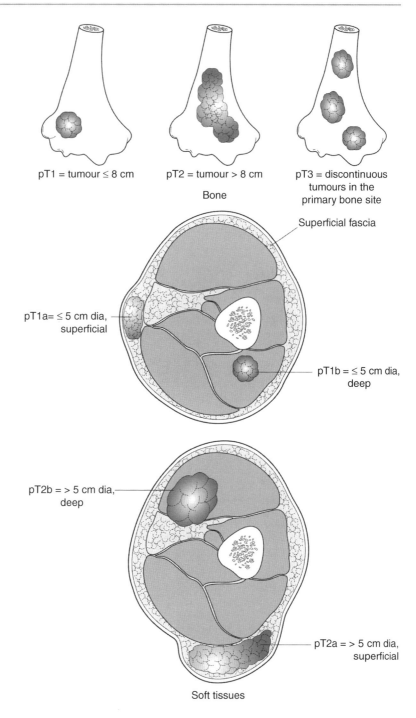

For pT1/pT2 optional descriptors are:

1. Beyond cortex to periosteum
2. Beyond periosteum to surrounding soft tissues
3. With extension to major vessels or nerves.

Stage grouping also incorporates histological grade: localised non-metastatic pT1/pT2 lesions are either stage I (low-grade) or II (high-grade), and pT3 cancers are stage III (any grade). Stage IV is nodal or metastatic disease of any pT or histological grade.

Many surgeons use the Enneking staging system: low-grade tumour (stage I) and high-grade tumour (stage II) which is either intracompartmental (A) or extracompartmental (B). Metastatic disease regardless of histological grade is stage III.

36.5 Lymphovascular Invasion

Present/absent.
　　Intra-/extratumoural.

36.6 Lymph Nodes

Site/number/size/number involved/limit node/
extracapsular spread.
　　Regional nodes: those appropriate to the site of
the primary tumour. Regional lymph node involvement is rare and cases in which lymph node status
is not assessed are considered N0 instead of NX.

pN0	No regional lymph node metastasis
pN1	Metastasis in regional lymph node(s).

　　Lymph node metastases are unusual with the
commonest mode of spread being *haematogenous*
resulting in pulmonary secondaries. Some sarcomas e.g. angiosarcoma, epithelioid sarcoma and
synovial sarcoma, may show lymph node spread.
Alveolar rhabdomyosarcoma can present in lymph
nodes or bone marrow as clinical lymphadenopathy
or erythroleucocytopaenia, and mimicking haematological malignancy or disseminated carcinoma.

36.7 Excision Margins

Distance (mm) to the nearest painted excision
margin.
　　Margins are superficial/deep, proximal/distal,
medial/lateral and can be an anatomical structure
e.g. fascia or periosteum. Resection can be *intrale-
sional or intracapsular* (within the tumour capsule
and submitted in fragments), *marginal* (through the
inflammatory tissue surrounding the tumour), *wide*
(with a cuff of normal tissue) or *radical* in extent.
The latter involves removal of the tumour and its
related compartment of soft tissues, with or without
the underlying bone, or amputation to include the
joint proximal to the tumour. Neoadjuvant chemotherapy with limb salvage surgery is used increasingly for various bone sarcomas.
　　A surgical margin clearance of <15–20 mm in
soft tissue sarcoma has an *increased risk of local*
recurrence unless further surgery or radiotherapy
is undertaken. This risk may be less if the margin
is bound by a fascial plane. For high-grade
tumour an even wider margin (20–50 mm) may
be desirable.

36.8 Other Pathology

Prostheses: allied to limb salvage surgery following wide local excision with preoperative neoadjuvant therapy.

　　Radio-/chemotherapy changes: necrosis/
inflammation and fibrosis in the primary tumour.
Similar changes are seen in metastases and also
tissue maturation phenomenon e.g. pulmonary
metastases of osteosarcoma resulting in nodules
of paucicellular osteoid.

　　Predisposing factors to sarcoma: Paget's disease of bone, childhood chemotherapy, prior irradiation, and some metallic orthopaedic surgical
implants can predispose to osteosarcoma.

　　Needle core biopsy and/or FNAC: can allow
categorization of soft tissue masses into benign
and malignant lesions in a majority of cases.
They can also exclude diagnoses such as *metastatic carcinoma, malignant lymphoma, multiple
myeloma and malignant melanoma* allowing a
more focused approach to the diagnosis of sarcoma. However, the pathologist must be aware of
the potential for sampling error with regard to
heterogeneity in tumour type and grade, and the
latter should only be commented on if it is high-
grade. The use of preoperative needle biopsy
with neoadjuvant treatment can impose limitations on the prognostic information in the resection e.g. necrosis induced by adjuvant therapy
invalidates traditional grading criteria.

Immunophenotype

Immunohistochemical markers can be applied to
formalin fixed paraffin embedded tissue to demonstrate a range of epithelial, neural, muscular, vascular and other mesenchymal antigens. They not only
reflect *cell lineage* (cytokeratins, EMA, desmin,
h-caldesmon, smooth muscle actin, S100, myoD1,
myogenin, CD31, CD34) but also protein expression

as a marker of *molecular changes* (TLE-1, INI 1, MDM2, CDK4). None is totally specific or sensitive, indicating that an assimilation of results (including negative ones) from a *panel of antibodies* is necessary. However for some soft tissue sarcomas a positive immunohistochemical profile is part of the definition of the tumour e.g. rhabdomyosarcomas, epithelioid sarcoma, clear cell sarcoma, desmoplastic small round cell tumour, and GISTs (gastrointestinal stromal tumours). It is also of use in diagnosing synovial sarcomas, undifferentiated retroperitoneal sarcomas and malignant vascular tumours. Metastatic carcinoma or malignant melanoma can be confidently excluded. Furthermore additional prognostic information can be given e.g. myogenic differentiation in a pleomorphic sarcoma, and strong myogenin expression in a rhabdomyosarcoma are adverse.

Antibody	Use
Cytokeratins	Synovial/epithelioid sarcoma
EMA	Synovial/epithelioid sarcoma
Desmin, myoD1, myogenin	Rhabdomyosarcoma
Desmin, h-caldesmon, smooth muscle actin	Leiomyosarcoma
Smooth muscle actin	Fibroblastic/myofibroblastic lesions
S100 protein	Malignant peripheral nerve sheath tumour, adipocytic and cartilaginous differentiation, clear cell sarcoma, synovial sarcoma.
CD99 (MIC-2), Fli-1	Ewing's sarcoma (plus PAS for glycogen)
CD99, TLE-1	Synovial sarcoma
DOG-1, CD117	GIST
INI 1	Epithelioid vascular tumours
Factor VIII, CD 31, CD 34	Angiosarcoma, epithelioid haemangioendothelioma
CD 34	Dermatofibrosarcoma, epithelioid sarcoma, solitary fibrous tumour (also CD99, bcl-2)
HMB-45	Clear cell sarcoma, PEComa.
HHV8	Kaposi's sarcoma
WT1	Desmoplastic small round cell tumour. It is also polyimmuno-phenotypic: cytokeratins/EMA/desmin and chromogranin/synaptophysin.
MDM2, CDK4	Atypical lipoma/liposarcoma
Bcatenin	Deep fibromatoses
ALK-1	Inflammatory myofibroblastic tumour

Chromosomal Analysis

Chromosomal analysis has gained increasing importance in *classification*, *prognosis* and *choice of treatment for a range of sarcomas* e.g. Ewing's sarcoma, PNET, synovial sarcoma, alveolar rhabdomyosarcoma, and desmoplastic small round cell tumour. Distinct molecular changes can warrant specific targeted therapy in dermatofibrosarcoma protuberans. Fresh tissue in a suitable transport medium was previously required for tissue culture although *reverse transcriptase polymerase chain reaction (RT-PCR) techniques* have been developed and are routinely used on formalin fixed, paraffin embedded tissue for most investigations. Examples are given in the Introduction, Tables 4 and 5.

Prognosis

Prognosis in soft tissue sarcomas relates to:
- Tumour size: >5 cm diameter.
- Grade: low-grade vs high-grade.
- Stage.
- Histological type.
- Site: superficial vs deep extremity vs retroperitoneum.
- Age: >50 years
- Adequacy of surgery.

The importance of excision margins is emphasised in soft tissue sarcomas where negative and positive margins in low-grade lesions are associated with 5 year recurrence rates of 2 and 28 % respectively. Current treatment of soft tissue sarcomas is wide monobloc resection with postoperative adjuvant radiotherapy to the operative site of high-grade lesions. With modern surgical techniques and adjuvant chemo-/radiotherapy average 5 year survival figures for soft tissue and bone based sarcomas are 70–80 %. *Prognosis varies with tumour stage, completeness of excision, histological type*, e.g. chondrosarcoma is better than osteosarcoma (60 %), and *grade*: grade I chondrosarcoma (78 %) vs grade III (22 %), myxoid liposarcoma (75 %) vs round cell (28 %), embryonal (botryoid/spindle cell: 85–95 %) vs alveolar (53 %) rhabdomyosarcoma. Grade of *response to preoperative chemotherapy* is also a very important indicator. Surgical excision of pulmonary metastases (20 % of sarcomas) is also helpful.

36.9   Other Malignancy

Metastatic carcinoma, malignant melanoma, malignant lymphoma (primary or secondary), multiple myeloma and leukaemia can all mimic soft tissue or bone sarcoma and immunohistochemical markers will be required to make these distinctions. *Malignant lymphoma* is usually of high-grade B cell type, solitary but occasionally multifocal. The cells are CD45/CD 20 positive with large irregular, multilobated nuclei. Fibrosis is present in 50 % of cases giving spindle cell (mimicking sarcoma) or compartmentalised (mimicking metastatic carcinoma) appearances. A minority are CD 30 positive with cytological features of anaplastic lymphoma and aggressive behaviour. *Metastatic carcinoma* to bone may be osteolytic (breast, lung, thyroid, renal) leading to pathological fracture or osteoblastic (prostate) in character. It can be focal or diffuse resulting in a leucoerythroblastic blood picture and extramedullary haemopoiesis. Rarely the bone marrow can show a granulomatous response as an indicator of micrometastasis (e.g. infiltrating lobular carcinoma of breast) which can be demonstrated by immunohistochemistry. Certain carcinomas tend to a preferred pattern of bone metastases e.g. thyroid carcinoma goes to shoulder girdle, skull, ribs and sternum. Metastatic disease is usually to the axial skeleton and rarely to the hands and feet.

Carcinoma

- Cytokeratins, CEA, EMA.

Malignant Melanoma

- S100, HMB-45, melan-A.

Leukaemia/Myeloid Sarcoma (Chloroma)

- CD34, CD43, CD68, CD117, myeloperoxidase, chloroacetate esterase, neutrophil elastase, tdt.

Multiple Myeloma

- CD138, κ/λ light chain restriction.

Specific Markers

- Thyroglobulin/TTF-1 (thyroid), CK7/TTF-1/napsin-A (lung adenocarcinoma), PSA (polyclonal)/PSAP (prostate), CA125 (ovary), ER/PR/GCDFP-15 (breast), SALL4/OCT3/4/PLAP/AFP/βHCG/CD 30/glypican-3 (germ cell tumours).

36.10   Comments on Retroperitoneum

The retroperitoneum contains the kidneys, adrenal glands, ureters, aorta, inferior vena cava, vessel tributaries, lymph nodes, nerve plexuses and autonomic ganglia. Due to its inaccessible anatomical location *tumours can attain a considerable size* before clinical presentation with *vague symptomatology*, or because of *pressure effects on adjacent structures* e.g. ureter. Investigation is by CT scan supplemented by ultrasound and MRI scan as appropriate. Arteriography may be used if resection of a large tumour is planned. Tissue diagnosis is by percutaneous CT guided needle core biopsy or FNAC. The commonest malignancies are periaortic lymphadenopathy due to nodal *malignant lymphoma* (diffuse large B cell lymphoma, follicular lymphoma or chronic lymphocytic leukaemia/lymphocytic lymphoma), or *metastatic disease* (testicular germ cell tumours, gastrointestinal, prostate, bladder, pancreatic or gynecological cancers). The need for a tissue diagnosis is determined by the availability of previous data, the nature and stage of the disease process at which the lymphadenopathy has arisen, and any further planned therapeutic management. Various clinical situations are: frozen section as a prequel to radical urological or gynaecological resection, needle core biopsy to establish a diagnosis, type and grade of malignant lymphoma, or, imaging with serum tumour markers to indicate surgery or radio-/chemotherapy in a patient with known prior testicular germ cell tumour. Kidney, germ cell and adrenal gland tumours are dealt with in their respective sections but primary tumours include:

Liposarcoma: especially well differentiated and sclerosing subtypes. Can attain a huge size encasing other structures and can be difficult to completely excise. May contain an aggressive and potentially metastatic dedifferentiated element comprising an abrupt junction between adipocytic tumour and high-grade spindle cell sarcoma.

Leiomyosarcoma: arising from the wall of the inferior vena cava or its tributaries and prone to cystic change when large. Tumour necrosis and size >10 cm are strong pointers to malignancy even if of low mitotic rate.

Malignant fibrous histiocytoma: exclude this pattern as an anaplastic component of other sarcomas (commonly liposarcoma), and also sarcomatoid renal cell or pelviureteric urothelial carcinoma.

Peripheral nerve tumours: neurilemmoma, neurofibroma, malignant peripheral nerve sheath tumours, paraganglioma, ganglioneuroma, neuroblastoma. Neurilemmoma (Schwannoma) can be large, cystic and show significant cytological atypia mimicking a sarcoma. Nuclear palisading and thickened hyalinised vessels are useful diagnostic pointers.

Ewing's sarcoma/PNET, rhabdomyosarcoma, desmoplastic small round cell tumour: usually in the abdominopelvic regions of children and young adults. Initial chemotherapy is more appropriate but may be supplemented by surgery which is the main modality in the other sarcoma types.

Resection specimens: can be large and complex with structures such as the kidney enveloped by tumour. For TNM7 staging purposes retroperitoneum is a deep structure. Due to the late presentation and difficulties in obtaining complete excision of retroperitoneal soft tissue sarcomas they have a *poor prognosis* with an *overall 25 % 5 year survival*. An operative wedge biopsy may be taken from non-resectable tumour if needle core biopsy has been inconclusive. Paraaortic lymphadenectomy is commonly performed for cervical cancer, high-grade endometrial cancer, radical prostatectomy, and cystectomy for urothelial cancer. Retroperitoneal lymph node dissection (RPLND) in testicular germ cell tumour is discussed in Chap. 33.

36.11 Comments on Adrenal Gland

Metastatic carcinoma in the adrenal gland, particularly from lung, breast and kidney, is *commoner than a primary neoplasm* and usually detected by CT scan during post surgical follow up. Adrenal gland is the fourth commonest site for metastatic carcinoma after lungs, liver and bone. Sometimes CT guided needle core biopsy or FNAC is used to make this distinction and to avoid progressing to surgical excision.

Otherwise, primary adrenal neoplasms variably present either as *an abdominal mass*, *an asymptomatic or incidental radiological mass* ("*incidentaloma*"), or are characterised by their *endocrinological symptoms and signs* and resultant *biochemical profiles*. Appropriate investigations include

- Serum cortisols, sodium and aldosterone: for an adrenocortical lesion
- 24 h urinary catecholamines: for an adrenal medullary lesion

Up to 20 % of adrenal mass lesions causing abnormal hormone secretion are without attendant clinical symptoms. *Some 80% are non-functioning adenomas* and they are usually <5 cm in size. *Phaeochromocytoma is a contraindication to biopsy* due to the risk of a catecholamine induced hypertensive crisis. CT/MRI scans can assess the size, characteristics and bilaterality of adrenal lesions helping to distinguish *hyperplasia* (secondary to hyperpituitarism and usually bilateral) from *adenoma* (usually solitary). However they are poor at designating benignity from malignancy apart from on the basis of size. *Adrenal carcinoma* cells are often dysfunctional or produce mixed hormonal effects, and the tumour reaches a significant size (*most are >5 cm/50–100 g*) before presentation. The best histological indicators of malignancy are *mitoses* (>5 cm/50 HPFs), *diffuse growth pattern, necrosis, fibrous bands* and *vascular invasion*, criteria that are used in the *modified Weiss scoring system*. The Ki-67 index is usually 5–20 %. However it can be difficult to distinguish an adenoma from a well differentiated adenocarcinoma and the term *adrenocortical neoplasm* may be used qualified by a morphological assessment of its likelihood to recur.

Spread of adrenal carcinoma is to lymph nodes, liver and lung sometimes with local retroperitoneal invasion into kidney and inferior vena cava. Nonfunctioning small (<5 cm) cortical lesions may be monitored by serial radiological CT scans. Otherwise, treatment is aimed at *complete local excision* which may be laparoscopic for small lesions but an open thoracoabdominal approach for a larger tumour. Note that laparoscopic specimens may be submitted as fragments making histological assessment of indicators for malignancy difficult. Capsular and any attached adrenal vein tissues should be sought and examined for tumour involvement or thrombosis. Overall *adrenal carcinoma* has a *35–65 % 5 year survival*.

Characteristic hormonal effects of adrenal cortical tumours are hypercortisolism (Cushing's syndrome), hyperaldosteronism (Conn's syndrome) and virilisation. Chest x-ray and CT chest examinations should also be done to exclude the possibility of a primary lung small cell carcinoma as a source of *ectopic ACTH* (adrenocorticotrophic hormone) causing bilateral adrenal cortical hyperplasia and a *paraneoplastic syndrome*.

Phaeochromocytoma is medullary in location, 3–5 cm in diameter and 75–150 g in weight, or larger, with a pale to tan coloured cut surface. It is usually unilateral and solitary, but if bilateral and multicentric can be associated with MEN2 A/2B, von Hippel Lindau disease and neurofibromatosis. Similar extra-adrenal paragangliomas are found elsewhere along sympathetic/parasympathetic nervous system sites in the retroperitoneum, mediastinum, carotid body, middle ear and urinary bladder. They have variable secretory capacity and functionality e.g. chemodectomatous head and neck paragangliomas. Radioisotope (MIBG) scan has a role to play in their detection. Adrenal phaeochromocytoma has a characteristic nested "Zellballen" pattern its cells secreting catecholamines and inducing paroxysmal symptoms of flushing, sweating, tachycardia, tremor and hypertension. *Surgical excision requires careful control of blood pressure to avoid a hypertensive crisis. Overall survival is 50 % with 10 % bilateral or extra-adrenal or malignant.* Malignant behaviour cannot be predicted histologically with metastases being the only reliable criterion. Spread is usually to lymph nodes, then the axial skeleton, liver, lung and kidney. Some morphological indicators of malignancy are: coarse cellular nodules, confluent necrosis, spindle cells, mitoses >3/10HPFs, abnormal mitoses, capsular and vascular invasion.

Neuroblastoma and ganglioneuroblastoma are characteristically seen in infants and children and are not further considered.

Immunophenotype of Adrenal Neoplasms

- *Adrenal carcinoma*: positive for cytokeratins (variable), vimentin, synaptophysin, inhibin, melan-A. CEA negative. Variable Ki-67 (MIB 1) proliferation index. Strong positivity for cytokeratin, EMA and CD10 would favour metastatic renal clear cell carcinoma, one of its main differential diagnoses.
- *Phaeochromocytoma*: positive for catecholamines, chromogranin, synaptophysin, neurofilament, cytokeratins (±) and intervening S100 positive sustentacular cells.

TMN7 Stage of Adrenal Cortical Carcinoma

pT1	Tumour confined to adrenal gland and ≤5 cm in greatest dimension
pT2	Tumour confined to adrenal gland and >5 cm in greatest dimension
pT3	Tumour of any size, locally invasive but not involving adjacent organs
pT4	Tumour of any size with invasion of adjacent organs: kidney, diaphragm, great vessels, pancreas and liver.
pN0	No regional lymph node metastasis
pN1	Metastasis in regional lymph node (s)

Other adrenal malignancy includes malignant lymphoma and malignant melanoma usually secondary to disseminated disease. Occasional benign lesions are ganglioneuroma, adrenal cysts, adenomatoid tumour and myelolipoma.

Bibliography

Allen DC. Histopathology reporting: guidelines for surgical cancer. 2nd ed. London: Springer; 2006.

Al-Nafussi A. Practical morphological approach to the diagnosis and differential diagnosis of soft tissue sarcomas. Curr Diagn Pathol. 2002;8:395–411.

Antonescu CR. The role of genetic testing in soft tissue sarcoma. Histopathology. 2006;48:13–21.

Athanasou NA. Colour atlas of bone, joint and soft tissue pathology. Oxford: Oxford University Press; 1999.

Brenn T, Fletcher CDM. Postradiation vascular proliferations: an increasing problem. Histopathology. 2006;48:106–14.

Bullough PG. Orthopaedic pathology. 5th ed. St Louis: Mosby Elsevier; 2010.

Coffin CM, Lowichik A, Zhou H. Treatment effects in paediatric soft tissue and bone tumors. Am J Clin Pathol. 2005;123:75–90.

Costa J, Wesley RA, Glatstein E, Rosenberg SA. The grading of soft tissue sarcomas. Results of a clinico-histopathologic correlation in a series of 163 cases. Cancer. 1984;53:530–41.

Coindre J-M, Trojani M, Contesso G, David M, Rouesse J, Bui NB, Bodaert A, de Mascarel I, de Mascarel A, Goussot JF. Reproducibility of a histopathogic grading system for adult soft tissue sarcoma. Cancer. 1986;58:306–9.

Coindre JM. Immunohistochemistry in the diagnosis of soft tissue tumours. Histopathology. 2003;43:1–16.

Dei Tos AP. Classification of pleomorphic sarcomas: where are we now? Histopathology. 2006;48:51–62.

Deyrup AT, Weiss SW. Grading of soft tissue sarcomas: the challenge of providing precise information in an imprecise world. Histopathology. 2006;48:42–50.

Dorfman HD, Czerniak B. Bone tumors. St Louis: Mosby Wolfe; 1998.

Fechner RE, Mills SE. Tumors of the bones and joints. 3rd series. Fascicle 8. Washington, DC: AFIP; 1993.

Fisher C. The comparative roles of electron microscopy and immunohistochemistry in the diagnosis of soft tissue tumours. Histopathology. 2006;48:32–41.

Fisher C. Immunohistochemistry in diagnosis of soft tissue tumours. Histopathology. 2011;58:1001–12.

Fisher C, Montgomery E. Biopsy interpretation of soft tissue tumours. Philadelphia: Lippincott, Williams and Wilkins; 2010.

Fletcher CDM. The evolving classification of soft tissue tumour: an update based on the new WHO classification. Histopathology. 2006;48:3–12.

Fletcher CDM, Unni K, Mertens F. WHO classification of tumours. Pathology and genetics. Tumours of soft tissue and bone. Lyon: IARC Press; 2002.

Gleason BC, Hornick JL. Inflammatory myofibroblastic tumours: where are we now? J Clin Pathol. 2008;61:428–37.

Guillou L. Pleomorphic sarcomas: subclassification, myogenic differentiation and prognosis. Diagn Histopathol. 2008;14:527–37.

Hahn HP, Fletcher CDM. The role of cytogenetics and molecular genetics in soft tissue tumour diagnosis – a realistic approach. Curr Diagn Pathol. 2005;11:361–70.

Holloway P, Kay E, Leader M. Myxoid tumours: a guide to the morphological and immunohistochemical assessment of soft tissue myxoid lesions encountered in general surgical pathology. Curr Diagn Pathol. 2005;11:411–25.

Hornick JL, Fletcher CDM. PEComa: what do we know so far? Histopathology. 2006;48:75–82.

Kempson RL, Fletcher CDM, Evans HL, Hendrickson MR, Sibley RK. Tumors of the soft tissues. 3rd series: Fascicle 30. Washington: AFIP; 2001.

McCarthy EF, Frassica FJ. Pathology of bone and joint disorders. Philadelphia: Saunders; 1998.

Miettinen MM. Diagnostic soft tissue pathology. New York: Churchill Livingstone; 2003.

Miettinen M, Fetsch JF. Evaluation of biological potential of smooth muscle tumours. Histopathology. 2006;48:97–105.

Mirra JM, Picci P, Gold RH. Bone tumours: clinical, radiological and pathological correlations. Baltimore: Lea and Febiger; 1989.

Nascimento AF. Rhabdomyosarcomas in adults: classification and differential diagnosis. Diagn Histopathol. 2008;14:538–45.

Pfeifer JD, Hill DA, O'Sullivan MJ, Dehner LP. Diagnostic gold standard for soft tissue tumours: morphology or molecular genetics? Histopathology. 2000;37:485–500.

Pringle JAS. Osteosarcoma: the experiences of a specialist unit. Curr Diagn Pathol. 1996;3:127–36.

Rossi S, Laurino L, Dei Tos AP. Desmoid-type fibromatosis: from morphology to molecular genetics. Diagn Histopathol. 2008;14:546–51.

Rossi S, Nascimento AG, Canal F, Dei Tos AP. Small round-cell neoplasms of soft tissues: an integrated diagnostic approach. Curr Diagn Pathol. 2007;13:150–63.

Sinha H, Peach AHS. Diagnosis and management of soft tissue sarcoma. BMJ. 2011a;342:157–62.

The Royal College of Pathologists. Cancer Datasets (Primary Bone Tumours, Soft Tissue Sarcomas) and Tissue Pathways (Bone and Soft Tissue Pathology). Accessed at http://www.rcpath.org/index.asp?PageID=254.

Unni KK, Inwards CY. Dahlin's bone tumors. 6th ed. Philadelphia: Lippincott, Williams and Wilkins; 2010.

Unni KK, Inwards CY, Bridge JA, Kindblom LG, Wold LE. Tumors of the bones and joints. AFIP atlas of tumor pathology. Series 4. Fascicle 8. Washington: AFIP; 2004.

Weiss SW, Goldblum SR. Enzinger and Weiss's soft tissue tumors. 5th ed. St Louis: Mosby; 2007.

West RB, van de Rijn M. The role of microarray technologies in the study of soft tissue tumours. Histopathology. 2006;48:22–31.

Retroperitoneum

Cullen MH, Stenning SP, Parkinson MC, Fossa SD, Kaye SB, Horwich AH, et al. Short-course adjuvant chemotherapy in high-risk stage I non-seminomatous germ cell tumors of the testis: a Medical Research Council report. J Clin Oncol. 1996;14:1106–13.

Parkinson MC, Harland SJ, Harnden P, Sandison A. The role of the histopathologist in the management of testicular germ cell tumour in adults. Histopathology. 2001;38:183–94.

Rosai J. Chapter 26. Peritoneum, retroperitoneum and related structures. In: Rosai J, editor. Rosai and Ackerman's surgical pathology. 10th ed. Edinburgh: Elsevier; 2011.

Sinha S, Peach AHS. Diagnosis and management of soft tissue sarcoma. BMJ. 2011b;342:157–62.

Stenning SP, Parkinson MC, Fisher C, Mead GM, Cook PA, Fossa SD, et al. Postchemotherapy residual masses in germ cell tumor patients: content, clinical features, and prognosis. Medical Research Council Testicular Tumour Working Party. Cancer. 1998;83:1409–19.

Adrenal Gland

DeLellis RA, Lloyd RV, Heitz PU, Eng C. WHO classification of tumours. Pathology and genetics. Tumours of endocrine organs. Lyon: IARC Press; 2004.

Hunt JL. Syndromes associated with abnormalities in the adrenal cortex. Diagn Histopathol. 2009;15:69–78.

Komminoth P, Perren A, van Nederveen FH, de Krijger RR. Familial endocrine tumours: phaeochromocytomas and extra-adrenal paragangliomas. Diagn Histopathol. 2009;15:61–8.

Lester SC. Chapter 11. Adrenal glands. In: Manual of surgical pathology. 3rd ed. Philadelphia: Elsevier/Saunders; 2010. p. 227–36.

McLean K, Lillenfeld H, Carracciolo JT, Hoffe S, Tourtelot JB, Carter WB. Management of isolated adrenal lesions in cancer patients. Cancer Control. 2011;18:113–25.

McNicol AM. Update on tumours of the adrenal cortex, phaeochromocytoma and extra-adrenal paraganglioma. Histopathology. 2011;58:155–68.

Singh PK, Buch HN. Adrenal incidentaloma: evaluation and management. J Clin Pathol. 2008;61:1168–73.

Stephenson TJ. Prognostic and predictive factors in endocrine tumours. Histopathology. 2006;48:629–43.

The Royal College of Pathologists. Cancer Datasets (Adrenal Cortical Carcinoma and Malignant Phaeochromocytoma/paraganglioma, Peripheral Neuroblastic Tumours) and Tissue Pathways for Endocrine Pathology. Accessed at http://www.rcpath.org/index.asp?PageID=254.

Volante M, Bollito E, Sperone P, Tavaglione V, Daffara F, Porpiglia F, Terzolo M, Berruti A, Pappoti M. Clinicopathological study of a series of 92 adrenocortical carcinomas: from a proposal of simplified diagnostic algorithm to prognostic stratification. Histopathology. 2009;55:535–43.

Volante M, Buttigliero C, Greco E, Berruti A, Pappoti M. Pathological and molecular features of adrenocortical carcinoma: an update. J Clin Pathol. 2008;61: 787–93.

Westra WH, Hruban RH, Phelps TH, Isacson C. Chapter 38. Adrenal glands. In: Surgical pathology dissection: an illustrated guide. 2nd ed. New York: Springer; 2003.

Part X

Ophthalmic Cancer

- Intraocular Malignancy
- Extraocular Malignancy

Ocular malignancy usually presents as an alteration in visual acuity and is rarely aspirated or biopsied due to potential tumour seeding. Occasionally, in the context of an appropriate clinical history, fine needle aspiration cytology (FNAC) is used for a solid intraocular tumour to distinguish between a primary tumour and metastatic carcinoma. Unless small and anteroequatorial, when a sight sparing local resection may be considered, treatment is usually by enucleation (removal of the globe with a short piece of optic nerve), or exenteration if significant extraocular spread is present. Exenteration is more usually reserved for extraocular malignancy e.g. of the eyelids and orbital contents.

37.1   Gross Description

Specimen

- FNAC/sectoral iridectomy/endoresection/ local resection of ciliary body and choroid/ evisceration/enucleation/exenteration.
- Weight (g).
- Anteroposterior, horizontal and vertical dimensions (cm).
  Length of optic nerve (mm).

Tumour

Site
- Bulbar conjunctiva/sclera/cornea: malignant melanoma, malignant lymphoma, squamous cell carcinoma.

- Iris/ciliary body/choroid: uveal melanoma.
- Retina/optic nerve: retinoblastoma.
- Anterior chamber/posterior chamber: posterior or equatorial – superior, inferior, lateral. Posterior lesions are of better prognosis than equatorial as they interfere with visual acuity and present earlier, whereas the latter can attain a larger size with potential for involvement of vessels in the sclera and Schlemm's canal. Iris malignant melanoma has a much lower mortality (10 % that of other uveal melanomas) due to earlier clinical presentation.

Size
- Length × width × depth (mm), but in particular maximum tumour thickness and scleral basal diameter (mm).

Appearance
- Nodular/plaque/diffuse/multicentric/pigmented/non-pigmented/haemorrhage/necrosis/calcification (retinoblastoma).

Edge
- Circumscribed/irregular.

37.2   Histological Type

Malignant Melanoma

- 80 % in the choroid and it is the commonest intraocular malignancy in adults. It elevates and detaches the overlying retina.

D.C. Allen, *Histopathology Reporting*,
DOI 10.1007/978-1-4471-5263-7_37, © Springer-Verlag London 2013

Retinoblastoma

- <3 years of age and 40 % familial, of which 90 % are multifocal and bilateral; retinoblastoma suppressor gene (Rb) 13q14 deletion. Also predisposes to risk of a subsequent second neoplasm, e.g. thyroid carcinoma in the treated radiotherapy field, or at other body sites e.g. osteosarcoma.

Metastatic Carcinoma

- Breast, lung, gastrointestinal tract (stomach).
- 10 % incidence at autopsy in disseminated carcinomatosis.
- Posterior choroid is the commonest site.

Leukaemia/Malignant Lymphoma

- 50 % of leukaemia patients at autopsy (infiltration and/or haemorrhage).
- Malignant lymphoma is usually secondary to extraocular disease.

Rare

- Medulloepithelioma, glioma, meningioma of optic nerve.

37.3   Differentiation

Malignant Melanoma

- *Spindle cell*: *better prognosis*
  - Slender cells, indistinct nucleolus, longitudinal fold in the nuclear membrane (spindle cell type A)
  - Nucleolar enlargement (spindle cell type B) is an adverse prognostic sign.
- *Epithelioid cell*: *worse prognosis*
- *Mixed (50%)*: defined as >10 % epithelioid cells and <90 % spindle cells. Small tumours tend to be spindle cell in morphology, and

large tumours spindle cell B and/or epithelioid in character.
- S100, HMB-45, melan-A positive, ± CAM 5.2.

Retinoblastoma

- Small round cells with basophilic nuclei and scant cytoplasm, calcification, mitoses and Homer Wright rosettes.
- Well differentiated: fleurettes and Flexner-Wintersteiner rosettes.
- Poorly differentiated: vascular pseudo-palisading necrosis, mitoses, apoptosis, and absence of rosettes.
- S100, NSE, synaptophysin, GFAP positive, high Ki-67 index.

37.4   Extent of Local Tumour Spread

Border: pushing/infiltrative.
Lymphocytic reaction: prominent/sparse.
Intraocular: ciliary body, iris, anterior chamber.
Transscleral/extrascleral spread: depth (mm).
Optic nerve invasion.

Uveal Melanoma of Choroid and Ciliary Body

TNM7 classification according to four size categories taking into account *maximum tumour thickness*, *scleral basal diameter*, and the presence and extent of *ciliary body* and *extraocular extension*. In clinical practice size is more accurately determined by fundus photography and high frequency ultrasound. Post fixation histology specimens are subject to tumour shrinkage and underestimation of dimensions. For further details related to tumour size see 8. Other pathology. Extraocular extension is diagnosed if the tumour grows outside the bulb with invasion of the orbit (commonest), optic nerve, outer eye muscles, lacrimal apparatus or conjunctiva. There is a tendency for *spread along the optic nerve with metastases to liver, lung, bone and skin.*

Retinoblastoma

- In bilateral cases the eyes are classified separately. The classification does not apply to complete spontaneous regression of the tumour.
- Endophytic, exophytic (subretinal) or retinal spread.
- TNM7 classifies retinoblastoma based on whether the tumour is confined to the eye with no optic nerve or choroidal invasion (pT1), shows minimal (pT2) or significant (pT3) optic nerve/choroidal invasion, or, optic nerve resection line/extraocular extension (pT4). There is a tendency for *spread along the optic nerve into subarachnoid fluid and brain with metastases to the cranial vault* (leptomeningeal/cerebrospinal fluid) and *skeleton* (pM1: bone marrow).

37.5   Lymphovascular Invasion

Present/absent.

Intra-/extratumoural.

Schlemm's canal of ciliary body to the conjunctival veins.

Vortex veins via the sclera: an adverse prognostic sign.

37.6   Lymph Nodes

Site/number/size/number involved/limit node/extracapsular spread.

Regional nodes: pre-auricular, submandibular, cervical.

pN0	No regional lymph node metastasis
pN1	Metastasis in regional lymph node(s).

37.7   Excision Margins

Distances (mm) to the nearest painted resection margin of the optic nerve (retinoblastoma), circumferential margins (iridectomy/local resection of ciliary body and choroid: malignant melanoma), or edge of the exenteration.

37.8   Other Pathology

Tumour Necrosis

- Spontaneous, or, secondary to FNAC or irradiation/cryotherapy/ photocoagulation.

Glaucoma

- Invasion of Schlemm's canal or secondary to FNAC.

Metastatic Malignant Melanoma

- Jaundice, hepatomegaly due to secondary deposits and a glass eye.

Prognosis

Malignant melanoma: has a *50% 15 year mortality rate*, but 66 % at 5 years for those with extrascleral extension. *Maximum tumour thickness, scleral basal diameter* and the *degree (≤5 mm or >5 mm) of extraocular extension* are the strongest prognostic indicators. *Cell type* is influential as 5 year survival rates are lower in epithelioid (25–35 %) than spindle cell B (66–75 %) lesions. Therefore a small (<7 mm) pure spindle cell A melanoma has a 5 year survival ≥95 %. *Local resection* of malignant melanoma may be considered if it is small (maximum dimension <1 cm) and anterior or equatorial in location. *Enucleation* is indicated for posterior melanoma, irrespective of its size, due to its interference with visual acuity.

Retinoblastoma: has a *90% 5 year survival*. The hereditary form is slightly worse, and 6–20 % of patients develop a *second malignancy after 10–15 years* e.g. osteosarcoma, rhabdomyosarcoma. Sporadic retinoblastoma is treated by *enucleation* (unless early, when radiation is used), and familial cases by enucleation and *selective radiotherapy* to the contralateral eye to treat any early metachronous lesions. Irradiation and *systemic chemotherapy* are reserved for cases with involvement of the optic nerve or soft tissue surgical margins.

Adverse prognostic indicators in malignant melanoma are:

- Old age.
- Tumour maximum dimension
  - Small: less than medium
  - Medium: 2.5 mm ≤ maximum thickness ≤10 mm, ≤16 mm basal diameter
  - Large: >10 mm thickness, or, >2 mm thickness and >16 mm basal diameter, or, >8 mm thickness with optic nerve involvement.

    In general tumour sizes up to 5, 10 and 15 mm have better, guarded and poor prognosis, respectively.
- Epithelioid cell type/nucleolar enlargement.
- Invasion of the ciliary body, anterior chamber, optic nerve, sclera, vortex veins and extraocular extension.
- Necrosis, mitotic activity, tumoural and extratumoural vascular invasion.

Adverse prognostic indicators in retinoblastoma are:

- Invasion of optic nerve, particularly its surgical margin.
- Invasion of sclera, choroid, anterior segment.
- Extraocular spread.
- Tumour size, multifocality and differentiation.

Bibliography

Barcroft JD. Histochemical technique. London: Butterworths; 1967.

Callender GR. Malignant melanocytic tumours of the eye: a study of histologic types in 111 cases. Trans Am Acad Ophthalmol Otolaryngol. 1931;36:131–42.

Font RL, Croxatto JO, Rao NA. Tumors of the eye and ocular adnexa. Atlas of tumor Pathology. 4th series. Fascicle 5. Washington: AFIP; 2007.

Ford AL, Mudhar HS, Farr R, Parsons MA. The ophthalmic pathology cut-up. Part 2. Curr Diagn Pathol. 2005;11:340–8.

Lee WR. Ophthalmic histopathology. London: Springer; 1993.

Lucus DR. Greer's ocular pathology. Oxford: Blackwell Scientific; 1989.

McLean IW, Foster WD, Zimmerman LE. Uveal melanoma: location, size, cell type and enucleation as risk factors in metastasis. Hum Pathol. 1982;13:123–32.

Shields CL, Shields JA, Baez KA, Cater J, De Potter PV. Optic nerve invasion of retinoblastoma: metastatic potential and clinical risk factors. Cancer. 1994;73:692–8.

The Royal College of Pathologists. Cancer datasets (Ocular Retinoblastoma, Conjunctival Melanoma and Melanosis, Uveal Melanoma). Accessed at http://www.rcpath.org/index.asp?PageID=254.

Extraocular tumours can present as an obvious nodule or plaque (eyelid, conjunctiva), swelling (lacrimal apparatus), proptosis or exophthalmos (orbital). Tissue diagnosis and treatment of eyelid and conjunctiva lesions usually involves primary local excision sufficient to remove the tumour but minimised to preserve function. Excision is by partial or full thickness wedge (eyelid) or strip (conjunctiva) resection, and these oculoplastic procedures may sometimes require intraoperative frozen section assessment of surgical margins. Incisional biopsy may be used to "map" the extent of a neoplasm prior to definitive resection. Exenteration is reserved for those tumours showing more extensive local spread which may be demonstrated by CT or MRI scans. Pleomorphic adenoma of the lacrimal gland is usually amenable to local excision via a lateral orbitotomy, but like adenoid cystic carcinoma may require more extensive surgery. Initial investigation of orbital tumours dictates planned management with avoidance of surgical excision of irresectable primary malignancies and metastatic tumours. Tissue diagnosis may be obtained by fine needle aspiration cytology (FNAC) or punch biopsy but often the latter is insufficient and a formal, deep, open biopsy via a lateral orbitotomy is required. Clinical assessment should consider various non-surgical possibilities e.g. metastatic carcinoma, malignant lymphoma, thyrotoxicosis and Wegener's granulomatosis. Surgery is geared towards excision of localised primary tumours e.g. cavernous haemangioma, pleomorphic adenoma, but exenteration, involving removal of the eye, surrounding orbital contents, eyelids, nasolacrimal apparatus ± orbital bone, may be required. The commonest indications for exenteration are malignant tumours of the eyelid such as basal cell, squamous cell or sebaceous carcinomas.

38.1 Gross Description

Specimen

- FNAC/punch or excision biopsy/exenteration.
  - Size (cm) and weight (g).

Tumour

Site
- Ocular adnexae:
  - Eyelid
  - Conjunctiva
  - Lacrimal apparatus.
- Orbit/retro-orbital tissues.

Size
- Length × width × depth (cm) or maximum dimension (cm).

Appearance
- Exophytic/verrucous/sessile/ulcerated/fleshy/infiltrative/pigmented.

Edge
- Circumscribed/irregular.

D.C. Allen, *Histopathology Reporting*,
DOI 10.1007/978-1-4471-5263-7_38, © Springer-Verlag London 2013

38.2   Histological Type

Adnexae

- *Basal cell carcinoma*: commonest, >80% of cases.
- Squamous cell carcinoma: 5–10 %.
- Sebaceous carcinoma: epithelioma (sebaceoma)/carcinoma.
- Merkel cell carcinoma: chromogranin/synaptophysin/cytokeratin (CAM 5.2, CK20) positive with a high Ki-67 index. An aggressive poorly differentiated/high-grade neuroendocrine carcinoma.
- Malignant melanoma: primary (de novo or origin in eyelid/conjunctional naevus, or, acquired conjunctival melanosis) or secondary.
- Malignant lymphoma: low-grade MALToma with indolent behaviour.
- Metastatic carcinoma: breast, gastrointestinal tract, lung.
- Lacrimal gland tumour: e.g. pleomorphic adenoma, adenoid cystic carcinoma and other salivary type neoplasms.

Orbit: Children

- *Embryonal (less commonly alveolar) rhabdomyosarcoma*, Burkitt's lymphoma.

Orbit: Adults

- Haemangioma, neurilemmoma, lipoma, nodular fasciitis, Langerhan's cell histiocytosis.
- Inflammatory pseudotumour: 20–40 years of age, sudden onset and painful but potentially steroid responsive.
- *Malignant lymphoma* (MALToma): the presence of lymphoid tissue in the orbit (not usual) is suspicious of neoplasia and up to 50 % are part of systemic disease.
- Haemangiopericytoma.
- Fibro-/osteo-/chondro-/liposarcoma, malignant fibrous histiocytoma, alveolar soft part sarcoma, malignant teratoma are all rare. *Fibrosarcoma/malignant fibrous histiocytoma is the commonest orbital sarcoma of adulthood.* There is an overlay with solitary fibrous tumour.

- Glioma or meningioma of optic nerve origin.
- Multiple myeloma/leukaemia.
- Metastatic carcinoma
  - *15–30% of orbital tumours.*
  - *Direct spread*: retinoblastoma; uveal melanoma; paranasal sinus carcinoma.
  - *Distant spread*: neuroblastoma; embryonal rhabdomyosarcoma; breast, lung, kidney, prostatic carcinoma, carcinoid tumour of lung or small bowel.
- Malignant melanoma: direct or distant spread.

38.3   Differentiation

Well/moderate/poor/undifferentiated, or, Grade 1/2/3/4.
- Carcinoma.
  Low-grade/high-grade.
- Lymphoma and sarcoma.

38.4   Extent of Local Tumour Spread

Border: pushing/infiltrative.
  Lymphocytic reaction: prominent/sparse.
  The TNM7 classification varies according to exact anatomical site and tumour type.

Adnexae

Carcinoma of eyelid is classified according to its size, involvement of the lid margin or full thickness, and adjacent structures as illustrated in Figs. 38.1, 38.2, 38.3 and 38.4. Maligant melanoma of eyelid is classified as for cutaneous melanoma. Conjunctival malignant melanoma has a separate classification based on the tumour radial extent, thickness and involvement of other tissues. Conjunctival carcinoma is pT1 (≤5 mm), pT2 (>5 mm), invades adjacent structures (pT3), or, the orbit or beyond (pT4).

Orbit

The TNM7 classification applies to sarcomas of soft tissues and bone.

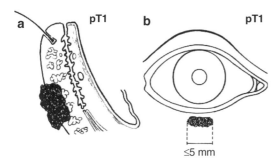

Fig. 38.1 Eyelid carcinoma (**a**) Not in tarsal plate or lid margin or (**b**) ≤5 mm (Reproduced, with permission, from Wittekind et al. (2005), © 2005)

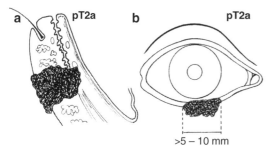

Fig. 38.2 Eyelid carcinoma. (**a**) In tarsal plate or lid margin or (**b**) >5–10 mm (Reproduced, with permission, from Wittekind et al. (2005), © 2005)

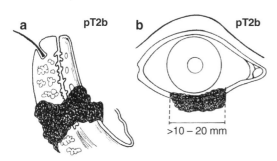

Fig. 38.3 Eyelid carcinoma. (**a**) full thickness eyelid or (**b**) >10–20 mm (Reproduced, with permission, from Wittekind et al. (2005), © 2005)

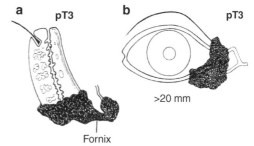

Fig. 38.4 Eyelid carcinoma. (**a**) Any tumour invading adjacent ocular or orbital structures, perinerural invasion, or requiring enucleation, exenteration or bone resection or (**b**) >20 mm (Reproduced, with permission, from Wittekind et al. (2005), © 2005)

pT1	Tumour ≤15 mm maximum dimension
pT2	Tumour >15 mm maximum dimension without invasion of globe or bony wall
pT3	Tumour of any size with invasion of orbital tissues and/or bony walls
pT4	Tumour invades globe or periorbital structures such as: eyelids, temporal fossa, nasal cavity/paranasal sinuses, or central nervous system (Figs. 38.5, 38.6, 38.7 and 38.8).

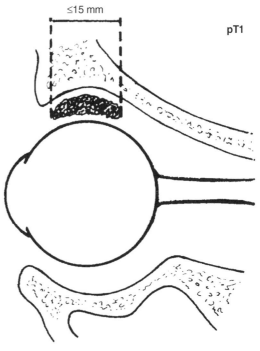

Fig. 38.5 Sarcoma of orbit (Reproduced, with permission, from Wittekind et al. (2005), © 2005)

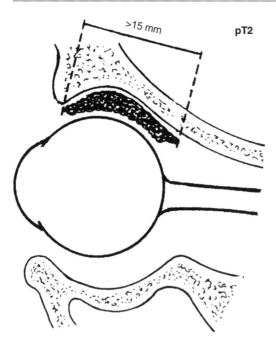

Fig. 38.6 Sarcoma of orbit (Reproduced, with permission, from Wittekind et al. (2005), © 2005)

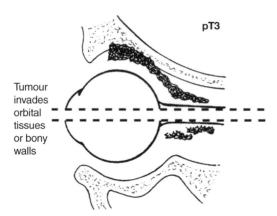

Fig. 38.7 Sarcoma of orbit (Reproduced, with permission, from Wittekind et al. (2005), © 2005)

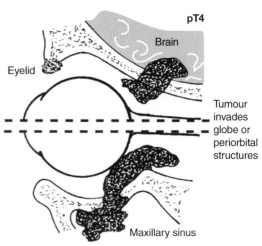

Fig. 38.8 Sarcoma of orbit (Reproduced, with permission, from Wittekind et al. (2005), © 2005)

38.6 Lymph Nodes

Site/number/size/number involved/limit node/extracapsular spread.

Regional nodes: pre-auricular, submandibular, cervical.

pN0	No regional lymph node metastasis
pN1	Metastasis in regional lymph node(s).

38.7 Excision Margins

Distances (mm) to the nearest painted excision margins.

38.8 Other Pathology

Mikulicz's disease (the pathology of which is similar to Sjögren's syndrome) is characterised by benign lymphoepithelial lesion (syn. lympho(myo-)epithelial sialadenitis), and in 10–15 % progression to develop low-grade malignant lymphoma of MALT type.

38.5 Lymphovascular Invasion

Present/absent.

Intra-/extratumoural.

Sun exposure, actinic keratosis and Bowen's disease are predisposing factors in carcinoma of the eyelid and conjunctiva.

Prognosis

Orbital tumours present with unilateral proptosis, the commonest types being *malignant lymphoma* and *metastatic carcinoma. Rhabdomyosarcoma* occurs in childhood, embryonal variants being of better prognosis than the alveolar type. A 50 % survival is achieved with chemo-/radiotherapy and resection is reserved for non-responsive cases. *Malignant fibrosarcoma/fibrous histio-cytoma* is the commonest type of sarcoma in adulthood with aggressive cases showing a 10 year survival rate of 20–25 %. It is treated by radiotherapy. Note that an orbital tumour may be the first presentation of an ocular tumour due to direct spread e.g. retinoblastoma or malignant melanoma.

The tissues behind the orbital septum are normally devoid of lymphatics and lymphoid tissue. *The presence of any lymphoid tissue at this site is therefore suspicious of malignancy.* Prognosis, which can be unpredictable, relates to the grade and stage of disease but is generally reasonably good (80 % survival). *Malignant lymphoma is the commonest adult orbital malignancy.* Tissues anterior to the septum show a wider range of antigen-driven reactive and low-grade neoplastic lymphoid proliferation. Treatment of malignant lymphoma is radio-/chemotherapy depending on the stage and grade of disease.

Immunophenotype

- *Malignant melanoma*: S100, HMB-45, melan-A.
- *Malignant lymphoma*: CD45, CD20, CD3; κ/λ light chain restriction; heavy/light chain immunoglobulin and T cell receptor gene rearrangements.
- *Carcinoma*: cytokeratins, EMA (note plasma cells can also be EMA positive).
- *Rhabdomyosarcoma*: desmin, myogenin, myo D1.

Bibliography

Barcroft JD. Histochemical technique. London: Butterworths; 1967.

Font RL, Croxatto JO, Rao NA. Tumors of the eye and ocular adnexa. Atlas of tumor pathology. 4th series. Fascicle 5. Washington: AFIP; 2007.

Ford AL, Mudhar HS, Farr R, Parsons MA. The ophthalmic pathology cut-up. Part 2. Curr Diagn Pathol. 2005;11:340–8.

Lee WR. Ophthalmic histopathology. London: Springer; 1993.

Lucus DR. Greer's ocular pathology. Oxford: Blackwell Scientific; 1989.

The Royal College of Pathologists. Cancer datasets (Ocular Retinoblastoma, Conjunctival Melanoma and Melanosis, Uveal Melanoma). Accessed at http://www.rcpath.org/index.asp?PageID=254.

Wittekind CF, Greene FL, Hutter RVP, Klimpfinger M, Sobib LH. TNM atlas: illustrated guide to the TNM/pTNM classification of malignant tumours. 5th ed. Berlin: Springer; 2005.

Index

Printed by Printforce, the Netherlands